Insights into Portuguese Medical History

Insights into Portuguese Medical History:

From the Birth of the Art of Asclepius

Edited by

Maria do Sameiro Barroso, Christopher John Duffin and João Alcindo Martins e Silva

Cambridge Scholars Publishing

Insights into Portuguese Medical History:
From the Birth of the Art of Asclepius

Edited by Maria do Sameiro Barroso, Christopher John Duffin
and João Alcindo Martins e Silva

This book first published 2022

Cambridge Scholars Publishing

Lady Stephenson Library, Newcastle upon Tyne, NE6 2PA, UK

British Library Cataloguing in Publication Data
A catalogue record for this book is available from the British Library

ISBN (10): 1-5275-8831-9
ISBN (13): 978-1-5275-8831-8

TABLE OF CONTENTS

List of Illustrations vii

Introduction xvii
Maria do Sameiro Barroso and Christopher J. Duffin

Contributors xxii

Chapter 1 1
Salus in West Roman Lusitania
José d'Encarnação

Chapter 2 17
Roman Medical-Surgical Instruments from the Archaeological Museum D. Diogo de Sousa, Braga
Maria do Sameiro Barroso

Chapter 3 58
Graeco-Roman Pharmacy and Medical- Surgical Tools from the Bühler-Brockhaus Collection
Maria do Sameiro Barroso

Chapter 4 81
The Emerald: A Magico-Medicinal Stone
Christopher J. Duffin

Chapter 5 179
Medical Aspects from Poussin's Plague
Carlos Lemos and Daniel Nunes

Chapter 6 198
History of Spectacles - Portugal in the Sixteenth Century
Maria do Sameiro Barroso

Chapter 7 262
Sanitary Precautions against the Plague in Portuguese Ports (14th-19th Centuries)
João Martins e Silva

Chapter 8 306
The Lazaretto Maritime of Lisbon and Other Health Structures and Procedures
João Martins e Silva

Chapter 9 367
Jacob de Castro Sarmento (1691-1762): A Brief Review
Christopher J. Duffin

Chapter 10 413
On Fevers and Other Foes of Humankind: A Collection of Medical Case Histories by the Physician Gaspar Lopes de Chaves (1729 – 1796)
Francisco Curate and Telmo António

Chapter 11 436
Two Centuries since the Isolation of Cinchonine: Bernardino António Gomes's Networks (1768-1823)
João Rui Pita, Maria Guilherme Semedo and Ana Leonor Pereira

Chapter 12 449
Pneumonic Influenza (Spanish Flu) in Portugal
António Trabulo

Chapter 13 463
Dr. Maria Ropala Cickersky (1881-1973), the First Romanian Woman Forensic Physician and her Portuguese Echo
Dana Baran

Chapter 14 490
Fernando de Almeida (1903-1979) - The Story of the Doctor who was one of the Greatest Portuguese Archaeologists
Carolina Moreira

Index... 506

LIST OF ILLUSTRATIONS

***Salus* in West Roman Lusitania**

Fig. 1.1. Fragmented votive shrine to Endovellicus (IRCP 508).
Fig. 1.2. Votive shrine to Salus (IRCP 290).
Fig. 1.3. Votive shrine to Salus (IRCP 375).
Fig. 1.4. Monuments' location. Map by José Luís Madeira.

Roman Medical-Surgical Instruments from the Archaeological Museum D. Diogo De Sousa, Braga

Fig. 2.1. Portrait of D. Diogo de Sousa. Tesouro-Museu da Sé de Braga.
Fig. 2.2. Map of Bracara Augusta in Frans Hogenberg, *Civitates Orbis Terrarum,* 1594.
Fig. 2.3. Detail from the "Ludovisi battle sarcophagus" or "Grande Ludovisi" sarcophagus. Ludovisi Collection, Rome.
Fig. 2.4. (a) Votive shrine wall of granite dedicated to Asclepius and Hygea. 2nd/3rd century AD. Inv. Nr. 1992.0686 (b) Handle with dog's head decoration. Copper alloy. 2nd century AD. Inv. Nr. 1992.0686.
Fig. 2.5. Female figurine. 2nd century AD. Inv. Nr. 2000.2666.
Fig. 2.6. (a) Leaf-shaped scalpel handle. Copper alloy. Inv. Nr. 2000.0672 (b) Bow shears. Iron. Inv. Nr. 2012.0876.
Fig. 2.7. (a) Conical hollow tube. Copper alloy. Inv. Nr. 1996.0297. (b) ear probe. Gilded copper alloy. 1st half of 4th century AD. Inv. Nr. 1991.2617 (c) Tweezers. Copper alloy. Inv. Nr. 2002.0028.
Fig. 2.8. Spoon-probe with olivary enlargement. Copper alloy. Inv. Nr. 1996.0547.
Fig. 2.9. (a) Ligula – fragmented item, bent shaft and broken tip. Copper alloy. Early 2nd century AD. Inv. Nr. 1998.1551 (b) Fragmented nail cleaner. Inv. Nr. 2008.0239.
Fig. 2.10. (a) Blue-green glass unguent/perfume bottle, conical body. Inv. Nr. 2009.0514. (b) Fragmented green-blue glass aryballus. 1st/2nd century AD. Inv. Nr. 2009.0515.
Fig. 2.11 (a). Transparent glass cup with broken rim and Snake-Thread decoration. Late 1st/early 2nd century AD. Inv. Nr. 2009.0419. (b) Fragment of iron strigil found at the excavation of S. Lázaro. Inv. Nr. 2009.0417.

Fig. 2.12. Translucent glass strigil. 3rd-4th century AD. Metropolitan Museum of Art, New York.
Fig. 2.13. Marble striated vase with snake handles. H. 175 mm, 2nd half of the 2nd century AD. Metropolitan Museum of Art, New York.
Fig. 2.14. Sarcophagus with a Greek Physician. Marble. Early 300s AD. Metropolitan Museum of Art, New York.
Fig. 2.15. Probe. Bronze. 4th century AD or later. Inv. Nr. 1998.1580. Entailing: Drawing of a metal syringe by Hero of Alexandria's Pneumatics.
Fig. 2.16. Digital radiology and CT scan of the probe Inv. Nr. 1998.1580.

Graeco-Roman Pharmacy and Medical- Surgical Tools from the Bühler-Brockhaus Collection
Fig. 3.1. (a) Greek marble votive thumb. Inv. Nr. 2016.0489 (b) Roman Campana plaque. Inv. Nr. 2016.0459.
Fig. 3.2. (a) Roman bronze balance. Inv. Nr. 2016.0549. 2nd-4th century AD (b) Roman bronze pharmaceutical sieve-spoon. Inv. 2016.0550.
Fig. 3.3. Set of five instruments. From left to right: large spatula (Inv. 2016.0568- L- 125 mm W. 46 mm.), tweezers (Inv. Nr. 2016.0569. L. 113 mm Max width 60 mm.), eyed needle, needle, spoon-probe (Inv. Nr. 2016.0572. L. 156 mm W. 22 mm.).
Fig. 3.4. (a) Roman small sardonyx bowl. Inv. Nr. 2018. 0070. (b) Parthian rock crystal unguentarium. Inv. Nr. 2018.0071 (c) Sassanid smoky quartz unguentarium. Inv. Nr. 208.0072.
Fig. 3.5. (a) Needle. Inv. Nr. 2016.0570 (b) Unknown tools (Tabanelli 1958 Tavolla LXXVIII) (c) Eyed needle. Inv. Nr. 2016.0571.
Fig. 3.6. Five probe cases from the Pharmacy and Health Museum. Double case at the upper left corner.
Fig. 3.7. (a) Portable probe case with three instruments inside and three loose instruments. Inv. Nr. 2016.0557 (b) Computerized Axial Tomography.
Fig. 3.8. (a) and (b) Digital Radiography.
Fig. 3.9. (a) Ear probe. Inv. Nr. 2016.0559 (b) Needle. Inv. Nr. 2016.0560
Fig. 3.10. (a) Cauteries from Pompei. Milne, 1907, Plate XV (b) Circular cautery. Inv. Nr. 2016.0558.

The Emerald: A Magico-Medicinal Stone
Fig. 4. 1. A specimen of Colombian emerald, Muzo Mine.
Fig. 4.2. The death of Pliny the Elder during the eruption of Vesuvius (79 AD). Boaistuau, P. (1560) Histoires Prodigieuses: "Prodigieuse mort

de Pline [dont le] corps fut mis en cendre [par les flammes du Vesuve]", Folio 64 verso.
Fig. 4.3. Statue honouring Garcia de Orta (c. 1501-1568), Lisbon.
Fig.4.4. Title page of Garcia de Orta's Colóquios dos Simples e Drogas da India published 10 April 1563.
Fig. 4.5. Apothecary jar for the storage of emerald fragments.
Fig. 4.6. Portrait of Theophrastus (c. 371 – c. 287 B.C.).
Fig. 4.7. Portrait of Albertus Magnus (Count Albert Bollstaedt; c. 1200-1280). Line engraving by T. de Bry (1597).
Fig. 4.8. Portrait of Hildegard von Bingen (c. 1098-1179). Line engraving by W. Marshall (active 1617-1650).
Figure 4.9. Entry for emerald (zamorat) in the Lapidario of Alfonso X (1221-1284). From Montaña (1881).
Fig. 4.10. Precious stones being washed out of Eden. Vincent de Beauvais' Speculum Historiale or "Mirror of History" (de Beauvais 1475?, fol. 54v).
Fig. 4.11. Aberdeen Bestiary, University of Aberdeen MS. 24, folio 101v.
Fig. 4.12. Entry for Smaragdus from the Hortus Sanitatis (1491).
Fig. 4.13. Image accompanying the entry for Smaragdus in the 1536 edition of Hortus Sanitatis.
Fig. 4.14. Portrait of Nicolas Culpeper (1616-1654), frontispiece to The English physitian (1652).
Fig. 4.15. Portrait of William Salmon (1644-1713). Line engraving by W. Sherwin, 1671.
Fig. 4.16. Portrait of Adrian von Mynsicht, (1603-1638). Line engraving by D. Diricksen.
Fig. 4.17. Zenexton from Croll (1664).
Fig. 4.18. L. smaragd. from the Corbyn Cabinet (Drawer 25 column 2 row 5), Museum, Royal Pharmaceutical Society.
Fig.4.19. Ceramic (faience) apothecary jar for Confectio de Hyacintho (18th century). The jar is marked with "C.De.Hyacint". Musée des Hospices Civils de Lyon Inventary number 2007.0.2478.M.
Fig. 4.20. Goa stone and holder, seventeenth century.

Medical Aspects from Poussin's Plague

Fig. 5.1. Nicolas Poussin, The Plague of Ashdod, 1630-31, oil on canvas (148 x 198 cm).
Fig. 5.2. Jacopo Tintoretto, St. Roch Healing the Plague-Stricken, 1549, oil on canvas 1549 (307 x 673 cm). Chiesa di San Rocco, Venice.
Fig. 5.3. Il Morbetto (The Plague of Phrygia), c. 1512, engraving (19.5 x 25.2cm).

Fig. 5.4. Angelo Caroselli, The Plague at Ashdod (after Poussin), 1631, oil on canvas (148 x 198 cm).
Fig. 5.5. Authored to Nicolas Poussin, The Philistines Struck by The Plague in the City of Ashdod, 1647-1660, oil on canvas (149,5 x 199 cm).

History of Spectacles — Portugal in the sixteenth century
Fig. 6.1. Saint Jerome. Wall painting by Ghirlandaio (1449-1494) in the church Ognissanti in Florence.
Fig. 6. 2. (a) Detail of fresco from by Tommaso da Modena depicting Cardinal Hugo of Provence wearing glasses. Serie dei Quaranta domenicani illustri, ex convento di San Niccolò, Sala del Capitolo, Treviso, 1352 (b) Detail of fresco from by Tommaso da Modena depicting Cardinal Nicholas of Rouen using a monocular lens.
Fig. 6.3. Portrait of Saint Paul with glasses. Ornamental letter from the Bible Historiale. 1st Epistle to the Romans. 14th century manuscript. Wellcome Images Collection.
Fig. 6.4. Death of the Virgin. Engraving by Martin Schongauer.
Fig. 6.5. (a) "The Death of the Virgin". Cleveland Museum (U.S.A.). (b) Detail. Apostle wearing rivet spectacles while reading a book.
Fig. 6.6. Master of the Saint Bartholomew Altarpiece, "Saints Peter and Dorothy", The National Gallery, London.
Fig. 6.7. Ludger tom Ring the Elder. The poet Virgil. Westphalian State Museum of Art and Cultural History, Münster.
Fig. 6.8 (a) and (b) "Adoration of the Magi" by Peter Bruegel and detail of man wearing spectacles attached to his cap. National Gallery.
Fig. 6.9. Jan van der Straet. Impressio Librorum, 1953.
Fig. 6.10. Jan van der Straet. Engraving on copper, 1953
Fig. 6.11. Folding spectacles (on the right); scissor spectacles and bow spectacles on the left. Germanic Museum, Nürnberg, Germany.
Fig. 6.12. Jan van der Straet. Spectacles, 1953.
Fig. 6.13 (a). Georg Bartisch. Title page. [Ophthalmodouleia] das ist, Augendienst, 1583. 6.13 (b). Cataract needles.
Fig. 6.14. Georg Bartish. Amulet containers. In [Ophthalmodouleia], das ist, Augendienst, 1583.
Fig. 6. 15. George Bartisch. In [Ophthalmodouleia], das ist, Augendienst, 1583.
Fig. 6. 15. Georg Bartisch. Chapter 3. [Ophthalmodouleia], das ist, Augendienst, 1583.
Fig. 6. 16. A scholar crazy for books in Sebastian Brant. Das Narrenschiff, 1872.

Jacob de Castro Sarmento (1691-1762): A brief review
Fig. 9.1 Jacob de Castro Sarmento (1691-1762). Mezzotint by R. Houston after R. E. Pine.
Fig. 9.2. Samuel Dale. Portrait of Samuel Dale, aged 78, line engraving 1737 by George Virtue.
Fig. 9.3. The Jerusalem Infirmary, Alias, a Journey to the Valley of Jehosaphat. Satirical print circa 1750.
Fig. 9.4. Title pages of the 1721 (English) and 1722 (Latin) editions of Sarmento's Dissertation on Smallpox.
Fig. 9.5. Lady Wortley Montagu (1689-1762). Line engraving by W. Findon, 1824, after J. Thurston after C. F. Zincke.
Fig. 9.6. Cinchona bark. Corbyn cabinet, Drawer 22 Column 1 Row 5, Royal Pharmaceutical Society Museum.
Fig. 9.7. "Quina quina". Plate from Sarmento (1756).
Fig. 9.8. Title page, Sarmento (1756).
Fig. 9.9. Title page, Sarmento (1735).
Fig. 9.10. Portrait of Herman Boerhaave (1668-1738).
Fig. 9.11. Portrait of Stephen Hales (1677-1761).

On Fevers and other Foes of Humankind: A Collection of Medical Case Histories by the Physician Gaspar Lopes De Chaves (1729 – 1796)

Two Centuries since the Isolation of Cinchonine: Bernardino António Gomes's Networks (1768-1823)
Fig. 11.1. Bernardino António Gomes (1768-1823). Biblioteca Nacional de Portugal.

Pneumonic Influenza (Spanish Flu) in Portugal
Fig. 12.1. 14 year-old girl suffering from tuberculosis of cervical tuberculosis lymphadenitis (scrofula) and cutaneous. Rodrigues, Rogério Palma. *Outão-Meio século de trabalhos e de memórias. A gripe pneumónica no Sanatório Marítimo do Outão.*
Fig. 12.2. Dr. Ricardo Jorge in the Municipal Bacteriological Lab in Oporto. Date: Before 1899. Municipal Archives from Oporto.
Fig. 12.3. Portrait of Amadeo de Souza Cardoso. Date: Before 1918.
Fig. 12.4. Amadeo de Sousa Cardoso "Unknown title" (Portrait of Physician). Calouste Gulbenkian Museum, Lisbon, Portugal.

Maria Ropala Cickersky, the first female Romanian Forensic Physician and her Portuguese Echo

Fig. 13.1. The photograph Maria Ropala offered to her niece, Gaby, in 1968, stating on the reverse that she was the first woman forensic doctor in Europe (autograph text).

Fig. 13.2. Diploma no. 264 of Doctor in Medicine and Surgery issued by the University of Iasi in Maria Cicherschi`s name, dated 15 December 1907. Pr. Bogdan signed it as dean of the Faculty.

Fig.13.3. (a) Dr. Ropala`s caricature illustrating a humorous 'Forensic Report' in a local magazine (The World), April 14th, 1935; b. Maria Cickersky Ropala's photo.

Fig. 13.4. Diploma of Forensic Physician of the Institute of Forensic Medicine and Psychiatry in Paris issued by the University of Paris in Maria Ropala`s name on 18 June,1928.

Fig. 13.5. Paris University. Faculty of Medicine. Institute of Forensic Medicine. Maria Cicherschy Ropala (white arrow), the only woman amidst her colleagues, exclusively men.

Fernando De Almeida - the story of the Doctor who was one of the greatest Portuguese Archaeologists

Fig. 14.1 Fernando de Almeida.

Fig. 14.2. Schematic representation of the horseshoe kidney, described by Fernando de Almeida. In: Sur L'Irrigation d'a reine en fer-à-cheval, Arquivo de Anatomia e Antropologia, 1934.

Fig. 14.3. The venous sinuses of the dura mater, their visibility to X-rays ("Os seios venosos da dura-máter, sua visibilidade aos raios X"). Egas Moniz (in collaboration with Abel Alves and Fernando de Almeida), Lisboa Médica, June 1932.

INTRODUCTION

The rich history of Portuguese medicine, ranging from Neolithic trepanned skulls to the country's unique contribution to the Age of Discovery by introducing the medical knowledge of Eastern *materia medica* into European medicine, has mainly been studied by Portuguese researchers. The 46th Congress of the International Society for the History of Medicine (Lisbon 3-6 September 2018) initiated a resurgence of interest in Portuguese medical history by both Portuguese and foreign researchers; the results of this new wave of research deserve the wider circulation that high-quality publications in English can bring about. The volume *Medical Heritage of the National Palace of Mafra,* published by Cambridge Scholars Publishing in 2021, paved the way for new insightful research. The current volume aims to bring together new studies by combining a Portuguese and international authorship, including medical doctors, geologists, archaeologists, anthropologists, historians and pharmacists, focusing on Portuguese medical history.

This book encompasses historical, epigraphic and archaeological research, exploring the rich mosaic of Portuguese medical history from Roman times up to the twentieth century, finishing with an outstanding medical doctor who was also an archaeologist and Director of the Lisbon National Museum of Archaeology.

The title, referring back to Asclepius, the Greek god of medicine, evokes the Greek influence embodied by the presence of Greek pottery, primarily vases discovered in archaeological excavations (Rocha Pereira, 2010). A tombstone dedicated to Asclepius, supposedly fashioned by a Greek freedman and found in Bracara Augusta, one of the most flourishing cities in the Iberian Peninsula during Roman times, establishes the thread traced in this book from Greek Medicine to that of present day Portugal.

In these times of new pandemics, an urgent reconsideration of the analogous experiences of the past has resulted in a meaningful reassessment and revitalization of the present. This mosaic of Portuguese medical history begins with an essay about the goddess *Salus* by **José d'Encarnação**, exploring the ancestral framework of religious beliefs and seeking appeals for godly cures in Roman funerary epigrams, highlighting the social and political concerns expressed in early times.

Further developing the relationship between archaeology and medicine in the Roman period in Portugal, **Maria do Sameiro Barroso** presents an innovative study of medical surgical instruments from Bracara Augusta. Framed within an archaeological context, this study sketches an overview of prevailing medical and surgical practice in the glamorous Roman settlement located in the present day city of Braga, and devised in the sixteenth century by Archbishop D. Diogo de Sousa, the patron of the Archaeological Museum. A second, complementary chapter on the Bühler-Brockhaus Collection completes an insightful overview of the materials used in ancient medical practice. Rare tools whose original functions challenge interpretation have been subjected to modern study techniques such as radiological investigation.

In an essay exploring ancient medical-religious traditions, **Christopher Duffin** presents an in-depth study of the medicinal use of emeralds–precious stones given special consideration by the Portuguese/Goan physician, Garcia de Orta (c. 1501-1568). Continuing his pioneering work on the use of geological materials in medicine, he provides yet another valuable contribution in an aspect of the history of the materia medica which, until now, has received very little attention in the literature.

Returning to the topic of pandemics, **Carlos Lemos and Daniel Nunes** explore Art History as a source providing a novel window into the study of ancient epidemics, focusing on the outbreaks of epidemic diseases and plagues.

Maria do Sameiro Barroso presents paintings and a sculpture of the earliest representations of spectacles in Portuguese Art History and a previously unpublished collection of the earliest spectacles found in Portugal following an overview of the use of magnifying beryls used as visual aids and the discovery and development of the earliest spectacles.

The socioeconomic disruption and, above all, the high mortality rate caused by the second pandemic of bubonic plague in Portugal were a constant source of concern for the monarchs who reigned from the fifteenth to the nineteenth century. In two detailed and comprehensive chapters, **J. Martins e Silva** considers how plague and other transmissible diseases were excluded from entry via Lisbon harbour and other Portuguese ports by the development of new norms and sanitary regulations exemplified by the lazaretto, health stations and the sanitary park.

Jewish physicians and their often tragic experiences with the court of the Portuguese Inquisition provide some of the most interesting chapters in Portuguese medical history. Jacob de Castro Sarmento (1690-1762), one of the most outstanding Portuguese physicians who fled to London and succeeded in becoming a Fellow of the Royal Society, is the subject of a biographical study by **Christopher J. Duffin**. Sarmento´s works included an account of variolation for smallpox, the introduction of Newtonian science in Portugal and a 'secret' recipe of a quinine-containing *Água de Inglaterra* ('Water of England').

Francisco Curate and **Telmo António** present another Jewish physician, Gaspar Lopes Henriques de Chaves (1729-1796), who managed to stay in Portugal and left valuable manuscripts reflecting his everyday activities. The authors investigate his unpublished collections of medical case histories as major sources of knowledge revealing medical practice and the physician's relationships with patients, providing a valuable contribution to the study of medicine in late eighteenth century Portugal.

Pharmacy studies are represented in this book by the chapter contributed by **João Rui Pita, Maria Guilherme Semedo and Ana Leonor Pereira** on the Portuguese physician Bernardino António Gomes (1768-1823), who isolated cinchonine from cinchona bark, engaging the French scientists Pelletier and Caventou in the study. Gomes stimulated the isolation of quinine, the alkaloid which was the mainstay in malarial treatment until the mid-twentieth century.

In a study of modern viral pandemics, **António Trabulo** recalls the catastrophe triggered by the Pneumonic Influenza (Spanish flu) of 1918-1919, focusing on the experiences and implications of the disease in Portugal, evoking Amadeo de Souza Cardoso (1887-1918), one of the most illustrious Portuguese contemporary artists, taken away by the virus.

The exciting topic of female physicians in the History of Medicine is the subject considered by **Dana Baran,** who presents an overview of the life of Maria Ropala Cickersky (1881-1973), the first female forensic physician in South-Eastern Europe and one of the earliest worldwide. Her personality and scientific work did not go unnoticed in Portugal. In 1936, the Portuguese assistant professor Carlos Ribeiro da Silva Lopes, from the Porto Faculty of Medicine and Institute of Forensic Medicine, emphasised a leading paper on the subject by Maria Ropala.

The volume is completed by the contribution of **Carolina Moreira** who considers Fernando de Almeida (1903-1969), a Portuguese gynaecologist and obstetrician, professor of the Lisbon Faculty of Medicine of Lisbon, who made a significant contribution to Neurology and research in collaboration with Egas Moniz (1874-1955), in the discovery of cerebral angiography. Fernando de Almeida also graduated in Historical and Philosophical Sciences, embarking on a highly successful new career in History and Archaeology, leading to his appointment as Director of the Lisbon National Museum of Archaeology, a post which he held from 1967-

1972, proving that a medical doctor can extend his cultural interests far beyond Medicine.

In short, this volume shows that the History of Medicine represents a confluence of multiple arts and sciences. The practice of Medicine is as complex as the human soul. Since ancient times, science has sought to elucidate the secrets of the human body through the dedication, shrewdness and wit that allowed the establishment of a system of medical reasoning based on empirical observation. *Tradition of Medicine,* also referred to as *On Ancient Medicine,* one of the earliest *Hippocratic writings* dating from the end of the fifth century BC, is surprising for its topicality:

> Medicine has for long possessed the qualities necessary to make a science. These are a starting point and a known method according to which many valuable discoveries have been made over a long period of time. By such a method, too, the rest of the science will be discovered if anyone who is clever enough is versed in the observation of the past and makes the starting point of his researches (Hippocrates, *Tradition in Medicine* in Lloyd 1894, 71).

Science and empathy stand as two leading characteristics. The ability to understand and share the feelings and emotions of other people, particularly during times of ill-health is the most fundamental, vital essence original to the development of Medicine, as stated by Sir William Osler (1849 –1919), one of the most brilliant physicians, sometimes known as 'The Father of Modern Medicine': *Medicine arose out of the primal sympathy of man with man: out of the desire to help those in sorrow, need and sickness* (Osler 1921, 6).

Citing Hippocrates (460-370 BC), Sir William Osler views the history of empathy as a complementary discipline of clinical medicine: *Where there is love of humanity there will be love of the profession* (Osler 1921, 62). Ultimately, cultivating an understanding of the past, the history of empathy is at the core of the History of Medicine.

Maria do Sameiro Barroso
Christopher J. Duffin

References

Lloyd, Geoffrey Ernest Richard (ed). 1983. *Hippocratic Writings*, Chadwick, John and Mann, William Neville (transl.). London: Penguin Books.

Osler, Sir William. 1921. *The Evolution of Modern Medicine. A Series of Lectures Delivered at Yale University of the Silliman Foundation in April, 1913.* New Haven: Yale University Press.

Rocha Pereira, Maria Helena de. 2010. *Greek Vases in Portugal.* Coimbra: Centro de Estudos Clássicos e Humanísticos da Universidade de Coimbra.

CONTRIBUTORS

Telmo António is an archaeologist (BA in History, discipline of Archaeology, Faculty of Letters of the University of Lisbon) at the Almada City Hall.

Dana Baran, MD, PhD "Grigore T. Popa" University of Medicine and Pharmacy, Iasi-Romania. Specialisation and publications in Histology-Cell Biology, Chronobiology, History of Medicine/ Pharmacy. Memberships: International Society for the History of Medicine (General Secretary); Balkan Medical Union; International Society of Chronobiology; Romanian Society for the History of Medicine (Vice President); Romanian Society for the History of Pharmacy History (Honorary member); Society of Physicians and Naturalists-Iasi; Romanian Society of Physician Writers and Publicists; European Academy of Sciences, Arts and Letters (Paris); Herald of the Panhellenic Society for the Dissemination of the Hippocratic Spirit (Athenes). National and international awards. Active professor emeritus.

Maria do Sameiro Barroso is a Medical Doctor, Family Medicine Specialist, Graduated in Germanic Philology, President of the Department of History of Medicine of the Portuguese Medical Association; invited lecturer in the History of Medicine at the Faculty of Medicine, University of Lisbon; researcher at the Centre for History, Faculty of Letters, University of Lisbon and Research Centre for Anthropology and Health (Centro de Investigação em Antropologia e Saúde - CIAS), University of Coimbra; Member of the International Society for the History of Medicine (ISHM), Societá Italiana di Storia della Medicina and British Society for the History of Pharmacy (BSHP); Advisory Board member of the Acta Medico-Historica Adriatica and Revista Portuguesa de Antropologia; Vice-President of the 46th Congress of the International Society for the History of Medicine, Lisbon 3-7 September 2018. She has authored numerous articles and book chapters indexed to SCOPUS, and is editor of the books Barroso, M.D.S., Duffin, C. J. and Sousa, G. (eds) (2020): *Medical Heritage of the National Palace of Mafra*, Cambridge Scholars Publishing, and Newcastle and Van Hee, R., Barroso, M.D.S, Galassi, F. M. (eds). 2020. *Asclepius in Lisbon. Selected papers from Lisbon 46th ISHM Congress 3-7 September*

2018, Vesalius XXVI June 2020 e-supplement. www.vesalius.org.uk- ISSN 1373-4857.

Francisco Curate is an anthropologist (PhD in Biological Anthropology, Faculty of Sciences and Technology, University of Coimbra). He is currently an assistant researcher at the Research Centre for Anthropology and Health (Department of Life Sciences, Faculty of Sciences and Technology, University of Coimbra) and teacher at the Superior School of Technology (Polytechnic Institute of Tomar). He is the author of several articles in the fields of palaeopathology, bioarchaeology and forensic anthropology and has been researching human skeletal variation, bone health and disease, and physical trauma in past populations.

José d'Encarnação is a retired full professor at the Faculty of Letters of the University of Coimbra (Portugal), in the area of Ancient History and Archaeology. He specialized in Latin Epigraphy, a field in which his work is internationally recognized, especially with regard to pre-Roman deities. He has over one thousand articles published in specialized magazines in Portugal and abroad. His graduate and PhD theses are: *Indigenous Divinities under the Roman Domain in Portugal* (1st edition, Imprensa Nacional, 1975) and *Roman Inscriptions of Conventus Pacensis* (1st edition, Coimbra, 1984). An Honorary Doctor at the University of Poitiers, he is an academic of merit of the Academia Portuguesa de História (Portuguese Academy of History), a member of the Real Academia de la Historia (Madrid) and Academia das Ciências de Lisboa (Academy of Sciences of Lisbon).

Christopher J. Duffin originally trained as a geologist and then completed an M.Sc. and a Ph.D. in Vertebrate Palaeontology and Comparative Anatomy at University College London. He has published extensively on a wide range of fossil groups, particularly sharks and their allies, is a multi-award-winning palaeontologist, and is co-author of *The Handbook of Paleoicththyology Volume 3D* (2010). A retired High School teacher, he was Senior Master, Director of Sixth Form, Head of Biology and Head of Critical Thinking at Streatham and Clapham High School in London. He holds a second Ph.D., this time in the History of Medicine from the University of Kingston. A long bibliography in the History of Medicine includes a number of edited volumes, such as *A History of Geology and Medicine* (2013), *Geology and Medicine: Historical Connections* (2017), *Amber in the History of Medicine* (2018), *Collection in the Space of Culture* (2019) and *Medical Heritage of the National Palace of Mafra* (2020). Chris is a Scientific Associate at The Natural History Museum in London, a

Research Associate at Bristol University and President of the British Society for the History of Pharmacy.

Carlos Lemos is a Medical Doctor and Clinical Pathology Specialist at Centro Hospitalar Lisboa Norte, E.P.E., and an invited assistant of Laboratory Medicine at the Faculty of Medicine of Lisbon University. He graduated from the Faculty of Medicine of Coimbra. He has authored several papers and lectures on Clinical Pathology, Bioethics and History of Medicine.

Carolina Moreira was born in Braga, Portugal, in 1995. She completed the Integrated Master Degree in Medicine at the Faculty of Medicine of Lisbon in 2020. In that same institution and under the guidance of Professor Vitor Oliveira, she presented a thesis entitled "D. Fernando de Almeida", the product of research into the life and work of the doctor and archaeologist. This thesis was initially presented as a poster at the 46th Congress of the International Society for the History of Medicine in September 2018 and later as an oral presentation on the Researcher's Day at the National Museum of Archaeology in April 2019. This research also resulted in an article for the magazine of the Portuguese Society of Anatomy published in July 2020. As a student, she was General Coordinator of RESSONÂNCIA, the official magazine of the Students' Association of the Faculty of Medicine of Lisbon and she has participated in several courses at the History Centre of the Faculty of Humanities of the University of Lisbon.

Daniel Nunes is a Medical Doctor and Clinical Pathology Resident at Centro Hospitalar Lisboa Norte, E.P.E. He graduated from the Faculty of Medicine of Lisbon University and has authored several publications on Clinical Pathology.

Ana Leonor Pereira, PhD in History (history of scientific culture). Professor at the Faculty of Arts and Humanities, University of Coimbra, Portugal (Department of History). Scientific Coordinator and Researcher of the History and Sociology of Science Group at the Center for Interdisciplinary Studies of the 20th Century at the University of Coimbra - CEIS20. Associate of the Biomedical Law Center, University of Coimbra. Her main research interests are history of science, history of medicine, pharmacy and health sciences, history of health sciences, history of Darwinism, history of scientific culture, and the history of culture. Vice-President of the Society for the Interdisciplinary History of Health. She is the author of several scientific papers published in national and international journals and many books and chapters of books. She has supervised and supervises several master's and doctoral theses and post-doctoral research in her scientific area.

João Rui Pita, PhD in Pharmacy (thesis in the history of Portuguese pharmacy, eighteenth to nineteenth centuries). Professor at the Faculty of Pharmacy, University of Coimbra, Portugal (Laboratory of Social Pharmacy and Public Health). Scientific Coordinator and Researcher of the History and Sociology of Science Group at the Center for Interdisciplinary Studies of the 20th Century at the University of Coimbra - CEIS20. Associate of the Biomedical Law Center, University of Coimbra. His main research interests are history of pharmacy and health sciences, the relationship between pharmacy and society and pharmaceutical ethics. President of the Society for the Interdisciplinary History of Health. He is the author of several scientific papers published in national and international journals and many books and chapters of books. He supervised and supervises several master's and doctoral theses and post-doctoral research in his scientific area. He has been awarded several national and international awards and distinctions. Member of the International Academy of Pharmacy History (Academie Internationale d'Histoire de la Pharmacie), since 2001.

Maria Guilherme Semedo holds a Master's Degree in Pharmaceutical Sciences from the Faculty of Pharmacy of the University of Coimbra. She is a PhD student in Pharmaceutical Sciences (specializing in Social Pharmacy) at the Faculty of Pharmacy of the University of Coimbra and a collaborating researcher in the Group of History and Sociology of Science and Technology at the Center for Interdisciplinary Studies of the 20th Century (GHSCT-CEIS20). She also holds a postgraduate degree in Herbal Medicines and Herbal Health Products. She has presented oral communications at national and international congresses and has published several articles in scientific journals. Her main research interests are Social Pharmacy, History of Pharmacy and the History of Science and Technology.

João Alcindo Martins e Silva graduated in Medicine from the Faculty of Medicine of the University of Lisbon, and holds a PhD in Medical Sciences (Physiologic Chemistry). He is a retired full Professor and Director of the Institute of Physiologic Biochemistry, former Dean (1994-2005) of the Faculty of Medicine of the University of Lisbon, retired Head Researcher of the Vascular Biopathology Unit of the Molecular Medicine Institute/ Faculty of Medicine of the University of Lisbon, former President of the Portuguese Society of Medical Education and co-founder and President of the Portuguese Society of Haemorheology and Microcirculation. He is a

Member of the NHMOM (Núcleo de História da Medicina da Ordem dos Médicos) (Portugal) and has published around five hundred articles in his scientific field and in medical education. He has written books and papers on the History of Medicine and contributed a chapter in the book of Barroso, M.D.S., Duffin, C. J. and Sousa, G. (eds) (2020): Medical Heritage of the National Palace of Mafra, Cambridge Scholars Publishing.

António Trabulo is a retired Neurosurgeon. He was Head of the Santo António dos Capuchos Hospital in Lisbon, Coordinator of the Teaching Committee of the Portuguese Society of Neurosurgery and President of the Board of Directors of the Neurosurgery of the Portuguese Medical Association. He has several publications in this area. He is an awarded writer who began his literary activity in 2002. He has published 25 books, including novels, short stories, biographies and essays in Portugal, Brazil, and Argentina. His most successful publication was the biography of the dictator Oliveira Salazar, ten editions having been sold out. He is the President of the Portuguese Society of Portuguese Writers and Artists. As a medical Historian, he collaborated on the volume *Medical Heritage of the National Palace of Mafra,* Cambridge Scholars Publishing, 2020.

CHAPTER 1

SALUS IN WEST ROMAN LUSITANIA

JOSE D'ENCARNAÇÃO

Abstract
After a general consideration of the concept of *Salus*, in its sense of physical and mental health (also meaning well-being and prosperity), I analyzed 15 Roman epigraphic documents containing the term. The informative content of each is synthesized to fit the word context. A shrine expressly offered to goddess *Salus* and other deities, conveying requests or thanksgiving, expresses this potentiality of divine spirits, regardless of specific characteristics, also benefiting from their great capacity to protect men in all aspects of their existence. Besides mentioning divinity, the epigraphic texts indicate the dedicator and the reason to have an inscription recorded. It is concluded that the (physical or spiritual) health concern covers all sectors of a population with no distinctions of gender or social class: men, women, slaves, and senators. On the other hand, it turns out that not only the goddess *Salus* is invoked since requests are also made to other Roman and even *indigenous deities.* The testimonies were found in urban and rural settings, although an expected urban political connotation is manifested. [1]
Key words: *Salus*, *pro salute*, Roman Lusitania.

---

[1] List of Text Abbreviations
CIL II = HÜBNER (Emílio), *Corpus Inscriptionum Latinarum – II*. Berlin: Berlin Academy of Sciences, 1869 e 1892.
HEp = Hispania Epigraphica, edited by Universidade Complutense de Madrid. Indica-se, geralmente, o número, a data da publicação e o número da inscrição.
HEpOL = *online* version of *Hispania Epigraphica,* edited by Universidade Complutense de Madrid, available at http://eda-bea.es/
IRCP = Encarnação, José d', *Inscrições Romanas do* Conventus Pacensis, Coimbra, 2013 [http://hdl.handle.net/10316/578]. [The number indicates the inscription number on the catalogue].

Resumo
Após uma consideração geral acerca do conceito de *Salus,* na sua acepção de saúde física e mental (bem-estar, prosperidade), analisam-se 15 documentos epigráficos romanos em que surge a palavra *Salus.* Sintetiza-se o conteúdo informativo de cada um, para se enquadrar o contexto em que o vocábulo surge: há o altar expressamente oferecido à deusa *Salus* e há os que veiculam pedidos ou acção de graças a outras divindades, o que prova essa virtualidade dos númenes de, independentemente de características específicas, usufruírem também dessa enorme capacidade de protegerem o Homem em todos os aspectos da sua existência. Os textos epigráficos – na medida em que, além da menção da divindade, indicam quem foi o dedicante e a razão por que teve a iniciativa de mandar gravar uma inscrição – permitiram concluir que essa preocupação pela saúde (física ou espiritual) abrange todos os sectores da uma população, sem distinções de género ou de classe social: homens, mulheres, escravos, senadores… Por outro lado, verifica-se que não apenas a deusa *Salus* é invocada, porque os pedidos são feitos também a outras divindades romanas e, até, a divindades indígenas. Além disso, os testemunhos encontram-se tanto em ambiente urbano como em ambiente rural, embora se adivinhe para o urbano uma sintomática conotação política…
Palavras-chave: *Salus, pro salute,* Lusitânia romana.

Introduction

When visiting the cathedral of Sienna on May 10, 1991, I was impressed by a pile of motorcycle helmets by the side of a chapel. The name of the patron saint - perhaps Saint Rafael – was thereby honoured by those who miraculously escaped and recovered from a severe accident.

The statue of Dr Sousa Martins (1843-1879), an outstanding medical doctor and thaumaturge at Campo dos Mártires da Pátria, in Lisbon, with its base overflowing with expressions of thanks for favours granted (naturally in the medicinal domain), also impressed me profoundly. Likewise, dozens of chapels in Portugal are filled with wax votive reproductions of human organs, indicating that, at that place, someone made a promise and received grace during a bout of serious illness. Ex-votos were also expressed in naive tables of miracles in which people resorted to charismatic temples in suffering or healing events, recounted by words and matching designs (on this subject, see Ribeiro et al. 1998).

Religion lies at the connection between the human and the divine, in the spiritual realm, whether we believe or not in the existence of another dimension. It would be challenging to penetrate people's "arcana" if these external signs as testimonies to people's experiences did not come to us. As a result, through the analysis of inscriptions that have come down to our time, perspectives will be rehearsed to understand better the role of *Salus* in the daily lives of those living two thousand years ago in the territory of western Roman Lusitania.

Firstly, I will consider the concept of *Salus* in a list of inscriptions selected as sources of information for this essay, ultimately trying to assess the meaning of these perspectives.

Salus

Joseph-Antoine Hild (1845-1914) was responsible for preparing an article on Salus for the classic *Dictionnaire des Antiquités Grecques et Romaines* (Hild in Daremberg & Salio 1969, 1056-1059). He begins by saying that, as with other "personified influences" in general, *Salus* has no relation to the health of an individual: its role assumes a predominantly political-social nature, promoting state welfare in peace and war.

It was common to believe that the State could only be "healthy" if the people were also healthy. As Hild warns, *Salus* could stand as equivalent to Fortuna (the goddess and personification of good luck) in her primary meaning, her invocation being reserved for critical life circumstances. Hence, in Portuguese, the Latin word *Salus* may have a double meaning, concerning both health and salvation! Holding drinking glasses, we toast "To our health!"; more informally, we exclaim "Let there be health!". Moreover, in the latter case, we end up including both people and organizations (state, government), promoting general and individual health.

Concerning the intimate nature of the Roman *Salus*, the Portuguese classicist Maria Helena da Rocha Pereira (1925-2017) notes that the Roman religion was "particularly fit to welcome personified abstractions among its gods" such as *Salus*. Moreover, she mentions the famous explanation of Cicero (106-43 BCE):

> *Again, there are the temples of Wealth, Safety, Concord, Liberty and Victory, all of which things, being so powerful as necessarily to imply divine governance, were themselves designated as gods.* (Cicerus, On the Nature of Gods, Book II, Chapter 23, Paragraph 61, translated by Rackham 1933, 183).

She also cites a confirmatory sentence by the classical philologist Viktor Pöschl (1910-1997):

They are divine powers that condition the action of man and, as divine powers, they are immutable and subtracted from the realm of what is changeable (Pereira 2002, 350).

Epigraphic testimonials

I will consider how these thoughts were expressed in the daily lives of the Romans from the western area of *Lusitania* (corresponding to the current area south of the Douro River in Portugal), by considering the epigraphic testimonies registering the word *Salus*, excluding monuments that otherwise fit into this salutary atmosphere either because of their text or because the invoked deity is likely to be endowed with these qualities.

Let us illustrate this idea with an inscription found at Elvas' ring (IRCP 572, HEp 14 2008 nº 451). Its current whereabouts are unknown; we know it exists since the Portuguese Renaissance humanist André de Resende (1498-1573) mentioned it, like the English knight John Breval (1680? - 1738), who visited Portugal and Spain in 1726 and became interested in the Roman inscriptions which he came across (Canto 2004, 265-364). The inscription reads as follows:

PROSERPINAE / SERVATRICI / C(*aius*) · VETTIVS · SIL/VANVS · PRO · EV/NOIDE · PLAVTIL/LA · CONIVGE · SIBI / RESTITVTA / V(*otum*) · S(*uum*) · A(*nimo*) · L(*ibens*) · P(*osuit*)

(To Liberating Proserpine – Caius Vettius Silvanus on behalf of Eunoide Plautilla, the spouse who was returned to him, put his vote of his own free will).

The inscription tells that Gaius Vettius Silvanus fulfilled his vow and willingly dedicated this headstone to Proserpine Servatrix. This epithet denotes not only passive protection, but it also accentuates an active "concern" over divine intervention in maintaining and preserving well-being. However, what particularly interests us in this context is why he made the dedication: *pro eunoide Plautilla coniuge sibi restituta.* Alicia Maria Canto's proposal of not reading in *eunois* an anthroponym but the Greek adjective that means "benevolent" or "sympathetic" (Canto 2004, 333-334) seems plausible. This highlights what comes next: that his wife, Plautilla, came back to him. We are quite accustomed to the fact that both old and current advertising campaigns favour ambiguity in order better to achieve their goals. In this case, what is meant by the phrase *back to him*? In a figurative sense, could it mean that someone who was deemed lost due to a fatal illness was saved and came back to the husband's arms by divine virtue? Or does it mean physical return after a marital deviation, or something else entirely?

What is certain is that Silvanus would have invoked Proserpine and, in his view, divine intercession solved the case. There is salvation, yes. This example introduces the concept of *salus* although the word does not figure in it.

In the inscriptions selected for this essay, the word *salus* figures, written in either upper or lower case letters, but with no pretensions to being an exhaustive study, since giving notice of all relevant considerations is beyond the scope of this essay and the new epigraphic findings contained therein. I will use the data provided by HEpOL, because it is assumed to be regularly updated. Any missing data should subsequently be easily integrated adding little to the conclusions that this selected inscription corpus provides.

1. In the inscription found in Meimoa, Penamacor (conventus Scallabitanus), it is highlighted that: *Pro salute imp(eratoris) Nervae Traiani Caes(aris) Aug(usti) Ger(manici) vicani Venienses campum consecraverunt* (To the health of the emperor Nerva Trajanus Caesar Augustus Germanicus – the Venien neighbours consecrated the field.) (Curado 1979, 145-148; HEpOL 16950).

We are facing the initiative of some *vicani* (neighbours) from a place whose indigenous designation remains and who do not hesitate, surely by means of an official act such as the consecration of a field, to toast the health of Emperor Trajan (reigned 98-117 AD), probably in year 98, since it was in October or November 97 that he was awarded the title of Germanicus.

We do not deny that the vote may have been sincere; however, what seems to be most noticeable is using a stereotyped formula, which tends to situate the initiative chronologically rather than making a sincere vote out of it.

2. The message that emperor Hadrian (reigned 117-138) sends to his freed procurator a metallis, Ulpius Aelianus regarding the ruling of the thermal baths of Vipasca (Vipasca II – IRCP 143, HEpOL 19 992), begins in this way: […] *Ulpius Aelianus suo salute* (To his Ulpius Aelianus – health! The usual greeting - "Cheers!" (In Portuguese "À saúde"-"To our health"), paralleled until recently by the usual expression "I hope it will find you in perfect health".

3. In Penamacor, a small votive shrine was dedicated to Victoria, *pro salute sua* (To the health of goddess Victoria). However, it is unknown who was the beneficiary of the vote, as the monument has been cut off (HEpOL nº 20 380). The presence of the deity Victoria seems to attribute a protective gesture to her that is now intended to be highlighted and thanked, more than to contain a future request.

4. From Torres Vedras possibly comes (Conventus Scallabitanus) the shrine consecrated to Salus–*Sal(uti) sac(rum)* – by Ap(pius) N(umisius?) Auca Piasirus after a promise (*ex voto posuit*) [HEpOL nº 20 283]. There is no doubt about the reconstitution Sal(uti); the dedicator's identification is not certain, however, mainly because it presents an unusual structure, making it impossible to guarantee its status as being that of a Romanized indigene.

5. Among numerous ex-votes dedicated to Endovellicus, I selected the one by L(ucius) Iulius Novatus, *pro salute Vivenniae Venustae Maniliae suae* (Lucius Iulius Novatus to the health of Vivennia Venusta Manilia) (IRCP 508, HEpOL nº 21 223 – Fig. 1.1).

We infer that Novatus summons the deity's protection for the well-being or physical health of a woman who is dear to him – he classifies her with the possessive "his". If the dedicator can be included in the list of Romanized indigenes (*tria nomina* with no mention of affiliation, which would not be postulated in this type of text), we find the manner of identification of the beneficiary strange, if we interpret Manilia as a well-known Gentile. Could it therefore refer to two Gentiles indicating an adoption? It does not look like it. By the possessive occurrence, we are tempted to see in Manilia a very personal form of affectionate treatment.

6. The ex-voto from Albia Pacina Fontano et Fontanae pro salut(e) Albi Fausti (Albia Pacina Fontano and Fontana to the health of Albus Faustus) comes from Bencatel [IRCP 438, HEpOL 21 239]. Faustus may be Pacina's patron, given the Gentiles' identity. Since we may consider both attitudes, the gratitude or the plea is made to a deity naturally protective of health. Fontanus is mentioned herein in both its masculine and feminine aspect, indicating Pacina's desire to embrace every detail of the deity's beneficence. The deity would be a spring of waters to which are attributed therapeutic properties. The choice of deity suggests that his curative action was manifested when drunk by the devotee instead of treatment in thermal baths. In addition to drinking, bathing was a healing procedure.

7. The investigation concluded that the ex-voto of Avitus Proculi f(ilius) to the Nymphs could have been identified for the first time at Saint Mary's church, in Monforte, in the Northeast of Alentejo, a territory of the Conventus Pacensis. However, its initial context is unknown, as can be deduced from the information José d' Encarnação and Maria José Gonçalves brought to light from mismatched references of ancient manuscripts (Encarnação & Gonçalves 2013, 255-276).

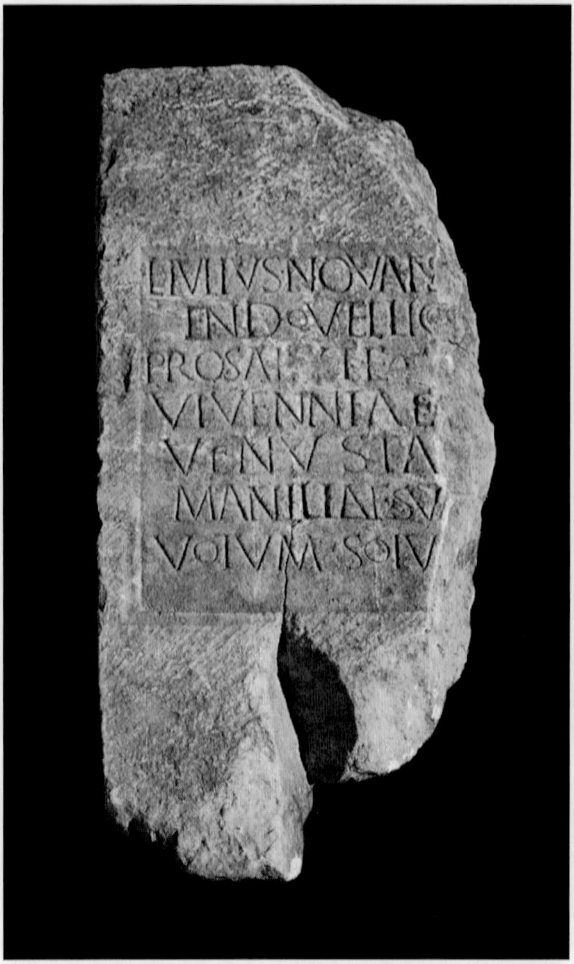

Fig. 1.1 Fragmented votive shrine to Endovellicus (IRCP 508). Reproduced with permission.

Because of the Nymphs' dedication, one might postulate, for example, the proximity of a watercourse or thermal spring dedicated to protective divinities. Therefore, the therapeutic qualities of the waters could be accessed, whether by being consumed as drinks or appropriated as thermal baths. Today, only Cabeço de Vide's pristine thermal baths near Monforte are extant.

What is certain is that Avitus consecrated *pro salute Flaccillae Flacci ucxoris suae* (to the health of Flaccillia Flaccus, his wife) to these Nymphs without a specifying epithet (because the ex-voto was placed next to the spring, such a specification was redundant). This means that the couple, identified with Latin names, still speaks in an indigenous way, capturing the Nymph's concrete meaning.

This being a family case, we feel tempted to attribute "health" as the intended meaning of *Salus*: Avitus invoked the Nymphs to cure some disease or acknowledged some particular grace which had been granted them.

8. According to tradition, a bronze plaque in the sands of Ribeira das Lampreias, near Alvega, containing the so-called *iusiurandum Aritiensium* (IRCP 647), proclaims the fidelity of the Aritium's inhabitants to Gaius Caesar Germanicus, Emperor Caligula (reigned 37-41 AD) in the year 37 AD. By this time, the rehabilitation of this putative successor to Emperor Augustus (reigned 27 BCE-14 AD) had taken place. It was to him, ultimately, after his death, that the Senate decreed sublime honours, consigned, for example, in the Tabula Siarensis [2] (González & Arce 1988).

Written to be proclaimed individually, the text says at a certain point: *neque liberos meos eius salute cariores habebo* (and, in my children, I will not cheer more than their health).

In cases where political plots led to murder, *Salus* should be understood as a protector of physical integrity, or well-being. In fact, the juror had already stated: *et si quis periculum ei salutique eius infert intuleritve armis bello internecivo terra marique persequi non desinam quo ad poenas ei persolverit* (and if someone threatens him, himself or his well-being, no I will not stop pursuing him, by weapons, in a deadly war, on land and at sea, until he is punished).

Although we have opted for the translation "well-being", in the context, the allusion to his physical integrity is quite clear, as stated.

9. News from 1842 reports that, in Lisbon's church of Saint Vicente de Fora, an epigraphic monument dedicated to Jupiter was found, an ex-voto placed there freely by *M(arcus) Iulius Primus pro salutem M(arci) Cassi Firmi* (Marcus Julius Primus to the health of Marcus Cassius Firmus). Priest Manuel da Gama Xaro (1800-1870) read it and transmitted it to the German archaeologist and epigraphist Emil Hübner (1834-1901) (CIL II 177); instead of *pro salutem*, the most usual form of words is *pro salute* (ablative); Hübner thinks that perhaps Xaro was mistaken, but there are other

---

[2] Document exhumed in the city of Siarium, in Andalusia, where the provisions voted by Rome's senate in 19 AD regarding the funeral honours to be paid to the Germanicus are discriminated.

testimonies, he added, of the use of the accusative: *quamquam similia reperiuntur*.

In this case, Jupiter is the divinity invoked, proving that, in reality, all the gods can be prayed to and thanked for having interceded in health issues.

There is no information concerning the possible kinship between the two characters mentioned since they are from different families – Iulia and Cassia, both dominant families at Olisipo; however, it is more plausible that the reference here should be to physical health.

10. From the sanctuary to the Sun, the Moon and the Ocean located in Vigia do Facho, in front of Praia das Maçãs (Colares, Sintra), where the Portuguese archaeologist and epigraphist José Cardim Ribeiro carried out important archaeological excavations, there is a specially dedicated inscription. This was made by Senator Decimus Iulius Caelianus, imperial legacy, "To the Eternal Sun and the Moon for the Eternity of the Empire and the Health of Emperor Caesar Lucius Septimius Severus Augustus Pius Felix, of Emperor Caesar Marcus Aurelius Antoninus Augustus Pius, [by Publius Septimius nobilissimus Geta] Caesar and Iulia Augusta, mother of the military camps" (Portuguese translation by Cardim Ribeiro 2019, 40).

In this testimony of official character, worship is carried out to SOLI AETERNO ET LVNAE PRO AETERNITATE IMPERI(i) ET SALVTE of the imperial family. Therefore, in this highly official connotation the word *Salus* is used in its greatest sense of generalized well-being, because, as recommended, the health of the government and their families will necessarily lead to the health and well-being of all their subjects.

11. António M. Dias Diogo and José Luís Neto brought to light (FE 285 = HEpOL nº 23 444), an intact granite votive band found in June 2000 in the parish of Mosteiro, municipality of Oleiros, with the following inscription:

PRO SAL / VTE M (- - -) · I (- - -) · C (- - -) · / SVI · P (osuit)

(has laid to the health of your Marco Júlio [?] C. [?])

The absence of a theonym "indicates", they wrote, "its placement in a sanctuary", an opinion that is shared by us. As for the interpretation that the three acronyms are the *tria nomina* of the prayer's "beneficiary", that also seems sensible – perhaps a M(arcus) I(ulius) C (?), here, of course, in the genitive; by mistake, however, they interpreted SVI as if it were SIBI, which it is not. Consequently, the ex-voto was dedicated to a deity unknown (to us) for his MIC health. In other words, *Salus* must be understood, in this example, as personal well-being. Further, it cannot be excluded that it refers to a craving for physical health. Note that representation by means of acronyms is not surprising in these circumstances; it is enough to see that, in the aforementioned plaques dedicated to Dr Sousa Martins, the beneficiary is often identified either with a common undifferentiated name or by acronyms. “*Nihil novi sub sole*”.

12. The very eroded limestone votive altar found at the villa of Milreu (Estoi, Faro) may have been ordered by a freedman named M. Acilius Balbus, *pro salute et reditu aeorum* (M. Acilius Balbus for their health and prosperity).

Both the divinity to whom it was dedicated and the identities of the beneficiaries are unknown; however, given the dimensions (it is 81 cm high), it seems to be an important monument and, therefore, it was recorded: “that the possible presence of the formula *pro salute et reditu eorum* suggests an ex-voto to an august deity, in honour of an imperial domus". In addition:

> It is an admissible hypothesis if we consider that at least three imperial portraits were found in the villa: Agrippina, Hadrian and Galienus (this one is from the 3rd century, at which time the monument can be reported by palaeography) (IRCP 2).

13. In the villa of Pisão, next to Beja, in a shrine of Trigaches marble, the slave Catulus willingly fulfilled a vow to *Salus*, for G(aio) Atilio Cordo n(ostro) [IRCP 290 – (Fig. 1.2)].

The ultimate meaning of this gesture cannot be overemphasized, especially because of the presence of the possessive our, demonstrating, without a doubt, the affection that the slave showed toward his master – whom, for this very reason, he prayed for a long healthy life sustained by divine intercession.

14. The same can be said about the granite shrine from São Bento do Mato (Évora), erected to *Salus* by *Canidius pro salute Acili Rufini* (To the health of Acilius Rufinus) (IRCP 375 = HEpOL 23722 – (Fig. 1.3).

There is apparently no explicit complicity here, and Canidius does not present himself as a slave – in fact, there is a chance that he may belong to the Canidii family, senators from Évora; however, the same vow is expressed that the deity will protect Acilius Rufinus and give him a long life.

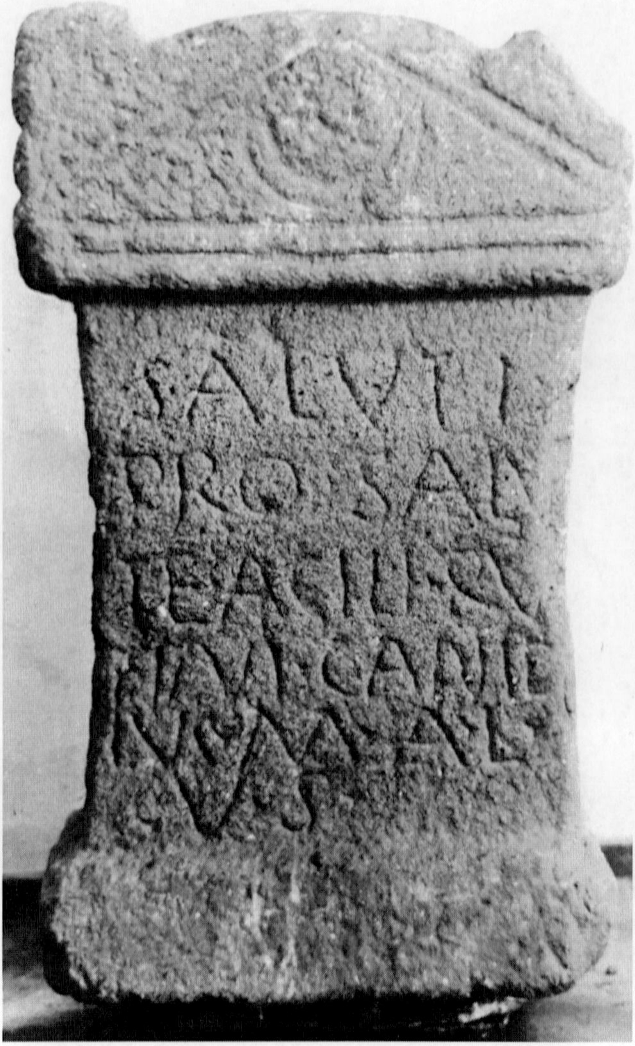

Fig. 1. 2. Votive shrine to Salus (IRCP 290). Reproduced with permission.

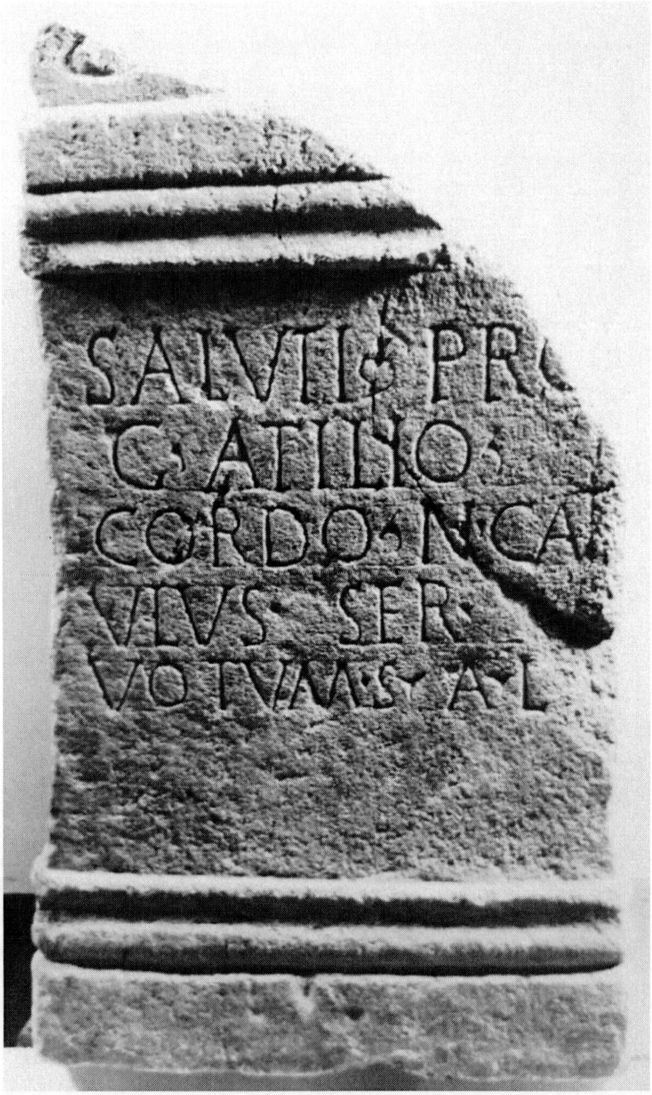
SALVTI PR
C ATILIO
CORDO NCA
VIVS SER
VOTVM S A L

Figure 1.3. Votive shrine to Salus (IRCP 375). Reproduced with permission.

15. A shrine found in S. Vicente da Beira (Castelo Branco) is housed in the Museum Tavares Proença Júnior, in Castelo Branco.

It is not possible to read the name of the dedicator, but it is known that – as a result of a promise – he ordered a shrine, 73 cm high, to Jupiter: *Iovi aram pos(uit) pro sua salute v(otum) l(ibens) s(olvit)* (He laid a shrine to Jupiter for his health and fulfilled the vow of his own free will).

As José Manuel Garcia strongly underscored: "Jupiter [...] is worshipped here for his salutiferous power since he will have granted his favours to those who, believing in his powers, thanked him for having this monument made" (Garcia 1984, 55).

Reflections

It is clearly impossible to reach extensive, valid conclusions from a sample of only 15 epigraphic documents, with various inherent limitations, especially if we take into account that the analysed space has been artificially delimited. It is a basic sample with inherent limitations.

Thus, in Vipasca II (nº 2), *salutem* is merely a greeting protocol.

The political connotation – an allusion to the health of the emperor or of the imperial domus – is, in turn, evident in the dedication of a campus in Trajan's time (nº 1); in the *iusiurandum Aritiensium* (nº 8), in a very expressive way; and in the dedication – which is very protocolar – to the Sun and the Moon by an imperial legacy (nº 10), in a sanctuary of obligatory pilgrimage, for how much we are told; also in Milreu (nº 12) the emphasis on pleasing the central power seems evident.

Dedications to the goddess *Salus* are extant from: Torres Novas (nº 4). The dedicator himself pleads on his own behalf; in the villa of Pisões (nº 13), a slave (?) invokes her for the sake of his master (really touching the presence of the possessive nostro); in the outskirts of Ebora (No. 14), the member of a well-known family (Senators Canidii) asks for a friend or family member.

In this salutiferous context, all the divinities are featured in a good way, we would say, starting from Jupiter, and invoked either for the health of the dedicator (nº 15) or for other reasons (nº 9).

The divine spirits related to the waters' beneficial properties occupy a prominent place in other areas of the Empire which were more fertile in terms of water springs. Here we have the case of Albia Pacina worshipping Fontanus in his double masculine and feminine qualities, possibly summoned for her husband (nº 6); and an invocation of Avitus to the Nymphs for the health of his wife (nº 7).

The ex-voto to Victoria (No. 3), made for the health of the dedicator himself, suggests a military environment. Victory will certainly help against diseases; however, good physical condition was essential to obtain it. And it was nearby that a campus – possibly military – was consecrated to the emperor's health! (nº 1).

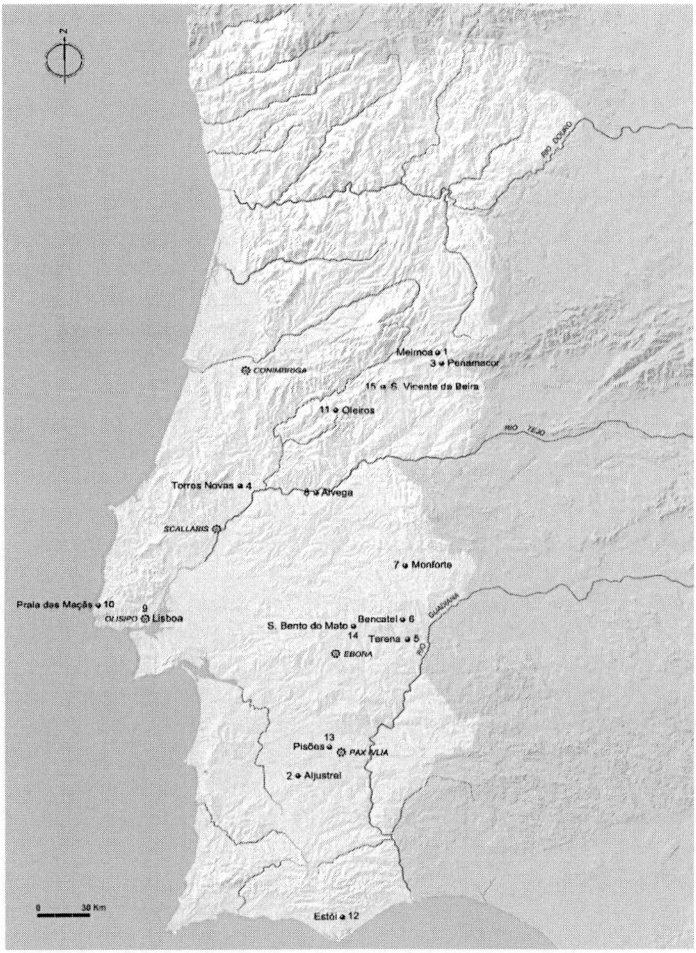

Fig. 1.4. Monuments' locations. Map by José Luís Madeira. Reproduced with permission.

From that same area around civitas Igaeditanorum, came title 11, to be placed in a sanctuary (of an indigenous deity?) for a family member's health. Note, again, the symptomatic presence of the possessive *suus*.

Of course, Endovelicus, an indigenous divinity, was also called to intervene on behalf of his Manilia (nº 5). The tenderness (marital?) keeps good credentials.

The inscriptions cover an entire population without social distinction - men, women, senators and slaves; both Roman and indigenous deities were appealed to in both urban and rural environments, with political connotations indicating the former (Fig. 1.4).

Conclusion

In early 2021, the world faced a physical health crisis: the deleterious consequences on the human body of the infection caused by the pandemic virus. Attention has also been paid – and with even greater concern, perhaps – to the severe consequences on mental health. This means that we face the concept of *Salus*, health, in its dual meaning – and who should decide which of the meanings is the fundamental one!

We were aware of both concepts as we worked through the inscription catalogue relating to the concept of *Salus* in this western territory of Lusitania: personal, physical health, and health synonymous with well-being and prosperity. When approaching these epigraphic monuments, it seemed that they were addressing situations where physical health was being threatened. Deeper analysis, however, revealed prominent spiritual or psychological dimensions were rather more numerous.

We should conclude that, like in Roman times, in his profound being, the perennity of Man, depending on a greater Force, goes over and over, along with feelings of helpless, facing invisible forces difficult to overcome, because they are so often wrapped in the fog of mystery...

Acknowledgement

The author is very grateful to Dr Maria do Sameiro Barroso for kindly translating the original Portuguese manuscript into English.

References

Canto, Alicia Maria. 2004. "Los viajes del caballero inglés John Breval a España y Portugal: novedades arqueológicas y epigráficas de 1726", *Revista Portuguesa de Arqueologia*, 7 (2): 265-364.

Cicero, Marcus Tullius. 1933. *De natura deorum*. Rackham, Heinemann, William (ed), Rackham, Harris (English translation). London: Harvard University Press.

Curado, Fernando Patrício. 1979. "Epigrafia das Beiras". *Conimbriga,* 18: 145-148.

Darenberg, Charles & Saglio, Edmond. 1969. *Dictionnaire des Antiquités Grecques et Romaines*. Graz: Akademische Druck-u-Verlagsanstalt.

Diogo, António Manuel Dias & Neto, José Luís. 2000. "Árula votiva de Vale do Souto, Oleiros". *Ficheiro Epigráfico* 63 2000 inscrição nº 285.

Encarnação, José d' & Gonçalves, Maria José. 2013. "Cilpes / CILPIS / Xilb / Silves? – Para uma discussão antiga um novo contributo. A inscrição de Silves evocativa do templo de Neptuno". *Espacio Tiempo y Forma* série II (História Antigua), 26: 255-276. http://hdl.handle.net/10316/25153

Garcia, José Manuel. 1984. *Epigrafia Lusitano-Romana do Museu Tavares Proença Júnior.* Castelo Branco: Museu de Tavares Proença Júnior.

González, Julián & Arce Javier (eds). 1988. Madrid: Consejo Superior de Investigaciones Cientificas. Centro de Estudios Historicos.

Pereira, Maria Helena da Rocha. 2002. *Estudos de História da Cultura Clássica* – II volume – Cultura Romana. Lisboa: Fundação Calouste Gulbenkian.

Ribeiro, Agostinho, Correia, Alberto & Borges, Dulce Helena Pires [eds], 1998. *Do Gesto à Memória – Ex-votos.* Lisboa: Instituto Português de Museus.

Ribeiro, José Cardim. 2019. *Escrever sobre a margem do Oceanus: epigrafia e religio no Santuário do Sol Poente (Provincia Lusitania).* (Sylloge Epigraphica Barcinonensis, Annexos III). Barcelona: Galerada.

CHAPTER 2

ROMAN MEDICAL-SURGICAL INSTRUMENTS FROM THE ARCHAEOLOGICAL MUSEUM D. DIOGO DE SOUSA, BRAGA[1]

MARIA DO SAMEIRO BARROSO

Abstract

Emperor Augustus (reigned 27 BC-14 AD) founded Bracara Augusta in 16 or 15 BC. The name derives from local indigenous peoples, the *Bracaros,* and Emperor Augustus. The Roman town, considered to rival other outstanding Roman capitals like Hispalis (currently Seville), is still awaiting thorough excavation. This essay selects a votive inscription dedicated to Asclepius and Hygeia to introduce the medical collection. The instruments, dated to between the 1st-4th century AD, were discovered at different archaeological sites in Braga and are housed in the Archaeological Museum D. Diogo de Sousa. Most tools rank among the common typologies of medical-surgical instruments from the Graeco-Roman world, some being rare or unique to the Portuguese territory such as a small scalpel handle and a pair of iron bow-scissors, bringing new insights into operations performed during Roman times. Most surgical tools were excavated at the Top of Cividade Hill which comprised buildings associated with baths and a theatre. Most tools were recovered from the deposits of later settlements, presumably being derived from the bath facilities. This discovery makes this collection particularly interesting. Only a few surgical instruments have previously been discovered in baths, where surgical operations seemed to

---

[1] Previous versions of this article we presented: "Roman medical-surgical instruments from the Archaeological Museum D. Diogo de Sousa in Braga" at the *Simposium Internacional Historia de la Cirurgía, Ciudad de México 9 y 10 de setiembre 2019*; *Bracara Augusta — Sob a protecção de Esculápio e Higeia* at III Jornadas Portuguesas de Paleopatologia. A saúde e a doença no passado, 2-3 de Novembro de 2012, Centro de Investigação em Antropologia e Saúde (CIAS) Departamento de Ciências da Vida, Universidade de Coimbra.

have taken place. No associated surgeon's tomb or physician's name has been identified so far. None of the instruments came from a specific medical-surgical context. Grave goods from Via XVII's necropolis include grooming tools, mainly balsamaria, an aryballos and a strigil. This instrument is also a medical device, whose function and symbolism in funerary contexts is reviewed.
Keywords: Bracara Augusta; Ancient surgical instruments; Roman baths; strigil; funerary practices

Resumo

O imperador Augusto (reinou de 27 a. C.-14 d.C.) fundou Bracara Augusta em 16 ou 15 a. C. O nome deriva dos povos indígenas locais, os Bracaros e do nome do imperador Augusto. A cidade, considerada rival de outras importantes capitais romanas como Hispalis (atualmente Sevilha), ainda aguarda escavações completas. Para este estudo, selecionámos uma inscrição votiva dedicada a Asclépio e Hígia para apresentar a colecção médica. Os instrumentos, datados entre os séculos I e IV d.C., foram descobertos em diferentes sítios arqueológicos de Braga e encontram-se no Museu Arqueológico D. Diogo de Sousa. A maioria insere-se nas tipologias comuns de instrumentos médico-cirúrgicos do mundo greco-romano. Algumas peças são raras ou únicas no território português, como é o caso de um pequeno cabo de bisturi e uma tesoura em ferro, o que acrescenta um novo conhecimento sobre as operações realizadas durante a época romana. Grande parte dos instrumentos surgiram em escavações no Alto da Colina da Cividade, constituído por edifícios associados a termas e a um teatro. A maioria das peças foi recuperada dos depósitos de assentamentos posteriores, presumivelmente provenientes das instalações do balneário. Esta descoberta torna esta coleção particularmente interessante. Apenas alguns instrumentos cirúrgicos foram descobertos anteriormente em complexos termais, onde as operações cirúrgicas parecem ter sido praticadas. Nenhum túmulo de cirurgião associado ou nome de médico foi identificado até agora. Nenhum dos instrumentos surgiu de um contexto médico-cirúrgico específico. Espólios funerários da necrópole da Via XVII incluem objectos de higiene, principalmente balsamários, um aríbalo e um estrígilo. Este é também um instrumento médico, cuja função e simbolismo em contextos funerários revemos neste estudo.
Palavras-chave: Bracara Augusta; Instrumentos cirúrgicos antigos; Balneários romanos; estrigilo; práticas funerárias

Introduction

The Archaeological Museum D. Diogo de Sousa was founded in 1918. It was a small museum housing archaeological remains from Bracara Augusta and religious and art collections which subsequently underwent many vicissitudes (Oliveira 1986, 171-195).

In 1980 it was revitalized. Its patron D. Diogo de Sousa (1468-1505) (Fig. 2.1) was a remarkable cleric and man of culture. Born in Évora, he studied Theology at the Universities of Salamanca and Paris. On his return to Portugal, he was appointed Canon at Évora (cónego eborense), and King John II (reigned 11-15 November 1477 and 1481-1495) nominated him Dean of the Royal Chapel. He participated in the tribute and obedience embassies to Pope Alexander VI (Papacy 1492- 1503) and Julius II (Papacy 1503-1513). He was Bishop of Oporto and Braga. During his visits to Rome, de Sousa became acquainted with the most elevated humanistic and artistic values of the Renaissance; these inspired his activities in the city where he was archbishop from 1505 until he died in 1532 (Silva 2011, 36-39).

Breaking through the medieval wall, he expanded the city with a building programme, creating new and airy squares that persist to the present day (Torres 2006, 35-44).

By this time, the city had expanded far beyond the Roman Bracara Augusta, appearing on the first map in Georg Braun (1541/2-1622) and Frans Hogenberg's work (1590?) *Civitates Orbis Terrarum*, as *Noua Bracarae Avgvste descriptio* together with Olisipo (Lisbon) and Conimbriga (Coimbra) (Braun and Hogenberg 1598). The presumed location of the Roman Forum was on the lower-left corner, according to Morais (*apud* Ribeiro 2015, 59) (Fig. 2.2). The excavation of the Roman town started in 1976 when archaeological remains came to light during construction works in the city of Braga (Lemos 2008, 203-239).

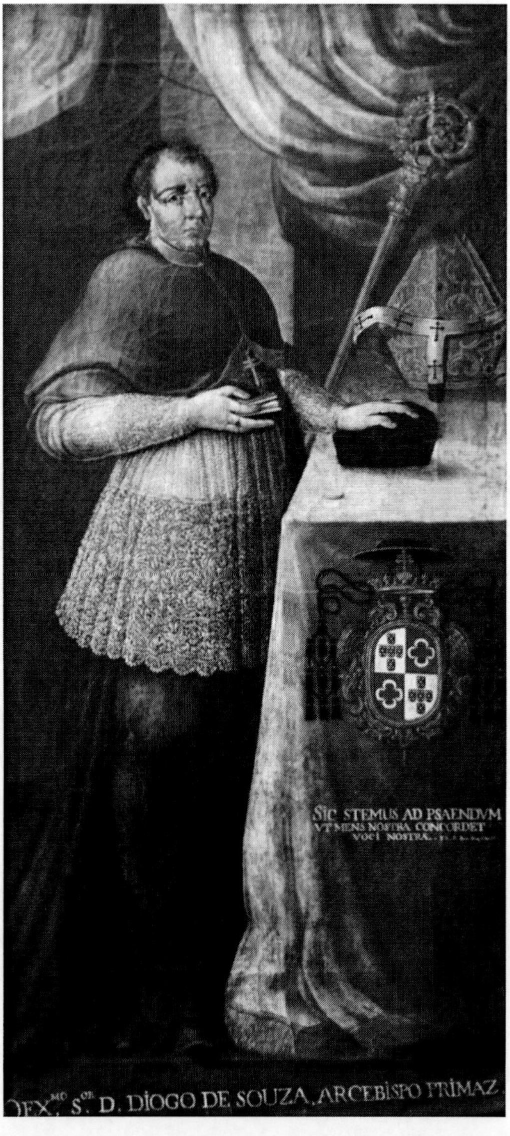

Fig. 2.1. Portrait of D. Diogo de Sousa. Tesouro-Museu da Sé de Braga. Public domain.

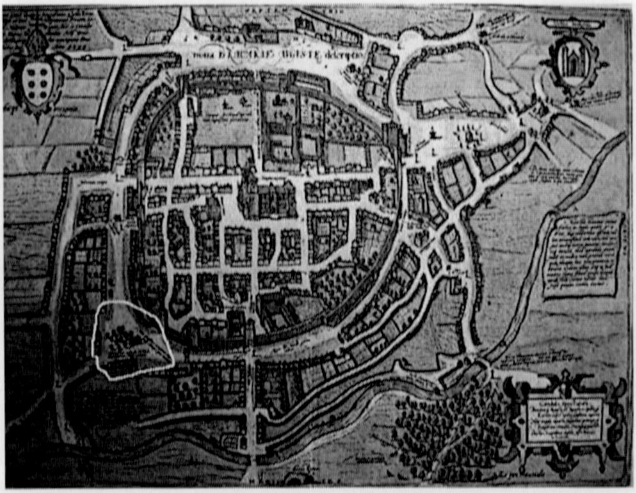

Fig. 2.2. Map of Bracara Augusta in Frans Hogenberg, Civitates Orbis Terrarum, 1594. Public domain.

Bracara Augusta

Bracara Augusta was founded by Emperor Augustus (reigned 27 BC- 14 AD) at the end of the Cantabrian Wars, around 16 BC, in the areas between the rivers Douro and Cávado, in Roman Gallaecia. The Bracaros, a Celtic tribe, had occupied the place. *Bracas were* the trousers worn by the Celtic population. Diodorus Siculus, an ancient Greek historian from the 1st century BC, described the physical appearance, clothing and religious and war rituals of the Celtic tribes from Gaul, referring to the *Bracas*:

> Their garments are very strange; for they wear partly coloured coats, interwoven here and there with divers sorts of flowers; and which they call Bracas. They make likewise their cassocks of blanket-work joined together with laces on the inside, and chequered with many pieces of work like flowers; those they wear in winter are thicker, those in summer ate more slender. (Diodorus Siculus translated by Booth, 1814, vol. II, Book V, chapter II, 315).

Bracae or Braccae were not items of clothing exclusive to the Bracaros. Diodorus refers to them as part of the peoples' clothing around Rome, such as the Medes, Persians, Parthians, Phrygians, Sacae, Sarmatae, Dacians, and Getae, Teutones, Belgae, Britons and Gauls. *Braccae* is the same as the

Scottish "breeks" and the English "breeches". These *Braccae* looked strange to the Romans because they were not part of Roman dress, clearly distinguishing the Greeks and Romans from the other peoples, at least during Republican times. Later, they become more familiar, although never coming generally into use (Smith 1859, 213).

The Roman historian Cornelius Tacitus (56-120 AD) still refers to the Roman general Aulus Caecina Alienus (died in 79 AD) when wearing bracas (Gallic clothes), marching through Italy, as being offensive to Roman clothing standards (Tacitus, *Annales* translated by Moore, 1962, volume II, chapter XX, 192).

Battles between the Gauls and Romans are part of battle field scenes depicted in Roman sarcophagi from the second and third centuries AD. The tradition was initiated in Greek sarcophagi from Hellenistic times with the 'Alexandre sarcophagus' decorated with battle scenes of Alexandre the Great (356-323 BC). Roman sarcophagi continued to depict the Romans as guardians of civilization against the Barbarians. Roman soldiers wear cuirass while Celtic (and Germanic tribes) wear breeches, as seen in the 'Ludovisi battle sarcophagus' from around AD 250–260AD depicting scenes from battles between Roman and Germanic soldiers (McCann 1978, 110-111) (Fig. 2.2).

The Bracaros seem to be the only people named after these pieces of clothing. They were fierce Celtic tribes whose cities (called castros) were first excavated by one of the earliest and most prominent Portuguese archaeologists, Francisco Martins Sarmento (1833-1899). He unearthed the castros of Citânias de Briteiros and Sanfins in Taipas, near Guimarães.

The discovery of pre-Roman settlements complemented the descriptions provided in the accounts of Strabo (63 BC-23 AD), the Roman geographer, providing detailed knowledge of the indigenous peoples living there (Espelosín 2007, 250-271). Concerning the names of the inhabitants in the inscriptions discovered during the excavations, Camal is the name of the chieftain of the warriors who did not know the meaning of fear (Vasconcellos 1885). Trousers would have been suitable for their riding activities. The wearing of trousers from the 1st millennium BC by the nomadic Scythians, originally from the steppes of Eurasia, was associated with horse riding (Clutton-Brock, 1992). Trousers were part of the rider's equipment, benefiting the adhesion between horse and rider and protecting the perineum and the horsemen's lower limbs, especially when spending much time on horseback (Barroso 2020, 1-6).

Roman authors like Strabo wrote about the Celtic tribe from the Northwest of Portugal, recounting how they slept under the stars and sacrificed bulls, singing prayers, praising the light and creation as simple, uncultured exalted devotees, fulfilling the rituals to their deities in their plenitude of worshippers of the sun (Espelosín 2007, 260).

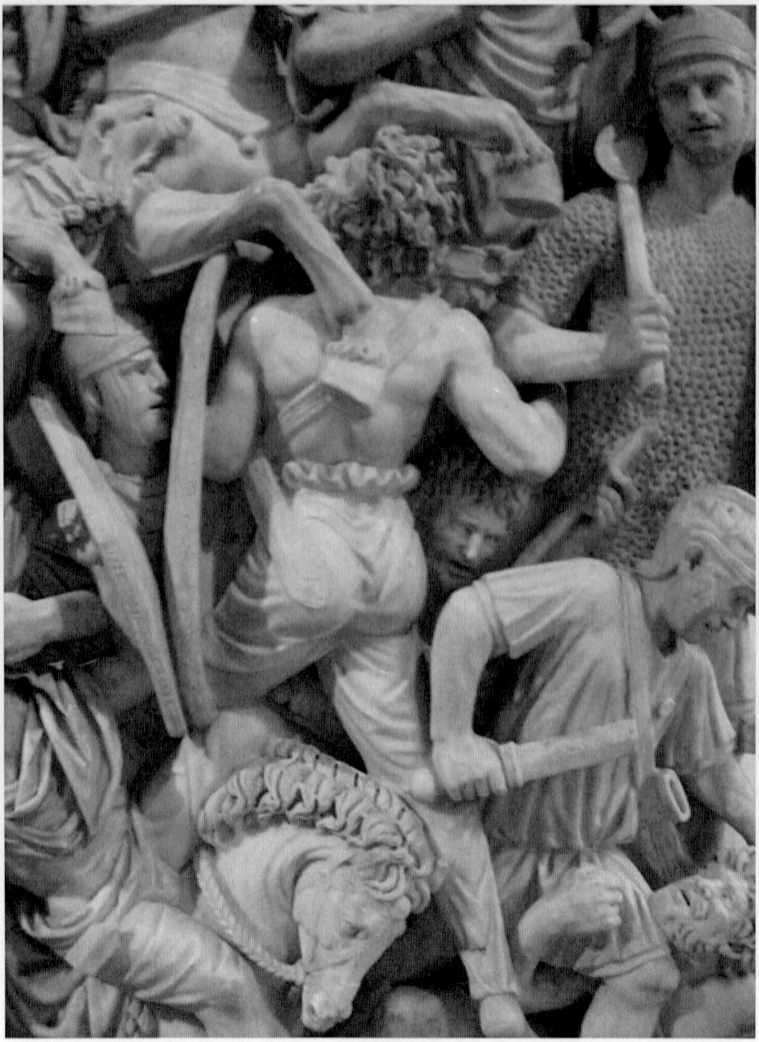

Fig. 2.3. Detail from the 'Ludovisi battle sarcophagus' or 'Grande Ludovisi' sarcophagus. Ludovisi Collection. Rome. Public domain.

José Leite de Vasconcellos (1851-1941), another prominent Portuguese archaeologist, founder of the National Musem of Archaeology in Lisbon, also medical doctor, linguist and poet, was a close friend to Martins Sarmento. He was very enthusiastic about Sarmento's findings, and recreated the everyday life of this tribe in a poem, bringing their story to light, as he states in the ending lines of a poem written on 26 June 1881, at the foot of Citânia de Briteiros:

> However, later on, I, as light of wit,
> Will spread sacred flashes in the dark...
> And Science will bring you to life
> Oh, barbaric soldiers![2]

The second name of Bracara Augusta derives from "Augustus", the given name of Emperor Augustus; the word means venerable, majestic, and consecrated by the augurs. Augustus embodied the noblest rites that presided over Rome's foundation as referred to by the celebrated poet Quintus Ennius (239-169 BC), as "renowned Rome was founded by august auguri" (Ennius, Annals, fr. 468-469 in Warmington 1935, vol. I, 177).

Bracara Augusta was also found in a sacred place often struck by lightning. Such practice was related to the cult of Jupiter, the god of the sky, thunder and the king of Roman gods. The city was devoted to the cult of the divine Emperor Augustus (Morais 2010, 15), reaching its maximum extent in the 2nd century AD (Morais 2010, 7). Bracara Augusta was counted among the four most magnificent cities by the Roman poet Decimus Magnus Ausonius (310-395 AD) in his book *Ordo Urbium noblilium* (*The Order of Famous Cities*):

> After these thou shalt be told, beloved Hispalis, name Iberian, by whom glides a river like the sea, to whom all Spain subjects all magistrates. Not Cordova, not Tarragona with its citadel contends with you, nor wealthy Braga, lying proudly in her bay beside the sea. (Gerald, Hugh, Evelyn-White (trans.) Ausonius, *The Order of Famous cities,* vol., chapter XI-XIV, 1919, 277).

---

2 Porém, mais tarde, eu, luz da inteligência,/No escuro espalharei clarões sagrados.../E há-de ressuscitar-vos a Ciência,/Ó bárbaros soldados! Vasconcellos 1885. English translation by the author.

Remains of the cult of Aesculapius in Bracara Augusta

1.Votive wall shrine

A votive wall shrine with an inscription dedicated to Asclepius and Hygea, the Greek names of Aesculapius and Salus, was found on the wall of a 16th-century house on D. Afonso Henriques Street, according to Rigaud de Sousa (Rigaut de Sousa 1978, 20). It was housed at the Biscainhos Museum until 16 December 1993. The capital and the base are very much deteriorated. Even so, ornamental traces are still visible in the pediment (Fig. 2.4a). Vasconcellos referred to this votive shrine as having been included in Aesculapius' cult in Rome settled by Greek freed men (Vasconcellos 1913, 164-65). In Rome, the *medicus* was frequently a slave or a freed man of Hellenic origin, and not a citizen of free origins (Alonso 2018, 119-137). The cult of Aesculapius was introduced into Rome in the 3rd century BC following an outbreak of plague. Asclepius had travelled in the form of a serpent, arriving by ship to Tiber Island where the first shrine to the Roman god Aesculapius was built (Künzl 2002, 24). Sextus Pompeius, Festus, a grammarian of the second century AD who copied fragments of the work *De significatu verborum* by the earlier grammarian Marcus Verrius Flaccus (c. 55 BC-20 AD), explained the reason for the choice of this place and highlighted some of the characteristics of Asclepius's cult, namely, the reasons for the presence of serpents and dogs in Asclepius' (Roman Aesculapius) cult:

> To Asclepius on the island [*sc.*, in the Tiber] a temple was built because sick people are aided by physicians particularly through water. The serpent is the guard of this temple because it is a most vigilant beast and his faculty is especially appropriate in safeguarding the health of invalids. Dogs are also used in this temple because he was nourished by the teats of a dog. He has a gnarled staff which signifies the difficulty of his art. He is crowned with laurel because this tree is full of many remedies. To him hens were sacrificed (Festus translated by Edelstein & Edelstein 1998, 361-362).

The great Roman encyclopaedist Plinius the Elder (23/24-79AD) pointed out the therapeutic effects of snakes by applying their entrails to help heal their bites. The healing properties of snakes could be the reason why they were sacred to Asclepius:

> Moreover, many remedies are believed to be obtained from a snake, as I shall report in proper order, and this is why it is sacred to Aesculapius (Pliny *NH* Book XXIX, Chapter XXII. 71, translated by Jones in Henderson 1963, 231).

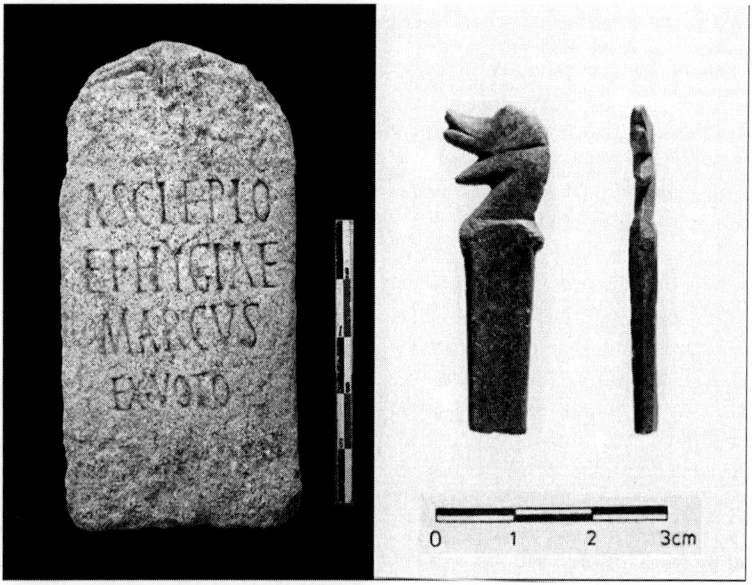

Fig. 2.4a. Votive shrine wall of granite dedicated to Asclepius and Hygea by Marcus. H. 780 mm Max Width 380 mm. 2nd/3rd century AD. Inv. Nr. 1992.0686. Photo credit: MDDS/Manuel Santos.
Fig. 2.4b. Handle with dog's head decoration. Copper alloy. L. 41 mm W. 14mm. 2nd century AD. Inv. Nr. 1992.0686. Photo credit: MDDS/Manuel Santos.

2. Handle decorated with dog's head

A handle decorated with a dog's head was discovered at the excavations in D. Afonso Henriques Street, located near the cathedral in the medieval town. The handle may have belonged to an object associated with the cult of Aesculapius or it might belong to a surgical instrument. Figure representation is rare on surgical instruments (Fig. 2.4b). The outstanding medical doctors and medical historians Theodor Meyer-Steineg (1873-1936) and Karl Sudhoff (1853-1938) reproduced a bronze scraper from the Hellenistic period decorated with a small figurine of Asclepius (Meyer-Steineg and Karl Suddhoff 1921, 90 fig. 55). Seven scalpel handles decorated with the bust of Heracles have been recovered, most from Pompeii.

Entailing labour and suffering, the myth of Heracles was an appropriate decoration for scalpels and other tools associated with pain (Bliquez 2016, 74). The handle may have belonged to a scraper since it presents no hole for insertion of the scalpel blade; it is impossible to make out any other typology because of the fragmentary nature of the specimen.

3. Female figurine

A female figurine discovered at the excavations of Colina do Alto da Cividade also presents challenges to interpretation. Such issues frequently occur with archaeological artefacts, as James Tschen- Emmons explains:

> Not everything survives, and so any picture we gain from artefacts is at best an incomplete picture. In recent decades archaeologists have also been keen to preserve as much from archaeological sites as they can, partially in hopes that future techniques will be better than those we possess now. At its best, archaeology is like working on a puzzle where many if not most pieces are missing. We get an idea of the past, but we cannot recover it completely. (Tschen-Emmonds 2014, xx).

The figurine was deemed to represent the local deity Tyche (or Cibele[3]) or Fortuna, the tutelary goddess of the city, since she wears a *corona muralis* with seven towers, holding an object first identified as a lituus (ritual stick used by the *auguri* to perform divinatory acts) under her left arm. A second crown, possibly belonging to another figurine, was excavated at the same locality (Morais 2010, 15-16) (Fig. 2.5). Giving cities the face of Tyche arises from the Greek habit of personifying cities, peoples and countries with the female figure of tutelary goddesses related to the cult of Tyche or Cibele.

Young protective goddesses were often depicted wearing a mural crown which replaced the cylindrical polos of the goddess Cibele (Allègre 1889, 190-92).

The female figure depicted presents an unusual facies. The ugly or unusual body features usually evoke retrospective studies of pathological images. One of these studies of mis-shapening representations collected in paintings, statues, reliefs, and coins in ancient history was carried out by the medical historians Mirko Grmek (1924-2000) and Dannielle Gourevitch (born in 1941). They succeeded in identifying conditions unknown in ancient times, this being the only source of knowledge about their existence. This approach should be complemented by the exegesis of ancient medical

---

[3] Anatolian Mother Goddess.

writings and paleopathology when available (Grmek & Gourevitch 1998, 28).

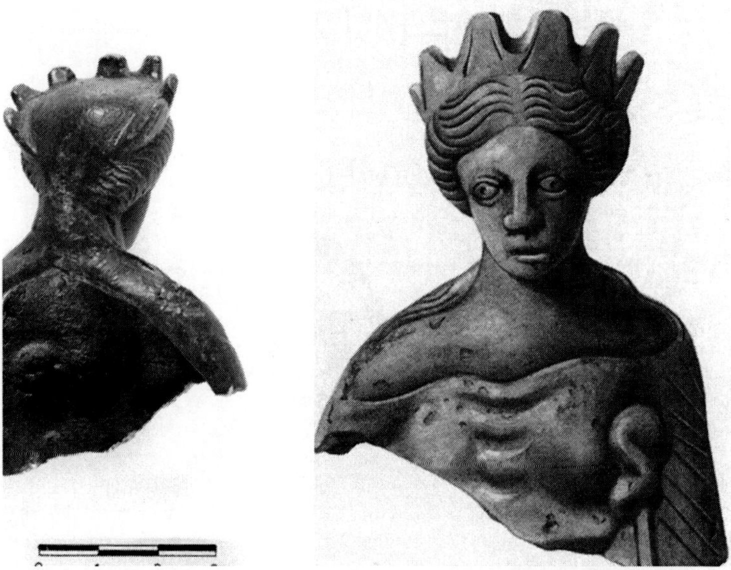

Fig. 2.5. Female figurine. Max height 70mm Max Width 49 mm 2nd century AD Inv. Nr. 1991.2666. Photo credit: MDDS/Manuel Santos.

The method can be considered when it is clear that the artist seeks to reproduce the model with a reasonable degree of fidelity since the artist would reproduce the pathological traits while observing the model. Manifest manufacturing defects are also excluding parameters. Identifying signs of a condition often leave little or no doubt as to the diagnosis. The medical interpretation of the hypothetical girl-goddess' anomalous face by the neurosurgeon, Dr António Trabulo, was as follows:

> The girl depicted in this figurine presents divergent strabismus, possibly by paresis of the right eye's internal rectus muscle, which presents exophthalmos (assuming the normal eye is the left). Besides, the temporal fossae are relatively convex, but not enough to diagnose hydrocephalus. The interorbital distance seems normal, and there is no reason to think about hypertelorism (increased distance between the orbits). The thickness of the wings of the nose may indicate African descent. In short, we observe

unilateral (right) exophthalmos with strabismus, tumour or congenital malformation standing as possible causes.

These facial abnormalities do not seem appropriate for a tutelary goddess symbolizing wealth and prosperity. A healthy face would be expected. Greek and Roman gods were usually depicted at the height of their imperishable beauty.

Further research by Armando Redentor has identified the object under her left arm as a serpent entwined around a rod, proposing the figurine as a personification of the goddess Salus (Greek Hygea) (Redentor 2011, I, 364-365). Morais et al. have hypothesised that the figurine could have been a syncretic deity wearing the crown of Tyche/Fortune combined with iconographic features of the goddess Hygea/Salus as indicated by the coiled serpent (Morais et al. 2013, 66).

Although this interpretation does not explain why she is wearing the mural crown, the relationship with the cult of Aesculapius seems very plausible.

Aesculapius and Graeco-Roman surgery and tools

Graeco-Roman medicine, extending from Hippocrates (460-370 BC) to Paul of Aegina (625-690 AD), the last Byzantine compiler, laid the foundations of rational medical thought, by explaining diseases by natural causes and by developing surgical procedures, mainly confined to the managing of traumatic conditions in earlier proto-medical approaches. As in the Greek world, the Roman Aesculapius continued to be an inspiring figure with characteristics of a humane medicine practitioner, being a reputed physician and surgeon. According to Gaius Iulius Hyginus (64-17 BC), a Roman writer born in the Iberian Peninsula:

> Chiron the Centaur, son of Saturn, first created the medical art of surgery after that of herbs; Apollo first created the medical art of ophthalmology; in the third place, moreover, Asclepius, son of Apollo, discovered „bedside“ medicine. (Hyginus, *Fabulae*, CCLXXIV, 9 in Edelstein & Edelstein II 1998, 186).

Marcus Tullius Cicero (106-43 BC), the Roman philosopher, summarized the legends of Aesculapius, and credited him with the invention of surgical materials:

> Of the various Aesculapi, the first is the son of Apollo, and he is worshipped by the Arcadians; he is reputed to have invented use of the probe and to have

> been the first surgeon to employ splints. (Cicero, *De Natura Deorum* III translated by Rackam, 1933, 341).

Greek physicians started to perform complex operations. Caius Cornelius Celsus (25 BC-50 AD), described a large number of surgical operations in his work *On Medicine*, frequently referring to the instruments used (Celsus, Books VII.VIII, Hendersen, 1938), together with other authors. Claudius Galenus (Galen) (129-200 AD) addressed the situation as follows:

> There is an operation for each part of the body, which we employ when we stitch up the eyelids and another completely different one for couching cataracts. There are three or four others bearing no similarity to one another, nor to those by which we cut away fractured bone from the skull, while in another part of the body (for example the arm or the forearm) we reduce and set and bind up fractures. Surgery for hernia is altogether distinct from such operations, just as surgery for varicose veins is from it, and just as the operation for bladder stone is from all those mentioned. For the majority of these interventions, we operate with a scalpel. On the other hand, to annoint the eyes or to reduce limbs or to put plaster on a part or two to employ a catheter properly or to apply a cupping vessel, requires no scalpel. These procedures are also completely distinct from one another and from all those aforementioned (Galen translated by Bliquez, 2016, 1).

In this text, Galen refers to simple procedures like applying cupping vessels or bloodletting, and procedures like lithotomy, a very dangerous surgical incision of the urinary bladder for removal of a calculus, only carried out in an attempt to save the patient's life when no further options remained (on this subject, see Barroso 2020 a, 192-196).

Victor Deneffe (1835-1908), one of the first surgeons devoted to the study of Graeco-Roman medical-surgical instruments, presented an insightful overview of the instruments and the operations performed by Graeco-Roman surgeons (Deneffe 1893, 11-18). Milne also related the mentions and descriptions of such instruments appearing in medical textbooks (Milne 1907). Around 120 different operations are recorded, at different times and places throughout the Roman Empire (Bliquez 2016, 1). Most surviving tools, dating from the 1st-4th century AD, were found either in funerary contexts or in consequence of natural disasters, such as the eruption of the Vesuvius in 79 AD (Künzl 2002, 58). Numerous instruments were found in the House of the Surgeon, currently housed in the Archaeological Museum of Naples. A fire at a physician's house in Rimini in the 3rd century AD also preserved 150 instruments. The house belonged to Eutyches, a military surgeon. Some typologies mentioned in medical texts such as the spoon of Diocles, devised to extract arrows, have never been found. (Domus Rimini).

Graeco-Roman medical-surgical tools in a funerary context

The study of Gaius Firminus Severus by Deneffe brought to light the relationship between Roman medical surgical instruments and funerary practices. By the end of the nineteenth century, the discovery of the tomb of the ophthalmologist Gaius Firminus Severus in Reims highlighted the practice of ophthalmology in Roman times. It was evident that the physician was most proud of his tools which had elegant decorations, also indicating his prestige and the high social status of his wealthy patients (Deneffe 1896, 12-13).

At that time, knowing nothing about asepsis, the physicians were not aware that decorative embellishments could harbour pathogens and consequently infect surgical wounds. Beautiful instruments, mainly handles (scalpel handles) with silver inlays and damascene decorations have been unearthed in the Roman city of Balsa, currently Tavira (Barroso 2014-2015, 341-373).

Among Gaius Firminus Severus‘ surgical tools, a fork appeared among the grave goods. Deneffe refers to funerary practices of the Romanized Gauls to figure out the meaning of this finding. Cadavers were cremated, purified by the fire. Bone ash and other remains preserved the eternal memory of the deceased in cinerary urns. The family members placed vases with small glass vessels containing the tears of both relatives and mourners hired for the funeral, together with bottles of perfume as signs of the deceased's memory around the urn. Plates of food and pitchers full of drink were also placed near the urn as travel supplies. At that time, people thought that the deceased would enjoy eating and drinking in the shadow's realm, surrounded by the things he liked when he was on earth. A coin to pay the ferryman, Charon, for crossing the Styx, the underworld river, was also placed in the tomb.

That tradition provides an important tool for dating the objects. The instruments of the profession were placed next to the deceased. Deneffe assumed that the main instruments would be selected: the most elegant, the most beautiful, the ones he cared about the most. There were gold and silver instruments in this tomb that probably were not the ones he commonly used. The fork was placed in the tomb to enable the deceased to consume food on his long journey (Deneffe 1893, 63-64, Pl. 4, Nr.13). Knives and spoons, among other objects, have also been found as grave goods in funerary practices in Northwest Europe from the 1st to early 3rd century AD (Pearce 2015, 223-248). These findings make it difficult to evaluate knives as surgical instruments.

In Roman times, in general, the deceased expressed pride in their profession in funeral inscriptions or depicted on tombstones. The tombs of *ornatrices*, for example, depicted combs and oil flasks (Kenrick 1858, 25, 29). Objects associated with grooming were depicted on tombstones to highlight the professions of barbers and hairdressers, depicting shears, combs and mirrors, or on tombstones of comb makers depicting combs. Such objects could also be depicted in on the tombstones of private individuals appearing to symbolize female virtue and status (Eckardt & Crummy 2008, 28). Tombs featuring physician's inscriptions date from the 4th century BC, in Greece, up to the 4th century AD throughout the Graeco-Roman world (Künzl 2002, 92).

Scalpel handles, probes, ear probes and tubes belong strictly to the surgical field. Scalpel handles often had the form of leaf-shaped spatulae. The different functions of the two sides of the instruments might have increased their functional range or, as Künzl has hypothesized, made them adaptablc and quick to manage in rapid operations performed without anaesthesia and involving high haemorrhagic risk (Künzl 2002, 51).

The following instruments leave no doubt as to the identification of a physician's grave: scalpels, lancets, dental forceps, bone elevators and chisels used in traumatology, as well as trepanation instruments, vaginal speculae, suction cups, cauteries, surgical needles and catheters (Künzl 2002, 35).

Scalpel handles survive preferentially because the blades, made of iron, are easily corroded over time. Probes, spatulae, forceps, and tweezers have frequently been discovered in excavations of Roman archaeological sites. Other implements, such as cataract needles, dental forceps, vaginal and rectal specula, bone levers, hooks, retractors, tubes, chisels, trepaning, lithotomy and embryotomy instruments have been found only rarely. Spatulae and spoon-probes were utilized in the preparation of medicines and topical application. Palettes, scoops and mixing rods are also part of that range of instruments. Bow scissors, tweezers and strigils were used in medicine and toiletry, frequently being found together in funerary contexts; toilet tools, however, are smaller and less elaborated.

Medical-surgical instruments from Bracara Augusta

All the medical-surgical artefacts housed in the Archaeological Museum D. Diogo de Sousa were found in excavations carried out from 1976 onwards.

Most came from Top of the Cividade Hill (Colina do Alto da Cividade), the highest place in the city located near the Forum where a theatre, baths, and a palaestra (area dedicated to the practice of sports) have been unearthed. The baths were built during the early 2nd century AD above an earlier building dating from the 1st century AD. The buildings related to the baths underwent refurbishment by the end of the 2nd and 3rd century. By the 4th century AD, they were no longer functional (Martins 2005, XVII). The theatre, next to the baths, was also built in early in the 2nd century AD. Just one-third of the building has been excavated so far (Ribeiro 2015, 141). Many grooming tools, mainly balsamaria, have been discovered at the necropolis of Via XVII (Lourenço 2012, 69). Just a few discoveries have been made at the other excavated necropolis. Four large necropoleis, located outside the city by the main exits, have been identified:

1- Necropolis of Maximinos at the Via XVI exit (Bracara-Olisipo) near the *Sinistra* Gate, occupying the West and Southwest of the city.

2- Necropolis of Via XVII in the Oriental part of the city, encompassing archaeological findings of the Post-office Building and Av. da Liberdade near the exit of Via XVII (Bracara-Astorga) by Acqua Flavis, currently Chaves.

3- Necropolis in the North, Campo da Vinha, connected with the exit either to Via XVIII (Bracara-Astorga) by the current Gallician city of Orense or Via XIX (Bracara-Lucus).

4- Necropolis in the South of the city, following the current Rodovia, corresponds to the exit connecting Bracara and Emerita Augusta by Egitania, currently, Viseu (Martins & Delgado 1998, 41-186).

Some instruments were recovered from a series of undifferentiated objects from different periods or dumps belonging to later settlements, making their exact dating equivocal. For this essay, we selected the most outstanding medical-surgical instruments from the Top of Cividade Hill and toilet tools from Via XVII's necropolis for study. The information on the tools, when unpublished, was provided by the files and information of the staff of the Archaeological Museum D. Diogo de Sousa, in collaboration with the Archaeological Department of the Minho University.

1. Scalpel handle (*Scalpellus)*

A tiny leaf-shaped scalpel handle of copper alloy provided with a slot where a replaceable blade was inserted was discovered in a later ditch associated with the abandonment of the theatre amongst a diverse association of material at the Top of the Cividade Hill (Fig. 2.6a).

Most surviving scalpels are similar to this one but larger. Small scalpels suited to eye surgery were relatively small (Bliquez 2016, 79). One such item figures among items belonging to Gallo-Roman ocular physicians (Deneffe 1896, Planche IV, nº 3). This typology is rare. So far, this item is the only one of its type discovered in Portuguese territory.

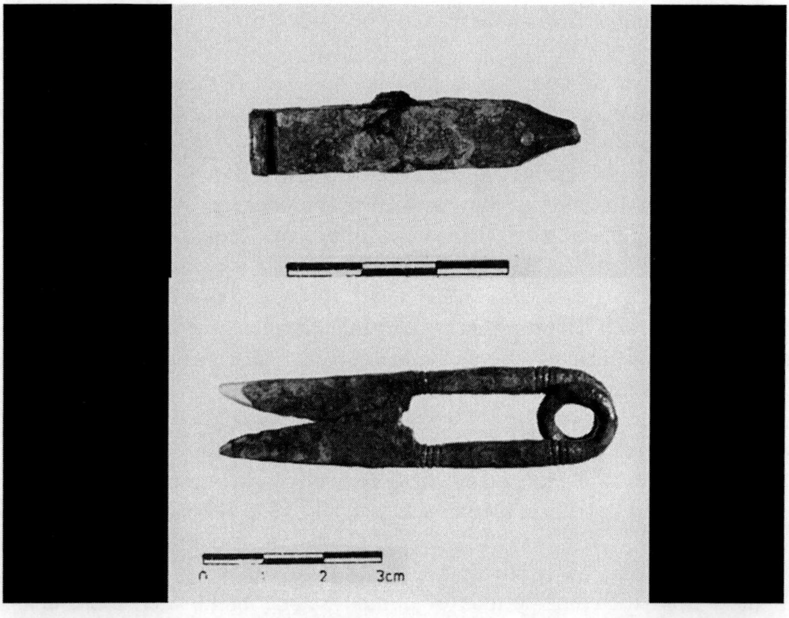

Fig. 2.6a. Leaf-shaped scalpel handle. Copper alloy. L. 44 mm; Max width 10 mm Inv. Nr. 2000.0672. Photo credit: MDDS/Manuel Santos. Fig.2.6b. Bow shears. Iron. Width 57 mm. Inv. Nr. 2012.0876. Photo credit: MDDS/Manuel Santos.

2. Bow shears (*Forfex)*

The pair of iron bow shears from Bracara Augusta is the only one known from Portugal to date. It is a well-preserved decorated piece, certainly for surgical use. The double knot makes it more robust and safer to use. It was found at a similar place as the scalpel-handle, at the Top of Cividade Hill, in a level filling associated with the abandonment of structures post-dating the theatre with Roman and medieval ceramic material (Fig. 2.6b).

Iron shears have been found in the Late Iron Age in Britain and the continent in male graves, with razors and weapons and female graves, being objects for personal grooming. In the Roman period, they appear in funerary context to cut human hair. They consist of pairs of connected separate iron blades each with a rounded handle. Considerable skill was required to operate the two unconnected blades. The twin blades were depicted in a series of tombs up to the 6th century AD. Barbers were proud of these tools which they chose to symbolize their profession (Eckart & Crummy 2008, 35).

Archaeological evidence also supports bow shears as surgical tools. A pair of bow shears is depicted in the relief of a hardware shop at Isola Sacra's necropolis in Ostia (2nd-4th century AD). Little is known about the manufacturers of medical-surgical instruments, this relief being a rare example in which bow shears are depicted among other medical-surgical tools (Künzl 2002, 54, fig. 70).

Iron/steel items have been excavated from the Casa del Medico Novo in Pompei and physicians' tombs in Landenburg, Nijmejen, Merida, Verona, Balcik, and Nea Paphos. They were used to prepare and cut sutures, ligatures, bandages and dressings in operations (Bliquez 2016, 107-108).

Perhaps the greatest risk to life was their use in Celsus' description of the cutting the omentum (a large sheet of fat that stretches over the intestines, liver, and stomach like an elastic apron) [4] when managing a perforated wound of the abdomen by a piercing weapon. This was a somewhat audacious procedure, which, retrospectively, is bone-chilling

[4] On the anatomy and physiology of the Peritoneum, see the following explanation: "Your peritoneum is a membrane, a sheet of smooth tissue that lines your abdominopelvic cavity and surrounds your abdominal organs. It pads and insulates your organs, helps hold them in place and secretes a lubricating fluid to reduce friction when they rub against each other. Your parietal peritoneum lines your abdominal and pelvic walls and your visceral peritoneum wraps around your organs."
https://my.clevelandclinic.org/health/body/22894-peritoneum#:~:text=Your%20peritoneum%20is%20a%20membrane%2C%20a%20sheet%20of%20smooth%20tissue,they%20rub%20against%20each%20other.
Accessed 17 August 2022.

because of the high risk of infection and consequent peritonitis leading ultimately to death:

> The omentum too must be examined, and any part that is black (dead) is to be cut away with shears; what is sound is returned gently into place in front of the intestines (Celsus Book VII, Chapter 16 translated by Spencer 1938, 387).

The egyptologist Sir Flinders Petrie (1853-1942) has reviewed metal shears and related objects such as knives, cutters, toilet tools and thread work, reporting rare ornamental specimens of metal shears dating prior to 300 BC, and appearing to be an Italian invention (Petrie 1917, 48 Plates LVIII and LIX).

3. Tube (*Xustra*)

Xustra are hollow conical tubes made of lead, bronze or tin designed to prevent contraction, adhesions and to convey medicines were found in Pompei, matching the descriptions of their use in operations on the rectum and vagina. Smaller tubes were inserted into the nostrils after abstraction of nasal polyps. These small tubes are frequently referred to as lead tubes (Milne 1907, 113-114). Not many of these tubes have survived to the present day. Three bronze tubes were discovered at Pompei (Milne 1907, 113, Plate XXXIX, 1). The hollow copper alloy tube, found in the excavation of São Paulo Street, being 59 mm long, diameter 5 mm, matches this description and is the only one found in Portugal (Fig. 2.7a).

4. Ear probe (*Auriscalpium*)

An ear probe whose handle is embellished with groove and cannelure decoration terminates in a sharp tip it is a particularly beautiful instrument from this collection. It was discovered at the Top of Cividade Hill and dates from the 4th century AD (Fig. 2.7b). Ear probes consist of a small circular scoop at one end and a sharp probe at the other. They were also utilized in eye surgery, as well as removing foreign bodies from the ear canal, and in the treatment of wounds (Barroso 2014-2015, 341-373).

Long thin rods provided with small ear scoop terminals were also utilized in urological procedures to remove bladder-stones from the neck of the bladder (Barroso 2020 a, 192-196).

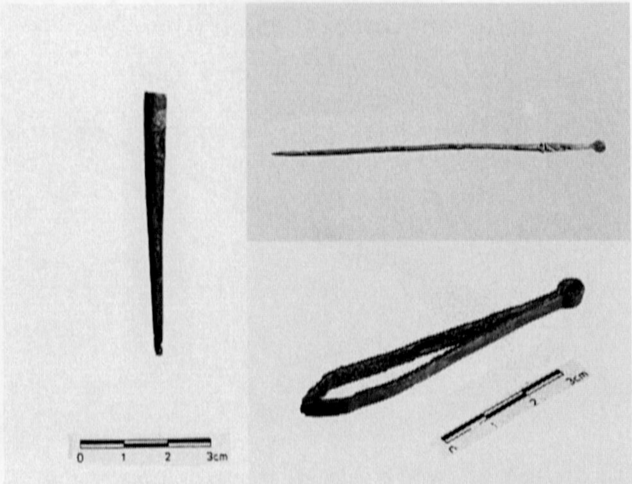

Fig. 2.7a. Conical hollow tube. Copper alloy. L. 59 mm D. 5 mm. Inv. Nr. 1996.0297. Photo credit: MDDS/Manuel Santos.
Fig. 2.7b. Ear probe. Gilded copper alloy. L. 120 mm D. of scoop 4 mm. 1st half of 4th century AD. Inv. Nr. 1991.2617. Photo credit: MDDS/Manuel Santos.
Fig. 2.7c. Tweezers. Copper alloy. L. 67 mm Width 24 mm. Inv. Nr. 2002.0028. Photo credit: MDDS/Manuel Santos.

5. Tweezers (*Vulsella)*

Small tweezers for cosmetic purposes or larger items with serrated jaws and incurved tips are amongst the most common surgical instruments found (Künzl 1983, 18). They are simple devices consisting of a strip of metal bent in on itself, followed by a straight unit with the jaws turned inwards (Milne 1907, 92, Plate XXVI, Nº 3). This is clearly evoked by the item from Bracara Augusta, which matches the description of grooming tweezers (Fig. 2.7c). These were found during the archaeological excavations at Santo António das Travessas Street. Milne reproduced a loop with three grooming objects suspended from it: tweezers, ear-pick and nail-cleaner. He called it a 'pocket-companion' (Milne 1907, 92, Plate XXVI, Nº 4). Toilet tweezers and surgical tweezers with beautiful decorations have been recovered from Balsa's Roman city (Barroso 2014-2015, 341-373).

6. Spoon-probe (*Ciathociscomele*)

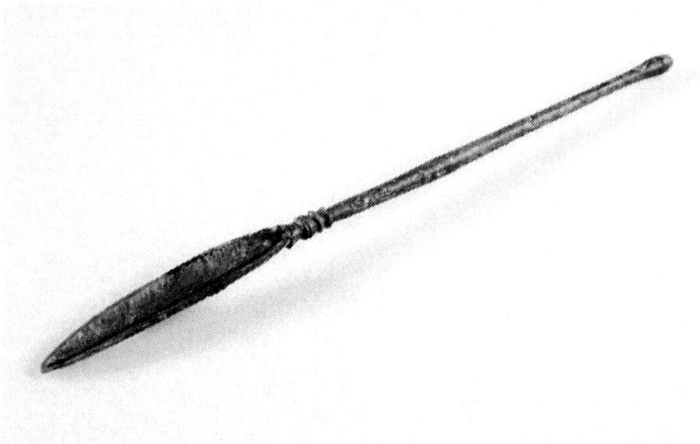

Fig. 2.8. Spoon-probe with olivary enlargement. Copper alloy. L. 160 mm Max width 10 mm. Inv. Nr. 1996.0547. Photo credit: MDDS/Manuel Santos.

Spatula-probes (*Spathomele*) are long rods with one extremity ending in an olive form and the other in a spatula. Spoon-probes (*Ciathociscomele*) are similar, the spatula being replaced by a spoon. The probe was used to introduce and examine cavities and wounds. The probe frequently had an olive-shaped tip and was used to mix liquids in a container and the spatula to spread the medicines over the affected areas (Milne, 1907, 58). The Bracara Augusta spoon-probe was recovered from the foundation ditch fill of a wall at São Paulo Street and dates from the 4th century AD (Inv. Nr. 1996.0547) The spoon scoop presents a dept groove three moulded rings on the shaft, terminating in the olivary tip, possibly having been used as a dropper (Fig. 2.8).

7. Toilet spoons (*Ligulae*)

Short or long-shafted ear scoops could be used to remove cerumen from the ear channel and extract cosmetics and perfumes from long-necked unguent bottles and apply them to the face or body. They commonly appear in domestic contexts, suggesting they were used mainly for grooming (Eckart & Crummy 2008, 39-40). They were also of medicinal use (Milne 1907, 63). The two specimens from Bracara Augusta present striated decorations of the shaft near the scoop (Fig. 2.9a).

8. Nail cleaner

Nail-cleaners were standard grooming tools but seldom made of bone like the specimen discovered at the necropolis of Via XVIII. A loop and large shoulders topped them, sometimes decorated with a leaf-shaped blade ending in pointed or bifurcated tips (Eckart & Crummy 2008, 121). The implement has broken extremities and bead moulding decorations. A bifurcated nail-cleaner with beautiful decoration, recovered from the excavations of Serpa and a portable set of a nail-cleaner ending in a pointed tip from Moutinho das Laranjeiras are housed in the National Museum of Archaeology in Lisbon (Barroso 2012, 115-122, fig. 8 and 9) (Fig. 9b).

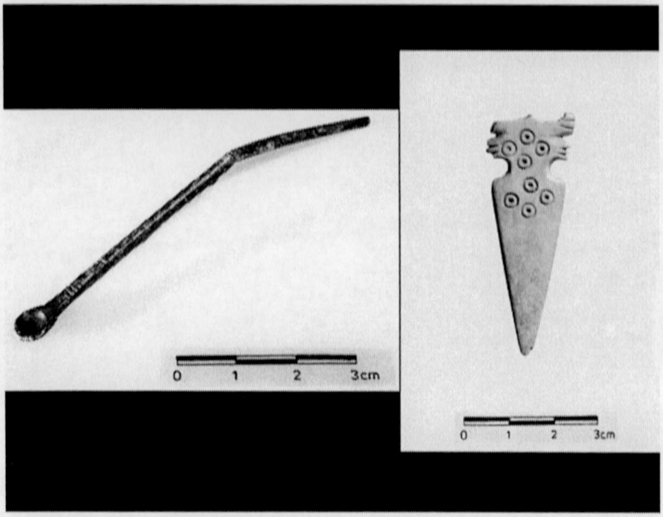

Fig. 2.9a. Ligula – Fragmented item, bent shaft and broken tip. Copper alloy. L. 82 mm Diameter of scoop 6 mm. Early 2nd century AD. Inv. Nr. 1998.1551. Photo credit: MDDS/Manuel Santos.

Fig. 2.9b. Fragmented nail cleaner. L. 50 mm W. 15 mm. Bone. Inv. Nr. 2008.0239. Photo credit: MDDS/Manuel Santos.

9. Perfume bottles

Small vessels in various forms, used either to contain oil to hydrate the skin after the bath or to store perfumes, were known as *aryballoi, alabastra, unguentaria* and *ampullae. Aryballoi* possess eyelets at the top and were suspended by a string or chain around the owner's neck, making it easier to carry to the baths. Olive oil was a common primary ingredient. Rose petals, tree resins such as styrax, cinnamon, and myrrh were popular scents and used medicinally. Selling perfumes was a profitable business, supplying temples, funerary clubs, public baths and general customers. The sellers were called *unguentarii or unguentariae,* since many were women (Tschen-Emmons 2014, 109-112).

Unguent bottles were the most common discoveries of glass in the cinerary tombs of the necropolis of Via XVII (Braga 2010, 89). Cinerary tomb INC100 is particularly interesting from the perspective of the toilet tools it contained, since a green-blue glass *aryballos,* broken at the neck, a blue-green glass unguent/perfume bottle, and a conical body were unearthed from the site along with two ceramic pots. The tomb, dated to the mid 2nd century AD, contained sandy silt, coal, ash and fragmented bones (Braga, 2010, File 35) (Figs 2.10a and 2.10b).

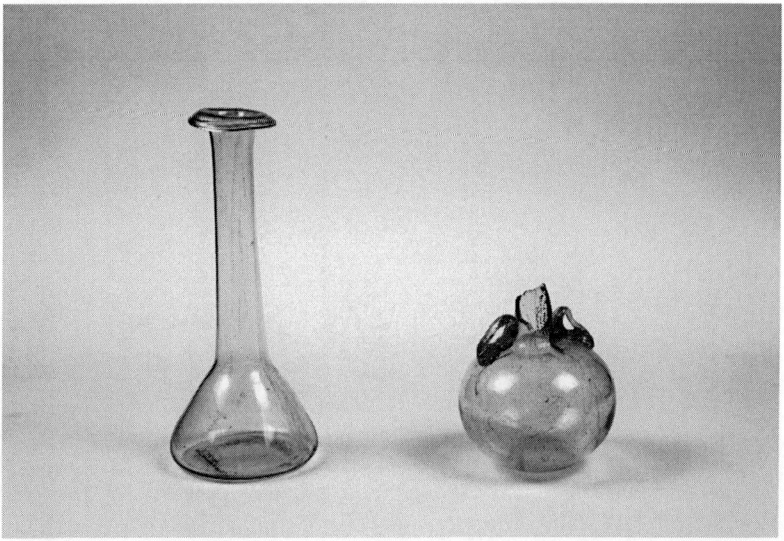

Fig. 2.10a. Blue-green glass unguent/perfume bottle, conical body. H. 165 mm D. 72 mm. Inv. Nr. 2009.0514. Photo credit: MDDS/Manuel Santos.

Fig. 2.10b. Fragmented green-blue glass aryballus. 1st/2nd century AD. H. 89 mm D. 74 mm. Inv. Nr. 2009.0515. Photo credit: MDDS/Manuel Santos.

10. Strigil

Sports were a leading activity in the ancient Greek world. Olympic games were held in honour of the god Zeus every fourth August from 776 BC to 395 AD at Olympia, a grassy plain with shady olive trees, poplars, vines and palm trees to the North of the river Alpheios. The festival, originating in funeral games honouring local heroes, attracted citizens from all over the Greek world. The river provided water for baths next to the *palaestra* framed for the athletes training. The athletes used to anoint themselves with olive oil to protect them from sunburn and accumulation of dust before going out to take part in the competitions. After exercise, they scraped off the oil, dust and sweat with the help of strigils before bathing themselves. Strigils were toilet tools consisting of a blade and handle (Swaddling 1980, 7-9). The athletes used to carry one or more strigils in a loop. They also used to carry an oil flask, the *aryballos*. The oil was sometimes bottled and sold as a medical treatment called *gloios* to relieve aches, pains and sprains (Strigil-Wellcome Image Collection).

The earliest mention of sport-related medicine appears in the manuscripts of Cnidian medicine, the earliest extant writings of Greek medicine (Grensemann 1975, Vorwort vii). Herodicus of Selymbria, a physician from the fifth century BC, is the father of Sports Medicine. He authored a manuscript discovered in 1893, *Anonymus Londinensis* IX 20-26, and his ideas are cited and commented on by later philosophical and medical authors (Grensemann 1975, 15-20; Georgoulis et al. 2007, 315-318). Georgoulis et al. summarized his relevance to medicine:

> Herodicus (fifth century BC) is the first person in the history of medicine who actually combined sports with medicine. He used to be a sports teacher, who later studied medicine and managed to succeed Euryphon in the medical school of Cnidos, one of the most prominent in ancient Greece, together with its neighbor medical school of Cos (Hippocrates' home). In Cnidos, Herodicus formed his own theoretical perspective of medicine. He considered, namely, bad health to be the result of imbalance between diet and physical activity and for this reason, he recommended strict diet, constant physical activity and regular training. He believed that this combination was the ideal way to maintain good standards of health, and he applied this type of treatment method to his patients. Unfortunately, Herodicus' works are lost today. (Georgoulis et al. 2007, 315-318).

However, due to insufficient knowledge of pathophysiology in times pre-dating Hippocratic medicine, Herodicus advised great efforts in patients with fever, which had hazardous consequences, as stated in Hippocratic writings:

> Herodicus killed fever patients with running, much wrestling, hot baths. A bad procedure. Fever is inimical to wrestling, walks, running, massage; that is trouble for them. Swelling of the blood vessels, redness, lividness, pallor, soft pains in the ribs. (Smith 1994, *Hippocrates VII, Epidemics 6, Chapter 3. 18,* 243).

Strigils were made of iron or copper and often carried together with oil flasks or *aryballoi.* Strigil blades had sharp edges to ease the scraping process, being curved for collecting dirt, oil and the other substances. They also played a prominent role in athletes' training and cleaning in the larger framework of comradely encounters and entertainment related to the musical and intellectual education provided at the *palaestra* (Eckardt & Crummy 2008, 37).

They have been mostly depicted in Attic red-figure vases related to the homoerotic or heterosexual experiences of the aristocracy, mainly with *hetaerae*, but were also used by women. There are also representations of strigils in funerary vases from the South of Italy (Kotera-Feyer 1998, 107-136). In Roman times, strigils appear in bathing and funerary contexts.

A beautiful transparent glass cup with Snake-Thread decoration, type Isings 85, with broken rim, and ceramic objects: a pot, a plate and an oil lamp, were also part of the grave goods.

A fragmentary iron strigil (the handle is missing) was also found in the cinerary tomb TAVL Nº 42 of the necropolis from Via XVII dated to the late 2nd/early 3rd century AD (Fig. 2.11). Strigils, unguent bottles, dishes, cups, bowls and other objects have been discovered as grave goods in Helshoven and Bocholtz, Limburg, the Netherlands in a tomb dating from the 2nd and early 3rd century AD (Pearce 2015, 243-244). Household and grooming grave goods have often been viewed as "evoking the domestic space in tombs considered as eternal homes for the deceased", according to Pearce (Pearce 2015, 127-238).

Strigils are rare discoveries in Portugal. An incomplete bronze strigil has been excavated from the baths of the Roman city of Conimbriga, near Coimbra. The handle is missing (Alarcão 1994,129, fig. Nrº 397). The fragmentary strigils from Bracara Augusta and Conimbriga are the only items excavated from Portuguese Roman archaeological sites.

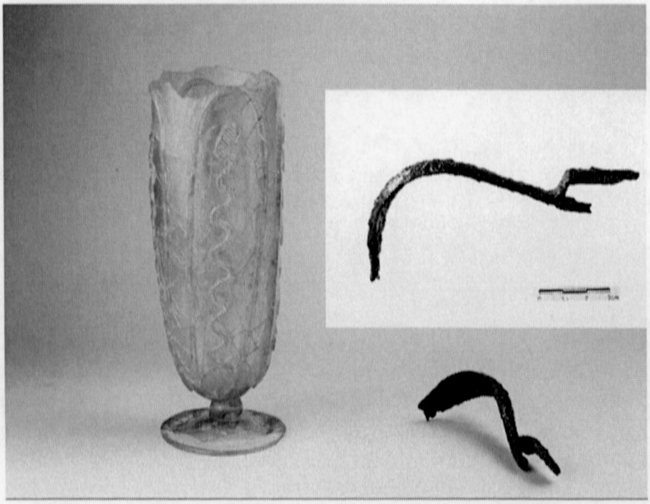

Fig. 2.11. Transparent glass cup with broken rim and Snake-Thread decoration. H. 206 mm D. 77 mm, Late 1st/early 2nd century AD. Inv. Nr. 2009.0419. Photo credit: MDDS/Manuel Santos

Four iron strigils and a small pair of bow-scissors were excavated from tomb N° 2315, dated to the 1st century AD, from the necropolis of Wederath, Belginum (Belgium), a place inhabited by romanized Celtic tribes. A strainer and a sieve of bronze for scooping and cleaning the wine, a ceramic pot and a very blue wine glass cup decorated with spherical motifs in relief, with broken indented rim were also part of the grave goods collection. The choice of these objects surprised the archaeologists who hypothesized that the deceased might have been a medical doctor of Celtic origin who had learned to appreciate body care and Roman wine drinking habits (Haffner 1989, 108-109, fig. 75). The wine glass cup from this tomb is surprisingly similar to the item from tomb 42 from Bracara Augusta.

Artistic representations of funerary rituals have been recorded as *Totenmahlen* (Funerary banquets) since the 6th century BC in the Graeco-Roman world, gods, heroes and unknown men being represented as enjoying the pleasures of the after-life in earthly existence. Typically, a bearded half-nude male figure is represented reclining on a *kliné* (couch), his right hand raising a *rhyton* (conical container in the shape of animal's head), a table before him displaying food, with a woman sitting before him. A serpent and a horse *protome* are also typically depicted together with a cupbearer and servants carrying offerings to the deceased (on this subject, see Barroso 2016-2017, 201-219). Epigraphic evidence points to the praising of wine-drinking associated with the baths in Roman times such as recorded in the epitaph of Gaius Domicius Primus from Ostia (Italy):

> I´m lying in this grave, I, the remarkable Primo. I have eaten oysters, I often drank Falerno wine! Bathing, wine and love have been my company until old age (English translation by the author).
>
> (*Hoc ego sum in tumulo Primus notabilissimus ille. Vixi Lucrinis, potabi saepe Falernum, balnia vina Venus mecum senuere per annos.*) (Encarnação 2012, 1-12).

Glass strigils also have been discovered in Roman tombs. Their fragility indicates that they were not used in the baths but fabricated as grave goods. A transparent yellowish-brown glass strigil, probably from a tomb, is housed in the Corning Museum of Glass. Five glass strigils were also found in Cologne (Germany) (Whitehouse 2003, 53-54). A glass strigil is housed in the Metropolitan Museum of Art, New York (Fig. 2.12).

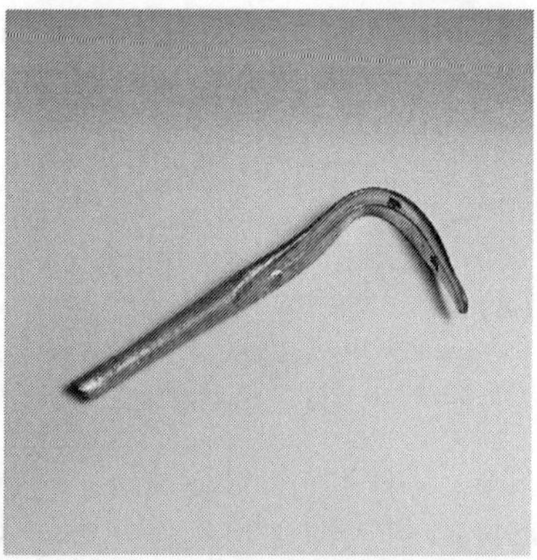

Fig. 2.12. Translucent glass strigil. L. 202 mm Max width: 27 mm. 3rd-4th century AD. Metropolitan Museum of Art, New York. Image in Public domain.

Between the 2nd and 4th century AD, strigils also decorated Roman marble vases and sarcophagi. A marble funerary vase, from the Antonin period, decorated with a strigilated pattern and handles in the form of intertwined serpents, substantiates its relationship with harmony after death in the chthonic world (Fig. 2.13).

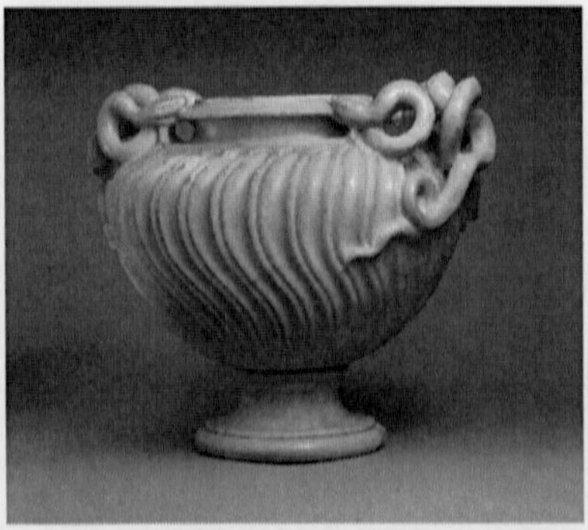

Fig. 2.13. Marble striated vase with snake handles. H. 175 mm, 2nd half of the 2nd century AD. Metropolitan Museum of Art, New York. Public domain.

Besides their primary function in hygiene care, strigils are medical-surgical instruments, being used to heat medicines and frequently applied to the ear and to stimulate an area of the body by rubbing (Bliquez 2016, 146). For Celsus, the strigil was the tool of choice when managing severe ear inflammation:

> It is desirable also to pour some medicament into the ear, and this should always be made lukewarm beforehand; and it is best dropped in from a strigil (Celsus Book VI, Chapter 7 translated by Spencer 1938, 229).

Caelius Aurelianus advised scraping the body with a strigil and dry massages as recovering manoeuvres in abdominal conditions (Drabkin 1950, Caelius Aurelianus, *On Chronic Diseases* IV, 881). Galen highly praised physical exercise and hygiene in preserving health, as stated in his book *Hygiene (De Sanitate Tuenda)*:

> But I have shown this in my works, and that those who were before continuously ill have kept free from disease by observing the rules of hygiene: this I show I have undertaken to write. For some I have forbidden to exercise at all, even with the most suitable exercises, wishing them to be satisfied with only the activities essential to life. And others, I have ordered to restrict the quantity of their exercise, in order to reduce the total to a minimum; and others to change merely the quality, or the order, or the time of their exercise; and others to change their entire regime. A similar giving precepts about baths, as not to bathe at all, or more than before, or less, and before meals only, or after meals, or with warmer water than before, or more

tepid, or colder, I have kept patients completely free from illness for many years. (Green, 1951, 187-188).

Nevertheless, he was aware of the hazardous consequences of overtraining:

Now, ulcerative fatigue (for we must begin with this) produces an annoying sensation on movement, as if the body were ulcerating, either the skin alone, when it is more moderate, or the underlying flesh, when it is more severe, or both together, when it is extreme. This is the fatigue symptom. Both the fatigue condition, on which the symptom is based, is an acidity of the thin and warm fluids, which erode and prick and sting the body. And this occurs sometimes from excessive exercise, as was shown in the book before this, and sometimes from some faulty secretion which has occurred without our realization. (…) (Green, 1951, 145-146).

We currently identify the acidity to which Galen refers to as an extremely low pH in the bloodstream caused by lactate build-up (especially L-lactate), provoking lactic acidosis when overtraining. Lactic acid is a by-product of energy-releasing anaerobic glucose metabolism and a waste product that leads to impairment of the body's oxidative metabolism, provoking muscle fatigue and soreness, and eventually the formation of microscopic muscle tears (on this subject, see Hargreaves 2020, 817-828).

Strigils appear as a symbol of balance and well-being associated with a healthy lifestyle and reliable preventive medicine support. In iconography, are highly emblematic symbols of the medical profession in antiquity.

In the strigilated sarcophagus from Ostia, dating from around 300 AD, the Greek physician is depicted with his scrolls (books), his basin for bleeding patients and his surgical instruments (Fig. 2.14).

Fig. 2.14. Sarcophagus with a Greek Physician. Marble. H. 213 mm L: 215.6 cm) Early 300s AD. Metropolitan Museum of Art, New York. Public domain.

11. Probe

An instrument resembling a syringe, or a syringe plunger (although the ringed shaft looks unlikely for that purpose) presents a most challenging interpretation (Fig. 2.15). It was recovered with items from different chronologies from the archaeological site of Fujacal, dating from the 4th century AD or later. This site encompassed an occupation period from the 4th century, when the Roman Wall of Bracara Augusta was erected, until the High Middle Ages (Pereira 2018, VII). Just one metal syringe from the Roman world, a *Pyoulcos,* has been excavated in Paphos, Cyprus, currently housed at the Archaeological Museum of Paphos (Bliquez 2016, 217-218).

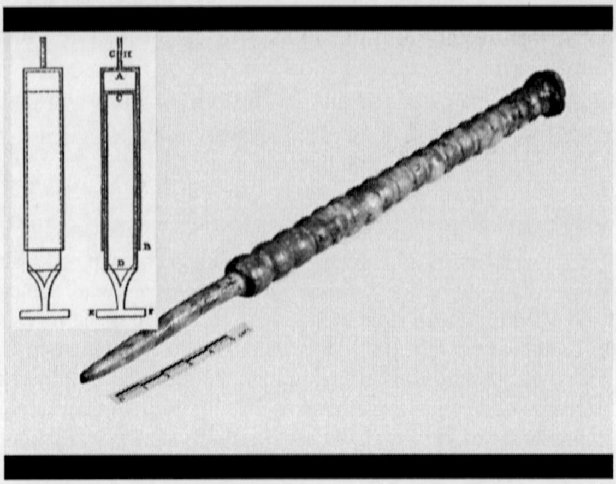

Fig. 2.15. Probe. Bronze. 4th century AD or later. Inv. Nr. 1998.1580. Photo credit: Manuel Santos. Entailing: Drawing of a metal syringe by Hero of Alexandria's Pneumatics.

Evidence supports knowledge of metal piston syringes in the Graeco-Roman world. Hero of Alexandria (10-70 AD), the Greek mathematician and engineer, described the device in his book *Pneumatics:*

> The instrument called a pyoulcus acts on the same principle. A hollow tube, of some length, is made, A B (fig. 57); into this another tube, CD, is nicely fitted, to the extremity C of which is fastened a small plate or piston, and at D is a handle, E F. Cover the orifice A of the tube A B with a plate in which an extremely fine tube, G H, is fixed, its bore communicating with A B through the plate. When we desire to draw forth any pus, we must apply the extreme orifice of the small tube, H, to the part in which the matter is, and

> draw the tube C D outwards by means of the handle. As a vacuum is thus produced in A B something else must enter to fill it, and as there is no other passage but through the mouth of the small tube, we shall of necessity draw up through this any fluid that may be near. Again, when we wish to inject any liquid, we place it in the tube A B, and, taking hold of E F, depress the tube C D, and force down the liquid until we think the injection is effected (Woodcraft 1851, 80).

According to Lawrence Bliquez, Galen gave notice of the existence and use of the *pyoulcos and* reported on its manufacture according to Hieron´s planning (Bliquez 2016, 217-218). The *pyoulcos* was used to aspirate liquids. A pig bladder was usually used to inject fluids by inserting a tip into the cavities (ear canal, uterus, anus). Dr Carlos Prates, a radiologist with expertise in Paleoradiology and principal chief radiology researcher of the Egyptian mummies from the National Museum of Archaeology in Lisbon (Lisbon Mummy Project), carried out a radiological study of the device. His report excludes the possibility of the device being a syringe or syringe plunger:

> Radiographic study of FEA12100277 - Elongated, ringed and pointed end piece from the Archaeological Museum of Braga D. Diogo de Sousa by Digital Radiography and CT Scan (figs 9, 10): Massive metallic piece, 27.3 cm long. Its density is very high at CT scan and reaches the measurement maximum (value of 3.071 U.H., limit value of the equipment for medical measurement) suggesting a probable bronze, copper and tin alloy. By this method, it seems homogeneous. However, in X-rays, it appears to consist of two components (artefact? - are we working with very high/real densities? See photo below) - a central metallic and very dense axis, varying in diameter harmoniously in its ring components, between 8 and 11 mm, as if by juxtaposed spheres, but without any identifiable separation between them. The termination extends, in continuity, by a pointed axis equally dense and elongated, with about 26 mm, but that is continued by another material, from this distance, very fragmented. Peripherally there is a less dense layer (it looks original, but we must consider a component of restoration material), which mirrors the same central annular shape, without identifiable separations and here with peripheral diameters ranging between 10 and 15 mm. It continues at the tip and most pointed area (through the piece outer lining), exhibiting a total length of about 7.4 cm. Its 2/3 distal are very fragmented and restored. There is a superficial loss of material from the fifth to the ninth ring, with further repair starting from the base.
>
> Between the base and the first ring, the third and fourth rings, there is an irregular crack of transversal repaired fragmentation. At the base, the opposite end of the tip, we observe a flattened finishing component as if with a "lid" of lowest density, slightly broader with about 19.5 mm diameter. It thus appears to be a piece of unique construction with a very dense core, and

with no internal cavity. Therefore, it is a piece of undetermined functionality (a probe or a piece for enlargement of any cavity, not necessarily medical? Veterinary? Or another type of work tool? Nevertheless, excluding the possibility of being a syringe (Carlos Prates / IMI-art / Affidea / Lisbon, 24 Nov 2019). (Fig. 2.16)

Since the device is not hollow, the possibility of it being a syringe or syringe plunger, which would also be hollow, is excluded. The instrument could be a probe, although no parallel seems to be found in human medicine, as far as we know. Veterinary surgical instruments look much like regular medical tools, except for the castration forceps used in the castration of horses and bovines which are specific to use in animals. Larger probes for the examination of wounds have been discovered (Künzl 2002, 75). Until some parallel can shed more light on this tool, we can only speculate as to its function.

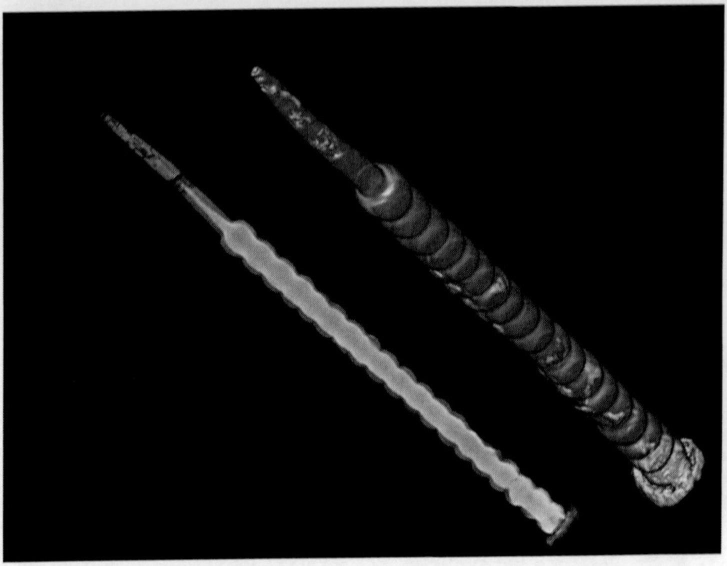

Fig. 2.16. Digital radiology and CT scan of the probe Inv. Nr. 1998.1580. Photo credit: IMI-art / Affidea.

The following table summarizes the tools as regards provenance and collection information.

Instruments from Bracara Augusta

Inv. Number	Instrument	Provenance	Material
1992.0686	Decorated handle ending in form of the dog's head	D. Afonso Henriques Street	Copper alloy
1991.2666	Bronze figurine	Top of Cividade Hill	Bronze
2000.0672	Leaf-shaped scalpel handle	Top of Cividade Hill	Copper alloy
2012.0876	Bow shears	Top of Cividade Hill	Iron
1996.0297	Conical hollow tube	São Paulo Street	Copper alloy
1991.2617	Ear probe	Top of Cividade Hill	Gilded copper alloy
2002.0028	Tweezers	Santo António das Travessas Street	Copper alloy
1996.0547	Spoon-probe with olivary enlargement	São Paulo Street	Copper alloy
1998.1551	Ligula	Top of Cividade Hill	Copper alloy
2008.0239	Fragmented bone nail cleaner	Necropolis of Via XVII	Bone
2009.0514	Blue-green unguent/perfume bottle	Necropolis of Via XVII	Glass
2009.0515	Fragmented green-blue aryballos	Necropolis of Via XVII	Glass
2009.0419	Cup with Snake-Thread decoration	Necropolis of Via XVII	Transparent glass
2009. 0417	Strigil with broken handle	Necropolis of Via XVII	Iron
1998.1580	Syringe/Probe	Archaeological site of Fujacal	Copper alloy

Most medical surgical tools have been found in tombs or houses of physicians. Regarding the material that has been excavated in Bracara Augusta, no physician's inscription or tomb has been discovered so far. The grooming tools from Via XVII's necropolis are related to medicine, but the funerary context is not a physician's tomb, and there are no primary medical-surgical tools. Neither has the Roman Domus excavation yielded any significant medical material so far. The instruments related to medicine and surgery have been recovered from Top of Cividade Hill's and excavations in the surrounding area, namely, a scalpel handle, bow shears, and a spoon-probe. The ear-probe has unusual decoration for this typology, but it demonstrates the characteristics of a surgical device. Tweezers and ligulae are grooming tools. The finding of surgical tools in this archaeological site may be explained by the fact that they originate from the baths building.

A close relationship between baths and health care is a well-established part of therapeutics. Massage and hydrotherapy are still helpful in physiotherapeutic treatments. In Roman times, the water temperature was also prescribed (on this subject, see Merten 1983, 101-113). The massagers (*unctores* or *alipta)* and *iatroalipta* (sports physicians; literally: a physician who cures by anointing) were members of the bathing staff (Merten 1983, 126-127). *Iatroalipta* were mentioned by Celsus:

> *Sanus homo, qui et bene valet et suae spontis est, nullis obligare se legibus debet, ae neque medico neque iatroalipta efere.*

> A man in health, who is both vigorous and his own master, should be under no obligatory rules, and have no need, either for a medical attendant or for a rubber and anointer.
> (Celsus, Book I Chapter I, translated by Hendersen 1938, 43).

Ernst Künzl has hypothesized that rooms associated with the Roman baths would have functioned as surgical rooms. Very little is known about the places where Graeco-Roman physicians carried out surgical operations. Their houses are possible candidates since many instruments have been found in excavations there. Not many surgical instruments have been found in baths excavations. However, baths, being quiet places with a water supply might have been suitable locations for conducting surgical operations. Surgical instruments discovered in a room at the baths of Colonia Ulpia Traiana, near Xanten, the capital of the Roman province Germania inferior (currently near Bonn, Germany) have also suggested baths as being likely locations. The excavated instruments were the following: two iron copper-alloy and iron scalpel handles with beautiful niello inlays; a circular iron handle decorated with three rings of a gold sheet with a small hole in which a cautery was possibly inserted (since cauteries were made of iron); two bone copper-alloy and iron surgical chisels with beautiful decorations of gold and niello. They were very well preserved, the bone chisels matching the Roman *scalprum planum* (Künzl 1986, 491-509, fig. 2, 3). These tools indicate complex bone operations, challenging to perform at home. Diverse medical tools have been found at the Trier Baths, such as ear-probes, mixing palletes, oculist seals, probes and spatula-probes; these also suggest the existence of medical activity, medicine preparation and ophthalmic care at the baths (Künzl 1986, 491-509, fig. 4, 5).

Bone chisels and elevators have been discovered at the Roman legion camp of Vindonissa (currently in Switzerland), a proper place for surgical management of traumatic bone injuries in soldiers (Künzl 2002, 42). Teeth or bone forceps and pharmacy tools were found in these places (Tabanelli 1956, 60, Tav. XV, XVI, XVII, XVIII). During Emperor Hadrian's time (reigned 117-138), bath facilities were reserved to assist patients from the public administration (Merten 1983, 63). The earliest Roman surgical instruments were found in the late republican Legionaries' camp of Cáceres el Viejo in Spain (Künzl 2002, 29).

Conclusion

The archaeological excavations of Bracara Augusta have unearthed interesting medical-surgical, and grooming devices some of which, like the probe, are difficult to interpret, and provide evidence that medicine and surgery were practised in the city just as in the towns of the Roman world. Some identified tools are either rare or unique in Portugal and add valuable information to the evidence supporting Roman surgery as practised in the Iberian Peninsula (on this subject, see Barroso 2020 c, 41-64). Baths are also rare places where surgical instruments have been discovered, suggesting the possibility that these facilities were exploited as surgical rooms. Since a large part of the Bracara Augusta still remains to be excavated, hopefully, more tools and specific surgical contexts will come into the light in the future.

Acknowledgements

I thank Dr Isabel Silva, Director of the Archaeological Museum D. Diogo de Sousa, Braga, for granting permission to study the medical-surgical and grooming tools of the Museum and for permission to reproduce associated images. I also thank Dr Maria José Sousa and the Museum staff for their kind support in the preparation of this essay. I thank Dr Francisco Sande

Lemos for fruitful exchange of ideas, Dr Antómio Trabulo for the medical reading of the bronze figurine, Dr Carlos Prates and IMI-art / Affidea for the radiological study of the syringe/probe instrument and Professor Martins e Silva and Professor Christopher John Duffin for their critical reading of the manuscript.

References

Alarcão, Adília. 1994. *Museu Monográfico de Conimbriga.* Lisboa: Instituto Português de Museus.

Alonso, María Ángeles. 2019. "Greek Physicians in the Eyes of Roman Elite (from the Republic to the 1st Century AD)." *Annales Universitatis Mariae Curie-Skłodowska Lublin – Polonia, Sectio F Historia,* 73: 119-137.

Allègre, Fernand. 1889. *Étude sur la déesse grecque Tyché.* Paris: Ernest Leroux Éditeur.

Barroso, Maria do Sameiro. 2012. "Cuidados de beleza e alguns objectos do período romano do Museu Nacional de Arqueologia." *Boletim de Estudos Clássicos,* 57: 115-122.

Barroso, Maria do Sameiro. 2014-2015. "Medicine, surgery, pharmacy, toilet, and other health care tools from the Roman city of Balsa (Tavira, Portugal) from the 1st at the 3rd century AD." *O Arqueólogo Português* Série V, 4/5: 341-373.

Barroso, Maria do Sameiro. 2016-2017. "Banqueting for Eternity – Two reliefs of the Lisbon National Museum of Archaeology." *O Arqueólogo Português,* [5] 6/7: 201-219.

Barroso, Maria do Sameiro. 2020a. "Herodotus and Hippocrates: two paradigms in interpreting castration among the Scythians." *Cadernos do GEEvH (Grupo de Estudos em Evolução Humana),* 9 (1): 1-6.

Barroso, Maria do Sameiro. 2020b. "Nephro-Urology in Graeco-Roman medicine. A solid catheter from the Lisbon National Museum of Archaeology." *Archives of Hellenic Medicine,* 37 (Suppl.2): 192-196.

Barroso, Maria do Sameiro. 2020c. "Lasting traces of Medical and Surgical Treatment in Ancient Portuguese Territory". 241-6 *In* Spani, G. & Varotto, E. (eds): *Malattie e medicina tra litteratura, storia e antropologia*. Holden, Massachussetts (USA): Quod manet.

Barroso, Maria do Sameiro. 2021. "Reading Graeco-Roman Medicine in the Light of its Medical-Surgical Instruments." 337-361 *In* Santos, A.L., Rola, A., Morais, C., Vasconcelos, C., Gomes, E., Rodrigues, I. T., Azevedo, J. & Rodrigues, S. (eds): *História da Ciência no Ensino.*

Revisitando Abordagens, Inovando Saberes. Coimbra: Imprensa da Universidade.

Booth, George (translator). 1814. *The fragments of Diodorus*. 15 books, 2 vol. London: Printed by W.M. Dowel for J. Davis.

Bliquez, Lawrence. 2016. *The tools of Asclepius, Surgical Instruments in Greek and Roman Times*. Leiden: Brill.

Braga, Cristina Maria Vilas Boas. 2010. *Rituais funerários em Bracara Augusta: o novo núcleo da Via XVII* . Thesis. Braga: Universidade do Minho.

Braun, Georg, & Hogenberg, Frans. 1598. *Civitates Orbis Terrarum*. Coloniae Agrippinae (No publisher) vol. 5-6 (Latin ed).

Celsus. *On Medicine.* 1938. Hendersen, Jeffrey (ed.), Spencer, Walter George (translator). Cambridge: Harvard University Press, 3 vol.

Cicero. 1933. *De Natura Deorum Academica.* Rackam, Harris (translator). London: Harvard University Press.

Clutton-Brock, Juliet. 1992. *Horse Power: A history of the horse and donkey in human societies*. London: The Natural History Museum.

Deneffe, Victor. 1893. *Étude sur la trousse d'une chirurgien gallo-romain du IIIe siècle*. Anvers: H. Caals Éditeur.

Deneffe, Victor. 1896. *Les Oculistes Gallo-Romains*. Anvers: H. Caals Éditeur.

Domus Rimini https://www.domusrimini.com/eng/the-surgeon-house/surgeon.php accessed 10 November 2020).

Drabkin, Israel Edward (editor and translator). 1950. *Caelius Aurelianus. On Acute Diseases and On Chronic Diseases.* Chicago: The University of Chicago Press.

Eckart, Hella & Crummy, Nina. 2008. *Styling the body in Late Iron Age and Roman Britain, a contextual approach to toilet instruments*. Montagnac: Éditions Monique Mergoil.

Edelstein, Emma Jeannette & Edelstein, Ludwig. 1998. *Asclepius. Collection and Interpretation of the Testimonies.* Baltimore, Maryland: The John Hopkins Press Ltd.

Encarnação, José d'. 2012. "Cidade, Gastronomia e Património/City, Gastronomy and Cultural Heritage." *Revista Memória em Rede, Pelotas.* 2 (7): 1-12.

Espelosín, Javier Goméz (translator). 2007. *Estrábon. Geografía de Iberia,* Madrid: Alianza Editorial.

Georgoulis, Anastasius; Kiapidou, Irini-Sofia; Velogianni, Lamprini and Stergiou, Nicholas. 2007. "Herodicus, the father of sports medicine." *Sports Traumatology, Knee Surgery and Arthroscopy*, 15 (3): 315–318.

Gerald, Hugh & Evelyn-White (translators). 1919. *Ausonius*. London: William Heinemann.

Green, Robert Montraville. 1951. *A Translation of Galen's Hygiene (De Sanitate Tuenda)* with Introduction by Henry E. Siegerist. Springfield, Illinois: Charles C. Thomas Publisher.

Gremek, Mirko & Gourevitch, Danielle. 1998. *Les Maladies dans l'Art Antiqúe.* Lyon: Fayard.

Grensemann Hermannn. 1975. *Knidische Medizin. Teil I: Die Testimonien zur ältesten knidischen Lehre und Analysen knidischer Schriften im Corpus Hippocraticum*. Berlin, New York: Walter de Gruyter.

Haffner, Alfred. 1989. *Gräber, Spiegel des Lebens. Zum Totenbrauchtum der Kelten und Römer am Beispiel des Treverer-Gräberfeldes Wederath-Belginum.* Mainz: Verlag Philip von Zabern.

Hargreaves, Mark & Spriet, Lawrence. 2020. "Skeletal muscle energy metabolism during exercise." *Nature Metabolism,* 2: 817-828.

Kenrick, John. 1858. *Roman Sepulchral Inscriptions. Their relation to Archeology, Language, and Religion*. London: John Russel Smith.

Kotera-Feyer, Ellen. 1998. "Die Strigils in der attish-rotfigurigen Vasenmalerei: Bildformeln und ihre Deutung." *Nikephoros,* 11: 107-136.

Künzl, Ernst. 1983. *Medizinische Instrumente aus sepulchralfunden der romischen Kaiserzeit.* Köln: Rheinland Verlag GmbH.

Künzl, Ernst. 1986. "Operationsräume in römischen Thermen. Zu einem chirurgischen Instrumentarium aus der Colonia Ulpia Traiana mit einem Auswahlkatalog römischer medizinischer Instrumente im Rheinischen Landesmuseum Bonn." *Bonner Jahrbuch*, 186: 491-509.

Künzl, Ernst. 2002. *Medizinische Instrumente der römischen Kaiserzeit im Römisch-Germanischen Zentralmuseum*. Mit einem Beitrag von Josef Riederer. Mainz: Römisch-Germanisches Zentralmuseum.

Lemos, Francisco Sande; Delgado, Manuela; Martins, Manuela. 1998. "Sondagens arqueológicas no Largo do Paço, Braga." *Cadernos de Arqueologia,* [2] 5: 67-76.

Lemos, Francisco Sande. 2008. "Antes de Bracara Augusta." *Forum* 42.43 Julho /Jan: 203-239.

Lisbon Mummy Project: https://artsandculture.google.com/exhibit/qgList1Ii30FLA?hl=pt-PT accessed November 28 2020.

Lourenço, Márcio Afonso. 2012. *Objectos do quotidiano de Bracara Augusta.* Thesis. Braga: Universidade do Minho.

McCann, Anna Marguerite. 1978. *Roman Sarcophagi in The Metropolitan Museum of Art.* New York: The Metropolitan Museum of Art.

Martins, Manuela & Delgado, Manuela. 1989-1990. "As necrópoles de Bracara Augusta. Os dados Arqueológicos." *Cadernos de Arqueologia, [2]* (6-7): 41-186.

Martins, Manuela. 2005. *As Termas Romanas do Alto da Cividade,* Braga: Unidade de Arqueologia da Universidade do Minho.

Merten, Elka Wilhelmina. 1983. *Bäder und Badegepflogenheiten in der Darstellung der Historia Augusta*. Bonn: R. Habelt.

Meyer-Steineg, Theodor & Sudhoff, Karl. 1921. *Geschichte der Medizin im Überblick mit Abbildungen.* Jena: Verlag von Gustav Fischer.

Milne, James Stuart. 1907. *Surgical Instruments in Greek and Roman Times*. Oxford, Massachusetts & London: Clarendon.

Morais, Rui. 2010. *Bracara Augusta,* Braga: Câmara Municipal de Braga.

Morais, Rui, Bandeira, Miguel, Pinho, Eliana Manuel. 2013. *Itineraria sacra. Bracara Augvsta Fidelis et Antica. Coimbra:* Imprensa da Universidade de Coimbra.

Oliveira, Eduardo Pires. 1986. "Documentos para a história do Museu D. Diogo de Sousa III." *Cadernos de Arqueologia* [2] (3): 171-195.

Pearce, John. 2015. "A 'Civilized' Death?" 223-248 *In* Rasmus, B.J., Prusac, M. & Roland, H. (eds): *Death and Changing Rituals. Function and Meaning in Ancient Funerary Practices*. Oxford and Philadelphia: Oxbow Books.

Pereira, Felipe Silos Moraes. 2018. *A Zona Arqueológica do Fujacal e os impactos urbanísticos e topográficos da construção da muralha romana de Bracara Augusta.* Thesis. Braga: Universidade do Minho.

Petrie, William Mathew Flinders. 1917. *Tools and weapons illustrated by the Egyptian collection in University College, London and 2000 outlines from other sources.* London: British School of Archaeology in Egypt.

Pliny the Elder. 1963. *Natural History* Books 28-32. edited by Henderson, J, (ed.), Jones, W.H.S. (trans.). Cambridge, Massachusetts & London,: Harvard University Press.

Redentor, Armando. 2011. *A cultura epigráfica no Conventvs Bracarauguvstanvs (Pars Occidentalis). Percursos pela sociedade brácara de época romana.* 2 vols. Coimbra: Universidade de Coimbra (Thesis de doutoramento policopiada).

Ribeiro, Jorge Manuel Pinto. 2015. *Arquitectura Romana em Bracara Augusta. Uma Análise das técnicas edílicas,* Thesis. Porto: CITCEM/Edições Afrontamento.

Rigaud de Sousa, José João. 1973. *Subsídios para a Carta Arqueológica de Braga*. Valladolid: Universidad de Valladolid.

Silva, Maria Manuela Ribeiro Conde. 2011. Inventariação de Retratos Pictóricos dos Bispos do Porto - Volume II. Thesis. Porto: Faculdade de Letras da Universidade do Porto.

Smith, Wesley Dean (editor and translator).1994. *Hippocrates VII. Epidemics* vol VII, Massachusetts, London: Harvard University Press.

Smith, William. 1859. *A Dictionary of Greek and Roman Antiquities*. Boston: Little, Brown, and Co.

Swaddling, Judith. 1980. *The Olympic Games*. London: British Museum Press.

Tabanelli, Mario. 1956. *Chirurgia Nell'Antica Roma*. Torino: Editrice Minerva Medica.

Tacitus, Cornelius translated by Moore, Clifford Herschel and Jackson, John. *Annales*. 1962. Cambridge, Massachussetts: William Heinemann LTD, IV vol.

Torres, Amadeu. 2006. "D. Diogo de Sousa no contexto cultural do Renascimento." *In D. Diogo de Sousa e o seu* Arcebispo de Braga (1505-1532). Braga 18-20 de Novembro de 2005. Braga: Càmara Municipal de Braga, Faculdade de Teologia.

Tschen-Emmons, James. 2014. *Artifacts from Ancient Rome.* Santa Barbara, California; Denver, Colorado; Oxford, England: Greenwood.

Vasconcellos, José Leite de. 1885. *Balladas do Occidente.* Porto: Livraria Portuense.

Vasconcellos, José Leite. 1913. *As Religiões da Lusitânia* (3 vol.) Vol. III. Lisboa: Imprensa Nacional.

Vasconcellos, José Leite. 1897. *Religiões da Lusitania na parte que principalmente se refere a Portugal.* Lisboa: Sociedade de Geografia de Lisboa.

Warmington, Eric Herbert. 1935. *Remains of old Latin; newly edited and translated* 3 Vol. I *Ennius and Cecilius.* London: Harvard University Press.

Wellcome Images Collection https://wellcomecollection.org/works/uawhk37b accessed 17 August 2021.

Whitehouse, David. 2003. *Roman Glass in the Corning Museum of Glass.* Vol 3. New York: The Corning Museum of Glass.

Woodcraft, Bennet (editor and translator). 1851. *The Pneumatics of Hero of Alexandria.* London: Taylor Walter and Maberly.

CHAPTER 3

GRAECO-ROMAN PHARMACY AND MEDICAL-SURGICAL TOOLS FROM THE BÜHLER-BROCKAUS COLLECTION

MARIA DO SAMEIRO BARROSO

Abstract

Private collections add valuable contributions to the assets of Portuguese Museums. Such is the case with the Bühler-Brockhaus Collection recently donated to the Archaeological Museum D. Diogo de Sousa in Braga. More than two hundred Mediterranean archaeological pieces collected by Marion Bühler-Brockhaus and Hans-Peter Bühler are mainly from Graeco-Roman times and include valuable pieces from the Near East and Etruscan civilizations. In this essay, we present the assemblage of pharmacy and medical-surgical tools, which includes rare and valuable pieces like a pharmaceutical sieve-spoon, a piercing eyed needle and a triple portable probe case, which was the subject of a palaeoradiology study.

Key words: History of collecting; Archaeology; Roman medical-surgical instruments; Palaeoradiology

Resumo

As colecções particulares acrescentam valiosos contributos ao espólio dos Museus Portugueses. É o caso da Coleção Bühler-Brockhaus recentemente doada ao Museu Arqueológico D. Diogo de Sousa em Braga. Mais de duzentas peças arqueológicas mediterrâneas coleccionadadas por Marion Bühler-Brockhaus e Hans-Peter Bühler são essencialmentemente da época greco-romana e incluem peças valiosas do Oriente Próximo e das civilizações etruscas. Neste ensaio, apresentamos o conjunto de instrumentos farmacêuticos e médico-cirúrgicos, que inclui peças raras e valiosas como uma colher-peneira farmacêutica, uma agulha de punção furada e um estojo portátil triplo de sondas que foi objecto de um estudo paleorradiológico.

Palavras-chave: História do colecionismo; Arqueologia; Instrumentos médico-cirúrgicos romanos; Paleorradiologia

Introduction

The taste for beauty, usually linked to religious rites and imagery, possibly begins at the dawn of history, enhancing the stimulus for collecting objects to which man attributes the most significant value. The Greeks and Romans valued and hoarded things to a degree of significance well beyond purposeful service. The dedicated, passionate collector, ascribing a particular value to the collected objects, emerged in the Western world during the late Middle Ages (Habsburg 1997, 7).

In the Renaissance, as the world began to open up, through the Age of Discovery, royal collections of art, jewellery, Natural History and all kinds of exotic, precious items garnered from all over the newly discovered world birthed the formation of so-called Kunstkammern - cabinets of art, wonders and curiosities. These cabinets constituted the embryos of modern museums or were integrated into later modern museum collections.

In addition to contributing value to museums' assets, private collections sometimes preserve rare or otherwise unknown objects. Such is the case with some pieces from the Bühler-Brockhaus Collection.

Graeco-Roman Surgery

Andreas Vesalius (1514-1564) included a letter to Charles V, Holy Roman Emperor (reigned 1519-1556), a preface to his work *De humanis corporis fabrica,* published in 1541-possibly the most significant Renaissance medical text. Here, Vesalius paid tribute to the Graeco-Roman medical legacy, which had laid the foundations of modern medicine and in which surgery emerged inseparable from medicine. He complained about the hazardous lack of the proper use of the hand, referring to surgery[1], a task practised by barber-surgeons and physicians, and not just by physicians, as in Graeco-Roman medicine. He also regretted that physicians no longer prepared their medicines as in Graeco-Roman times:

> But in bygone times, that is to say [in the West after the Gothic deluge and [in the East] after the reign of Mansor at Bochara in Persia, under whom, as we know, the Arabs still lived as was right on terms of familiarity with the

[1] "Surgery" and "Chirurgia" derive from Greek word "Kheirourgia". "Kheiron", Latin "Chiro", means "Hand".

> Greeks, medicine began to be sore distempered. Its primary instrument, the employment of the hand in healing, was as so neglected that it was relegated to vulgar fellows with no instruction whatsoever in the branches of knowledge that subserve the art of medicine. For it is indeed above all other things the wide prevalence of this hateful error that prevents us even in our age from taking up the healing art as a whole, makes us confine ourselves merely to the treatment of internal complaints, and, if I may utter the blunt truth once for all, causes us, to the great detriment of mankind, to study to be healers only in a very limited degree. For when, in the first place, the whole compounding of drugs was handed over to the apothecaries, then the doctors promptly lost the knowledge of simple medicines which is absolutely essential to them; and they became responsible for the fact that the druggists' shops were filled with barbarous terms and false remedies, and also that so many elegant compositions of the ancients were lost to us, several of which have not yet come to light; and, finally, they prepared an endless task for the learned men, not only of our own age, but for those who preceded it by some years, who devoted themselves with indefatigable zeal to research in simple medicines; so much so that they may be regarded as having gone far to-restore the knowledge of them to its former brilliance (Vesalius, translated by Farrington, 1932, 1357-1136).

Surgery was learned from textbooks, and surgical skills from peer-assisted learning, as is the case nowadays. However, Graeco-Roman surgical instruments are difficult to study since we have no drawings to work from. Galen (AD 130-210) explains that surgical tools were devised by physicians, who made wax models, which were passed on to blacksmiths who produced the instruments themselves (Singer &Van de Eijk, 2013, 78-79).

No images figure in textbooks, and no instrument sale catalogue has been preserved if they ever existed. Therefore, information concerning surgical tools must be drawn from descriptions in medical treatises. Frequently, the authors of such works confine themselves to just mentioning their use (Künzl 2002,48). Instruments recovered from archaeological excavations complete the information provided in medical texts. Instruments depicted on reliefs, coins and funerary tombs provide valuable information on the shapes of complete tools. Some instruments like spatulae or knives are similar in construction, whether used for painting, household, or medical purposes. Studies on the context of the findings (in a house or tomb of a surgeon, for example) provide more accurate evidence about their intended use. When no information on the context is available, the possible medical functions of some objects are much less certain.

Hans-Peter Bühler and Marion Bühler-Brockhaus

Hans-Peter Bühler and Marion Bühler-Brockhaus, who belong to the publishing family responsible for Brockhaus Dictionaries, which is so crucial in the study of German, share a passion for art, archaeology and collecting. The familial kinship with the descendants of the great composer Richard Wagner (1813-1883) extends their artistic relationships to the most sublime achievements in music history. In Archaeology, their ancestors also played an essential role in the almost mythical publication of the early works of Heinrich Schliemann (1822-1890) on the discovery of the ruins of Troy (on this subject, see Costabile 2019, 8-11). Their passion for archaeology and ancient history stimulated life-enriching travels and, finally, brought them to Portugal, where they were enchanted by the ruins of Tróia on the banks of the River Sado. The couple moved from Munich, where they owned an Art Gallery, to Setúbal in 2006. They founded a cultural foundation, the Buehler-Brockhaus Foundation, in 2008, to which they donated an extensive part of their assets. In 2019, after a friendly and fruitful relationship with the Director and Curator of the Archaeological Museum D. Diogo de Sousa in Braga, Dr Isabel Cunha e Silva and Dr Maria José de Carvalho e Sousa respectively, they donated over two hundred valuable archaeological assets to the Museum.

The Graeco-Roman Culture is predominant in the Collection, including pieces from the archaic period, Cyprio-archaic, Greek, Etruscan, Hellenistic, Roman, Eastern Roman Empire, Egyptian, Phoenician and from the Near-East.

The Collection includes some attractive items of toiletry and pharmacy containers, such as beautiful glass unguentaria and balsamaria, including aryballos, and three pieces from semi-precious stones: a Roman oval sardonyx bowl, two unguentaria (a Parthian rock crystal unguentarium), and a quartz Sassanid smoke quartz unguentarium). All are infrequent items, denoting Peter Bühler's interest and study of gemstone vessels (Bühler 1966; Bühler 1973). A green marble anatomical ex-voto in the form of a thumb is also rare. A Roman Campana Plaque depicting a poppy capsule used in a ritual context is also of interest. This essay will discuss the ensemble of pharmacy and medical-surgical tools and other objects related to medicine and pharmacy, such as the two crystal balsamaria and the sardonyx plate, the anatomical ex-voto, and a plaque indicating the use of poppy in a ritual context.

The tools from the Bühler-Brockhaus Collection

Most tools from the Bühler-Brockhaus collection were undoubtedly used in pharmacy, medicine and surgery. Some can be dated; others cannot. In addition to a green marble ex-voto, as part of the magical-religious healing process and an intriguing plaque depicting an opium capsule in a cult context, we will consider pharmacy tools for the preparation and storing of medicines, followed by surgical tools. A balance and a pharmacy sieve-spoon are emblematic for weighing, measuring and sieving the doses of the substances to be prepared, as well as a small sardonyx dish or mixing bowl and two rare rock crystal balsamaria; pharmacy tools are scarce, and unusual-coloured marble are rarely found among objects related to medicine.

Ancient cult objects

1. Greek marble votive thumb

Anatomical ex-votos, expressing a healing request to a health deity, are some of the iconographical resources about diseases in the ancient world. Most anatomical ex-votos, made from marble or terracotta, were dedicated to Asclepius in the Greek world. Others were dedicated to other healing deities like Amphiaros. A large number of these structures was found in the Athens Asclepieion. Those models were later disseminated in Rome (Santrot et al. 2011, 46-61).

A marble stele low relief found at the Acropolis in Athens presents the patient, identified by an inscription as Lysimaclides, carrying a votive of a leg, suffering from venous insufficiency, identified by a long varicose vein (Grmek & Gourevitch 1998, 294, fig. 231). A Roman ex-voto depicts another sign of varicose insufficiency: an oedematous foot with a varicose vein (Penso 1984, 286, fig. 153).

The Greek marble thumb in the Bühler-Brockhaus Collection, dated to the third/fourth century BC and coming from Taranto, Magna Grecia, points straight up, with decoration lines close to the nail base and the knucklebones in the lower part (Catalogue 2019, 21, fig. 8). Signs of the disease that would be behind are not evident (Fig. 3.1a).

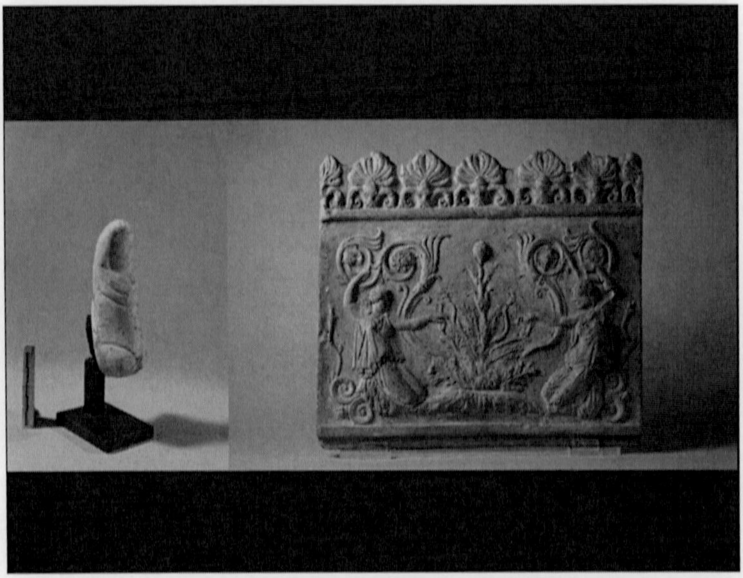

Fig. 3.1a. Greek marble votive thumb. Inv. Nr. 2016.0489. H. 95 mm.
Fig. 3.1b. Roman Campana plaque. Inv. Nr. Inv. 2016.0459. H. 400 mm W. 440 mm.
Photo credit: MDDS/Manuel Santos.

2. Roman Campana plaque

Poppy (*Papaver somniferum* L.) is one of the most important medicinal plants in the whole History of Pharmacy. The red, pink or white flowering annual plant produces a milky sap containing over forty highly potent alkaloids. The milky juice from the herb of oblivion, according to Ovid, emerges from the unripe seed capsule after the surface has been scratched. When the milky sap hits the air, it coagulates into a brown mass, the raw opium. The discovery of opium production was not, as is often wrongly assumed (Rätsch 2014, 315), in Southeast Asia, but in Stone Age Central Europe.

Poppy was also used in ritual contexts. In the Minoan civilization, poppy capsules were symbols of healing, fertility, wealth and immortality (Askitpoulou et al., 2002, 23-29). A clay figurine of the "Poppy Goddess", with hands raised either in greeting, blessing or prayer and which may symbolize her appearance on earth in human form, is crowned with three opium poppies (Sakelarakis 1985, 91).

In Greece, the cultic use of poppy has been documented in mystery cults of vegetation gods during the seasons, consecrated, namely, to Aphrodite, Demeter and Dionysus. Their sacred plants were the pomegranate, poppy, cereals and grapevine (Rätsch 2014,33).

In an Idyll by Theocritus, a Greek poet from Sicily (c.300-after 260 BC), speaks of a calming draught at the bedside and Demeter at her alter, holding a poppy in each hand:

> Such a draught that ye Nymphs that day made seam for us bedside
> Harvest Demeter's altar, upon whose mound of corn
> May it be mine once more to plant the great fan, while she sits
> And smiles upon us, holding sheaves and poppies in each hand
> (Theocritus, Idyl VII, translated by Trevelyan 1947, 29).

Roman Campana reliefs were decorative terracotta plates produced from the middle of the first century BC to the first century AD. They are named after the Italian collector Giampietro Campana (1808-1880), who published some of these reliefs for the first time (Clay plaque Mvsei Vaticani). The Campana plaque from the Bühler-Brockhaus Collection displays a poppy at the centre, associated with feelings of happiness, abundance, fertility and well-being related to the Peace achieved by Emperor Augustus (reigned 27 BC-14 AD), celebrated in Ara Pacis Augustae (Altar of Augustan Peace), and dedicated to Pax, the Roman goddess of Peace. The catalogue description reads as follows:

> Remains of white engobe and reddish colour. The symmetrical composition depicts a luxuriante Akanthus plant with a poppy capsule in its middle. The plant is flanked by two kneeling *peplophoroi* on each side, bending forward to touch the Akanthus. The cultic act of kneeling reveals them to be servants of a deity, presumably of vegetation. Scrolling tendrils in the background refer to plaques of the Ara Pacis Augustae in Rome dated about 10 BC. *Campana* reliefs means a group of Roman clay tablets which served as ornaments for temples, as well as for public and private buildings (Catalogue 2019, 128, fig. 112) (Fig. 3.1b).

Pharmaceutical tools

1. Balance

The balance comprises a sliding weight, a suspension (which is missing) and three hooked arms of unequal length (Catalog 2019, 151, Image 136) (on pharmacy balances, see Barroso 2014-2015, 341-373) (Fig. 3.2a).

2. Sieve-spoon

A pharmaceutical sieve-spoon is a rare instrument. Some tools used to prepare and apply medicines double up in their functions, such as spatula-probes or spoon-probes. Pharmaceutical spoons usually consist of a spoon and a handle or a probe used as a mixing rod (on this subject, see Barroso 2014-2015, 341-361, fig. 18 and 19).

Greek and Roman medical authors mention reports on the use of sieves or strainers, sometimes necessary for preparing medicines, referring to this tool as a *cribum* or *cribellum.* Sometimes, household sieves might be also be used for this purpose.

A medical (or pharmaceutical) sieve was mentioned by Marcellus Empiricus (Bliquez 2016, 269-271). Marcellus Empiricus, also known as Marcellus Burdigalensis (Marcellus of Bordeaux), was a physician from Gaul who lived in the fourth or fifth century AD. He gave a recipe for a powder of quince apple, which had passed through a medical sieve (*cribello medicinali*) when dealing with diseases of the male genital system and hernias (Marcellus, 33, 9, in Helmreich 1889, 342).

Sieves or spoons also appear among grooming objects, combined with toothpicks, implying an association with tableware, to pass the wine, which contained grape seeds in ancient times (Eckart & Crummy 2008, 164, fig. 107). In this case, sieves were spoons with grooves. According to the Scottish surgeon John Stuart Milne (b.1871- ?): “There are large numbers of sieves and strainers in bronze and earthenware in the Naples Museum” (Milne 1907, 165).

Sieves and strainers must have taken several forms. The sieve-spoon from the Bühler-Brockhaus Collection seems to be a pharmaceutical tool tailored to measure and strain the same amount of medicine. “Very rare, this is an example of two different items merged into a single piece”, as underlined in the Catalogue (Catalogue 2019, 151, fig. 137) (Fig. 3.2b).

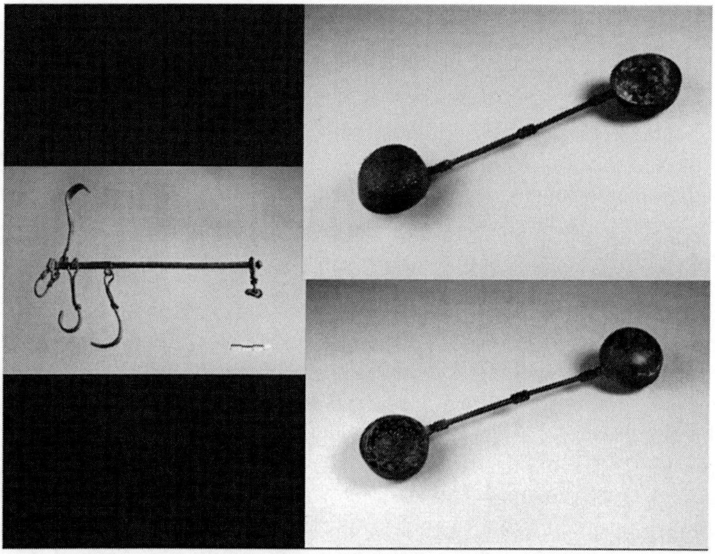

Fig. 3.2a. Roman bronze balance. Inv. Nr. 2016.0549, L. 210 mm. 2nd-4th century AD.
Fig. 3.2b. Roman bronze pharmaceutical sieve-spoon. Inv. 2016.0550 L. 280 mm Photo credits: MDDS/Manuel Santos.

3. Spoon-probe

A set of five bronze instruments, dating from the 2nd-4th century AD, was acquired at Tessier-Sarrou, Drouot, Paris, 2015 (Catalogue 2019, 151, fig. 139). Some were also used in the preparation of medicines (Fig. 3.3a).

A spoon-probe (*ciathiscomele)* belongs to a wide variety of instruments in which a spoon is combined with a probe (Fig. 3.3b - 1st from right to left). These instruments had multiple applications in medicine and pharmacy - to mix, measure and apply medicines (Bliquez 2016, 126), among other uses (on this subject, see Barroso *Roman Medical-Surgical Instruments from the Archaeological Museum D. Diogo de Sousa, Braga,* this volume).

The spatula-probes were also multi-purpose instruments in which a spatula was combined with a probe (on this subject, see Barroso *Roman Medical-Surgical Instruments from the Archaeological Museum D. Diogo de Sousa, Braga,* this volume).

4. Spatula

The spatula from the Bühler-Brockhaus collection is larger than usual and is not combined with a probe. Occasionally, spoons are just combined with a handle. An oval spatula from Pompeii is a rare example of such an instrument (Bliquez 1994, 137, ILL 62: No. 115) (Fig. 3.3. - 1st from left to right). However, when dealing with spatulas, probes, spatula-probes and spoon-probes, we must keep in mind that:

> The spatulas, scoops, spoons and swab-sticks that were commonly used in the home and in the shop were also the probes utilized by a physician. For this reason these items ought never to be identified as instruments of surgery (a common practice in publications of minor objects) unless they are found in the company of articles created only or primarily as surgical tools: e.g. specula, cauteries, cupping vessels, scalpels and the like (Bliquez 2016, 109).

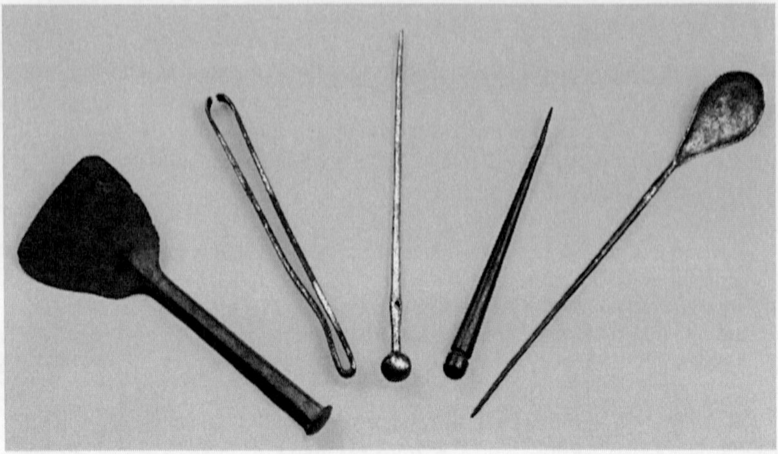

Fig. 3.3. Set of five instruments. From left to right: large spatula (Inv. 2016.0568- L- 125 mm W. 46 mm.), tweezers (Inv. Nr. 2016.0569. L. 113 mm Max width 60 mm.), eyed needle, needle, spoon-probe (Inv. Nr. 2016.0572. L. 156 mm W 22 mm.). Photo credit: MDDS/Manuel Santos.

5. Roman small oval chalcedony-sardonyx bowl

A small chalcedony-sardonyx bowl from this Collection, as Hans Peter Bühler noted, appears to have been used to prepare medicines. Marble mortars and pestles were widely used to grind vegetable or mineral medicinal ingredients. Small plates of the same material would receive the ground substances. The bowl was carefully carved to preserve the white part of the stone toward the bottom of the bowl (Catálogo s.d., 46, fig. 24) (Fig. 3.4).

When discussing materials used to prepare and preserve medicines, Pliny the Elder (23/24-79 AD) refers to an onyx marble (layered calcedony) in the preparation of unguents:

> Many people consider that for the preparation of unguents there is little to choose between onyx marble and the "lygdinus" (possibly marble even whiter than most of the Parian marble, but perhaps not marble at all), which is found in Paros in pieces no larger than a dish or mixing bowls, although in early times it was normally imported only from Arabia. (Pliny, *NH* Book XXXVI, Chapter XII, § 8, translated by Eichholz, 1962, 48-49).

6. Parthian small rock crystal and Sassanid smoke quartz unguentarium

Balsamaria were usually made of coloured glass, terracotta, and lead rock crystal containers are rare. Some Roman rock crystal pharmacy tools have come down to us, such as a rock-crystal silver spoon from the first half of the first century AD, housed at the New York Metropolitan Museum of Art, which provides the following information:

> The Romans treasured vessels made of rock crystal, and quite a number of small scent bottles belonging to the Early Imperial period are known. There is, however, no parallel for the use of rock crystal for a utensil such as this spoon. (https://www.metmuseum.org/art/collection/search/257437 accessed February 26, 2022).

An inhumation tomb from the second century AD, discovered in Saint-Médard-des-Pres, Fontenay-le Comte, Vendée, France (former Roman province of Gaul Aquitaine) was thought to have belonged to an artist (a painter). The chemical analysis of the substances remaining in the flasks revealed materials used to treat eye disorders. Therefore, it was concluded that the tomb belonged to a female pharmacist or physician who dedicated herself to preparing eye medicines. Two small crystal shovels, some bowls and two marble and alabaster mortars were found among numerous balsamaria, bronze rectangular boxes to store medicines and two bronze spatula-probes (Santrot et al. 2011, 46-61).

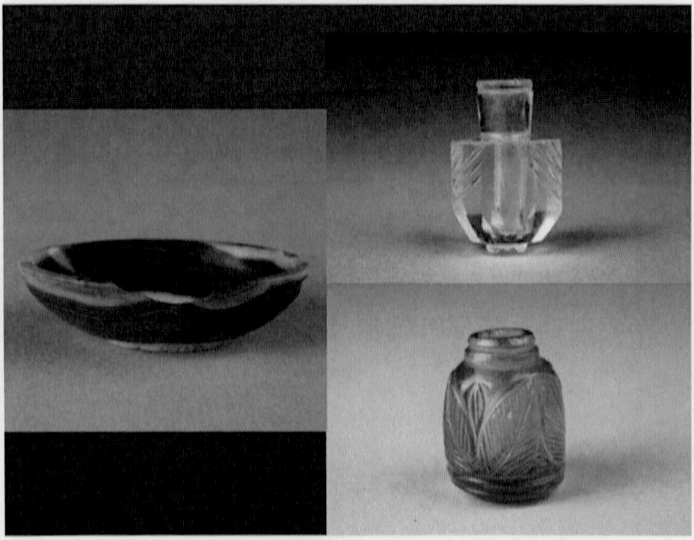

Fig. 3.4a. Roman small sardonyx bowl. Inv. 2018. 0070. H. 14 mm. Diameter. 50 to 30 mm.
Fig. 3.4b. Parthian rock crystal unguentarium. Inv. Nr. 2018.0071. H. 41 mm.
Fig. 3.4c. Sassanid smoky quartz unguentarium. Inv. Nr. 208.0072. H. 30 mm. Photo credits: MDDS/Manuel Santos.

Rock crystal balsamaria are also known from other regions. Two rock crystal flasks of this Collection dating to the fourth/fifth century AD display faceted polish, a characteristic of Sassanian art (Catálogo s.d. 46, fig. 25 and 26) (Fig. 3.4b).

A beautiful rock crystal unguentarium from Amlash, according to information from the previous owner, is described as having eight facets, four with triple hollow-ground corrugation and standing on four tiny feet. The remains of a reddish substance still adhere to the interior wall (Catalogue 2019, 24, fig. 20). An analysis of the remains would disclose the composition of the contained product.

A Sassanid smoky quartz unguentarium from Parthia, in north-eastern Iran, presents relief decorations in the form of incised leaves in the body (Catalogue 2019, 21, fig. 21) (Fig. 3.4c).

Surgical instruments

1. Tweezers

Tweezers are frequently found in medical and grooming contexts. They have different shapes. The pair of tweezers from the Bühler-Brockhaus Collection is quite plain: flared and straight-sided, made from an undecorated continuous strip of copper alloy, folded to form plain blades. This specimen is flared towards the grips, matching the drawing provided by Eckart & Crummy (2008, 148, fig 9). However, the tweezers from the Bühler-Brockhaus Collection have serrated grips, usually found in tweezers for medicinal use (Eckart & Crummy 2008, 148).

Medical tweezers, like probes, are the "mechanical substitute for fingers" (Bliquez 2016, 233). Small specimens with serrated grips were utilized in eye surgery (Bliquez 2016, 238) (Fig. 3.3d- 2nd from left to right).

2. Needle

Needles, mounted on a shaft and terminating in a probe, also existed, the cataract needles being the most emblematic (Bliquez 2016, 154). Curved or straight needles for stitching wounds with wool, animal, or even human hair were also used for other purposes, listed by Bliquez:

> Aside from introducing various types of threading into position for ligating blood vessels or for positioning tissue, blood vessels and even eyelashes for incision, excision, or removal by some other means, needles acted as lancets, probes, retractors, directors and cauteries (Bliquez 2016, 147).

For this reason, we find needles with other shapes, not used for suturing but for puncturing or cauterising. Such is the case with the needle in the Bühler-Brockhaus Collection (Fig. 3.5a). A needle with a similar purpose is figured along with a set of unknown instruments from Pompeii in Tabanelli (1958 tavola LXXVIII, 1st from right to left) (Fig. 3.5b). Cataract needles, the most important of this typology, were better understood after the discovery of four specimens in the river Saôn at Monbelet in Roman Gaul (Künzl 1982, 89). These needles highlighted the operation of cataract couching in Roman times and described by the great Roman encyclopedist Aulus Cornelius Celsus (c.25 BC-c. 50 AD) in his work *De medicina* Book VII, 18 (Celsus translated by Spencer 1938, 397).

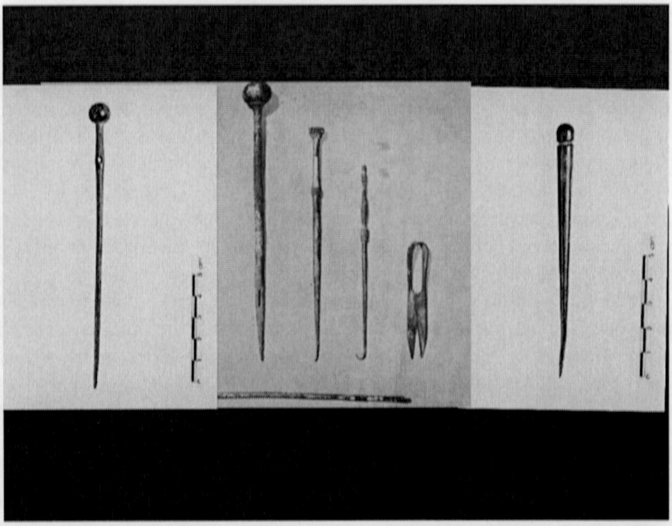

Fig. 3.5a. Needle. Inv. Nr. 2016.0570. L 132 mm Max width 11 mm. Photo credit: MDDS/Manuel Santos.
Fig. 3.5b. Unknown tools (Tabanelli 1958 Tavolla LXXVIII).
Fig. 3.5c. Eyed needle. Inv. Nr. 2016.0571. L. 103 mm Max width 7 mm. Photo credit: MDDS/Manuel Santos.

3. Eyed-needle

An eyed needle from the left of the same Tabanelli's plate with a round handle in the upper shaft is similar to the needle from the Bühler-Brockhaus Collection (Fig. 3.5c). These needles were used for threading and suturing within cavities (Tabanelli 1958 tavolla LXXVIII) (Fig. 3.5b).

4. "Triple" portable probe case

Rectangular boxes divided in two sections, one for holding instruments such as scalpels and the other for medicines, have also been found. Cylindrical cases to carry a set of instruments, mainly probes, have also been unearthed in archaeological excavations. They are usually unique (Milne 1907, 198-199).

Portable cases for carrying instruments and medicines were first mentioned by Hippocrates (c.460-c.360 BC), when giving useful advice for medical practice:

> You must practise these things in medicine with all reserve, in the matter of palpation, anointing, washing, to ensure elegance in moving the hands, in the matter of lint, compresses, bandages, ventilation, purges, for wounds and eye troubles, and with regard to the various kinds of these things, in order that you may have ready beforehand instruments, appliances, knives and so forth. For lack in these matters means helplessness and harm. See that you have a second physician's case, of simpler make, that you can carry in your hands when on a journey. The most convenient is one methodically arranged, for the physician cannot possibly go through everything.
>
> Keep well in your memory drugs and their properties, both simple and compound, seeing that after all it is in the mind that are also the cures of diseases; remember their modes, and their number and variety in the several cases. This in medicine is beginning, middle and end (Hippocrates, *Decorum*, translation by Jones VIII, IX, 291-293).

A set of probe cases from the Lisbon Pharmacy and Health Museum displays a double probe case and four probe cases with a unique compartment, one still keeping the chain[2] (Fig. 3. 6.).

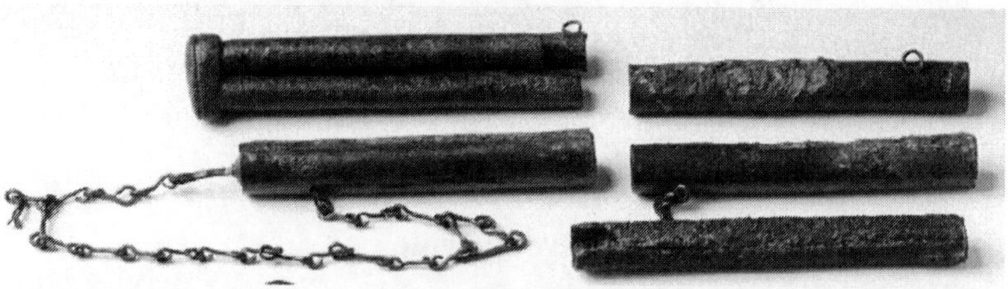

Fig. 3.6. Five probe cases from the Pharmacy and Health Museum. Double case at the upper left corner. Reproduced with permission.

One of the most fascinating pieces from the Bühler-Brockhaus Collection is composed of three tubular containers. They house three instruments-probes and needles are inside. Melting by fire could be a possibility (Fig. 3.7.a). However, no distortions caused by fire are apparent.

Therefore, a Computerized Axial Tomography (Fig. 3.7.b) and a Digital Radiography (Fig. 3. 8ª and 3.8b) were produced by Carlos Prates, a

---

[2] Detail of Inv. 010636
https://www.museudafarmacia.pt/collection/ficha.aspx?lang=PO&a=0&pa=&id=2198 accessed 22 August 2022.

radiologist, also interested in palaeoradiology. Surprisingly, his report reads as follows:

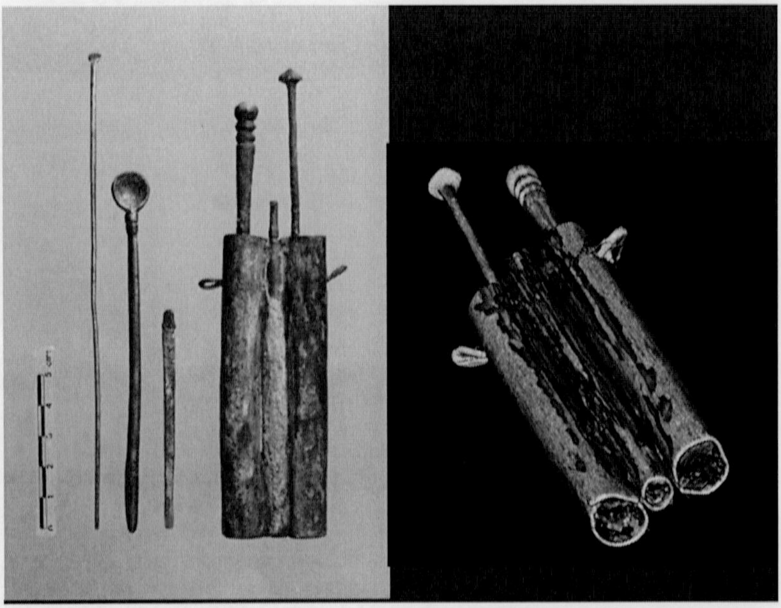

Fig. 3.7a. Portable probe case with three instruments inside and three loose instruments. Inv. Nr. 2016.0557. Dimensions of the set: H. max 214 mm; W. 48 mm. Dimensions of the triple case: H. 96 mm; W. 35 mm.
Fig. 3.7b. Computerized Axial Tomography.
Photo credits: IMI-art / Affidea

Radiographic Study of 2 pieces by Digital Radiography and CAT (from the Archaeological Museum of Braga D. Diogo de Sousa) Carlos Prates / IMI-art / Affidea / Lisbon, 24 Nov 2019

FEA17010376: Triple "Case", with instruments and side clamp rings

For correlation, we designate container 1 as the one with the most horizontal side clamp ring and the probe with the upper decorated end, two as the central one and three as the one with the upper angled clamp ring.

Three tubular containers:

Juxtaposed and very high-density metal, with artefacts, and compatible with bronze (value of 3,071 U.H., limit of equipment for medical measurement) – probable bronze, copper plus tin.
Containers 1 and 2 present average thicknesses, ranging from a minimum of 7 to 8 mm and a maximum of 16 to 17 mm. The central container may have a very tenuous lower overall thickness but is very similar.

The 3 cylindrical containers were constructed from a metal sheet, rolled and hammered in a longitudinal joint area.

The joining lines have central topography, hidden in the junction of the 2 lateral components with the central one, while that of the central container is in contact with container 3.
The central joining of the tubular containers does not reveal welding or dense metallic material, and a preserved interface of low density always seems to be preserved – at least of a much lower density than metal (some glue? Some other kind of material?).
Strangely, the bottom of the cylindrical containers (although looking like bronze, very similar to the material of the tubular walls in the photo) the X-Ray and TAC images do not reveal a dense lid or plate structure with a density similar to the walls. Strangely it almost looks like termination of much less density, either non-metallic or open.
The side fixing clamp rings penetrate inside the sidewalls of the cylinders, crimped by their internal ends, internally as small spikes.

Three "probes" inserted into the tubular containers:
All have a similar metallic density (and maximum, in the Computerized Axial Tomography (CAT) evaluation), held in place by a residual and irregular internal structure, with very different densities, from negative (fats) to medium and very high, even similar to metallic ones.

Description of the containers:
Container 1 — looks like a probe or needle, with a total length of 10.1 cm, a distal gauge, at the tip, of 2 mm with a blunt end, gently widening to the top worked by clamp rings and terminal spherical end. At the top of the shaft, it has a 4.5 mm calibre. The top three-ring clamps are similar at 5.6mm and a 7mm ball on top. The most cranial ring cramp, just below the spherical end, has a side-to-side perforation, more noticeable on CAT.
Container 2 — similar piece, length 8.6 cm, without top decoration. The lower end is also relatively blunt but more tapered than container1. It has a maximum proximal gauge of about 3 mm. Its upper

8 mm is narrower, with 1.7 mm, as if representing a "handle" (another attachment component?).
Container 3 — is the most tapered and most extended piece at 10.7 cm, looking more like a needle, with a total length of 10.1 cm medium gauge of 1.3 to 1.4 mm. Top with quadrangular configuration, accessible to observation.

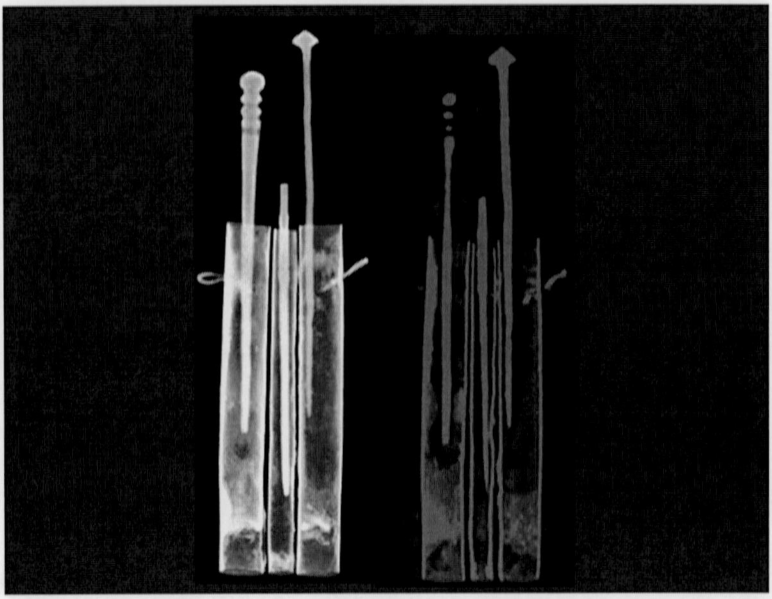

Fig. 3.8a and 3.8b. Digital Radiography.
Photo credits: IMI-art / Affidea

The radiological studies were most helpful in understanding a very rare "Triple" portable probe case. Three other tools were not attached to the set.

5. Ear probe

Ear probes are frequent discoveries at archaeological sites (on this Subject, see Barroso, *Roman Medical-Surgical Instruments from the Archaeological Museum D. Diogo de Sousa,* this volume). Being multifunctional instruments, this long and thin specimen, found in a portable case may be an example of what Milne called an "Ear specillum for wounds" (*specillum vulnerarium*), in which the ear probe could be combined with a probe or a scoop, but on a larger scale (Milne 1907, 68) (Fig. 3.9a).

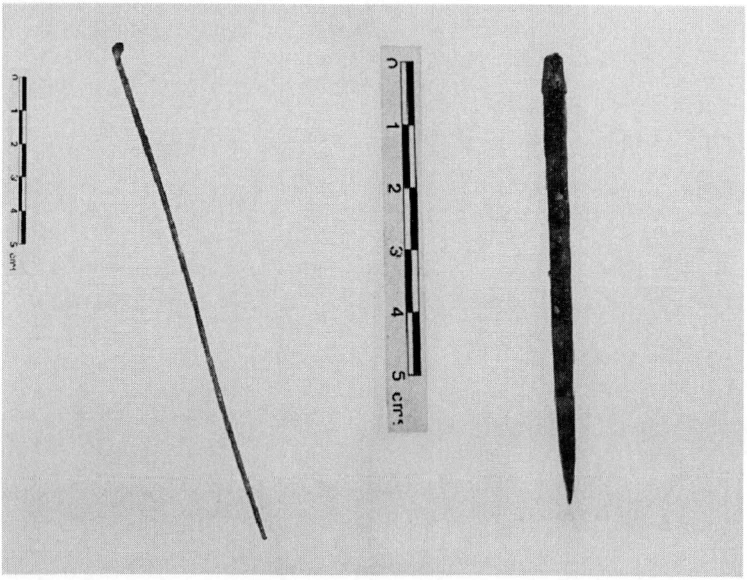

Fig. 3.9a. Ear probe. Nº Inv.: 2016.0559. H. max.: 155 mm. Width: 4,5 mm. Thick: 2 mm
Fig. 3.9b. Needle. Nº Inv.: 2016.0560 – H. max.: 71 mm. W: 4 mm Thick: 3 mm.
Photo credit: MDDS/Manuel Santos.

6. Needle

Another instrument from this portable case features the typology of puncturing needles described above in the five instruments set (Fig. 3.9b).

7. Circular cautery

Cauteries and scalpels were widely used as surgery lancing and cauterizing tools, mainly to staunch bleeding, eliminate diseased and necrotic tissue and drain abscesses. Cauteries, made from iron or bronze, were devised into different shapes, according to the purpose and extension of tissue which it was necessary to necrotize. Milne presented four types of cauteries from

Pompeii. One is circular, matching one found in the triple portable probe case described above (Milne, 1907, Plate XV. Nr. 4) (Fig. 3.10 a and 3.10.b).

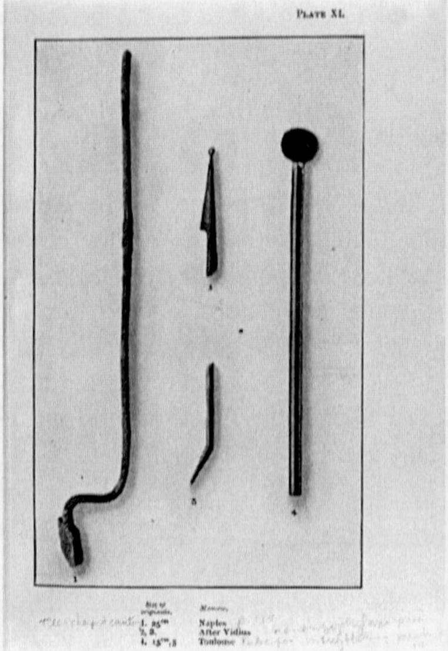

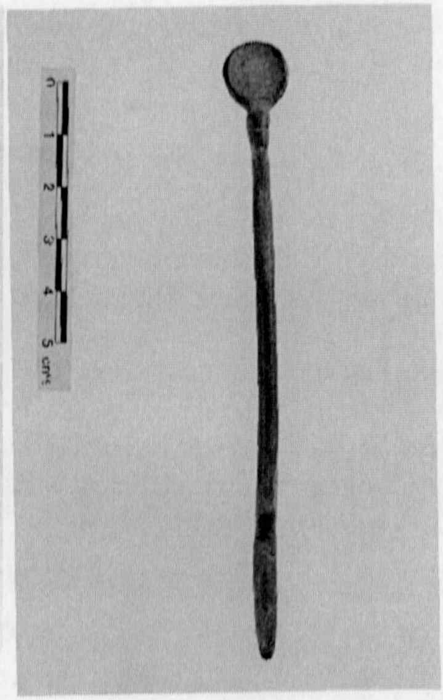

Fig. 3.10a. Cauteries from Pompei. Milne, 1907, Plate XV.
Fig. 3.10b. Circular cautery. Nº Inv.: 2016.0558. H. max:118 mm W: 13 mm. Thick: 4,5 mm.
2016.0571. Photo credit: MDDS/Manuel Santos.

Hippocrates referred to surgery as the last resort when all other therapeutic interventions did not work:

> What drugs will not cure, the knife will; what the knife will not cure, the cautery will; what the cautery will not cure must be considered incurable (Hippocrates, *Aphorisms,* Section VII, 87 in Lloyd 1894, 236).

We wonder if Hippocrates' aphorism means that cauterizing would get better results because, as we know now, it was a more aseptic procedure than lancing. Heat kills the pathogenic micro-organisms of which the ancient physicians were not aware. The aphorism also focuses on the importance of Graeco-Roman surgery, mostly carried out in emergency conditions in a desperate effort to avoid the patient's death:

"Desperate cases need the most desperate remedies" (Hippocrates, *Aphorisms,* Section I, 6 in Lloyd 1894, 206).

That is why Vesalius paid tribute to the Graeco-Roman heritage and we modern doctors to our pioneering ancestors.

Conclusion

Although the pharmacy and medical-surgical instruments of the Bühler-Brockhaus Collection are not represented in large numbers, they contain some very rare pieces. The pharmaceutical sieve-spoon, the eyed needle and the triple portable probe case significantly enrich and complement the collection of instruments from the Bracara Augusta excavations found in the Archaeological Museum D. Diogo de Sousa, in Braga, thanks to the collectors and patrons that added such value to the Museum and current knowledge concerning Ancient Medicine and Graeco-Roman tools.

Acknowledgements

I thank Dr Isabel Silva, Director of the Archaeological Museum D. Diogo de Sousa, Braga, for granting permission to study the medical-surgical and grooming tools of the Museum and for permission to reproduce associated images. I also thank Dr Maria José Sousa and the Museum staff for their kind support in the preparation of this essay. I thank Dr Carlos Prates and IMI-art / Affidea for the radiological study of the "Triple" portable probe case, Dr. João Neto, Director of the Pharmacy and Helath Museum for the kind permission to reproduce the portable probe case images, and Dr Christopher J. Duffin for the critical reading of this essay.

References

Askintopoulou, Helen, Ramoutsaki, Ionna A., Konsolaki, Elina. 2002. "Archaeological evidence of the use of opium in the Minoan world" 23-29. In *International Congress Series*, Volume 1242.

Catálogo de exposição Museu de Setúbal. Convento de Jesus. s.d. *Arqueologia. Colecção Bühler-Brockhaus.* Setubal: Fundação Bühler-Brockhaus.

Barroso, Maria do Sameiro. 2014-2015. "Medicine, surgery, pharmacy, toilet, and other health care tools from the Roman city of Balsa (Tavira, Portugal) from the 1st at the 3rd century AD." *O Arqueólogo Português* [5], 4/5: 341-373.

Bliquez, Lawrence. 1994. *Roman Surgical Instruments and Other Minor Objects in the National Archaeological Museum of Naples.* Mainz: Verlag Phillip von Zabern.

Bliquez, Lawrence. 2016. *The tools of Asclepius, Surgical Instruments in Greek and Roman Times*. Leiden: Brill.

Bühler, Hans-Peter. 1966. *Antile Gefässe aus Calcedonen.* Dissertation. Maximilian Universität zur Würzburg.

Bühler, Hans-Peter. 1973. *Antike Gefässe aus Edelsteinen*. Mainz: Philipp von Zabern.

Catalogue. 2019. *The Bühler-Brockhaus Collection. Ancient Mediterranean Art. Greco-Roman World. Donation to the Museu de Arqueologia D. Diogo de Sousa, Braga.* Setúbal: Fundação Buehler-Brockhaus.

Celsus. *On Medicine.* 1938. Hendersen, Jeffrey (ed), Spencer, Walter George (translator). Cambridge: Harvard University Press, 3 vol.

Clay plaque. Mvsei Vaticani https://m.museivaticani.va/content/museivaticani-mobile/en/collezioni/musei/museo-gregoriano-egizio/sala-iv--l_egitto-e-roma/lastra-campana.html accessed 9 March 2022.

Eckart, Hella & Crummy, Nina. 2008. Styling the body in Late Iron Age and Roman Britain, a contextual approach to toilet instruments. Montagnac: Éditions Monique Mergoil.

*Farrington, B*enjamin.1932. "The preface of Andreas Vesalius to De Fabrica Corporis Humani 1543". *Proceedings of the Royal Society of Medicine*, 25 (9): 1357-1366.

Grmek, Mirko & Gourevitch. 1998. *Les maladies dans l'art antique.* Paris: Fayard.

Hippocrates. 1959. Spencer, W. G. (translation) Volume II, Cambridge: Harvard University Press.

Jutta Costabile; Jutta. 2019. "Nulla vita sine arte" 8-11. In Catalogue. 2019. *The Bühler-Brockhaus Collection. Ancient Mediterranean Art. Greco-Roman World. Donation to the Museu de Arqueologia D. Diogo de Sousa, Braga.* Setúbal: Fundação Buehler-Brockhaus.

Künzl, Ernst. 1982. *Medizinische Instrumente aus sepulchralfunden der romischen Kaiserzeit.* Köln: Rheinland Verlag GmbH.

Lloyd, Geoffrey Ernest Richard (ed). 1983. *Hippocratic Writings*, Chadwick, John and Mann, William Neville (transl.), London: Penguin Books.

Marcellus. 1889. Helmreich, Georg ed. *De medicamentis liber.* Lipsia: Teubner.

Milne, John Stuart.1907. *Surgical Instruments in Greek and Roman Times.* Oxord: Massachussetts, London: Clarendon.

Penso, Guiseppe. 1984. *La medicine Romaine. L'art d'Esculape dans la Rome antique.* Paris: Les Éditions Roger Dacosta.

Pliny the Elder. *Natural History.* 1962. Edited by Jeffrey Henderson. Translated by Eichholz. D. E., Books 36-37. Cambridge, Massachussetts, London: Harvard University Press.

Rätsch, Christian. 2014. *Heilpflanzen der Antike. Mythologie, Heilkunst und Anwendung.* Aarau und Münschen: AT Verlag.

Sakelarakis, Yannis. 1985. *Heraklion Museum.* Athens: Ekdotike Athenon S. A.

Santrot, Jaques; Wible, François; Touwaide, Alain; Cazanove, Olivier de. 2011. "Médicaments et pharmacologie". *Arqueo-Thema 16. La medicine à l'époque romaine*, setembre-octobre; 46-61.

Singer, Peter & Van de Eijk, Philip (eds). 2013. *Galen: Psychological Writings*, Cambridge; Cambridge University Press.

Tabanelli, Mario. 1958. Lo stumento chirurgico e la su storia. [Forli]: Romagna Medica.

Trevelyan, Robert Calverly. 1947. *A translation of the Idyls of Theocritus. Cambridge:* Cambridge University Press.

Von Habsburg, Géza.1997. *Fürsterliche Kunstkammern in Europa* (Original *Princely Treasures,* The Vendome Press, New York), German translation by Von Gemmingen, Stuttgart: Kohlkammer GmbH.

Chapter 4

The Emerald: A Magico-Medicinal Stone

Christopher J. Duffin

Abstract
The history of the medicinal uses of emerald from pre-scientific times to the mid-eighteenth century is investigated here for the first time. The main source of the gemstone from classical times to the sixteenth century was Egypt, after which the rich deposits of emeralds yielded from Colombian mines began flooding the import market in the Iberian Peninsula and Goa. The *smaragdus* of classical texts certainly included emerald, but probably also referred to prase, malachite and green tourmaline, with which it was relatively easily confused. Potential therapeutic properties are ascribed to the stone right from their first mention (as being good for the eyes) by Theophrastus. The opinions of medieval authors, particularly Albertus Magnus and Pseudo-Aristotle, shaped later suggestions as to the therapeutic value of emeralds through lapidary texts to the medical works of early modern writers. The gem was commended as an amulet against epilepsy, poisoning, fevers, ague and as an aid to controlling childbirth. It was a focal component in some compound medicines and included with many other ingredients in others. Prominent examples of emerald-containing compound medicines include the gem electuary of Johannes Mesuë and the seventeenth century Goa Stone imported to Europe from the Portuguese colony. Explanations for the therapeutic mode of action of the gemstone ranged from channelling the energy from the stars to the magnetic extraction of poisons from a person's body. Potential tests of authenticity included holding the gem in the line of sight close to a toad or snake; a genuine, high-quality specimen would cause the toad to burst or its eyes to liquefy, and the snake's eyes to pop out of their sockets. The emerald was used to test for the presence of poison, neutralise it, and to treat a wide range of diseases, some of unknown aetiology, but also including epilepsy, ocular disorders, fevers, plague, melancholy, vertigo and the bloody flux. It was also believed

to generate higher personal qualities in an individual, such as eloquence and sexual probity.
Key words: Emerald; Egypt; Colombia; Smaragdus; Gem Electuary; Goa Stone; Plague; Epilepsy; Poison

Resumo
A história do uso medicinal da esmeralda desde os tempos pré-científicos até meados do século XVIII surge neste capítulo, sendo investigada pela primeira vez. O Egipto foi a principal fonte da pedra preciosa, desde a Antiguidade Clássica até ao século XVI, até as ricas jazidas de esmeraldas provenientes das minas colombianas começarem a inundar o mercado de importação na Península Ibérica e Goa. A *smaragdus* dos textos clássicos incluía seguramente a esmeralda, mas, provavelmente, também se referia à opala prase, à malaquite e à turmalina verde, com as quais era relativamente fácil de confundir. Potenciais propriedades terapêuticas são atribuídas à pedra desde sua primeira referência (como boa para os olhos) por Teofrasto. As opiniões de autores medievais, particularmente Alberto Magno e Pseudo-Aristóteles, enquadraram as indicações posteriores quanto ao valor terapêutico das esmeraldas, desde os textos dos lapidários até às obras médicas dos primeiros escritores modernos. A pedra preciosa foi recomendada como amuleto contra a epilepsia, o envenenamento, as febres e a malária, e como adjuvante no trabalho de parto, tendo sido um ingrediente fundamental de alguns compostos medicinais, e incluído em outros com variados ingredientes. Exemplos notáveis de compostos medicamentosos, contendo esmeraldas, incluem o electuário de pedras preciosas de Johannes Mesuë e a Pedra de Goa do século XVII, importada para a Europa da colónia portuguesa. As explicações para o modo de acção terapêutico variavam desde o aporte da energia das estrelas até à extracção de venenos por uma espécie de acção magnética. Testes de possível autenticidade incluíam segurar a pedra na linha de visão junto a um sapo ou uma cobra. Uma pedra genuína e de alta qualidade faria o sapo explodir ou provocaria a liquefacção dos olhos que lhe saltariam das órbitas. A esmeralda foi usada para testar a presença de veneno, neutralizá-lo e tratar um amplo espectro de doenças, algumas de etiologia desconhecida, mas nas quais se incluíam também a epilepsia, problemas oculares, febres, peste, melancolia, vertigem e hemorragias. Acreditava-se também que dava origem a qualidades pessoais superiores, tais como a eloquência e a integridade sexual.
Palavras-Chave: Esmeralda; Egipto; Colômbia; *Smaragdus*; Electuário de gemas; Pedra de Goa; Peste; Epilepsia; Veneno

Precious and semi-precious stones in medicine

From the modern perspective, outside of crystal therapy, the use of precious and semi-precious stones in medicine seems quite strange. Historically, though, lithotherapy-the medicinal use of rocks, minerals, fossils and earths-has a long and well-established pedigree. Indeed, their use was common in Egyptian, Babylonian, Assyrian, Sumerian, Hindu, Chinese, Tibetan and European medicine traditions (e.g. Kunz 1913). Precious and semi-precious stones, probably by virtue of their exoticism, rarity and mineralogical characteristics (especially hardness, durability, often deep and intense colours, crystalline form and diaphaneity) were often afforded particularly high status as therapeutic agents. Although often sceptical concerning the properties claimed for such materials, Pliny the Elder (A.D. 23-79) did much to establish belief in them by faithfully recording elements of their folklore from Roman tradition and the writings of his antecedents and contemporaries. Much of the lore which he introduced into his *Naturalis Historia*, written around A.D. 77, is magico-medicinal in nature. A foundational and revered text, much of the information which he presented was repeated relatively uncritically in the succeeding centuries. New observations and suggestions were added from medieval Arabic writers and the Western lapidary tradition (Duffin 2013a). Whilst much of this magico-medicinal information continued to be propagated in early modern times, the amuletic use of geological materials slowly declined and they tended to become incorporated into compound medicines designed, successfully or not, to treat diseases physiologically.

The history of use of geopharmaceuticals is a somewhat neglected area of study, generally being part of broader overviews of the history of geological materials (e.g. Kunz 1913, 1915; Lecouteux 2011), although some more detailed studies have been produced recently (e.g. Duffin 2008, 2013c; Bogdasarov & Bogdasarov 2016; Barroso 2019).

So far as precious and semi-precious stones in particular, are concerned, Führer (1956) and Pazzini (1939) have produced useful overviews and early modern lapidary medicine has been tackled in a Ph.D. thesis (Harris 2009). Individual minerals have also received some recent attention, particularly Amber (Duffin 2013e, 2015b), Malachite (Barroso 2017), Lapis lazuli (Duffin 2014) and Rock Crystal or Quartz (Duffin 2020a). Once rendered into a very fine powder (levigated), precious and semi-precious stones could be mixed with various liquids (usually alcohol or specialised herbal waters) and/or binding agents and either applied to the body surface in emplasters, ointments, liniments and unguents, or taken internally in pills, troches, lozenges, lohochs, electuaries etc. The wide range of materials used in this way is illustrated by the list of ingredients added to restorative sick dishes (see below): gold coins, pearls, diamonds, rubies, sapphires, turquoise, emerald, coral, amber, jasper, jacinth, onyx, crystal (quartz) chalcedony, sardonyx, chrysolite, beryl, topaz, chrysoprase and amethyst (Duffin 2012, 83).

The purpose of this paper is to give an overview of the historical uses of emerald (including references to *smaragdus*) as an item of *materia medica*, with a particular emphasis on English early modern pharmaceutical literature. As will be clear from the following, this precious stone was used extensively in a wide variety of ways and delivery vehicles to treat a surprising diversity of conditions. It was part of the stock-in-trade of the apothecary, as surviving drug jars indicate (Fig. 4.5).

Emeralds

The cyclosilicates or ring silicates are a group of silicate minerals in which interlinked SiO_4 tetrahedra are closed to form a ring. The interstices between adjacent rings may accommodate more unusual elements. Minerals containing closed rings each with six SiO_4 tetrahedra include the Beryl group, whose chemical formula is $Be_3Al_2(Si0)_6$. Trace quantities of chromium and/or vanadium in the crystal lattice give rise to the green colour that is typical of Emerald (Fig. 4.1). Other gem varieties of Beryl include Aquamarine, Heliodor and Morganite which are blue, yellow and pink respectively although, as might be expected, there are colour gradations between the mineral species depending on the balance of appropriate cations in the crystal lattice (Duffin 2006, 21; Giuliani & Groat 2019). The geological formation of emeralds requires a source of beryllium, which is a very rare crustal component (coming 98th in terms of crustal abundance), and chromium/vanadium. There are three main geological occurrences of emeralds: (1) as new crystal growths due to the interaction of metasomatic fluids with desilicated pegmatites; (2) high level Be-rich crustal evaporitic brines interacting with Cr-rich sediments; (3) in metamorphic rocks such as schists, due to interaction with circulating, deeper crustal fluids (Giuliani et al. 2019).

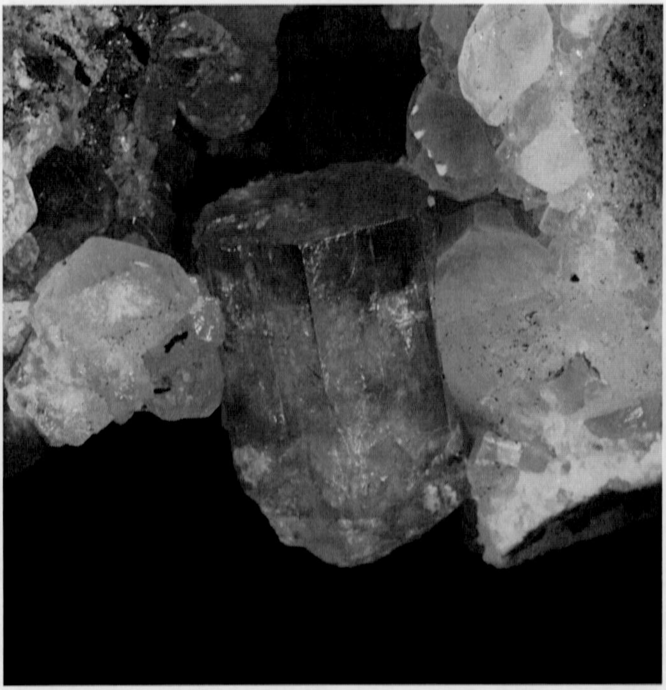

Fig. 4.1. A specimen of Colombian emerald, Muzo Mine. Image courtesy of The Arkenstone iRocks.com.

With a hardness of 7.5 to 8.0 on Mohs' Hardness Scale, emerald crystallises in the hexagonal crystal system and has a colourless streak. Crystals are transparent to opaque and are typically a rich green colour. Pliny the Elder (Fig. 4.2) was particularly impressed by the green colour, noting that, compared to all other things "it surpasses them all in pleasant verdure" (Holland 1636, 611). Thomas Nicols (fl. 1650) expands on this sentiment, stating that emerald has "so excellent a viridity" that its' colour will "overcome the meadows glorie, by the glory of that spring of viriditie which it hath in its self: The largenesse of the meadow it will overcome with the amplitude of its glory, wherewith farre above its greatnesse it doth feed the eie: and the virescencie of the meadow it will overcome with the brightnesse of its glory, which in it self seemeth to embrace the glorious viridity of many springs" (Nicols 1652, 91).

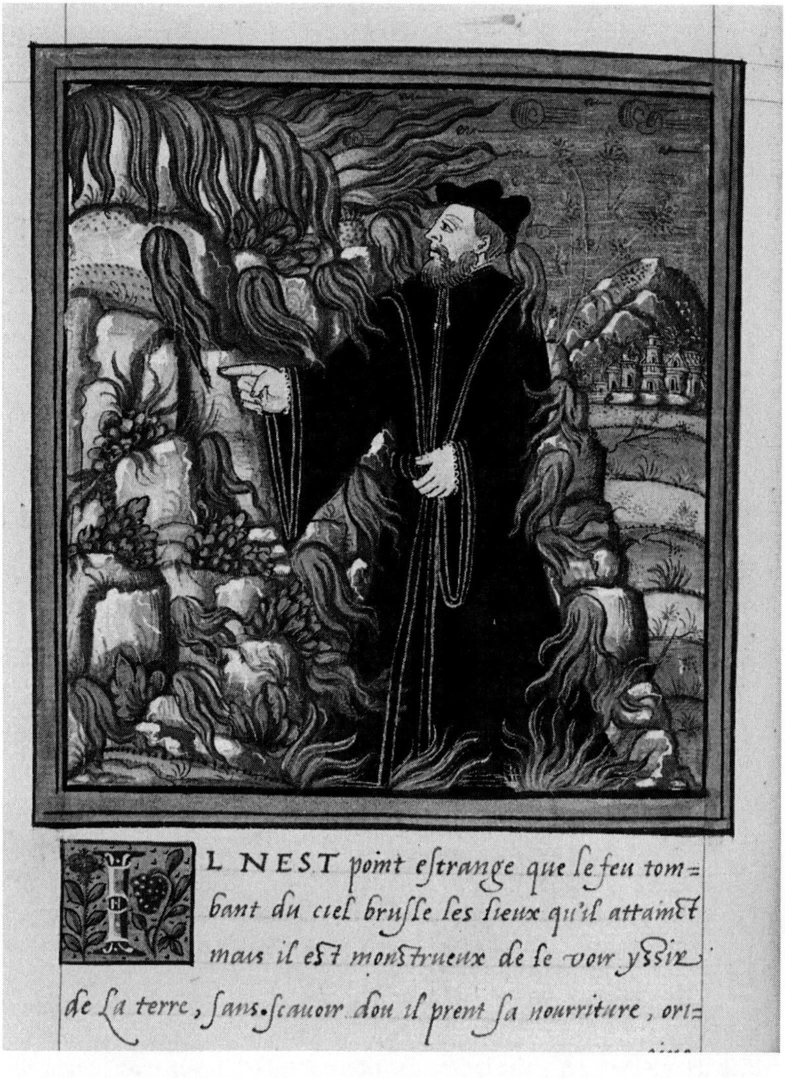
IL NEST point eſtrange que le feu tom=
bant du ciel bruſle les lieux qu'il attainct
mais il eſt monſtrueux de le voir yssir
de la terre, ſans ſcauoir dou il prent ſa nourriture, ort=

Fig. 4.2. The death of Pliny the Elder during the eruption of Vesuvius (79 AD). Boaistuau, P. (1560) Histoires Prodigieuses: "Prodigieuse mort de Pline [dont le] corps fut mis en cendre [par les flammes du Vesuve]", Folio 64 verso. Reproduced by kind permission of the Wellcome Library, London.

Provenance

Pliny lists twelve contemporary types of emeralds from ancient and classical times, mostly associated with distinct production areas; the most important three, in his estimation, were Scythia, Egypt and Bactria. The Scythian emeralds were allied in folklore with the Arimaspians, a cyclopian race often identified as living in the Ural Mountains. The association seems to be a conflation with the story of the gold-guarding griffins (Mayor & Heaney 1993). Nevertheless, the tale is propagated through some early modern literature (Nicols 1652, 94).

In Pliny's time, Bactria embraced an area that includes present-day Iran and Afghanistan. The source of the Bactrian emeralds mentioned by Pliny is unknown, but it is interesting to note that modern commercial exploitation of emeralds has taken place in the Panjshir Valley area of the Hindu Kush Mountains in Afghanistan (Bowersox et al. 1991).

It is generally agreed that the Egyptian deposits mentioned by Pliny accounted for most of the emeralds coming into circulation in classical times, although it has been suggested that the Romans also worked deposits at Habachtal near Salzburg in Austria (Sinkankas 1981, 371-377; never very productive, the area has been worked sporadically for emeralds since the late eighteenth century). Historical Egyptian emerald mining sites are known from several localities near (within about 15km of) the best known and most ancient mine at Wadi Sikait in the Eastern Desert. This locality, sometimes referred to as Montanus Smaragdus, probably began production toward the end of the Ptolomaic Period in the first century B.C., although it was also actively exploited in Roman and Byzantine periods (1st to 6th centuries AD). Production at other sites in the area continued until the sixteenth century (Harrell 2004).

The Cordillera Oriental (Eastern Ranges) of the Colombian Andes yielded emeralds to local indigenous peoples in pre-Columbian times; Colombian emeralds were being worshipped, widely traded through Mexico and South America, and used ceremonially and for personal adornment when the Spanish arrived in the early sixteenth century. In 1537, the Spaniards took over the operational Chibcha Indian mine near Chivor, using the Indians as an enslaved workforce. In 1564, the Muzo and Caijma Indians' mine some 7 km to the West was forcibly added to the Spaniards' productive emerald holdings. Together, these two mines yielded high grade, gem quality emeralds which fed the European and Indian markets through early modern times (Keller 1981). Colombia is still the largest producer of emeralds today.

Etymology

The Ancient Greek word *smaragdos* (Latin: *smaragdus*) refers to a green gem. In Vulgar Latin this became *esmeraldus* which, through the Old French *esmeraude* and Middle English *emeraude*, resulted in the English name emerald. Pliny's identification of twelve different varieties of *smaragdus*, together with the general meaning of "green gem" mentioned above, means it is eminently possible that minerals in addition to emerald were included in that titular umbrella in early references. Other possible mineral candidates also known from green varieties include tourmaline, prase (a variety of quartz) and peridot (chrysolite), together with the hydrated copper carbonate mineral, malachite (especially considering Pliny refers to *smaragdus'* occurrence in copper mines) (Meadows 1945). Several early modern writers insist that emeralds are meant when referred to as *smaragdus*. Sebastian Münster (1489-1552), the German scholar and cartographer, published his *Cosmographia*, the earliest German-language description of the world, in 1544 (Münster 1544). The English translation of selections from the original 1553 by Rycharde Eden, records *smaragdus* from the "Iland of Gyaua" stating that the gem is "ye true Emerode" (Eden 1553, unnumbered page). Likewise, the anonymous translator of Albertus Magnus' (c. 1200-1280) *Book of Secrets* in 1560 indicates that *smaragdus* is "in Englishe speache an Emeraude" (Magnus 1560, unnumbered page).

Garcia de Orta

Along with the Spanish colonisation of large parts of the "New World", the Age of Exploration (or Discovery) also saw the westward expansion of the Portuguese Empire during the sixteenth century, resulting in the colonisation of parts of present-day Brazil, Uruguay and Venezuela. As noted above, the Spanish were having increasing success in annexing and exploiting mineral deposits from the indigenous population in the northern part of South America. Portugal sought similar riches and despatched several expeditions to search for mineral wealth, particularly in Brazil; emeralds were amongst the minerals for which there was a specific focus in the various expeditions into the Brazilian hinterland of 1568, 1573, 1591 and 1588-1596 (Guimarães 1981; Machado & Figueirôa 2001, 11). There seemed to be early success when an expedition led by Sebastião Fernandes Tourinho (fl. second half of the sixteenth century) discovered gold and emeralds in the province of Minas Gerais in 1573 (Reys 2014). Unfortunately, it is generally agreed that the reported emeralds were actually green tourmalines and no significant emerald sources were uncovered by the expeditionary programmes. Note that modern discoveries of emeralds in Brazil began in 1912. Minas Gerais is still an important mineral-producing area including, ironically, yielding some emeralds.

All was not lost, however. The Portuguese excelled at establishing trading routes throughout their Empire and it was not long before an intracontinental system of staging and trading posts was funnelling a wide range of trade goods derived from natural resources across the Atlantic to Lisbon. The imported items of trade included a wide range of South American gemstones, of which emeralds must have constituted a significant fraction.

The Portuguese presence in India was established several decades before their burgeoning interest in South America (Duffin 2010, 22). Trade routes back to Portugal were quickly established and Lisbon rapidly became an expanding import hub for goods, including a variety of gems, from Goa. By the time high quality emeralds and other precious stones were entering the port from South America, the lapidary trading and artisanal processing legacy of Goan exports was ready and able to cope with the new influx of raw materials. The city hosted an active and diverse collection of jewel-processing tradesmen (cutters, polishers, drillers, goldsmiths) and merchants, at least partly focused in the "lower downtown" area of Lisbon on the Rua dos Ourives or "Goldsmith's Street" (currently the "Rua do Ouro"; Lane 2010, 98). The Inquisition was introduced in Portugal by King D. João III (1502-1557; reigned 1521-1557) in 1536. Jews were expected to convert to Catholicism which, in practical terms, meant that many of the lapidary traders and artisans in Lisbon were *conversos*. Besides supplying a domestic and European market for gems, significant quantities of high-quality Colombian emeralds were shipped to trading posts in Goa to feed an enthusiastically buoyant market amongst the Mughal nobility (Babb 2013, 51).

Apothecaries' shops were particularly abundant (nine in total) in the Rua Nova (Gschwend & Lowe 2015, 114), and acted as a second focal destination for a wide range of materials from both India and the New World.

Living at points of entry for imported gems and other goods gave residents a certain advantage when it came to intercepting new materials for study, consideration, collection and incorporation into personal collections and Kunstkammern. In the case of Goa, this meant Garcia de Orta (c. 1501-1568; Fig. 4.3) (Boxer 1963). Born in Castelo da Vide to parents of Spanish Jewish heritage (but forcibly converted to Christianity in 1497), de Orta studied in Spain (arts, philosophy and medicine at Alcalá de Henares and Salamanca), returning to Portugal following his father's death to practice

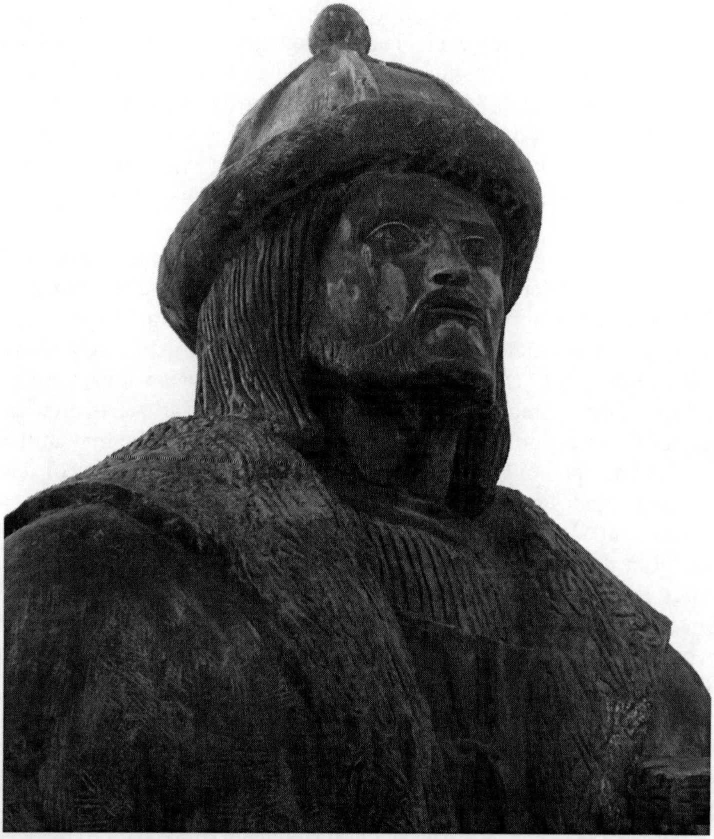

Fig. 4.3. Statue honouring Garcia de Orta (c. 1501-1568), Lisbon. Author's photograph.

medicine. He continued his work in Lisbon from 1526, where he was also briefly appointed to a lectureship at the university in 1532 and served as royal physician to D. João III. As the Portuguese Inquisition gathered pace and intensity, the *Cristão Novo* (new Christian) *converso* (see above) de Orta sailed to Goa as Chief Physician to the fleet, arriving in September 1534. He remained there until his death, keeping up with a busy medical practice, travelling widely and maintaining a rich correspondence. He is probably most famous for his publication-*Colóquios dos Simples e Drogas da India* ("Conversations on the simples, drugs and materia medica of India") (Fig. 4.4). Written in Portuguese, published in 1563, only seven years after the introduction of the first printing press in Goa, and riddled with typographical errors, it is constructed in the style of a dialogue, emulating the approach of one of his literary heroes, the Italian physician Antonio Musa Brasavolus (1500-1555) (Brasavolus 1536).

¶ Coloquios dos ſimples, e
drogas he couſas mediçinais da India, e
aſsi dalgũas frutas achadas nella onde ſe
tratam algũas couſas tocantes amediçina,
pratica, e outras couſas boas, pera ſaber
cõpoſtos pello Doutor garçia dorta : fiſico
del Rey noſſo ſenhor, viſtos pello muyto
Reuerendo ſenhor, ho liçençiado
Alexos diaz : falcam deſenbar-
gador da caſa da ſupricaçã
inquiſidor neſtas
partes.

¶ Com priuilegio do Conde viſo Rey.

Im preſſo em Goa, por Ioannes
de endem as x. dias de
Abril de 1563. annos.

Fig.4.4. Title page of Garcia de Orta's Colóquios dos Simples e Drogas da India published 10 April 1563. Public domain.

The *Colóquios* is acknowledged to be a pioneering work on tropical medicine and natural history, covering many aspects of exotic botany. Written in a didactic style, the 57 colloquies or conversations reveal de Orta to be an erudite scholar with diverse interests, making wide use of the expertise provided by an enormous network of helpful informants (Loureiro 2008) and ready to challenge falsehood wherever possible. He is known to have possessed an extensive library (Ficalho 1886) and the imaginary conversations in the Colloquies clearly illustrate the focus, depth and breadth of his active reading. As both a physician and a mercantile ship owner standing at the cultural, intellectual and trading crossroads of the East and the West, he was uniquely placed to offer insights into the goods that passed through his hands.

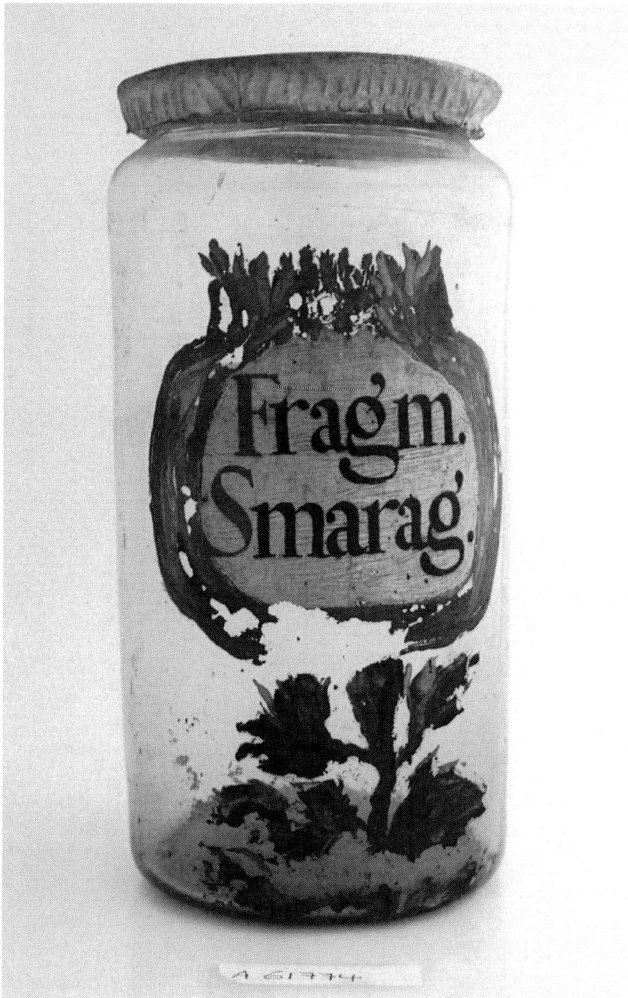

Fig. 4.5. Apothecary jar for the storage of emerald fragments. Reproduced by kind permission of the Wellcome Library, London.

De Orta records a lively discussion between himself and Ruano, a new arrival in Goa with the Portuguese annual fleet from Lisbon. The conversation takes place between two equals with matching educational backgrounds but differing levels of experience; Ruano seeks a greater understanding of the imported drugs he is using in Lisbon and peppers de Orta with questions. In the ninth Colloquy, de Orta nails his colours to the mast-in medical matters he is more concerned with truth born of experience than the weight of opinion of classical authors, writing "Do not try to frighten me with Dioscorides or Galen, because I merely speak the truth and say what I know" (Orta 1913, 60).

Colloquy 21 records a servant girl interrupting the discussion about elephants to announce the arrival of Andrea, a *lapidario* from Milan (Orta 1913, 187), who has located a possible buyer for two emeralds in de Orta's possession; Orta is thus identified as a gem trader. Precious stones were ideal items of intercontinental trade on account of their high commercial value, easy transportation and possibly concealment from authorities; Goa was destined to become a crucial centre for gem trading (Cunha 2001).

The 44th Colloquy concerns precious stones. Here, Orta is able to display his understanding that emeralds are rare, commanding high prices, and that the whereabouts of Asian mining sources was unknown (i.e. the Scythian and Bactrian sources of Pliny cited above), and to offer his opinions regarding the etymology of the stone in different languages (Orta 1913, 358); in the latter case he reveals the depth of his reading by referring to the works of the tenth century Assyrian physician Mesuë, Christophorus Georgius de Honestis (c. 1320-1392), Serapion the Younger (twelfth or thirteenth century Arabic writer) and the Salernitan physician Mattheus Silvaticus (c. 1280-c.1342), all of whom included information concerning the magico-medicinal properties of emeralds and other precious stones in their various works.

Considering his mercantile and medical commitments, Orta's position regarding the supposed magico-medicinal "virtues" of precious stones is of interest. Whilst he accepted that loadstone (magnetite: *pedra de cevar*) and carnelian were both efficacious in stopping haemorrhages and that those "who eat it [loadstone] in small quantity to prevent them from growing old and to preserve their youth" (Orta 1913, 342, 351) he notes that, regarding diamonds:

> As for their employment in physic, it is not the custom to use these diamonds; yet I have seen Gentio ["heathen", i.e. Indian] doctors who give them to break the stone, administering with a syringe. But it is not given inwardly, as there is an error among the people that it is poison because of its great penetration, and boring the entrails (Orta 1913, 343).

Indeed, his generally stated position seems to be that "if they [their healing virtues] are not contrary to reason, they may be true" (Orta 1913, 349).

Ruano raises the question of South American emeralds: "A modern doctor says that our emeralds of Peru are of much more use for medicinal purposes" (Orta 1913, 359). De Orta's riposte was that the imported gems were false (which is untrue) and that his guest should be "on your guard against them" (Orta 1913, 359).

Thus, apparent from a few very specific instances, de Orta's approach to the question of magico-medicinal properties inherent in precious and semi-precious stones was either to dissimulate or argue against their existence; he clearly could see little therapeutic value in their use and was reticent to endorse their employment in medical treatments. For further background discussion on this point see Loureiro (2013).

Medical applications

1. Classical references

The earliest mention of *smaragdus* seems to be that of Theophrastus (c. 371-c. 287 B.C.; Fig. 4.6), Aristotle's student and successor at the Peripatetic School in Athens. A man of wide-ranging interests, his enormously diverse *oeuvre* contains the earliest work dedicated to a consideration of stones and minerals-*Peri Lithon*. Suggested as having been written near the end of the fourth century BC, when Theophrastus was middle-aged, it is the only surviving source quoted by Pliny, and has been suggested as comprising student notes taken at one of the philosopher's lectures (Caley & Richards 1956, 4). Despite its position as a foundational geological text, Theophrastus' work was not translated into English until Sir John Hill did so in 1746 (Duffin 2018). Citing specimens of *smaragdos* as being small and rare, Theophrastus makes the observation that "It is also good for the eyes, and for this reason people carry seals made of it, so as to see better" (Caley & Richards 1956, 4, 50, 100). This is the only observation in the whole volume made by Theophrastus concerning the medicinal effects of the stones which he discusses.

Neither Dioscorides nor Galen seem to mention *smaragdus* in their writings, contrary to certain suggestions in appeals to classical authorities by a number of later writers. Damigeron, a second century lapidarist, introduces some new, largely non-medical properties ascribed to the emerald: its usefulness for "watery divination", its ability to influence business ventures, improve body and speech (so long as the bearer remains chaste while wearing it), clear or protect from storms, and maintain personal freedom. Damigeron closes with the observation that, mounted on a brooch and suitably placed "it will adorn you and your belongings, and you will see the power of the stone given to it by God" (Tahil 1989, 14).

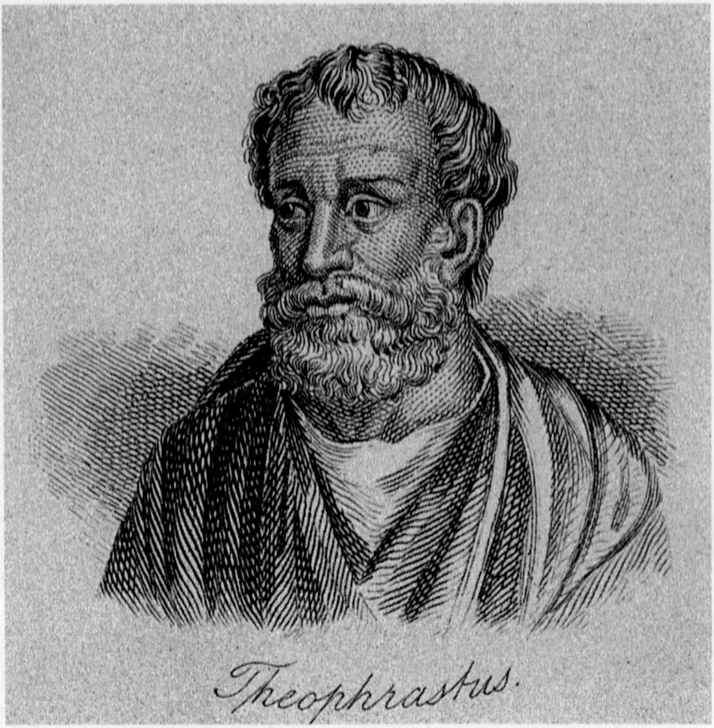

Fig. 4.6. Portrait of Theophrastus (c. 371-c. 287 B.C.). Reproduced by kind permission of the Wellcome Library, London.

Pliny the Elder (Gaius Plinius Secundus; AD 23/24–79; Fig. 4.2), who famously died in the eruption of Mount Vesuvius, collected a great deal of Roman folklore and information concerning precious stones gleaned from written sources, most now lost. His entry for the emerald in his *Historia Naturalis*, written around AD 77 concentrates on the classification and possible sources of the gem. Concerning potential therapeutic actions, he focuses on its supposed efficacy with regard to vision, considerably amplifying the information given by Theophrastus. His entry, in the first English translation of Philemon Holland (1552-1637) is as follows:

> Besides, there is not a gem or precious stone that so fully possesseth the eie, and yet neuer contenteth it with sacietie. Nay, if the sight hath bin wearied and dimmed by intentiue poring vpon any thing els, the beholding of this stone doth refresh and restore it againe, which lappidaries well know, that cut and ingraue fine stones; for they haue not a better means to refresh their eies than the Emeraud, the mild green that it hath doth so comfort and reuiue their wearines and lassitude. Moreouer, the longer and farther off that a man looketh vpon Emerauds, the fairer and bigger they seem to the eie, by reason that they cause the reuerberation of the aire about them for to seeme green: for neither Sun nor shade, ne yet the light of candle, causeth them to change and lose their lustre: but contrariwise, as they euer send out their own raies by litle & little, so they entertain reciprocally the visual beams of our eies; and for all the spissitude and thicknesse that they seeme to haue, they admit gently our sight to pierce into their bottome: a thing that is not ordinary in water. The same are shaped many times hollow, thereby to gather, vnite, and fortifie the spirits that maintain our eie-sight (Holland 1634, 611).

Note the comment concerning the emerald causing the air to reverberate around it, an effect that implied the presence of a hidden, occult force able to confer upon the stone magico-medical properties which, in this case, would strengthen the sight. He also notes that "Nero the Emperor was wont to behold the combats of fencers and sword-plaiers in a faire Emeraud." It is not entirely clear as to whether Nero was using the emerald as a lens through which to watch the gladiatorial games, or whether the text means something else (Holland 1634, 611). For further discussion on emeralds as lenses see Barroso (this volume).

In the third century AD, the Latin grammarian Gaius Julius Solinus refers to emeralds in the section of his *Collectanea rerum memorabilium* ("Collection of Curiosities", also known as Polyhistor) dedicated to the Arimaspians. Living in Scythia, a region reputed to abound in gold and gems, Solinus develops the theme of the emerald-guarding Gryphons first introduced by Pliny. Matriculating from Jesus College, Cambridge in 1552, the prolific Elizabethan translator of Latin works, Arthur Golding (c. 1536-1606), turned his attention to Solinus. In the words of his translation (Golding 1587, unnumbered page) the Gryphons are "a most fierce kinde of foule, and cruell beyond all cruelnesse" which tear apart visitors to their lands in a bid to protect their precious materials. They are "creatures made of purpose to punish the rashnesse of couetous folke". Noting that their lands are "the natiue soyle of the Emerawdes", Solinus goes on to note that "The eye canne beholde nothing more pleasaunt, nor nothing more wholesome than them, first they glister gréene aboue the moyste grasse, and aboue the hearbes that are in the Ryuers". Indeed, they "refresh the eyes that are wearyed with beholding other thinges. For they relieue and sharpen the sight that was dymmed or dulled w[t] the glosse of another stone".

2. The Early Encyclopaedists

Isidore of Seville (Isidorus Hispalensis; c. 560–636), Bishop of Seville, presented a summary of ancient and contemporary knowledge arranged through the 20 books which make up his *Etymologiarum* ("Etymologies"). Seemingly first published in 1472, a total of eleven incunabular editions of the text are known to exist (Duffin 2013a, 16). Book XVI, *De Lapidibus et Metallis* concerns "Stones and Metals" and contains a brief entry for *smaragdus*. This essentially repeats the information provided by Pliny– comments on the superb green colour causing the surrounding air to reverberate with its power, the outline classification of emeralds by provenance and quality, and their soothing quality on the eyes (Barney et al. 2006, 322).

A similar pattern is maintained throughout the encyclopaedic works produced by western authors from the sixth century onwards. See, for example, the following:

(a) Arnoldus Saxo (fl. late twelfth–early thirteenth century), *De gemmarum virtutibus* or "On the Virtues of Gems") in his *De finibus rerum Naturalium* ("On the Boundaries of Nature"; c. 1220), 38d (Stange 1905, 75).
(b) Vincent of Beauvais (also Vincentius Bellovacensis and Vincentius Burgundus; c. 1190–1264), *Speculum Naturale* ("The Mirror of Nature") (de Beauvais 1478?, unnumbered page).

Rabanus Maurus Magnentius (c. 780–856) who eventually rose to the post of Archbishop in his hometown of Mainz is believed to have written *De Universo* between 842 and 847. Heavily reliant on Isidore of Seville's earlier work, in turn derived from Pliny, Maurus brings a theological dimension to bear when considering the emerald. He interprets the stories about the Arimaspians and emerald-guarding gryphons in terms of Christian allegory. The emerald is seen as the soul "always vigorous in the faith" resisting the temptations of the world (represented by Scythia itself). The gryphons attack the Arimaspians, signifying the dedicated Christian, focused with one-eyed intensity on spiritual riches, and digging up "the gem of faith and other virtues". The purpose of these unclean spirits in bird-like form is to "rip from us the seed of divine word" (Throop 2009, 171).

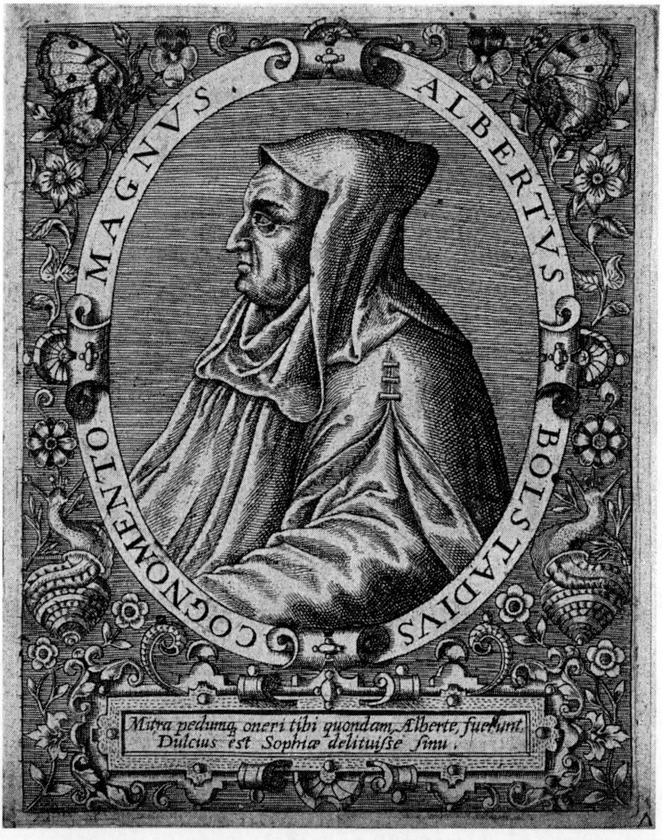
ALBERTVS BOLSTADIVS
COGNOMENTO MAGNVS ·
Mitra pedumq; oneri tibi quondam, Ælberte, fuerunt.
Dulcius est Sophiæ delituisse sinu.

Fig. 4.7. Portrait of Albertus Magnus (Count Albert Bollstaedt; c. 1200-1280). Line engraving by T. de Bry (1597). Reproduced by kind permission of the Wellcome Library, London.

Albertus Magnus (c. 1200-1280; Fig. 4.7), the son of the Count of Bollstädt in Bavaria, joined the Dominican Order in the 1220s. He was a popular teacher and highly influential writer; he is credited with having produced an enormous number of titles, although some of these are surely pseudepigraphical (falsely attributed). For our purposes, his most important contribution, *De Mineralibus* ("Book of Minerals"; Magnus 1476), was probably written around 1262. Here, his entry for *smaragdus* indicates (rather surprisingly) that the stone is not rare. He repeats the information concerning the colour of the stone, its ability to "tinge the air around it with its own greenness", its provenance (including a spurious record from Britain, probably a corruption of *Bactriani*; propagated in later literature–see, for example, Lonicer 1679, 722; Pomet 1748, 172), and its association with gryphons. He does introduce some new observations:

> "it has been found by experience in our own time that this stone, if it is good and genuine, will not endure sexual intercourse: because the present King of Hungary [probably Bela IV, reigned 1235-1270] wore this stone on his finger when he had intercourse with his wife, and as a result it was broken into three pieces. And therefore what they say [of this stone] is probable-that it inclines the wearer towards chastity. They say, too, that it increases wealth, and confers persuasive speech in [pleading] cases; and suspended from the neck, cures hemitertian fever and epilepsy. [...] They say also that it improves the memory, and averts tempests, and is good for divination; and therefore it is sought after by magicians" (Wyckoff 1967, 119-120).

Magnus includes a test for the wonder-working emerald, somewhat incongruously, in his *De vegetabilibus et plantis* (Lib. VI, tract. ii, cap. I; Jessen 1867, 475; Thorndike 1923, 547):

> An emerald was recently seen among us, small in size but marvellous in beauty. When its virtue was to be tested, someone stepped forth and said that, if a circle was made about a toad with the emerald, and then the stone was set before the toad's eyes, one of two things would happen. Either the stone, if of weak virtue, would be broken by the gaze of the toad; or the toad would burst, if the stone was possessed of full natural vigour. Without delay things were arranged as he bade; and after a short lapse of time, during which the toad kept its eye unswervingly upon the gem, the latter began to crack like a nut and a portion of it flew from the ring. Then the toad, which had stood immovable hitherto, withdrew as if it had been freed from the influence of the gem.

Slightly later, the Paduan physician Pietro Tommasi (see below) commented that "The emerald is undoubtedly a very effective gem: due to the power it releases, the toad's eyes that are fixed on it are liquefied" (Tommasi 1968, 79).

The Book of Secrets (*Liber Secretorum Alberti Magni virtutibus herbarum, lapidum and animalium quorumdam*), now generally ascribed to Pseudo-Albertus Magnus and first printed around 1480, repeats some of this information. In a section head appealing to anyone who "wolde make anye man's witte sharp and quicke" it encourages the reader to take an emerald because "it maketh a man to vnderstande well, and geueth to hym a good memory, augmenteth the ryches of hym that beareth it, & yf any man shall holde it vnder hys tung, he shall prophecy anone" (Magnus 1560, unnumbered page).

As will be seen below, the new themes introduced by Albertus Magnus and Pseudo-Albertus were to be taken up enthusiastically by later writers, incorporated into the overall lore attributed to the stone, and form the basis for derived therapeutic properties in early modern times.

Konrad von Megenberg (1309–1374), cathedral canon and member of the town council at Ratisbon, seems to have modelled his *Buch der Natur* ("Book of Nature"), written around 1349, on the approach of Thomas of Cantimpré. Megenberg's comprehensive survey of natural history is believed to be the first to be written in vernacular German. He picks up some of the information provided by Albertus Magnus and conflates it with other beliefs, as in "whoever wears the stone [if they are] chaste and honourable is safe from falling sickness". Megenberg also emphasises the ability of the stone to increase one's property, make you agreeable in temperament, and attract blessing. In terms of sexual probity, he indicates that the emerald "calms unchaste desires", going on to explain that, therefore "The emerald is the symbol of chastity, because this keeps the human body green, that is, healthy and pure. This virtue surpasses all other human virtues […] It brings grace before God, men and angels and bears the image of our Lord Jesus Christ on it" (Kirnbauer 1960, 54-55; my translation).

Georgius Agricola (Georg Bauer, 1494–1555) was apothecary and physician at St Joachimstahl (now Jáchymov) in northwest Bohemia (now Czech Republic; 1527–1530), before moving on to Chemnitz where he served as town physician. Published the year after his death, *De Re Metallica*, subsequently became an influential text on mineralogy. In it, he expands some of the themes from Albertus Magnus, writing, for example, that

> If either a man or a woman wears this gem during cohabitation and it touches the flesh, even when set in a ring, it will be shattered. It combats epilepsy as though it were a deadly enemy until it either overcomes the lesser power of the disease or is overcome by a greater power. In the former case the stone remains whole and intact but in the latter case it is fractured into many small pieces. For this reason kings and priests suspend it from the necks of boys and wear it in rings in order to test whether it will have the power to expel this horrible disease (Bandy & Bandy 1955, 126).

3. Sources from the Arabic tradition

Medieval Islam fostered a vibrant scholarly community with strong ties to the West, especially the Hellenic School. Strong and innovative medical and lapidary knowledge were often combined in the texts produced (Duffin 2013a, 14). Precious stones were highly regarded and are cited in a diverse contemporary literature (Amar & Lev 2017).

Ruano makes the following request of Garcia de Orta: "It is very desirable that you should tell me about the emerald, the best stone of all" (Orta 1913, 357). Not for the first time, this provides de Orta with the opportunity to display both his broad knowledge of the literature and his facility with languages–he seems to have been a polyglot, proficient in a number of languages, including an understanding of Arabic. In his reply to the query, de Orta states "the name of an emerald in this country and in Persia is *Pachec* and in Arabic *Zamarrat*. Serapio, in the chapter on emeralds, has *Zabarget* instead of *Zamarrat*, but it should not be *Zabarget*, as the Pandetarian shows" (Orta 1913, 358). The French linguist and translator of oriental languages, Jean-Jacques Clément-Mullet (1795-1865) provides the transliteration *zeberdjed* (Clément Mullet 1868, 65), noting (incorrectly) that this in turn is a translation of the term *zouroud* according to the Islamic philosopher Abu Nasr Al-Farabi (c. 872-950/1; also known as Alpharabius), who served at the court of Sayf al Dawla al Hamadani (916-967) in Baghdad. Other transliterations include *zamarrud* (Said 1989, 140) and *zumurrudh* (Huda 1998, 103).

The emerald was amongst the most highly prized precious stones in Islamic culture (Amar & Lev 2017, 378), appearing in the works of a wide range of authors including Pseudo Aristotle (ninth century), Ibn Abi Ramtha al-Tamimi (tenth century), Yuhanna ibn Masawaih (777-857), Abu Rayhan Muhammad ibn Ahmad al-Biruni (973-1048), Ahmad ibn Yusuf al-Tıfachı (1184-1253), al-Akafanı (1286-1348), Ibn al-Baytar (d. 1248), Zakariyya al-Qazwını (1203-1283) and Abu al-Abbas Ahmad al-Qalqashandı (1355-1418). Unfortunately, many of these volumes are available in Arabic only (see Steinschneider 1895 and bibliography in Amar & Lev 2017).

Perhaps the earliest volume accessible to me is by Pseudo-Aristotle, the name given to a group of authors whose works were originally ascribed to Aristotle himself, but which have subsequently been found to be pseudepigraphic. Sometimes referred to as "Aristotle's Lapidary", there has been much discussion over its origins and linguistic history (Klein-Franke 1970). A German translation was provided by Julius Ruska (1867-1949), in which the emerald is indicated as coming exclusively from "the land of the West" and found associated with gold deposits. Medicinally, it is reported as having a cold and dry nature in terms of Aristotelian element classification. The therapeutic properties of the gem are described as follows:

> Its specific effect is that it helps against deadly poison when taken against injury from creeping worms that bite or sting. If a quantity equivalent to eight grains of barley is rubbed off [the stone] and ingested by those who have drunk poison before that poison works in them, with God's help it will save them from death, and they will not lose their hair and skin. The emerald is a pure green stone; the noblest are the most strongly green-coloured. If you let your gaze rest on it, the weakness disappears from his eyes, and whoever wears it in a necklace or as a signet ring it will keep epilepsy at bay if you put it on before a seizure occurs. It is also worn around the newborn when it is born (Ruska 1912, 134-135).

Some of these remarks were repeated by the Syrian Christian physician from Baalbeck (Roman Heliopolis; now in modern-day Lebanon), Costa ben Luca (Qusta ibn Luqa; 820–912). Luca is famous as a translator of Greek texts, collected during his travels in the Byzantine Empire, into Arabic. His treatise on the efficacy of amulets, *De physicis ligaturis*, was translated into Latin by Arnald de Vilanova who noted that many ancient writers ascribed the efficacy of amulets not to any inherent natural property, but to a hidden virtue or occult power. While not prepared to deny the truth of this belief, he first considers that the beneficial results might be psychological. He notes from Pseudo-Aristotle that emeralds ward off epilepsy, "wherefore we often prescribe to nobles that their children should wear this stone hung about the neck lest they incur this infirmity" (Thorndike 1923, 656).

The polymathic and polyglot scholar, Al-Biruni, came from the Birun area of Chorasmia in west Central Asia, served at Gorganj as part of a nexus of high-quality intellectuals, eventually moving to Ghazni where he became court astrologer and was able to travel widely. His book on minerals has been described as "the most complete medieval text of mineralogy" (Said 1989, xxiii). Al-Biruni's text contains several similar ideas to those found in Pseudo-Aristotle, such as the suggestion that *zabarjad* and *zamarrud* are synonymous, although they are presented in much expanded form. If a ninth century date for Pseudo Aristotle is secure, a matter of some controversy, a certain amount of borrowing must have taken place by Al-Biruni.

Al-Biruni refers to the emerald mines in Upper Egypt, together with many tales and much lore concerning the gems, freely quoting from a range of Arabic scholars. One such legend, propounded by Abu Nasr al-Utbi (died 982) and defended by the statement that "God has conferred upon everything a specific attribute and characteristic", is that the emerald makes snakes blind. This claim was tested extensively by al-Biruni in a number experiments over a nine month period, the results leading him to conclude "despite the consensus of the authorities, I found this claim to be wrong" (Said 1989, 146).

In his commentary on al-Biruni's book, Said provides some additional useful information concerning the contemporary use of emeralds (Said 1989, 273). He indicates that, medicinally, the gems were considered to be cold in the second and dry in the third degree. Mohammad Hossein Aghili Khorasani Shirazi wrote *Makhzan al-Adviyeh*, a twelfth century AH (seventeenth to eighteenth century Gregorian) volume in Persian concerning simple medicines (Ardakani et al. 2018). It records that the emerald acts as an exhilarant, cardiac and cephalic (brain) tonic employed to treat gastric ailments, epilepsy, pleurisy and "agitation" (Said 1989, 273).

Said (1989) further provides details of some emerald-containing compound drugs. *Khamiras* are semi-solid fermented confections in which various decoctions or powders are added to a sugar or honey base. They are generally employed as cardiac, cephalic (brain) or general tonics. As its name suggests, *Khamira Zamarrud* is just such a tonic based upon the incorporation of emeralds into the mix. Additional ingredients include gold and silver foils, lapis lazuli, ambergris, silkworm (*Bombyx mori*) and various other materials. Used as a cardiac stimulant, anodyne and tranquillizer, the recipe was subsumed into the Unani System of Indian medicine during the late sixteenth century (Ahmad et al. 2010, 98).

Triturated emerald also appears together with silver foil, pearls, green agate, mineral bezoar, ambergris and nine herbal ingredients in *Khamira Gaozaban Ambari Jawahardar* (Said 1989, 290). In addition to strengthening the heart and brain, it is also used as an eye tonic. Interestingly, the recipe has been transported into Unani medicine minus the emeralds, pearls, agate and mineral bezoar, but with the addition of gold leaf to the recipe (Ahmad et al. 2010, 96).

Triturated emerald also joins mineral bezoar, pearl, sapphire, green agate, ambergris, cowrie shell and a range of other ingredients in *Khamira Nazli Jawahar wala* (Said 1989, 293). The Unani version of the recipe is, once again, different; this time the emerald is retained but the sapphire and agate are replaced with rubies (Ahmad 2010, 97).

Kushtay are medicinal calx, mineral or metallic powders that have been heated and sometimes mixed with non-mineral ingredients. The name *Kushta* comes from the Persian word for "kill" or "conquer", the idea being that this is how they overcome the affliction they are being used to treat (Aslam et al. 1979, 279). *Kushta zamarrud* is emerald-based; the gems are finely ground, sieved and triturated, and mixed with Damask Rose Water and cakes of cow dung (Said 1989, 311). It was commended as a tonic for both the liver and the heart, a bronchodilator, and to relieve excess urination.

In Unani medicine it has been deemed appropriate as a treatment for diabetes, a clear link with the symptom of excess urine production (Hamiduddin et al. 2019). A study of *Kushtay* being imported and prescribed to the local population of Bradford in the late 1970s revealed that the precious stones had been replaced with calcite and quartz-based mineral components (Aslam et al., 1979, 281).

The final recipe quoted by Said (1989, 316-7) concerns *Kushta Marjan Jawaharwala*. This seemingly versatile preparation contains ten ingredients, amongst which are oyster shell, carnelian, ruby, green agate, cow dung and gold and silver foils. Triturated and mixed together in Damask Rose Water, it was commended both as a cardiac tonic and stimulant, plus being an anti-catarrhal agent and analgesic.

The slightly later (circa 1243) treatise by Ahmad ibn Yusuf al-Tıfachı, the traveller and judge in Cairo and Tunis also has an entry concerning emerald. Following some discussion on the origins, provenance, qualities and defects of the gem, he considers some of its characteristics. Amongst these he includes the strange relationship between the stone and snakes previously cited by al-Biruni. In this instance he highlights a property exclusive to the emerald that could be used to distinguish a genuine stone from a fake; if a snake looked at a genuine emerald it would cause their eyes "to pop out of their sockets on the spot" (Huda 1998, 105). Like al-Biruni, al-Tifachi claims to have tested the statement personally, but his supposed results were dramatically different to those of the earlier writer. Al-Tifachi's account is as follows:

> I had acquired a pure *zhubabi* emerald [the most valuable, expensive and best quality kind] that I wanted to test using the eyes of snakes. Therefore, I hired a man to catch a snake, which he did, and I put it in a large basin. I took a piece of wax, stuck it at the end of an arrow, and glued the emerald on it, then I approached it from the eyes of the snake, which started leaping first at the arrow, moving furiously, trying to get out of the basin. As the emerald neared its eyes, I heard a light noise, as if one was killing a nit on his nail, and I saw that the eyes of the snake had bulged considerably, and it roamed perplexed in the basin, not knowing which direction to turn to nor wanting to get out. Most of its movements had become still, and its strength had abandoned it completely (Huda 1998, 105).

Huda (1998, 105) further records that a lapidary dating from 1282 and written by Bailak al Qabadjaqi (dates unknown) refers to a similar episode (original source not traced in this study).

In terms of the therapeutic applications of the stone, al-Tifachi repeats the assertion that it strengthens the eyesight and that, worn as an amulet around the neck or in a ring it protects the wearer from epilepsy so long as it is employed before disease manifests itself. He expands this idea, however, in an echo of Pseudo-Aristotle, by stating that "for this reason, the sages used to order kings to make their children wear this stone around their neck at birth, in order to prevent the occurrence of epilepsy" (Huda 1998, 106), perhaps indicating high prevalence of paediatric seizures in the population.

He has an entry concerning the use of emerald as an anti-poisoning agent which is very similar to that expressed in Pseudo-Aristotle, with the addition that wearing an emerald would cause all poisonous animals to be repelled. In addition, al-Tifachi introduces the idea that emerald is effective "against blood discharges and against the affliction called dysentery if it is hung over the liver and the stomach externally" (Huda 1998, 106). He goes on to claim first-hand success with this treatment in cases where the patient was close to death. Al-Tifachi also indicates that, hung on the upper arm, an emerald can be used talismanically to exploit its general protective powers, and that when tied to the thigh it could be used to hasten childbirth. This latter property is more usually ascribed to the *aetites* or Eagle Stone (Duffin 2012).

Ruano says to Garcia de Orta "It is very desirable that you should tell me about the emerald, the best stone of all, which is an ingredient in the lectuary de gemis". Once again, de Orta is able to demonstrate his knowledge of the literature: "The intention of Mesue was to enter emerald in this composition, though Cristofero de Honestis, the commentator of Mesue, felt differently" (de Orta 1913, 357-358). The pair are here referring to the gem electuary, or *Electuarium de Gemmis*, a compound, precious stone-based syrup or julep invented by Mesuë the Younger, often known as Pseudo-Mesuë, Maswijah al-Marindi or Johannes Mesuë of Damascus (died 1015) (Duffin 2013b). No original version in Arabic has so far been discovered, leading some authors to consider that the main works normally ascribed to Mesuë might have been produced in Latin at Bologna or Padua, perhaps by Peter of Abano (1250-1316) (Duffin 2013b, 85). The more conservative view is that the work survives only in Latin versions from lost Arabic originals, produced during the intense period of translation, often carried out at dedicated scriptoria (such as that at Toledo) toward the end of the thirteenth century.

The recipe for the gem electuary is found in both of the two main publications ascribed to Mesuë–his *Canones Universales* and his *Antidotarium*, both first published in the second half of the fifteenth century but republished several times, often with associated commentaries, during the fifteenth and sixteenth centuries (e.g. Mesuë 1497, leaf 44; Sylvio 1553, leaf 142). The medicinal paste incorporates emeralds together with several other precious and semi-precious stones (sapphire, red chalcedony, garnet, amber), gold and silver, plus a wide range of additional animal and herbal ingredients (see Duffin 2013b, Table 1, 88-90 for full details and an analysis of the components). Initially conceived as an antidote to poisons, the gem electuary was enthusiastically adopted by the medical community, especially in early modern times. Sometimes used as a stand-alone mixture but also incorporated with additional components, it evolved into a treatment used to protect against or treat an enormous range of conditions: nightmares, gynaecological disorders, plague, psychological disorders, urogenital problems etc., as well as being utilised as something of a cure-all with generally strengthening powers, especially for the heart (see details in Duffin 2013b).

4. Hildegard von Bingen

The Benedictine Abbess, Hildegard von Bingen (c. 1098-1179; Fig. 4.8), also referred to as Hildegardis Bingensis, led a very productive life as a visionary, mystic, healer, linguist, poet, artist, musician, composer, biographer, theologian and preacher. As a female author in medieval times, she is one of a very select few. Her collected medical writings appear in the *Liber subtilitatum diversarum naturarum creaturarum* ("The Book of the Subtleties of the Diverse Natures of Creatures") (c. 1152–c. 1163 AD). This, in turn, contains two works-the *Liber simplicis medicinae* ("Book of Simple Medicine"), also referred to as the *Physica*, and the *Liber compositae medicinae* ("Book of Compound Medicine"), also known as *Causae et curae* ("Causes and Remedies") (Duffin 2013a, 17; Brigo et al. 2018). The latter volume, which presents a descriptive inventory, in nine books, discusses therapies based on elements gleaned from the natural world; known from a handful of fourteenth and fifteenth century manuscripts (see Otlewska 2012, 316) it contains a section on stones–the first of the 26 entries is dedicated to emeralds.

Hildegard has an interesting view on the source of therapeutic power in precious stones (for further background see Otlewska 2012). Her argument is framed in the terms of her theology:

> The devil abhors, detests, and disdains precious stones. This is because he remembers that their beauty was manifest on him before he fell from the glory God had given him, and because some precious stones are engendered from fire, in which he receives his punishment. By the will of God, the devil was vanquished by the fire into which he fell, just as he is vanquished by the fire of the Holy Spirit when humans are snatched from his jaws by the first breath of the Holy Spirit (Throop 1998, 137).

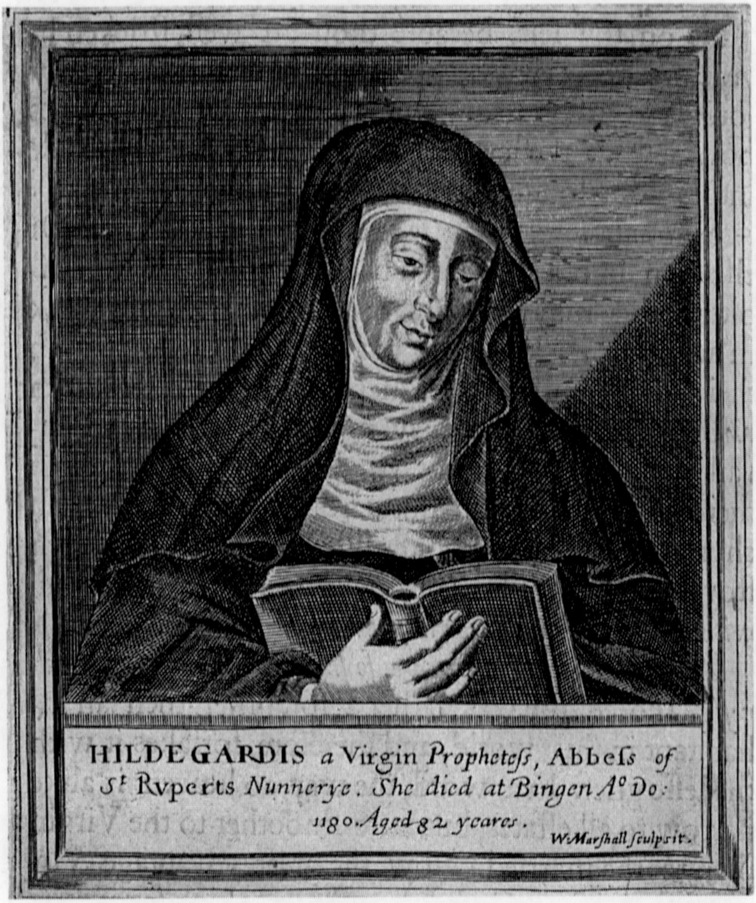
HILDEGARDIS a Virgin Prophetess, Abbess of
St Ruperts Nunnerye. She died at Bingen Ao Do:
1180. Aged 82 yeares.
W.Marshall sculpsit.

Fig. 4.8. Portrait of Hildegard von Bingen (c. 1098-1179). Line engraving by W. Marshall (active 1617-1650). Reproduced by kind permission of the Wellcome Library, London.

Despite subscribing to the prevailing notions of humoral medicine and the Aristotelian elements, Hildegard's explanation for the means of action of emerald in effecting a cure are based on her ideas concerning the origins of precious stones. She envisages the sun-heated mountains of the East (perhaps in the Garden of Eden) interacting with rising river waters to produce a froth which, when the waters recede, dry and harden to stone. They then "take their colours and powers in accordance with the time of day and the temperature. Drying and hardening, they become precious stones and fall onto the sand, just like flaking fish scales" (Throop 1998, 137) before being washed to other countries. She applies this idea to the emerald, specifically, indicating that it grows in the early morning at sunrise when "the natural vigour of the earth and grasses is especially lively, the air still cold, the sun hot". She concludes that "the emerald is powerful against all human weakness and sickness, since the sun readies it, and since all its matter is of the vitality of the air" (Throop 1998, 138).

Hildegard sees this origin, born of the heat of the sun, as investing the stones with therapeutic power; the emerald interacts positively with the patient's condition by bringing about physiological change through its heating action, utilising the stored energy which it has received from its birth by solar heating. This process is illustrated by reference to the remedial action of emerald when placed in the mouth of sufferers from plague and other ailments:

> Whence, one who ails in his heart, stomach, or side should have an emerald with him. It will heat up his flesh, making him better. If this person is so beset by pestilences which cannot restrain their commotions, he should place an emerald in his mouth, so it becomes wet from his saliva and the saliva heats up from the stone. He should repeatedly place it on, and take it from, his body. The sudden pestilential attacks will cease, without a doubt (Throop 1998, 137).

Like earlier authors, Hildegard associates the emerald with the treatment of epilepsy, but her applications have a novel twist. Instead of wearing the emerald as an amulet, it should be placed in the mouth and reinforce the action of the stone by uttering a prayer once the stone has been extracted:

> When someone tormented by epilepsy falls, put an emerald in his mouth while he is lying prostrate. It will revive his spirit. After he gets up and takes the stone from his mouth, he should look at it intently, and say, "Just as the breath of the Lord filled the whole earth, so may his grace fill the house of my body, so that it can never be moved." He should do this in the morning for the next nine days, and he will be cured. He should always have that stone with him and look at it every morning while saying those words, and he will be healed (Throop 1998, 139).

The prayer was an important part of the healing process so far as Hildegard was concerned; she used it here and elsewhere in her writings as a means of getting the patient to take personal responsibility and become fully invested in promoting a cure by actively engaging in the healing process by ensuring that their spiritual state before God was assured, offering no impediment to His working power through the stone.

The stone is similarly effective against headache, but the means of application is slightly different:

> One who has great pain in his head should hold it near his mouth and warm it by his breath, so that it becomes damp from his breath. He should rub it, so dampened, on his temples and forehead. Then he should put it in his mouth and, holding it in his mouth for a little while, he will be better (Throop 1998, 139).

The person who was suffering from an excess of phlegm and saliva (perhaps including respiratory diseases such as colds, influenza, catarrh etc.) could also use the emerald, again in a novel way. An emerald was placed on top of a linen cloth covering a metal bowl. Heated wine was then poured over the stone and through the cloth into the bowl. This process was repeated several times. Treatment then involved drinking the wine mixed with ground broad beans: "It will purge his head and diminish the phlegm and saliva" (Throop 1998, 139).

The final application of emerald recommended by Hildegard concerned a situation where someone was being eaten by worms (skin parasites?). Her suggestion was to: "place a linen cloth, with an emerald on top, over the wound. He should tie over it other small pieces of cloth, so that the stone grows warm. If this is done for three days, the worms will die" (Throop 1998, 139).

5. Western lapidaries

Lapidaries, or books about stones, were particularly popular in medieval times. Some broader works have lapidary sections in them, as is the case with many of the authors dealt with above in the section on early encyclopaedists.

Although not the earliest of the lapidaries, that produced under the direction of Alfonso X el Sabio (Alfonso X The Learned, King of Castile, León and Galicia, 1221–1284) is very distinctive. The text, originally ascribed to Abolays and supposedly translated by him from Chaldean into Arabic, was translated into Castilian around 1253. Certain elements are evocative of the Arabian texts considered above. The entry for emerald (*zamorat*; Fig. 4.9) is placed under the sign of Taurus and records its ability to resist poisons and any injuries sustained from venomous animals. If a person has been poisoned, it is recommended that he take a drachm of pulverised emerald in either wine or water, and the entry gives the reassurance that he will not die, and in a reiteration of Pseudo-Aristotle, his hair will not fall out and his skin will not slough off.

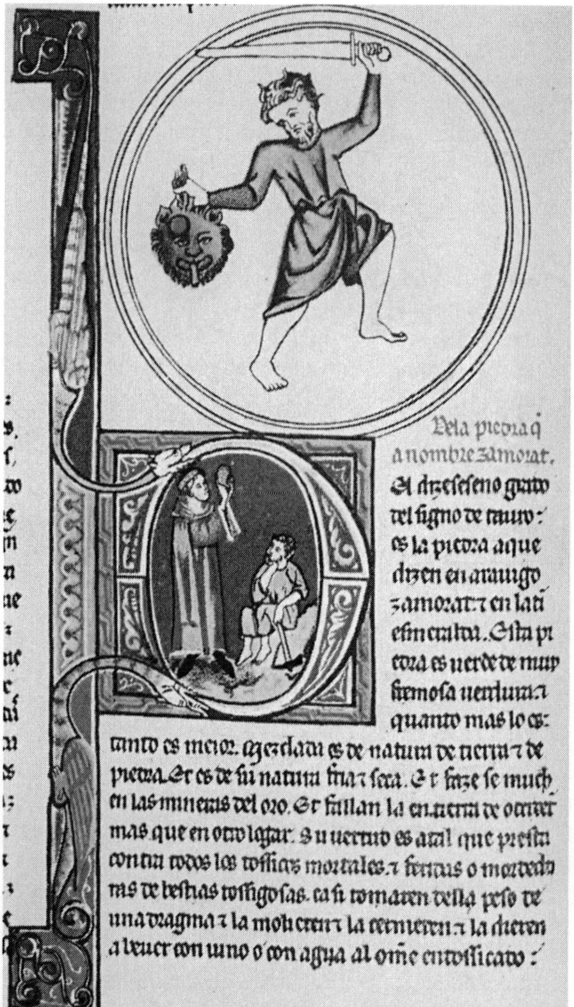
Dela piedra q̃
a nombre zamorat.
El dizeseseno grado
del signo de tauro:
es la piedra a que
dizen en arauigo
zamorat. & en lati
esmeralda. Esta pi
edra es uerde de muy
fremosa uerdura. &
quanto mas lo es:
tanto es meior. Esmeralda es de natura de tierra & de
piedra. Et es de su natura fria & seca. Et faze se much
en las mineras del oro. Et fallan la en la tierra de occident
mas que en otro logar. Su uertud es atal que presta
contra todos los tossigos mortales. & feridas o mordedu
ras de bestias tossigosas. ca si tomaren della peso de
una dragma & la molieren & la cernieren & la dieren
a beuer con uino o con agua al ome entossicado:

Figure 4.9. Entry for emerald (zamorat) in the Lapidario of Alfonso X (1221-1284). From Montaña (1881) (author's collection).

There is the familiar advice to wear an emerald to ensure safety from epilepsy, here referred to as "the demon". Children are commended to wear it tied to their left upper arm or their left thigh "before the disease gets old" (Bahler & Gatto 1997, 56).

Marbode, Bishop of Rennes (also Marbodus Gallus; c. 1036–1123), famous for his Latin poetry, probably wrote his lapidary around 1090. It discusses 60 individual stones in 732 lines. The entry for the emerald, at 38 lines, is one of the longest accounts. After repeating much information from Pliny, Marbode details the magico-medicinal properties of the stone as follows (in Charles King's rather free verse translation; King 1861, 396-7):

Of mighty use to seers who seek to pry
Into the future, hid from mortal eye.
Wear it with reverence due. 'Twill wealth bestow
And words persuasive from they lips shall flow.
As though the gift of eloquence inspired
The stone itself or living spirit fired.
Hung round the neck it cures the ague's chill,
Of falling sickness, dire mysterious ill;
Its hues so soft refresh the wearied eye,
And furious tempests banish from the sky:
So with chaste power it tames the furious mood
And cools the wanton thoughts that fire the blood.

Marbode's lapidary, surviving in many manuscript copies and derivative texts, served as something of a model for later lapidaries dating from the eleventh through to the sixteenth century, most of which see the stones arranged in alphabetical order.

Perhaps the most succinct statement is found in Richardoune's Verses (B.M. Additional Manuscript 34360; MS. E), a moralising work which dates from the late fifteenth century. Lines 36 to 37 of this rather short (56 line) work, which focuses "upon Christs being ye true stone upon ye Cross", records "many stones ther ben of vertues commendable", and says of one of these: "The grene smaragde that is medicinable / Ayenste tempeste, sikenes and fantasy" (Evans & Serjeantson 1933, 61).

Several medieval English lapidaries take up the Christian allegorical theme introduced by Hrabanus Maurus in his *De Universo* (see above), with the Arimaspians ("aropiles" in the London Lapidary and "Arimples" in the North Midland Lapidary) representing "veray cristen men" (London Lapidary folio 124v; Evans & Serjeantson 1933, 21) seeking the emerald, the wonderful green colour of which "be-tokenes ye grenes of gud fayth, for ye gud patriarkes & ye gud profettes wer so fynly gretly grennhed, yerfor yai haue ye gret Ioy of heuen" (North Midland Lapidary, folio 47; Evans &

Sejeantson 1933,41). "The gryffons signifien ye deueles to whom thei feighten ayeins" (London Lapidary, folio 124v; Evans & Serjeantson 1933, 21); the North Midland Lapidary refers to them as "fendes" (fiends; North Midland Lapidary, folio 47; Evans & Sejeantson 1933,41). Both lapidaries commend those who don emeralds to think on this picture, elevating the wearing of them to an act of meditation.

The London and North Midland Lapidaries both have the Biblical book of Revelation, which lists the emerald as being one of the four foundation stones of the city walls of the New Jerusalem (Revelation 21, 19), in view whilst discussing the gem. They indicate that the precious stones are found in the "waters of Paradise". The Lapidary of Sidrac (13th century; Duffin 2015a) takes this idea a little further and even presents the gryphons fishing for gems in the rivers flowing out of Eden. This quotation comes from an English translation of the Lapidary known from only a single volume in the British Library (Duffin 2015; Anonymous 1528?, unnumbered page), reproduced here because of its rarity and relative inaccessibility :

> The finest Emeraudes come out of the lande of Beheste [Holy Land or Promised Land] / and out of the flode of Paradyse terrestre […] There is a maner of beestes that be called Gryffons/ that kepeth these stones Emeraudes/ on the floode that cometh from paradyse terrestre into the lande of Beheste. And these maner of bestes have. iiii. feet and. ij. iyen/ & the body before lyke an Egle/ and behynde lyke a Lyon. And a maner of folks that be named Arymples that haue but one iye in the forhede/ And they seke & fynd these Emeraudes/ and when they go for them/ they be all armed/ and so they seke the said stones in the sayd floode of Paradise terrester/ and there they fynde them. And the said Gryffons flye all about and seke these sayde folks/ that have but one iye in the forhede: and they do theyr power to take away the stones fro them/ for they be right fearse & angry with them/ that they bere them away/ but these sayd folks be so armed/ that the sayd fowle Gryffons may do them no harme.

This picture of gemstones being washed out of "Paradise terrester" is captured in an image illustrating a copy of Vincent de Beauvais' *Speculum Historiale* or "Mirror of History" (de Beauvais 1475?, fol. 54v; Fig. 4.10). In line with the Biblical explanation of the banishment of Adam and Eve from the Garden of Eden (Genesis 3, 24), the image shows the angel with his sword of flaming fire protecting the garden's border, while the waters of the River Girshon flow from the garden itself, carrying precious stones with it. Thus, in addition to the intrinsic value of emeralds as rare, costly and exotic stones with impeccable colour, there is now the added concept that they are invested with power that emanates directly from the presence of God, the source of all healing. This is somewhat reminiscent of the virtue

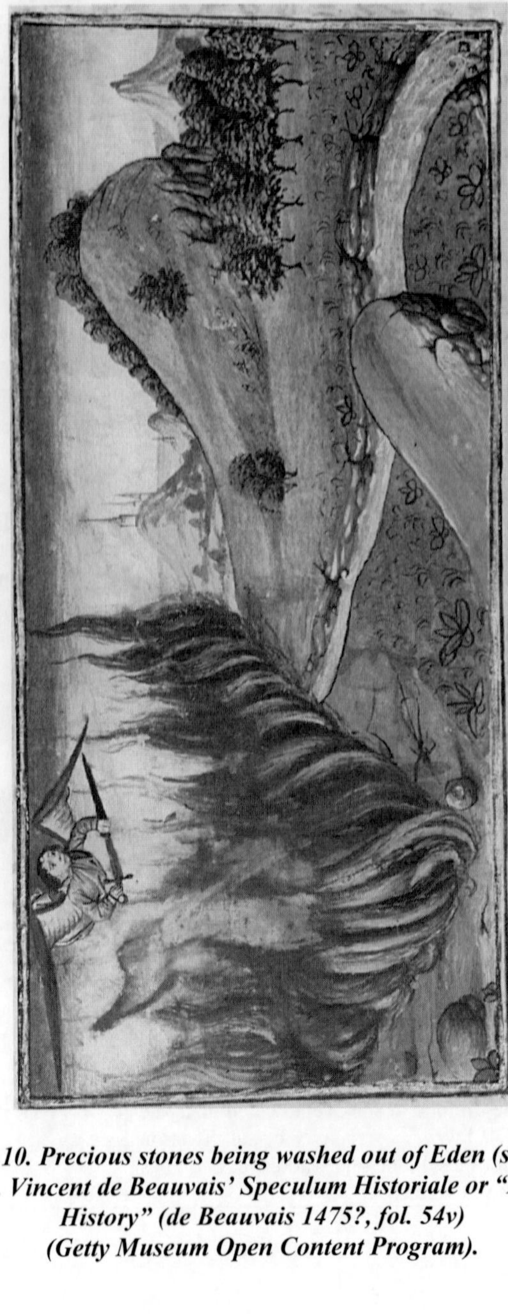

Fig. 4.10. Precious stones being washed out of Eden (see top right corner). Vincent de Beauvais' Speculum Historiale or "Mirror of History" (de Beauvais 1475?, fol. 54v) (Getty Museum Open Content Program).

ascribed to the unicorn horn, the beast being believed to enter the Garden of Eden to feed and thus maintain the therapeutic and alexipharmic power of the alicorn (Duffin 2017).

The idea of Edenic gems being washed out of Paradise into the wider world may have its origin in the twelfth century tales of Prester John, the legendary Christian Patriarch and ruler over a lost Christian Kingdom. The Letter of Prester John records a visit to Rome during the time of Pope Calixtus II (1119-1124) in which he spoke "of memorable matters of his Indian region that were unknown to the Romans", including the gold and gems forming the bedload of the River Physon flowing out of Paradise (Thorndike 1923b, 239).

The London Lapidary even goes so far as to say, mistakenly, that Saint John records the presence of gryphons guarding these stones in his apocalyptic writings (London Lapidary, folio 124v; Evans & Serjeantson 1933, 21).

With this supposed Edenic provenance in mind, it is perhaps no surprise that the Christian Medieval English Lapidaries all agree that God is the source of all the virtues ascribed to the stone. The descriptions of those qualities represent a fairly stable account, representative examples of which are given below for the purposes of illustration (Evans & Serjeantson 1933, 21, 40, 85, 121).

Hit encreseth richesse, & hit maketh worde of man dredful, & is moche worth for ye goute & ayeins tempeste & / lecherye. & wittes wele that he that bereth emeraude aboute hym, the more he shal loue his body in clennesse, & ye lesse wille to seye vilanies & the more loue to thenke on his solle, & to be of better berynge & to loue gode werkys, for god to this stone yave suche vertues.	London Lapidary First half of the fifteenth century
[…] & he wald knaw by vertu of ye ston what thyng yt he wald seche; & also yt ston incresses a man ryches, & sal do a man spek in gud tempour;& also he helles a man of a sekenes yt is cald ennentesce; & also he is myche worth a-gayns tempest & a-gayns lyghthinge;& knaw it well yt he yt beres a emeraud upon hym ye mor he sal loue to kepe his body in chast, & ye lesse / he sal loue to spek velany, and glady he sal ber hym-self fayr, & ye gladlyer he sal thynk on ye saule, & mor he sal loue gud warkes, & he yt has yis ston he has yes vertus.	North Midland Lapidary Fifteenth century

It encresseth ryches & maketh word of man dredfull. Also is myche worse azens the gowte & azens tempest & azens lechery, & it is gode souerenly for ye syzte to be-holdyn. Wit it wel, he that bereth it upone him ye more he schal led his body in clennes, & the les to loue unclennes bothe of body & soule, & he schall haue the mor loue to thinke one his soule, & the more yo loue clene beryng, & the mor to loue gode workys. Also this ston bereth him from tempest.	Peterborough Lapidary Late fifteenth century
This stone multiplieth a mans goods; if he bere it on him & keepe it cleene, it maketh him to be of word & fortune wyse. It is good for the knawing gowt of a man, it mendeth the sight of a man, & doth a-way great tempests of wethers. It voydeth lechery, For God gave it such vertue;/ And to a man that kepeth it, his body and members should be euer cleane and withour euell. It must be set in gold of ye best and bore on ye right side of a man.	Sloane Lapidary Late sixteenth century
The vertue of this stone is, that they wch weare or carrye this stone aboute them, it makethe them encline to Chastytie, for Albertus magnus reportethe, that yf this stone be good, right, & trewe it will not suffer a man to deale wth a woman: for A certaine kinge of Hungariae thatraigned in his tyme, being in deling wth his wyfe in that arte, hadd this stone in a ringe uppon his finger, & because of this acte, the stone brake in three peces./ it encresethe riches, gyvethe wordes to persuade in causis, & hanged aboute the necke it healethe sharpe aques, & the falling sicknes, it helpethe a weake sighte, & Comseruethe the eyes/ it makethe a good memorye, & puttethe awaye tempestes & stormes, & preuaylethe to devine, for the wch it is of the Magiciens soughte for.	Goldsmith's Lapidary 1604

The Aberdeen Bestiary (Fig. 4.11), written and illuminated in England circa 1200, is slightly unusual in that it also contains a short lapidary section. After some comments on the green colour, and its provenance, the Bestiary records that it:

> does not change its colour on account of the sun, moon or shade. It is so even that you can look through it, as Nero used to do; you can use it to find things under water. It brings wealth if it is worn chastely; it endows you with persuasive eloquence if it is worn on the neck. It cures fever; it gets rid of the hemitertian fever and epilepsy; and it banishes storms and wantonness' (Aberdeen Bestiary fol. 101v; Figure 11).

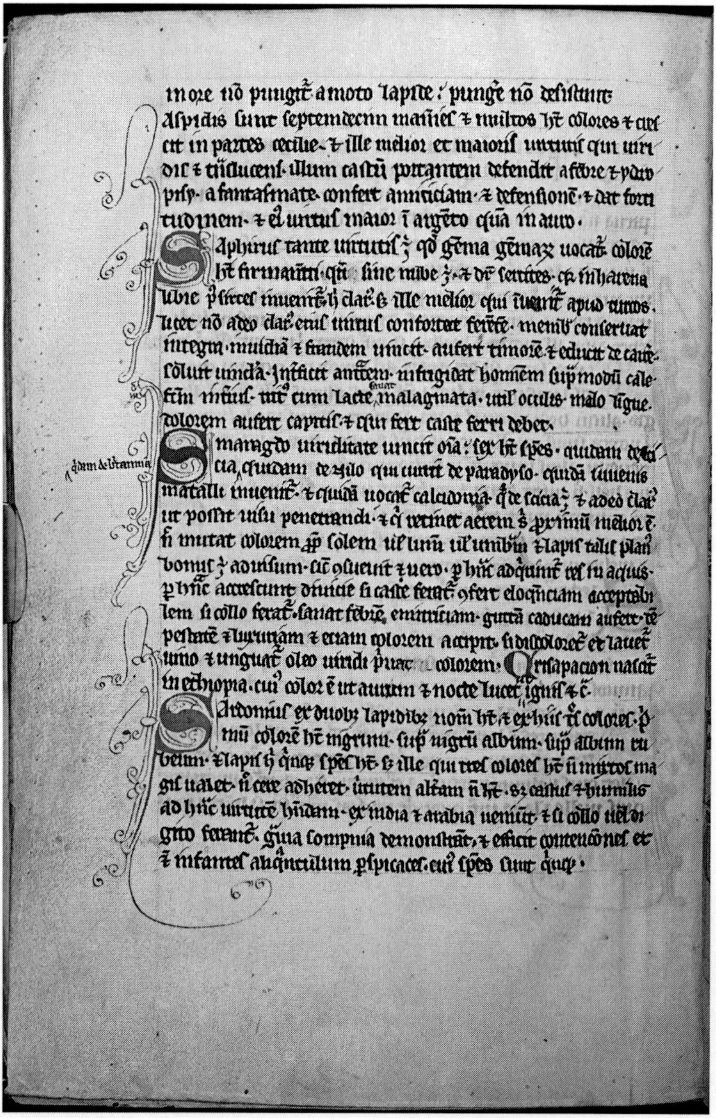

Fig. 4.11. Aberdeen Bestiary, University of Aberdeen MS. 24, folio 101v. Reproduced by kind permission of Aberdeen University.

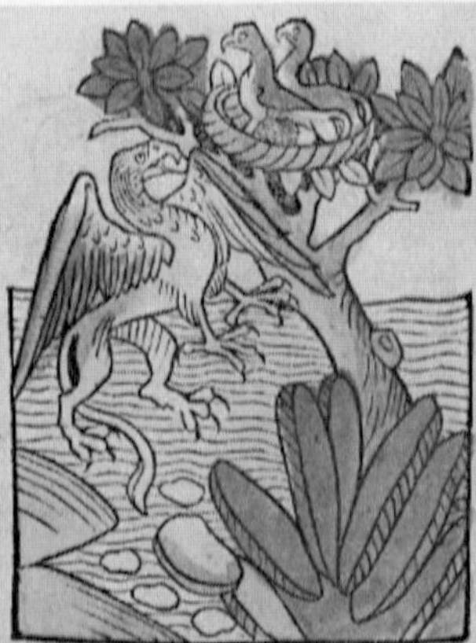

Ca. cxiiij.

Smaraldus. alias ſmaragdus Albertus ĩ lapidario ſuo de ſmaraldo. Smaraldus lapis eſt precioſior multis alijs ⁊ non rarus. Et color eius eſt viridiſſimus tranſlucens ita ꝙ vicinum aerem ſua viriditate ſigurare videatur. Et melior eſt planicies ſuperficiei quia tunc vna pars non obumbrat aliam. Melior tamen eſt qui nec lumine nec vmbra variatur. Huius planiciei ⁊ colorum varietatum dicũt eſſe diuerſitates. xij. eo ꝙ aliquando fel nigrum ꝑ modum virgularum admixtum habet. Hij ſunt a locis ſcotici ⁊ britanici ⁊ biliaci. ⁊ qui in venis eris naſcuntur. ⁊ maculoſi quidam. ⁊ quidam calcedonici eo ꝙ admixturaꝫ habẽt cum illo lapide. Meliores autem ſunt ſcotici. Et ferũt quidam ꝙ illi de nidiſ griffonum auferuntur qui lapidem hunc cum crudelitate magna cuſtodiunt. Dixit aũt vnus de grecia veniens veridicus. ⁊ curioſus experimẽtator. ꝙ hic lapis naſcitur in rupibus que ſunt ſub aqua maris. ⁊ ibi inuenitur. Rationale etiam eſt ꝙ in venis eris in perſpicuo quidem ad eris ſubſtantiam non veniens naſcitur eo ꝙ rubiginis eris habet viriditatem.

Operationes.

A Quando ſmaraldus ponitur ĩ potu conuenit venenis mortiferis. ⁊ morſibus venenoſis ⁊ punctionibus habẽtibꝰ aculeum. B Qui ergo dederit in potu de limatura eius pondus. viij. granorum ordei illi qui ſumpſit venenũ anteꝙ̃ feceritimpreſſionem liberat eũ a morte. ⁊ non cadẽt capilli eius neqꝫ excorienẽ et eſt ſua euaſio. et ille qui aſſiduat aſpicere ipſum preſeruat eius viſum a nocumentis. ⁊ conſeruat eum incolumẽ. C Et q̃ defert ipſum in anulo. preſeruat eam ab epilẽtia quãdo ducit cum digito anꝙ̃ ſuꝑueniat. D Et propter hanc cauſam docemus reges ꝙ ſuſpendant eos in collo filiorum quando naſcuntur ſtatim ne ſuperueniat eis epilentia E Et idem auctoritate Raſis. Taberzet vel feruzegi. i. ſmaraldꝰ conuenit leproſis quando ſumitur ĩ potu limatura eius. Et ſi cadat aſpectus tiri ſuper lapidẽ ſmaraldi diſſoluunẽ oculi eiuſ ⁊ liqueſcunt. F Dyaſcorides caplo de ſmaraldo Smaraldus portatus augꝫ ſubſtantiam habens perſuaſionẽ in omni negotio corꝑe ⁊ ſermone caſtos letoſqꝫ facit ſubuenit et in tempeſtatibus. Sculpiẽ in eo ſcarabeus ⁊ pertundiẽ aurea fibula. G Albertus in lapidario ſuo capitulo de ſmaraldo. Expertũ eſt noſtris temporibus ꝙ hic lapis ſi vere viridiſ ⁊ bonus eſt retinet coitum propter quod rex vngarie qui nr̃is regnabat temporibus cum in digito in hora coitus cũ vxore ſua habebat in coitu. in tres partes diuiſus eſt. H Et ideo probabile eſt q̃d dicitur ꝙ hic lapis geſtantem ſe ad caſtitatem inclinat. I Unde auget opes ⁊ incantatus dat verba perſuaſoria. ⁊ ꝙ collo ſuſpenſus curat emitriteum ⁊ caducos morbos. K Expertum autem eſt ꝙ viſum debilẽ confortat. ⁊ oculos conſeruat. L Et bonam facit memoriã ⁊ tempeſtatẽ auertit. Et valet diuinantibus propter quod queritur a magis.

Fig. 4.12. Entry for Smaragdus from the Hortus Sanitatis (1491). By kind permission of the Countway Medical Library.

The *Hortus Sanitatis* or "Garden of Health", first published in 1491, contains a section on stones entitled *de Lapidibus*. Dr Johann Wonnecke von Caub (Johannes de Cuba; dates unknown) is believed to have been the author of this large compendium of *materia medica*, almost all derived from the natural world. The first edition of the text was published in Latin by Jacob von Medenbach in Mainz, but a number of later printings, pirated editions and translations are known, a measure of its considerable popularity (Duffin 2013a, 22; 2020b). The emerald has a relatively long entry in the list of 144 stones. The volume draws extensively on the work of earlier authorities, as indicated by the suggestions to take 8 grains in a suitable beverage to eliminate poison, to wear it in a ring against epilepsy, that it preserves vision and a good disposition, increases the bodily health and good speech of a chaste person, and can be used in the treatment of leprosy (Fig. 4.12).

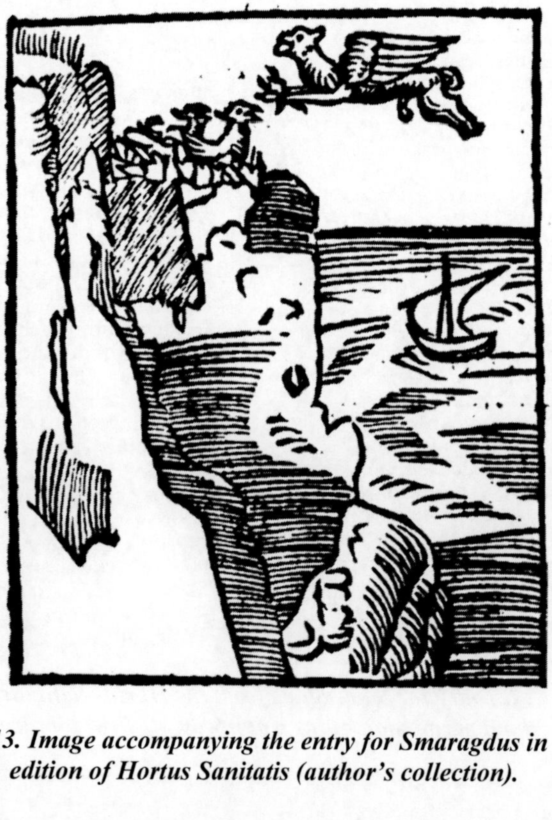

Fig. 4.13. Image accompanying the entry for Smaragdus in the 1536 edition of Hortus Sanitatis (author's collection).

The latter is ascribed to the famous Persian physician Abū Bakr Muḥammad ibn Zakariyyāʾ al-Rāzī or Rhazes (c. 864-925/935) (original not traced in this study). The image accompanying the entry for *smaragdus* in the 1491 edition depicts an eagle returning to its nest in the branches of a tree; the image is used elsewhere in the same section to depict *aetites* (*De Lapidibus* cap. x), and *Hexacontalitus* (cap. l) (de Cuba 1491). The 1536 edition of the Strasbourg printer, Matthias Biener (also known as Apiarus; fl. 1533-1553), however, depicts a gryphon flying to its nest high on some sea cliffs, an acknowledgement of the tale surrounding the Scythian emeralds and an image unique to this entry (Fig. 4.13; de Cuba 1536).

Camillus Leonardus (fl. 1500) dedicated his *Speculum Lapidum* or "Mirror of Stones", first published in 1502, to his Master Caesar Borgia (1475-1507). This work is rather intermediate between works of the earlier lapidary tradition and later early modern scientific texts (Duffin 2013a, 29) in that it focuses on mineralogical information, rather than enumerating many magico-medicinal properties for the stones which he considers. In the case of the emerald, for example, he is content to reiterate the observation that it is restful for the eyes (Leonardus 1502; 1750, 225).

6. Early modern medical texts

The invention of the printing press around 1450 triggered a revolution in the dissemination of knowledge. Multiple copies of classic texts could be produced both rapidly and relatively cheaply. Translations into vernacular European languages meant that knowledge was no longer the sole preserve of those educated in Latin and Greek. A veritable army of new authors was ready to share its experience, erudition, knowledge and insight to both a broad and a highly specialised readership. The sixteenth and seventeenth centuries saw an enormous boom in the production of medical texts and commentaries. Drawing from the wells of earlier wisdom, early modern authors began to modify, adapt and extrapolate items of *materia medica* from the strict bounds of ancient wisdom to contemporary medical problems such as the seemingly regular appearance of plague. Traditional simples were employed in novel ways to new situations, compounded together to form newly invented medicaments and newly appraised in the light of experience; classical authors and their ideas came under critical scrutiny as never before and the long-held theories of disease and its treatment began to be replaced with new explanations based more on experience than tradition. Hippocratic humorism and Aristotelian philosophy were slowly eroded as Neo-platonism and empirical observation led inexorably to the various threads of the scientific revolution and its increasingly sophisticated new ways of working, culminating in a maturing appreciation of the scientific method. This section will examine how, in terms of the variety of its application, the pharmaceutical use of emerald blossomed until its eventual extinction from *materia medica* cabinets in the eighteenth century.

Improvement of sight

The use of emerald to bring rest to the eyes has been a constant theme since Theophrastus first introduced medicinal properties for the gem in the third century BCE. There are relatively few mentions of emerald being used in this regard in the large numbers of English early modern medical books used in the present study, and all repeat the information provided by earlier authorities. Stephen Batman (died 1584) produced an English translation, with additional comments, of Bartholomew the Englishman's *De Proprietatibus rerum* ("On the Nature of Things") in 1582, whilst he was serving as domestic chaplain to Lord Hunsdon. He states, for instance, that emerald "comforteth feeble sight" (Batman 1582, 265), while Newton (1580, unnumbered page) indicates that "The Emeraulde burned, and beaten to Powder, helpeth the dimnesse of ye sight". Nicols (1652, 95) states that "This stone is good to recreate the sight", while Turner (1657, 90) states that it "strengthen and quickens" it. Nicolas Culpeper (1616-1654; Fig. 4.14) is unusually non-critical, being happy to record that emerald "helps the sight" (Culpeper 1659, 264). Lovell (1661, 74) indicates that it "doth mightily recreate the eyes".

An interesting side note to the tale of emerald lenses concerns a pair of eyeglasses with teardrop-shaped lenses (dated to the seventeenth century) set in a later (nineteenth century) diamond-studded frame which were withdrawn from an auction sale at Sotheby's on 27 October 2021, having failed to make the £3 million pound sale estimate (https://www.thetimes.co.uk/article/bidders-fail-to-see-value-in-3m-emerald-spectacles-ws0gkdsp3). The importation of high-quality emeralds from Colombia into India by merchants such as Garcia de Orta, mentioned above, led to Goa being established as a premier trading centre. This coincided with an increasing level of Mughal appreciation for the gem (Dirlam et al. 2019). Something of a precedent was set by Charles V of France (1338-1380) in whose treasury is recorded several green "bericles" (beryls) set in frames as spectacles (Holmes 1934, 200).

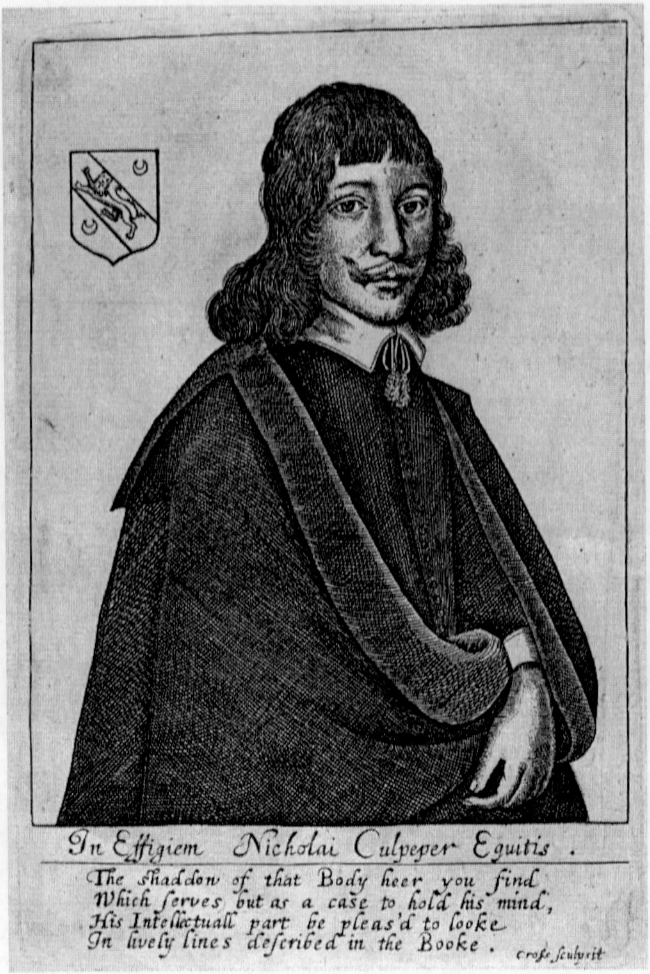
In Effigiem Nicholai Culpeper Equitis.
The shaddow of that Body heer you find
Which serves but as a case to hold his mind,
His Intellectuall part be pleas'd to looke
In lively lines described in the Booke.
crosse sculpsit

Fig. 4.14. Portrait of Nicolas Culpeper (1616-1654), frontispiece to The English physitian (1652). Reproduced by kind permission of the Wellcome Library, London.

Epilepsy

Emeralds have been associated with epilepsy since at least the time of Albertus Magnus in the thirteenth century. His recommendation that it be worn around the neck as an amulet against the disease is repeated by many early modern authors (e.g. Batman 1582, 265; Culpeper 1649, 74; Rattray 1658, 34). William Salmon (1644-1713; Fig. 4.15), a self-styled "Professor of Physick", recognises emerald as only one out of a plethora of possible amulets against the disease: "and about the Neck you may hang *Xenechtons* or *Amulets,* made of Peony seeds and roots, Elks hoof, Coral, Jasper, Emeralds, *Lapis Chelidonius,* Vervain, Ox horns, Antimony, Camphir, and other things of like nature" (Salmon 1681a, 355).

Christopher Wirtzung (c. 1500-1571), a German physician and polyglot (Lier 1898, 521), was convinced that it was the olfactory impact of certain herbal amulets, like those listed by Salmon, that made them effective in controlling epilepsy, unlike the superstitious basis of reliquaries and certain other medicines from folk medicine:

> In this falling sicknesse are some things highly commended of all the famous Phisitions, to be hanged about the necke, and they alleage thereto also certaine reasons and experiences, wherewith they do proue and shew, that they that weare them about the necke, do not fall, and omitting it, their disease presently returneth. This is also no misbelief, like as the common people thinketh: but it is the smell or sauour, which doth most vehemently withstand this euill, and therefore is the same at no hand to be omitted. Some write also, that the red Corall and the Emerald hath the same vertue, which experience must teach vs. [Then follows a list of, to him, suspicious items] [...] These things for the most part are accounted as gospel of old doting women: [...] but these remedies following are of better estimation, and of a more secret or hidden vertue, to wit; Bryonie worne about the necke: also Thyme, Hyssope, Rue, and Southernwood worne likewise in the bosome, for by reason of their smell they may haue some effect (Wirtzung 1605, 157).

The Tudor paediatrician, Thomas Phayre (c. 1510-1560), was convinced that the wearing of precious stones next to the skin was always beneficial:

> But it is good in all tymes, to beare about you preciouse stones, (yf ye haue them) speciallye a iacincte, a rubie, a garnet, an emeralde , or a saphyre, whiche hath a special vertue agaynst the pestilence, & they be the stronger, yf they be borne vpon youre naked skinne, chieflye vpon the fourth finger of the left hande, for that hath greate affinitie with the hert aboue other membres (Phayre 1550, unnumbered page)

In addition to wearing the jewel around the neck, Jean de Renou (also known as Renodeus; 1568-c.1620), Royal Physician to a succession of French Kings and a doctor at the Faculty of Medicine in Paris, claims it was a "preservative" against epilepsy when worn in a ring, due to its "eximious faculties" (Renou 1657, 413).

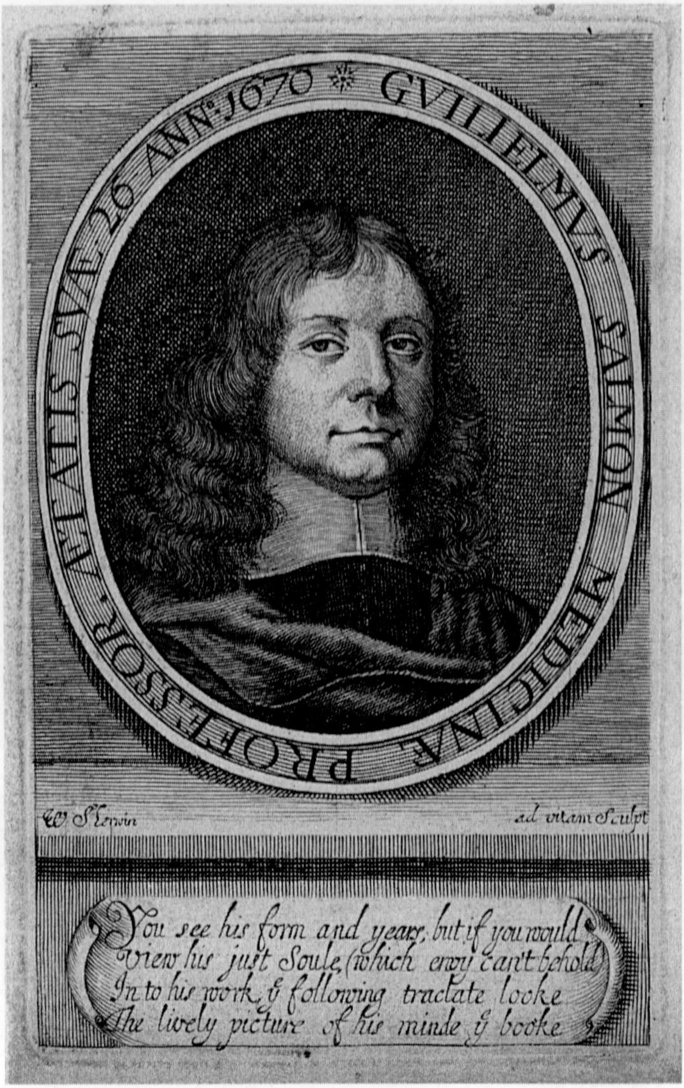
GVILIELMVS SALMON MEDICINÆ PROFESSOR · ÆTATIS SVÆ 26 ANNo 1670
W Sherwin
ad vitam Sculpt
You see his form and years, but if you would
View his just Soule, (which envy can't behold)
In to his work & following tractate looke
The lively picture of his minde & booke

Fig. 4.15. Portrait of William Salmon (1644-1713). Line engraving by W. Sherwin, 1671. Reproduced by kind permission of the Wellcome Library, London.

Certain aspects of their action in the treatment seem to be conflated with earlier tales of emeralds being broken during sexual intercourse. The theologian, Thomas Burnet (1635?-1715), indicates that:

> Among the amulets, the emerald is especially recommended. Even when worn on the fingers, all authors assert that it prevents epilepsy, and that it possesses the ability, so that if the disease is so severe that it cannot be overcome by a jewel, it can be broken off into pieces, and therefore either destroyed by the disease, or broken, as it were, conquered by the powerful battle (Burnet 1673, 315).

This echoes the sentiment that the emerald is engaged in a struggle or battle against epilepsy, as first presented by Georgius Agricola (see above). In the words of one writer "The Smaragdus not only drunk, but if it be hanged about the neck, it wars and expels the Falling-sickness as an enemy" (Anonymous 1664, 134).

Nicolas Culpeper (1659, 264), who elsewhere supported wearing emeralds prophylactically, makes the statement that "taken inwardly, it cureth the Falling sickness". Robert Johnson (b. 1640?), about whom very little is known, presents a medicine for internal use which comprises many of the items worn amuletically against the disease, as if delivering the occult healing virtues of these components directly to the body's tissues. His recipe is as follows:

> Take the Roots of Peony, Valerian, of each half an ounce; the Moss that groweth upon a Man's skull, the triangular Bone of a Man's skull prepar'd, Missletoe of the Oak, Elks-hoof, the Seeds of Peony, sweet Fennel and Annise, of each two drachms; red Coral, whitest Amber, and Emerald prepar'd, of each one drachm; white Sugar the weight of them all, let them be reduc'd into a fine powder.You may give a Child twenty grains of this powder with a little Oil of sweet Almonds, so soon as it is born, which may happily preserve it from Convulsions, and Epileptick fits (Johnson 1684, 34).

Lorenz Scholz von Rosenau (also Laurentius Scholzius; 1552–1599) was the son of a Breslau pharmacist. He studied medicine at Wittenberg, Padua and Bologna. His research into the plague earned him a Bohemian peerage with the title "Scholz von Rosenau". He is probably most famous for his translations and collections from Greek and Arabic writers, and for his collections of letters from prominent contemporary physicians (Cohn 1891, 229-230).

A letter which he received from Johannes Crato von Krafftheim (1519-1585) on 4 August 1561 (whilst in Vienna, serving as personal physician to Emperor Ferdinand I) and published in his *Epistolarum philosophicarum* cites the use of emerald in an anti-epileptic powder (Scholz 160, column 217). In addition, the recipe contained powdered rock crystal, precious red coral and oriental pearl mixed in a solution of Dandelion Water ("*aq. Taraxi*"; the scientific name for the common Dandelion is *Taraxacum officinale*). This was administered to two patients. He records that although the patients were each delivered from the epileptic seizure, both of them later died (see also Salmon 1683, 171; Burnet 1673, 315). His conclusion was that rock crystal (see Duffin 2020) was unsafe to use, and that the medicinal emerald in common use was either ineffective or fake ("*Smaragdus quo vulgo utuntur, non est verus*"), actually consisting of the green mineral, prase, imported from Peru. The medicament was hailed as "Caesar's secret against the falling sickness" (Scholtz 1610, column 216; Salmon 1683, 171).

The causes of epilepsy were not understood during early modern times. A rough classification of types of epilepsy emerged, based on supposed origins. One of these was an infestation in the patient of intestinal worms. Thomas Willis (1621-1675) was a pioneering anatomist, neurologist and psychologist and founder member of the Royal Society, originally from Great Bedwyn in Wiltshire. Willis treated "a Child being miserably afflicted with Convulsions that he seemed to be just dying" with purging medicines (*Mercurius dulcis* or Calomel-Hg_2Cl_2–and Resin of Jalap, tuberous roots of *Ipomoea purga* which contain the powerful cathartic compound called convolvulin). He made the connection with worms because he examined the stools which the patient produced and found that they contained twelve worms; following the purge, the patient "presently grew well" (Willis 1684, 27). The purge had apparently both rid the disease of its source and consequently ameliorated the condition (see also Temkin 1994, 208, 247, 251).

William Salmon suggested an emerald-containing recipe specifically to treat worm-induced epilepsy:

> Take Elks-hoof prepared, six drams: Mans skull prepared, four drams: Ox horns prepared, Diamoschu dulcis, red Coral, Pearls, Emeralds, Crystals, all prepared, Terra sigillata, of each two drams: seeds of Nigella, of Rue, of Peony, white Ditany, Nutmegs, Misletoe of the Oak, salt of Harts-horn, of each one dram: roots of Peony, Harts-horn prepared, Pea-cocks-dung, Scordium, Marjoram, Coralline, of each three drams: Musk and Ambergrise,

> of each half an ounce: mix all in a fine pouder: Dose from half a dram to a dram, in black Cherry Wine (Salmon 1683, 352).

Notice once again that the recipe is a compound of many simples, each with their own reputation for treating epilepsy.

Further suggestions from William Salmon includes a powder made from "Male-peony" root, emerald and human skull bone. Credited as being "a powerful remedy", if powder of castor sacs (castoreum) is added "it not only powerfully roots out the Epilepsy but the Apoplexy also" (Salmon 1683, 319). The author credits the recipe to Jacob Horst (1537-1600), Professor of Medicine at the University of Helmstadt (original not found in this study).

Salmon (1681a, 363) also provides recipes for three emerald-containing antiepileptic powders and an electuary for the same purpose. Each is compounded from a wide range of ingredients in which simples commonly used against epilepsy feature prominently-peony, oak misteltoe and elk hoof, for example.

The short-lived German alchemist, Adrian von Mynsicht, (1603-1638; Fig. 4.16), was quite enthusiastic about including powdered emeralds in his various medical recipes. He provides two opium-based suggestions for treating epilepsy (Mynsicht 1682, 71-72). One is a draught comprising a mixture of Betony syrup, Waters of Lavendar and Lime, Camphor, Oils of Amber and Hartshorn, and Elixir of Peony. The other is a bole or large soft pill which contains Peony flowers which have been vitriolated (i.e. mixed with sulfuric acid or converted to a sulfate), Oil of Rosemary and species Dialunae. The latter (*Silberspecies* in German; Zedler 1743, column 1277-1278) was a complex preparation invented by Mynsicht and containing, among other ingredients, seeds and roots of Peony, cinnabar, peacock dung, red coral, castoreum, musk and ambergris. Emerald was added to both of these preparation as a confection, presumably meaning ground to a powder with added sugar, honey or syrup.

Johann Heinrich Zedler (1706-1751), a Leipzig publisher and bookseller records recipes for at least 64 different powders for use against epilepsy, some with several variants, in his monumental work, *Grosses vollständiges Universal-Lexicon aller Wissenschafften und Künste* (Great Complete Encyclopedia of All Sciences and Arts), published in 68 volumes over the course of 25 years (1731-1756). Ten of these recipes employ emerald as one of their ingredients (Zedler 1741, columns 1494-1509; see Duffin 2022).

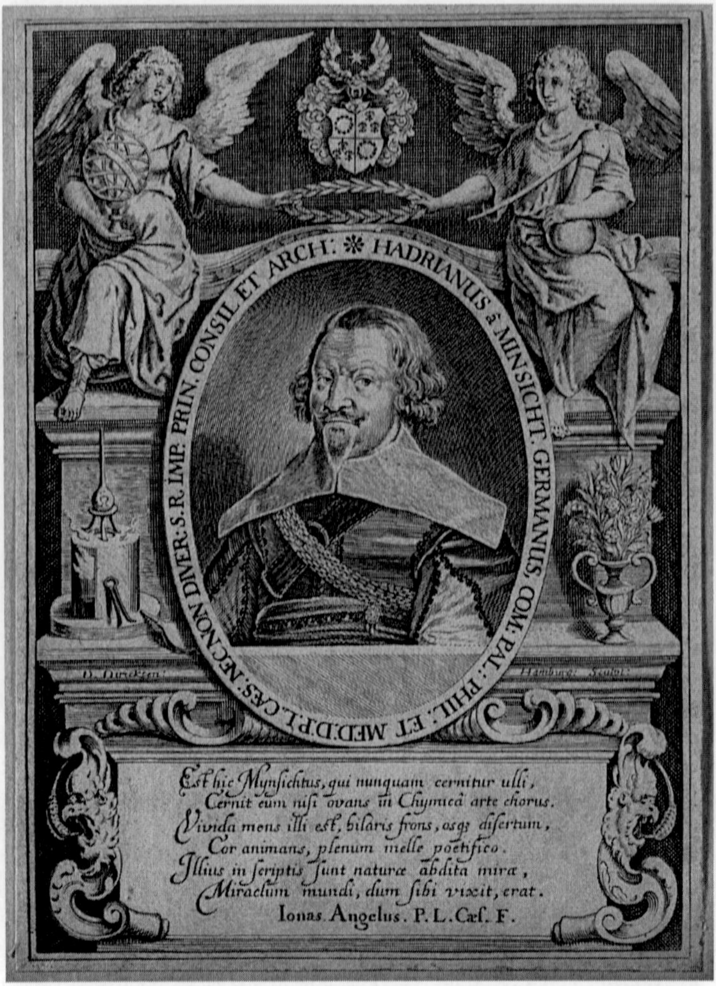
HADRIANUS à MINSICHT. GERMANUS. COM: PAL: PHIL: ET MED: D: P: L: CÆS: NEC NON DIVER: S.R. IMP. PRIN. CONSIL ET ARCH:
Est hic Mynsichtus, qui nunquam cernitur ulli,
Cernit eum nisi ovans in Chymicâ arte chorus.
Vivida mens illi est, hilaris frons, osq; disertum,
Cor animans, plenum melle poetifico.
Illius in scriptis sunt naturæ abdita mira,
Miraclum mundi, dum sibi vixit, erat.
Ionas Angelus. P. L. Cæs. F.

Fig. 4.16. Portrait of Adrian von Mynsicht, (1603-1638). Line engraving by D. Diricksen. Reproduced by kind permission of the Wellcome Library, London.

Resisting poison

Alexipharmic medicines are those which act as antidotes to poisons, either combating or expelling the toxic agents in some way. Interest in poisons and their potential treatment dates back to classical times with the writings of the Greek physician Nicander of Colophon (fl. second century BC).

Moses ben Maimon or Maimonides (1138–1204) was a Sephardic Jew from Cordoba. Both a physician and a rabbi, he fled Andalucia in exile when it fell to the Berber Muslim Almohads, moving to Morocco, Israel and Egypt. In his treatise on poisons and their antidotes, written in 1198, he has a particular entry for the emerald in his section on simple remedies, taken internally against snakebite and used as a substitute for terra sigillata in theriac:

> Emerald acts as a simple antidote against poisoning only when it is juicily green, translucent and reduced to a fine powder. In such a condition, 9 grains of it should be taken in cold water or in wine. Ibn Zohr, the Master, said this remedy had been sufficiently proven and admits of no doubt. It serves as an antidote against poisons which are forced out by it through vomiting, the way terra sigillata acts and serves as a substitute for the latter (forming part of the theriac) when it is unobtainable (Muntner 1966, 17).

The Italian physician, Pietro d'Abano (1257-1316), a Professor of Medicine at Padua, suffered at the hands of the Inquisition, being accused of atheism and heresy; he is believed to have died in prison before his trial had ended. D'Abano was at the forefront of championing the ideas and writings of medieval Islamic scholars such as Avicenna (c. 980-1037) and Averroes (1126-1198). His famous treatise on poisons (*De venenis, atque eorundem commodis remediis*; d'Abano 1537) refers in several places to the alexipharmic use of emeralds. In an interesting link with prase, one of the green minerals commonly confused with emerald, he states that the former is "the matrix [womb] and palace" of the emerald, since he says the two are often found together (d'Abano 1537, 26). He states that, when administered as a powder in some form of drink, emerald could be relied upon to expel all poisons, as "I tested many times" (Rankin 2021, 35). D'Abano also cites a non-medical test which has echoes of that applied to snakes by al-Biruni and al-Tifaschi, considered above, but using toads as a substitute. If a toad gazes on the best sort of emeralds, "his eyes rattle at its presence" ("*ipsius oculi crepitant ad præsentiam ipsius*"; d'Abano 1537, 28). If merely kept on the table, the emerald was believed to weaken the presence of any poison in the food or drink, but if held in the mouth it releases the patient from the power of the poison (d'Abano 1537, 28). D'Abano also suggested its use in cases of poisoning with specific toxins; in the case of poisoning with Loadstone (Magnetite), emerald should be administered in wine three times over a nine-day period; those suffering from Aconite poisoning (Monk's Hood, Wolf's Bane or "The Queen of Poisons") should take two drachms of emerald in wine, because "they will die unless they receive the emerald" (d'Abano 1573, 38, 48). Those who have the "tail end of the deer" will be prone to accidents unless they have taken a draught of emerald. The stone was also used to treat those who had been poisoned with the blood of a toad, or by the bite of a serpent (d'Abano 1573, 64, 66).

It is clear from d'Abano's chief work, *Conciliator differentiarum philosophorum* [*et*] *medicorum,* written in 1303 and first published in 1471, that he was a committed student of astrology. He espoused the opinion that God does not interpose himself directly in the affairs of men, but acts through a series of mediums, particularly celestial bodies, which he saw as "the first causes of happenings in this world" (Thorndike 1923b, 891). Indeed, his stated opinion was "that precious stones and medicines have marvellous and occult virtues which cannot come from the qualities and natures of the elements (constituting them)", and that, instead, they were invested with healing power through the medium of the stars (d'Abano 1521, *Differentia* LX, 85-87; Thorndike 1923b, 893). Likewise, he deemed that an understanding of the science of astronomy was "absolutely essential to medicine".

Guillaume de Grimoard (1310-1370) reigned as Pope Urban V from 1362 until his death. He commissioned a treatise on poisons in the first decade of his service as pontiff (Rankin 2021, 41). The manuscript, now held at the Vatican Library (Marra - *Opusculum quod dicitur Sertum Papale de Venenis*) contains several recommendations for the use of emerald, some clearly based on d'Abano's work.

Pietro Tommasi (fl. early fifteenth century) probably gained his doctorate in medicine from Padua in 1402 (Gibbs 2020, 102). His *Consilium de universali praeservatione contra venena* ("Advice Concerning Universal Preservation from Poison") recommended, as had some earlier authors, a four-fold approach to the whole problem of poisons; choosing servants carefully, recognising early warning signs of any who might be planning to poison their masters, means of detecting poisons and the application of universal remedies in the event that successful poisoning had taken place. In the latter case, he cites several emerald-containing recipes, and in terms of prevention he recommends that if the emerald is "held in the mouth before taking poison, [it] causes the latter to lose the power to kill", and that placing an emerald on the table "takes away much of its effectiveness from the poison" (Tommasi 1968, 79). Amongst the emerald-containing recipes promoted by Tommasi is the *Confectio Magisterialis*. In addition to fragments of emeralds, the recipe called for garnet, sapphire, jacinth, gold and silver leaf, red coral, *os e corde cervi* (Stag's heart bone), raw silk, cockroach and a range of herbal ingredients, all of which were rendered together into a powder (Tommasi 1968, 90). He also cites a non-laxative pill which was recommended to various popes. The powdered ingredients included snake meat, deer heart bone, unicorn horn, pearls, emerald, sapphire, jacinth. Gold leaf, musk, amber and a few seeds and roots. The powder was moistened with the juice of Hypericum and bound together using Juniper Gum (Tommasi 1968, 92).

Some authors of medical works from the sixteenth and seventeenth centuries are content to reiterate the idea that emeralds resist poisons without further comment (e.g. Banister (1575, 105– "The Smaragde stone, colde and drie, driueth away venim"). Nicolás Monardes (1493-1588), the Spanish physician from Seville who wrote about many of the new herbal, zoological and mineral (including emeralds) imports from South America, merely stated that emeralds provide a "marvellous medicine against all venom" (Monardes 1580, 113, 125).

Gaspar de Morales (fl. late sixteenth century), a Zaragoza-born Aragonese apothecary completed his *De las Virtudes y Propriedades maravillosas de las piedras preciosus* ("Of the wonderful virtues and properties of precious stones") in 1598; the Vatican placed it on the list of banned books and the Spanish Inquisition confiscated as many examples of it as they could find, making it a very rare book today. In his entry for the emerald, de Morales (1605, lib. 2, cap. 4, fol. 101-102) records a statement by Avenzoar (1094-1162) that, having sampled a poisonous plant, he effectively cured himself by placing one emerald in his mouth and placing another specimen on his stomach (original source not found in this study).

Culpeper (1654, 153) opines that some stones are more precious than others, and that, "Those which are more precious, alter by a quality Manifest or Hidden. […] By the second manifest quality they resist Poyson and Inchantment". Slightly later (Culpeper 1659, 84), he explains that, while amulets themselves made up of poisonous components (such as powdered toad, arsenic and quicksilver) "draw the venomous poyson to themselves, by the similitude of their own substance", "the greatest hope of health and security, is in medicines that resist poyson, out of which those are to be selected which by long experience have been approved", amongst which he lists the emerald. Jonstonus (1657, 111) indicates that emerald, "hath wonderful vertue; It is an Enemy to poysons and bitings of venemous beasts; and it breaks, if they overcome it". Lovell (1661, 74) states that "it cureth venemous bitings".

A few authors give further details as to how the emerald might be used. Rattray (1658, 41) writes: "The emerald, if it is in the hand of the one to whom the poison is offered, immediately loses its greenness and takes on a different colour". Nicols (1652, 96) quotes Avenzoar (1094-1162) as saying "it is good against poysons, and that six grains of its powder in a convenient water is an excellent Cordiall".

Salmon (1681, 191) offers the following advice in cases of food poisoning:

> If you apprehend any danger by Meat or Drink that has been taken, the following Pouder is good: Take Harts-horn, one dram: Coral both sorts, of each two scruples: Emeralds prepared one scruple: Bezoar-stone, half a scruple: leaves of Gold, to the number of nine: mix them, and make a Pouder: which may be taken in the Emulsion of Citron seeds, in Carduus water.

Other authors recommend emerald as a defence against specific poisons. The famous French Barber-surgeon, Ambroise Paré (c. 1510-1590), subscribed to the belief that the loadstone (magnetite) was poisonous: "The Load-stone makes them mad that take it inwardly" (Paré 1634, 810). His suggested antidote was "the powder of gold and an emerald drunk in strong wine". The otherwise obscure "W.R." agrees as to the toxic nature of magnetite and recommends a treatment regimen consisting firstly of inducing vomiting, secondly by applying an enema "If it indeed descends to the intestines", and finally employing pulverised emerald administered in a glass of wine (W.R. 1663, 51). Although pessimistic concerning the outcome of poisoning by Aconite ("Such is the malignity and venemous nature of this Hearb, that if present remedy be not used, no Antidote is of sufficient force to allay or resist it, but in short time kills them that have taken it"), he nevertheless commends the use of emeralds to treat it (W.R. 1663, 70). He also suggests the use of emerald (also rock crystal and terra sigillata) in cases of poisoning by Euphorbium. The use of an antidote is clearly desired as his description of the symptoms which the patient can expect shows:

> If the Juyce, Gumm, or otherwise [of Euphorbium is] taken into the Body, irregularly, or in too great a quantity, causeth an extraordinary heat in the Tongue, Mouth, Jawes, Stomach, and bowells, exciting intolerable paines by corroding and gnawing those parts: it provoketh Vomit, nauseousness and Hiccop; inflameth the whole body, with inextinguishable thirst; bringeth cold sweats, sownding fits, grievous Dysenteries, and at length Death it self (W.R. 1663, 96).

Although remarking that poison from the skin of a toad is relatively weak for animals found in colder climes, Jonstonus (1678, 153) describes the symptoms produced as follows: "One poysoned swells, looks wan, sighs, is shortbreathed, and taken with seed-flux; sometimes with the bloodyflux, inflammation of throat, and giddinesse". He includes emeralds in the list of antitoxins given to treat the poisoned patient.

Finally, it is worth noting an allusion to emeralds (*smaragdus*) as a type of dragonstone, which was also used as an alexipharmic. A manuscript of the Alexander Romance (circa 1420-5; *Le livre et la vraye hystorire du bon roy Alixandre* [Royal MS 20 B XX, f. 73r]) illustrates a battle between Alexander the Great and dragons bearing green stones on their heads (for further details see Pymm and Duffin 2020, 31). A Middle English translation of an explanatory passage from MS Worcester Cathedral F.172 indicates that the green stones are emeralds.

Plague and Pestilence

Providing a rational explanation to account for observations regarding the plague according to humoral theory, where a disease-state came about because of an imbalance of the humours, became extremely difficult. This was because plague was no respecter of humours-it killed sufferers of every humoral complexion. Catastrophic events became the explanation of choice for most physicians (Rankin 2021, 45), giving way to a general appreciation that a poison was at work in the bodies of plague patients. Indeed, the Italian physician Gentile la Foligno (died 1348) called plague "the most venomous of all poisons" (Foligno quoted in Rankin 2021, 45; see also Gibbs 2019). This meant that prophylactics and therapies formerly employed against poisons could now be applied to the plague. In turn, this led to emerald, both as a simple medicine and as a component in novel compounds invented by early modern physicians, being praised as efficacious in a wide range of therapeutic contexts. The influential French physician, Lazare Rivière (Riverius; 1589-1655), for example, provided instructions for manufacturing his Essence of Emeralds, concluding that it is "a most potent Cordial against Poison, and malignant, pestilential Fevers; and succors all Diseases of the Brain, as Madness, Apoplexies and the like" (Rivière 1685, 18). As a result, some early modern medicines began to take on the status of wonder drugs-therapies that could be applied to a wide, if not universal range of conditions.

Rivière's receipt for the Essence of Emeralds was the model for producing similar preparations of other precious stones. Emerald fragments were pulverised with Nitre (potassium nitrate, KNO_3) and then calcined in a glass vessel. The mixture was then "dulcified" or sweetened with warm water. The whole process of addition of reagents, calcination and dulcification was repeated another twice. The final powder was then placed in a crucible and kept in a high temperature glass or reverberatory furnace for a period of six days. Spirit of Salt (Hydrochloric Acid, HCl) was then added and the mixture placed in a hot bath for twenty days and the process repeated until the powder was completely dissolved in the liquid. This was then allowed to "digest" in a stopped vessel for a further month. Light distillation would then yield a tincture, whose virtue was "augmented" by the addition of Spirit of Wine (alcohol) (Rivière 1685, 18-19).

He also provided instructions for emerald-based pills against pestilential diseases, but which also had wider applications:

> Take wash'd Aloes, Saffron, Myrrh, of each half an Ounce, Oriental and Occidental Balsam, of each half a Drachm, six bones of Harts-heart: Unicorns-horn, Emeralds, Oriental Bezoar, Pearls, and Coral prepar'd, wood of Aloes, of each ten Grains, Ambar-grise five Grains; our Tincture of Ambar-grise; of Ambar, and Magistry of Tartar, of each, as much as will form a Mass of Pills, where take one of half a Drachm weight; going to bed, twice a week. These mundify the Blood, corroborate the Head and Stomach, help pains of the Heart, comfort all the Spirits, revive youth and retard old age (Rivière 1685, 108).

Traditional emerald amulets also received something of a makeover. As mentioned above, Thomas Phayre (1550, unnumbered page), acknowledging that both emerald and sapphire had special efficacy against pestilence, explains that they are stronger "yf they be borne vpon youre naked skinne, chieflye vpon the fourth finger of the left hande, for that hath greate affinitie with the hert aboue other membres". George Thomson (1666, 158), one of the small number of physicians who remained in London through the time of the Great Plague (Duffin 2016, 35), recounts a novel use of those two gems which were:

> often drawn in a Circle about a Bubo or Carbuncle placed directly against the Sun-beams or light, as (Helmont advises) do magnetically extract the virulence and malignity in the body, as is evident by a blackness arising from those fuliginous cauterizing Atoms that exhale.

Michael Ettmüller (1644-1683) takes this advice a little further, explaining that drawing a circle around the Bubo was intended to stop it spreading wider. Having thus supposedly contained bubonic expansion, the tip of the swelling should be touched with Butter of Antimony (Antimony trichloride; $SbCl_3$) in order to encourage scab formation, and then treated with one of a variety of plasters, cataplasms or ointments (Ettmüller 1699, 278).

Paracelsus (Philippus Aureolus Theophrastus Bombastus von Hohenheim; 1493-1541) wrote several treatises concerning the plague, a disease which he must surely have had first-hand experience of (Hedesan 2018; Gunnoe 2019). Amongst these, *Zwey Bücher von der Pestilentz und jhren zufällen* ("Two Books concerning the Plague and its Effects"), written around 1529 is a standalone piece, and *De Peste libri tres* ("Three Books on the Plague") probably written around 1531-1535, is generally believed to be pseudepigraphical (Khan 2020). In these texts, Paracelsus began to integrate his understanding of the plague into his overall medical viewpoint. Espousing a three-fold origin for the plague (via ingested food and drink, through astral influence, and imagination), Paracelsus nevertheless emphasises a connection with astrological observations which reveal the interdependence and interactions of the microcosm (man) and the macrocosm (heavens). He suggested that the evil intentions and activities of man so poisoned the heavens, that their response was to reflect that poison back onto mankind by star-mediated infection (see further details in Gunnoe 2019). In terms of treatment, Paracelsus introduces the idea of *Zenexton*, defined elsewhere as a "preservatory Amulet against the plague" and "a preservative Pomander against the Pest" (Helmont 1664, 767, 1144).

Clearly, protection and cure against maladies caused by personally-direeted, astrally-mediated power from the heavens would require a specialised means of intervention. The *Zenextons* also harnessed astrological power. Oswald Croll (1563-1609), an alchemist and follower of Paracelsus, provided details for the construction of the specialist holders for carrying amuletic cakes produced according to a precise recipe. The holders (Fig. 4.17) were to be of steel or gold (decorated with precious stones in the latter case), on which a serpent and a scorpion were to be engraved at astrologically auspicious times: "The Sculpture of the Instrument must be made at the certain position of the Celestials, *viz. Sol* and *Luna* entring the Sign *(b) Scorpio:* At the same time also the Pentacles must be scaled, or at least, when *Luna* attains the Sign *Scorpio;* for so the superiors with inferiours in sympathical undissolvible union are conjoyned and united" (Croll 1670, 136). Some *Zenextons* could be quite simple in content, reflecting Paracelsus' somewhat surprising incorporation of folk remedies into his writings-quicksilver or arsenic enclosed in a hazel nut (filbert) and hung around the neck, for example. Croll also provided specialist recipes for cakes of material (which he referred to as "constellate amulets or pentacles", reflecting their astrological thrust). These contained the first menstrual blood of young girls, white and red arsenic, Dittany root, Tormentil, pearls, coral, hyacinth, emerald and crocus together with 18 carefully sun-dried toads. He advises stopping the nostrils when pulverising the toads, and also adding musk or amber to the mixture to help diminish the offensive smell. Hanging the *Zenexton* from

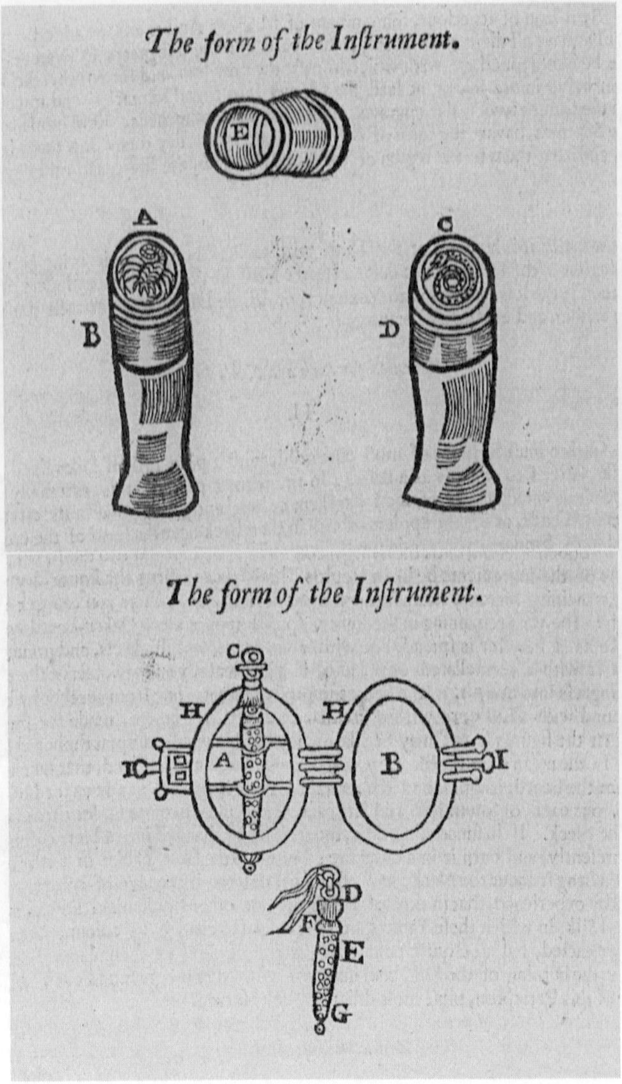

Fig. 4.17. Zenexton from Croll (1664). Reproduced by kind permission of the Wellcome Library, London.

the neck by means of a silk cord so that it lay over the heart ensured that it "not only preserves from the Pestilence, but hinders whereby the body is the less infected with Venomes, or Astrale Diseases" (Croll 1670, 136). He explains that the cakes attract "the venome from within, and externally consumes it" (Croll 1670, 136).

Van Helmont (1664) gives a little further explanation and discussion. Noting that many of the components of contemporary cures for plague might themselves be defiled by receiving seeds of contagion from the macrocosm, he indicates that "a preservative Amulet requires, that in it self it be wholly undefileable" (Van Helmont 1664, 1145). Precious stones seemed to fit the bill because of their intense colours, their various light-dependent properties, and the fact that they could be used to inscribe circles around buboes to encourage their detoxification (Van Helmont 1664, 1146). He was a little suspicious of the real ability of gems to act as "Zenexton or preservative pomander from stones" in the specific case of plague, however. Van Helmont refers to Paracelsus' preference for the therapeutic use of dried toads; holding complete specimens against buboes in the groin supposedly caused the toad to swell, a sure sign that it was drawing the poison from the diseased lymph nodes by a magnetic attraction. Van Helmont was unable to confirm these observations from his own trials with dried toads however, and had to conclude that Paracelsus' opinion was "ridiculous". He did, however, embrace the use of differently prepared dried toads (which had worm infestations in their eyes) as Zenexton.

William Kemp (dates unknown) ascribes "the most perfect Amulet" against plague to Rhenanus (presumably Beatus Rhenanus or Beatus Bild; 1485 –1547). It was designed to "be moist, and as it were sweat, at the approach or presence of the Pestilential venom, and they are then to be dried at the fire, or over a fume". The mixture combined a series of expensive gems with simples that were themselves poisonous, so that the whole would exploit both the exoticism and the sympathetic action of like components against the pestilential poison.

> Take (saith he) of white and yellow Arsenick of each half an ounce, the powder of dried Toads two ounces, *Mercury* sublimed, Wheat Flowre, the Roots of Dittany, of each three drams, Saffron, the Fragments of Jacynth and Emerald, of each one scruple, make them all into powder, and with Gum Dragon dissolved in Rose-water, make them into Cakes, and dry them as aforesaid.

A rather similar recipe, but with the addition of Tormentil root, pearls, red coral, Ambergris and Musk, is given by Salmon (1683, 710).

Kemp felt compelled to instruct his readers not to eat the anti-pestilential cakes, but instead to sew them into silk bags that could then be hung about the neck by a ribbon in such a way that they lay over the heart in the centre of the chest. He made the comment that "I have known some of these worn in the City of Bristol, in the time of the Plague, and the parties sometimes would have little pimples like the Itch, rise about the breadth of the Amulet in their Breast, which they did rub and scratch, but never had the Plague, and are alive till now" (Kemp 1665, 63).

Kemp also usefully summarises the various contemporary theories as to the mode of action of amulets in protecting the bearers against disease:

(1) The presence of amulets containing poisonous materials hanging over the heart makes it accustomed to their presence so that when the poison of plague or other disease comes along, it is not so easily overwhelmed.
(2) Being mostly made up of materials classified as hot, amulets tend to "dry up noxious humours, and disperse offensive vapours" (Kemp 1665, 61).
(3) The amulets encourage the vital spirits resident and concentrated in the heart to unite and strengthen themselves, so that they are primed to resist any further poison.
(4) Amulets intercept and neutralise any poisonous vapours that might be present before they enter the body. They do this by means of sympathetic attraction. Alternatively, if the poison is already present in the body, the amulet draws it out by means of attraction.

Fully convinced of the medical effectiveness of taking vinegar-based medicines (Kemp 1665, 86), the author goes on to recommend two emerald-containing mixtures for cases of plague. The first calls for seven grains each of Bezoar and emerald, plus three grains of Jacinth, pulverised and dispersed in vinegar. The liquid should then be taken, followed by a further drink of unadulterated vinegar for good measure. The second receipt requires the addition of powdered *os e corde cervi* to the mixture. Kemp makes the interesting comment that authentic bezoar was hard to obtain and commonly the subject of fabrication: "there be those in the World that have done as great matters as counterfeit them" (Kemp 1665, 79). Indeed, the Goa Stone was manufactured, distributed and exported by Portuguese Jesuit apothecaries in Goa directly because of the shortage of bezoar stones entering the marketplace (Duffin 2010a, 2010b; Barroso 2020; see further details below). Even the Goa stones themselves were subject to rather crude fakery (Duffin 2013d, 13). Kemp further states that the precious stones then available were "but the spare and crust of them" (Kemp 1665, 79). A survey of eighteenth century *materia medica* cabinets in the UK reveals that the original specimens of *smaragdus*, unsurprisingly, are now lost. An exception is provided by the Corbyn Cabinet (Drawer 25 column 2 row 5), held by the Museum of the Royal Pharmaceutical Society in London (see Duffin 2019 for background). The specimens included here under *L. smaragd.* are not emeralds, but a variety of tinted quartzes (mostly rose, prase and amethystine; Fig. 4.18) suggesting that substitution for authentic emeralds might have been common practice. This fits well with the later observation of Sir John Hill (1716-1775), who noted that "Our Druggists ought to sell us for medicinal Uses the Chippings and Fragments of this Stone, or those small Emeralds which are fit for no other Purposes though genuine. But instead of this, they keep under the name of this Gem, fragments of coloured crystals and Spars which are found in Abundance about the Mines of Copper and Iron" (Hill 1751, 292). The consequence of his mistrust of the authenticity of available bezoar stones and precious stones meant that Kemp "would be loath to venture my life on their operation, neither do I perswade others to relie upon them" (Kemp 1665, 79).

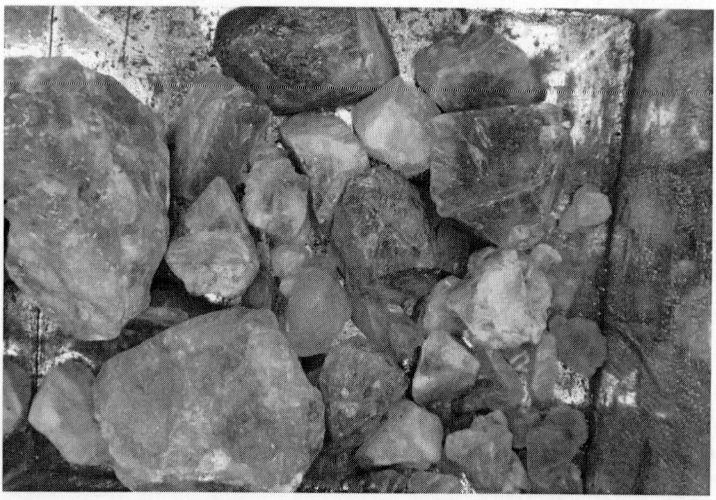

Fig. 4.18. L. smaragd from the Corbyn Cabinet (Drawer 25 column 2 row 5), Museum, Royal Pharmaceutical Society. Author's photograph.

The Secrets of Alexis of Piedmont seemingly gave rise to a whole genre of Books of Secrets which continued to be published through the seventeenth and eighteenth centuries (Eamon 1994). This very popular volume went through hundreds of editions and was translated into many languages. It was ascribed to Alessio Piemontese (also Alexius

Pedemontanus). The Secrets were published by the sixteenth century Italian mathematician, cartographer and alchemist, Girolamo Ruscelli (1518-1566), and first appeared in an Italian edition of 1555. Many authors believe that Alexis of Piedmont was a pseudonym of Ruscelli's, although a case has recently been made for the two gentlemen being separate authors (Bela 2016). First translated into English in 1558, the volume contains a "soueraigne pouder agaynst the venyme of the plague for ryche men and for prynces" (Ruscelli 1562, 47-48; see also W.J. 1665, unnumbered page):

> Take Saphyre, Hyacinthe, Smaragdus, of one of these, or two, or of all, one Dragme: of Pearles, Bole armenicke of the best, the seedes of Oxalis, of eche two Dragmes: of the scraping of Iuorie two scruples, of Unicornes horne a scruple, of the seedes of Ocimum halfe a scruple, yellowe or redde sanders: Agallochi or Xilaloes of the best. Doronici, Cynamom exquisite, saffron, of eche three graynes, Muske syxe graines. Make hereof a fyne pouder. You maye leaue out the Muske for them that loue it not.

Culpeper (1649, 173) presents a recipe for the *Confectio de Hyacintho* (Fig. 4.19), or Hyacinth Confection, seemingly first introduced by Royal College of Physicians; the receipt occurs in the first edition of the *Pharmacopoeia Londinensis* published in 1618 (Royal College of Physicians of London 1618, 79). In this context, "Hyacinth" refers not to the plant of that name but to the precious stone, often referred to as jacinth. Modern mineralogy identifies this stone as a reddish-brown variety of zircon, but in older literature a variety of stones might fall under this title, including sapphire. The recipe contains numerous costly ingredients:

> Take of Jacinth, red Corral, bole Armenick, earth of lemons [probably referring to Terra Lemnia], of each half an ounce, the berries of Kermes, the roots of Tormentil and Dictamni, Citron seeds husked, the seeds of Sorrel, Purslain, Saffron, Mirrh, red Roses, all the sorts of Sanders, Bone of a Stags heart, Hartshorn, Ivory of each four scruples, Saphire, Emerald, Topas, Pearls, raw Silk, the leaves of Gold and Silver, of each two scruples, Camphire, Musk, Amber greece, of each five grains, with syrup of Lemmons make them into a Confection according to art.

Acclaimed as a cordial, it was recommended as being "exceeding good in acute feavers, and pestilences, it mightily strengtheneth and cherrisheth the heart". Popular for a long time, it was incorporated into numerous pharmacopoeias, but its range of application and the degree of admiration for it was fading by the late eighteenth century. Vitet (1778, 538), for example, noted that the mixture was "so unworthy of celebrity" and "does not enjoy all the virtues attached to the substances which enter into its

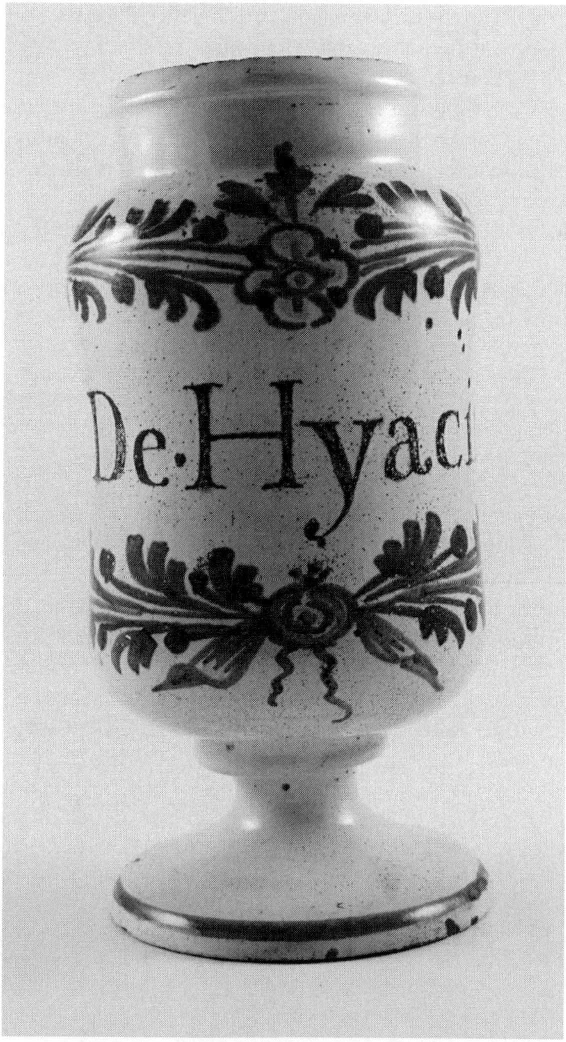

Fig. 4.19. Ceramic (faience) apothecary jar for Confectio de Hyacintho (18th century). The jar is marked with "C.De.Hyacint.". Musée des Hospices Civils de Lyon Inventary number 2007.0.2478.M (© Musée des HCL, Aurélie Troccon et Manon Mauguin 2014). CC-BY-SA 4.0.

composition". By then, it was relegated to occasional use in treating diarrhoea, vomiting and children's colic. Moyse Charas (1619-1698) remarked on the cutting of corners by apothecaries in producing a sub-standard confection sold as the real thing:

> They never seek after the true fragments of Jacinths or other precious Stones, the Oriental Pearls, nor the Bone in the Deer's-Heart; but being perfect cheats sell for considerable rates, that which is good for nothing but to fill their own Pockets (Charas 1678, 147).

He further remarks on the particular ability of the mixture to kill worms. Culpeper (1649, 177) also reports on Pietro Matthioli's (1501-1577?) "great Antidote against Poyson and Pestilence". This enormous recipe contains over 100 plant products, 12 materials derived from animals, 2 geological components (one of which is emerald) and 10 compound medicines (including theriac, mithridatium and the gem electuary); this represents redundancy of components on a massive scale! The many ingredients were mixed together in over eight pounds of honey. This must have been an impressive and complex medicine to manufacture, but the often acerbic and critical Culpeper seems happy to recommend it as being "excellent for those uses" (Culpeper 1649, 177).

Culpeper reverts to type in the 1653 edition of his translation and commentary on the *Pharmacopoeia Londinensis*. The emerald-containing Spirit of Lavendar, based on a gallon of Lavendar flowers in three gallons of Spirit of Wine, with many aromatic flowers, leaves and woods added to the mix, was criticised on the basis of cost and difficulties in gathering herbal ingredients which came into season at different times. His comment is that the task is "almost, if not altogether, as hard as to piss down Pauls" (Culpeper 1653, 64). Emeralds and other precious stones were also incorporated into the recipe for *Pulvis Bezoardicus Magistralis,* a powder which also contained nutmeg, bezoar stones from both South America and the East, musk and unicorn horn. Culpeper's comment was that it is "a great Cordial to revive the body, but it will bring the purse into consumption" (Culpeper 1653, 124). The *Species confectionis Liberantis* also contained emerald and was assessed as being "exceeding good in pestilential Feavers and preserveth from ill airs, and keepeth the humors in the body from corruption, it cools the heart and blood, and strengtheneth such as are oppressed by heat", but was "out of the reach of a vulgar mans purse" (Culpeper 1653, 124).

Primarily used against "Plague, Epidemical diseases, and all kinds of Poison", Adrian von Mynsicht's *Aurea Hadrianea* ("Golden" on account of its perceived excellence as a medicament) was also commended against "Epilepsies, Apoplexies, Hemicrania's, Cephalalgia's, Vertigoes, Convulsion, Palsie and Melancholy. It is a present help in the Asthma, pains of the Heart,

Spleen and Liver, Dropsies, spitting of Blood, the bloody Flux, Colick, Sciatica, Gout; and all kinds of Feavers either Quitidian, Tertian, or Quartan" (Mynsicht 1682, 61). The recipe combined emeralds with a range of herbal and zoological simples, compound medicines such as Venice Treacle, Mithridatium and *Confectio Alkermes*, plus alchemical preparations such as Jovial Bezoar.

Rotulae Zedoarticae pro Pueris or Zedoary Rowls for Children were small round cakes based on Zedoary or White Turmeric (*Curcuma zedoaria*). They were esteemed to be "good against the Contagion of the Plague, and defend and preserve the body from being hurt by any malignant and infectious Air" (Culpeper 1653, 136-137). Combined with amber, terra sigillata, Jacinth, Elk horn, Magisteries of red Coral, Oriental Pearl and Crab's Eyes (*oculi cancrorum*), plus a range of roots, seeds and herbal oils, prepared emerald was mixed with a pound of sugar dissolved in Waters of Roses and Water-lily flowers.

Robert Midgley translated the Latin text of the Geneva physician, Theophilus Bonet (1620-1689), into English. Suggesting a complex recipe for "a truly royal medicine" in cases of pestilential fever, Bonet prescribed one drop of the concoction daily for patients suffering from plague. He also suggested:

> adding 1 drachm of this Powder; Take of Hartshorn, Unicorns-horn, each 1 scruple, *Terra sigillata* half a drachm, Pearl, Emerald, each half a scruple, Camphire 7 grains; 5 grains of Bezoar-stone may be added; and every 3 hours 1 scruple of this powder may be given with Water of Water-lily, Sorel, *&c.* and when the Patient has taken it, let him Sweat (Midgely 1686, 239).

Hectic fevers were so-called because they involved relatively wide temperature swings (about 1.4°C), often over a fairly short time period. Although non-diagnostic, they have sometimes been taken to suggest pyogenic infections, although they are known to be associated with a range of other conditions (Dall & Stanford 1990). Non-specific, they were associated in early modern times with a range of infectious diseases, including the plague. Several authors mention the use of emerald in such cases, but Culpeper (1649, 161) goes a little further by providing a recipe for *Species confectionis liberantis*:

> Take of the roots of Tormentil, the seeds of Sorrel, Endive, Coriander prepared, Citrons of each a drachm and an half, the three sorts of Sanders, white Dictamni, of each one dram, Bole Armenick, Terra Lemnia of each three drachms, Pearls both sorts of Corral, white Amber, Ivory, Spodium, bone of a Stags heart, both sorts of Been (or in leiu of them, the roots of

> Avens and Tormentil) Angelica roots, Cardamoms, Cinnamon, Mace, wood of Aloes, Cassia lignea, Saffron, Zedoaary of each half a drachm, Penidies, Sugar Candy, raw silk torrified, Emeralds , Jacinth, Granate of each two scruples, the flowers of water Lillies, Bugloss, and red Roses of each a scruple, Camphire seven grains, Musk and Amber greece, of each three grains, beat them into pouder according to art.

He concludes that this medicament is "exceeding good in pestilential feavers, and preserveth from ill airs and keepeth the humours in the body from corruption, it cools the heart and blood, and strengtheneth such as are oppressed by heat, to conclude, it is a gallant cool cordial though costly" (Culpeper 1649, 161).

George Bate (1608-1669; Bruce-Chwatt 1983) graduated from Oxford and went on to treat Charles I (1600-1649), Charles II (1630-1685) and Oliver Cromwell (1599-1658) and his family; he was also one of the founding members of the Royal Society of London. The *Pharmacopoeia Bateana*, originally written in Latin, was produced in English translation by William Salmon (1694). It contains a recipe for emerald-containing *Pulvis Pannonicus rubeus* (Red Hungarian Powder) which was credited with having "great Power in curing malign, contagious, and pestilential Fevers". The powder also contained gold leaf, Terra Lemnia, ruby, sapphire, jacinth, red and white corals, pearls, spodium, cinnamon, red sanders, Sorrel seeds, Cloves, Saffron, Citron Peel, Stag's heart bone and Ivory (Salmon 1694, 823). Moyse Charas commended the recipe as being:

> us'd in Malignant Fevers, and all Epidemic Distempers, and against all sorts of Poysons. It prevails wonderfully against the Small-pox, for it expels the malignity forth, and strength'ns the Noble-parts. They usually dissolve it in some Cordial-water, sweetn'd with Syrup of Gillow-flowers, Lemons or Granates, and take it fasting from half a scruple to half a dram. The Tablets tak'n one in a morning fasting, produce almost the same effect against Pestilential-Air (Charas 1678, XXX).

Cordial

Cordial medicines were popular in early modern times and were believed to invigorate and strengthen the body, particularly the heart. Precious stones were commonly promoted as possessing strengthening or restorative properties; they were also often commended for raising the spirits. Emerald was amongst the long list of precious and semi-precious stones which Monsieur Chiquart, Master Chef of Amadeus VIII ("The Peaceful"; 1383-1451), Duke of Savoy, added to his "Restauratives" or "sick-dishes" (Ms. S

103 Bibliothèque Supersaxo, Bibliothèque cantonale du Valais, Sion, Switzerland; dated 1420; Duffin 2012, 83).

Emerald is commonly listed in early modern texts as a cordial medicine which could comfort or revive the spirits (e.g. Bacon 1638, 132; Nicols 1652, 96). William Bullein (c. 1515-1576) presents a cordial, emerald-containing recipe called *Diamargaritum frigidum.* Renou ascribes this receipt to the twelfth century Salernitan physician, Matthaeus Platearius, and reproduces it in his own work, but minus the emerald (Renou 1657, 599). In addition to emeralds, Bullein notes the use of sapphire, jacinth, ambergris, gold, musk, red and white corals and a range of herbal ingredients (Bullein 1579, 5).

The use of emeralds and certain other simples for this purpose was not without its critics, however. Gideon Harvey (1636 or 1637-1702), for example, wrote that "the addition of tosted raw Silk, the fragments of Sapphir, and Emeralds, and of the bone of a Stags Heart, to the *Species Cordiales,* is a most senseless Superstition, never received into the belief of the least rational, except Physicians" (Harvey 1689, 142).

Melancholy

Often considered to be caused by an excess of black bile, one of the four humours, melancholy was one of the four temperaments. It was marked by despondency, depressed mood, low spirits and fearfulness often expressing itself through poor appetite, abulia (lack of will or initiative), sleeplessness, irritability and agitation. John Pechey (1655-1716) gives a recipe for a "temperate cordial species" or *species cordiales temperatae* which was commended to treat melancholy and revive the spirits. Replete with expensive ingredients, it was prepared as follows:

> Take of the wood of Aloes, of the spodium of Ivory, each one dram, of Cinnamon, Cloves, bone of a Stags Heart, of the roots of Angelica, Avens, Tormentile each a dram and an half, of prepared Pearl six drams, of raw silk tosted, of both the corals, each two drams, of Hyacinths, Emeraulds , and Saphyrs, each half a dram, of Saffron one scruple, of the leaves of Gold and Silver, each ten; Ambargrease, and Musk, each half a dram, make a powder according to art (Pechey 1694, 53).

The dose to be taken was a scruple to half a dram (see also Culpeper 1653, 121 and Culpeper 1649, 151 who says it is "questionlesse a great cordial, a great strengthener, both of the heart and brain").

Other than this specific medicine, most authors merely list the emerald as being therapeutic in cases of melancholy (e.g. Lovell 1661, 74; Le Fevre

1662, 96; Mynsicht 1682, 62, 73; Salmon 1681, 230, 354; Anonymous 1664, 126).

Diseases of the Brain

The emerald is cited as an effective therapeutic agent in a range of conditions, loosely associated together here as diseases of the brain.

Claims that it strengthens the memory date back to the writings of Albertus Magnus, and are commonly repeated, mostly without any further comment in early modern texts (e.g. Lovell 1661, 74; Culpeper 1649, 74; Renou 1657, 413; Magnus 1483, unnnumbered; Magnus 1560, unnumbered; Batman 1582, 265; Gaule 1657, 221; Culpeper 1659, 264). It is a pity that most sources give little further detail concerning the condition of forgetfulness, making it difficult to judge its origin. Memory loss can be related to a range of medical conditions (e.g. some disorders of the liver, kidneys or thyroid, head injuries, alcohol abuse, poor diet, brain infections and tumours), as well as being part of the normal aging process, dementia and certain emotional problems.

Hannah Woolley (1622-c.1675) began writing books on household management after the death of her husband in 1660. She commends an emerald-containing, lavender-based "Palsie-water". Additional ingredients include a long list of herbal simples, powdered, steeped in ethanol and which, following a six-week period of "digestion" in a sealed container, is filtered. The emeralds and some additional ingredients are then added, hung "in a Sarsenet Bag in the water, being well sewed that nothing go out". Her praise for the drink is effusive and she gives a long list of conditions in which it useful:

> Swoundings and Weaknesses of the heart, and decaying of Spirits in all Apoplexies and Palsies, also in all pains of the Ioints coming of Cold, for all Bruises outwardly bathed and dipped Clothes laid to; it strengtheneth and comforteth all animal, natural and vital Spirits, and cheareth the external Senses, strengtheneth the Memory, restoreth lost Speech, and lost Appetite, all weakness of the Stomach, being both taken inwardly, and bathed outwardly; it taketh away the Giddiness of the Head, helpeth lost Hearing, it maketh a pleasant Breath, helpeth all cold disposition of the Liver, and a beginning Dropsie; it helpeth all cold Diseases of the Mother; indeed none can express sufficiently; it is to be taken morning and evening, about half a Spoonful with Crums of Bread and Sugar (Woolley 1670, 26).

A second recipe designed to treat a variety of diseases of the brain is given by von Mynsicht (1682, 129). His *Rotulae Smaragdinae* or "Rowls of Emerauld" contain many of the ingredients listed here in other preparations-calcined Elk horn, Peony seeds, Citron seeds, Dittany root, Kermes berries, Saffron, Oak Mistletoe, Magisteries of Pearl, Coral and Hyacinth, oils of Amber, Rosemary and Lavendar, for example. These components were mixed together in a specific Water of his design. His assessment was that:

> They wonderfully preserve from the Apoplexy, Epilepsie, Palsie, &c. They correct the Vertigo, and take away the debility of the Brain, sharpen the Memory and Sense, comfort the Head, refresh the Spirits, support and relieve the Faculties of the Mind, debilitated by study and continual cares, which are dangerous to the Animal Faculties.

Likewise, vertigo or the sensation of dizziness, is a symptom associated with numerous medical conditions (e.g. some migraines, benign paroxysmal vertigo, labyrinthitis, vestibular neuronitis and Menière's Disease). The origin of the belief that wearing an emerald, either in a ring or over the heart would combat the condition (Culpeper 1649, 74; 1659, 256) is not entirely clear. Several authors provide pharmaceutical recipes for medicines claiming to ease the symptoms of vertigo, often as one of a number of conditions. Pechey (1694, 484), for example, specifies an emerald-containing mixture which also includes Doronicum root, Sarsaparilla, St. Benedict's Thistle, Castoreum, and Betony, amongst others. Andromachus' Theriac and other preparations are also added for good measure.

Adrian von Mynsicht's *Aurea Hadrianea* or "Golden Hadrianean"-so-called because of its "value and excellence"-is an enormously complicated recipe. It calls for standard preparations of compound medicines such as Theriac, Mithridatium and Confectio Alkermes, various Magisteries and alchemical preparations (e.g. Jovial Bezoar) together with a range of over 30 additional ingredients, mostly of herbal origin. Emerald is also added. Mynsicht recommended it for a wide range of diseases:

> Epilepsies, Apoplexies, Hemicrania's, Cephalalgia's, Vertigoes, Convulsions, Palsie and Melancholy. It is a present help in Asthma, pains of the heart, Spleen and Liver, Dropsies, spitting of Blood, the bloody flux, Colick, Sciatica, Gout; and all kinds of Feavers either Quotidian, Tertian or Quartan (von Mynsicht 1682, 62).

His wonderfully named Marmelada Cephalica or "Marmelade for the Head" supposedly "roborates the Brain, and resists all the affects thereof. It is also happily given in the Apoplexy, Epilepsie, Vertigo, Lethargy, Palsie, Trembling" (von Mynsicht 1682, 162). The recipe called for *Diacydonium* (Electuary of Quince), *Diamoschu dulce* (Sweet Powder of Musk), *Diamoschu Diambrae* (Powder of Ambergris), together with Peony root,

Walnuts, Nutmeg, Amber, Marjoram and Rosemary plus, of course, emeralds.

Finally, his *Confectio Cephalica* contained emerald, a range of herbal ingredients, plus amber, coral, pearls, Salt of a Man's Skull, and Stag's heart bone. The ingredients were dissolved in *Aqua Apoplectica*, a Water of his own invention designed to treat "dangerous diseases of the head" (von Mynsicht 1682, 221). He noted that it deserved the soubriquet "Water of Philosophers" because of its wonderful virtue. The confection was claimed to be "good for all, or at least the most dangerous diseases of the Head, which it takes away and happily cures. And is very agreeable to Suffocations, Vertigo, Apoplexy, Epilepsie and Lunacy, and was only invented to dry the humidity of the Brain" (von Mynsicht 1682, 169).

William Drage (1637?-1669) (1664, 200) presents a recipe, similar to that provided by Von Mynsicht (see above) for an emerald-containing compound recommended for vertigo and which contains, amongst other ingredients, Peacock Dung.

Fluxes

Flux is a medical archaism which refers to any flow or discharge of fluid. Astringents are medicines that produce contraction or constriction of mucous membranes and are sometimes used to target and reduce the discharge of mucous secretions and blood. Emerald is identified as an astringent by Lovell (1661, 74), who goes on to say, therefore, that "being drunk it stoppeth all fluxes of the belly, and bloud, especially the dysentery, either arising from a sharp humour, or poyson". Such was the power of its healing virtue that, when applied to the outer surface of the abdomen "it doth undoubtedly stop all dysenteries, and flux of the hemorrhoides". Yarwood (dates unknown) (1683, 91) gives a little more detail; amongst the various brief recipes which he recommends, he suggests that Tincture of Emeralds, whose manufacture is considered above (Rivière 1685, 18-19), is excellent.

Culpeper (1653, 94) provides a more detailed recipe with emerald as its focal ingredient, for similar use:

> After that the fragments of *Emeralds* have been purely calcin'd by ignition and extraction in water of juice of Bugloss, and then triturated or ground to an Alkohol upon the Porphyry stone with the same water and dryed, it may be administred in Bolus or Pill, with Conserve of Marigold flower from iiij. *gr.* to x. against all manner of Lasks of the Belly and bloody Fluxes: but chiefly against Dysentery, either proceeding from erosion of the Entrals, or from some malignant matter.

"Lasks" in this text is derived from an old Northern French term "lasque" derived from "lasquer" meaning to loosen. "Lasks of the Belly" therefore indicates diarrhoea. The "bloody flux" refers to the presence of blood in rather loose faeces and probably often indicates amoebic dysentery. Culpeper also promoted the idea that keeping an emerald in the mouth would help to control nosebleeds, and that holding against the chest would help to mitigate the bloody flux and "Emrods" (haemorrhoids) (Culpeper 1653, 95).

The French alchemist, Nicolas le Fèbure (also Nicolas le Fèvre;1615 - 1669), served as Demonstrator of Chemistry at the Jardin du Roi in Paris, and later, in England, was Professor of Chemistry to Charles II, as well as Apothecary in Ordinary to the Royal Family in 1660. In 1662 he wrote of a "chymical" preparation of emerald, the instructions for production being as follows:

> Take fragments of Emerald the greenest and cleanest you can meet with, beat them to pouder in a steel-Mortar, and searce the pouder through a fine linnen Searcer fitted in a Box, which in the *French* shops is called *Cicotriner;* or it is as good to triturate them into an impalpable pouder, which put in a Matrass, pouring upon it of the volatile spirit of Urine having yet its phlegm, to draw the colour, and the spirit being sufficiently coloured, draw it off and pour on other until it takes no more colour; then filtrate the Tincture through a Cotten, and put them into a Cucurbite to draw off the Spirit, till you have the bottom in the consistency of an extract, upon which pour very good spirt of Wine; then stopping the Vessel with a Blindhead, lute it, and in the vapour of Balneo put it to extract, digest and circulate untill the spirit be ting'd with a high green, after this draw back again the half or two thirds of the spirit with a slow heat, and you shall have an *Elixir* or essence of *Emerald* left.

In addition to treating Melancholy, Phrensie (Madness), Hebetation (stupidity or dullness), swooning, post-infection weakness and palpitations, he accounted this medicine as being "a soveraign Remedy against Dysentery and all other kinds of flux of the belly, red and white Courses of Women, Emrods and Hemorrhagy" (Le Fèbure 1662, 96).

Adrian von Mynsicht can also be relied upon to have a medical receipt dedicated to this topic. His *Species Diasuccini* was a powder compounded from white amber, Magistery of red coral, Nutmegs, Oriental bole, Crocus martis (ferrous sulfate, $FeSO_4$), Dragons blood, Styrax, Hart's horn, opium, seeds of Rose and Plantain, flowers of Wild Poppy, Cloves, Saffron, Cinnamon and Mace. He acclaimed it as "the only healing medicine in all Dysenteries and Fluxes of Blood by stool", explaining that it "restrains and obtunds the viscous and tartarous salts which erode the Bowels, and doth disqueit the ordure of the Guts" (von Mynsicht 1682, 98).

Likewise, his *Marmelada Stegnotica* or Astringent Marmelade, which included emeralds and many of the same ingredients that are found in his *Species Diasuccini* (above), "stays a Loosness although old, and in a wonderful manner helps Dysenteries and pains in the Guts: It stays the immoderate flux of the Terms and Piles, and all fluxes of humors from the Head to the lower parts" (von Mynsicht 1682, 167).

Jacinths, emeralds and sapphires are all featured in a recipe given against "defluxions of humours" from the head causing catarrhs and coughs (Salmon 1683, 190). Salmon further notes an emerald-containing recipe originating with Platearius against all types of flux and describes emerald as being an "interceptive" because of its supposed astringent property (Salmon 1683, 232).

Excessive menstrual bleeding (*Mensium Fluxus Immodicus*) was targeted firstly by bleeding, then applying cupping glasses to the breasts, followed by giving purging and vomit-inducing medicines, according to John Tanner (c. 1636-1715). He then suggests that the following, rather different emerald-containing preparation should be tried:

> Take the Shells of two new layd Eggs burnt; Frankin-cense, Mastick, of each, half an Ounce: Pearls and red Corall prepared, and Amber, of each, two drachms: Haematites and Emerald, of each, half a Scruple: Barly meal fine sifted, two Pugills: the Whites of four Eggs, and chalybiated Water, enough to make the Powder into two Cakes; bake them in an Oven, so hard, that they may be beaten to Powder; give, of this Powder, half a Drachm, or a Drachm in the Morning, in Broth made of Sheeps feet or Calves feet (Turner 1659, 322)..

Leprosy

Michael Psellus (1017 or 1018-1078), a Byzantine monk, cites the use of emerald and water in a poultice or cataplasm in the treatment of leprosy ("*Cum aqua impositus ut cataplasma leprosos adjuvat*"; Psellus 1745, 33). Considering how socially significant and well-established Leprosy (known to the Ancient Greeks as *elephantiasis graecorum*) was in Western Europe in medieval and early modern times, it is rather surprising to discover how few texts reiterated al-Rhazes' advice, presumably derived from Psellus, cited in the *Hortus Sanitatis* (1491). The only account I have come across reads: "Anoynted wyth water, and wyth gumme Arabicke, it [*smaragdus*] helpeth the Leaper" (Newton 1580, unnumbered page).

Sleep disorders

The fourth century compilation of magico-medicinal lore known as the *Kyranides* was originally produced in Greek, but complete or partial translations have been made into Latin, Arabic, French and German. An English version was published in 1685. The writer recommends that

> The Emerauld is a green precious Stone. Engrave therefore upon it the Bird *Harpe,* and under its feet a Sea-Lamprey, and under the Stone enclose the Root of the Herb, and wear it, against Disturbance, and Dreams, and Stupidity. It causes Rest to Lunaticks, and to them that are troubled with the Colick. And it is better, if the Fat of the Sea-Lamprey be put underneath: For this is Divine (Anonymous 1685, 18).

Adrian von Mynsicht refers to specially formulated emerald pills or *Pilulae Smaragdinae* which, in addition to driving away poisons and comforting the spirits, were supposed to "drive away grievous and terrible dreams (which otherwise debilitate the body by breaking the rest) and procure sleep". The recipe for the pills is as follows (von Mynsicht 1682, 120):

> Take Emeraulds *prepared a dram and a half, Sulphur of the Moon dryed two scruples, Hyacinth prepared half a dram, Magisteries of Oriental Pearls and of red Corals of each a scruple.* Mix them, and with Syrup of Citron rinds and Nutmegs make a mass for Pills; from which mass make small Pills with Oyl of Aniseeds, and gild them with silver.

A scruple of the mixture taken at bed-time was the recommended dose.

Cholera

The only reference I have come across claiming that emeralds are useful in the treatment of cholera is that of the Leipzig physician Michael Ettmüller. A well-travelled student, he held the chairs of botany and surgery plus anatomy at Leipzig University. He was succeeded by his son, Michael Ernst Ettmüller (1673–1732), who published his father's collected works in 1708. The abridged English version of his *Opera omnia* contains a description of the symptoms of the disease; the sufferer could expect to suffer "vicious humors are impetuously thrown out both upwards and downwards, with a violent Pain in the Stomac and Belly, distention of the Hypocondria, Heartburnings, Thirst, Perplexity of the Breast, a swift and sometimes small pulse, frequent swoonings, unquietness, tossing, a Coldness in the outer Parts, Cold sweats especially upon the forehead, prostration of strength, and at last Convulsions and Hiccoughs" (Ettmüller 1699, 112). Ettmüller indicates that "Alexipharmacal Medicines" are called for in these cases and he lists emerald amongst the items he considers suitable, together with prepared rock crystal and terra sigillata.

Smallpox and Measles

Ettmüller is likewise the only source I have discovered commending the use of emeralds for these diseases. In this instance he provides the following receipt:

> Take of Plantan-Water an Ounce; Eye-bright and Rose Water, of each half an ounce; prepar'd Emerald, twelve grains; prepar'd Pearls, six grains; Camphyr, three grains; Saffron, four grains. Mix and drop it into the Eye. Some choose to drop into the Eye, a drop or two of the Fat of Vipers (Etmüller 1699, 271).

The means of administration seems a little incongruous, perhaps, for the diseases being experienced.

Diabetes

Once again, I have found only one source referring to the use of emeralds in the context of this disease. Yarwood (1683, 105) describes diabetes thus:

> It is commonly call'd unmeasurable Pissing, for the Retentive faculty is so weak, that whatsoever is drank by the Patient is sent forth again by urine as it was taken, there is an unquenchable Thirst, heat in the Bowels, Leanness, and if it be not suddenly cured 'tis deadly, bringing the Patient into a Consumption.

His recommended treatment is to administer ten grains of Tincture of Emeralds (for which he provides no manufacturing instructions) in Malaga wine. Salmon (1681b, 735) agrees that the Tincture and essence of Emerald is the most superior medicine to apply in such cases.

Obstetrical and gynaecological conditions

One group of early modern texts recommends the use of emeralds to control childbirth and to prevent abortion. The English midwife, Jane Sharp (c. 1641-1671), suggests that while prayer is the chief remedy for barrenness, encouraging conception can be achieved by avoiding all those things that might prevent it, such as certain meats and drinks (especially the Dutch drink called "Stum"), and taking care not to eat Ivy berries. Prospective mothers are also warned to avoid wearing both sapphires and emeralds (Sharp 1671, 180).

This is perfectly logical when one considers the recommendations of other authors concerning the use of emerald. John Jonston (1603-1675), the Polish physician of Scottish heritage for example, records that "It is said, to further womens labour, tyed to the hips; and to hinder it, laid to the belly" (Jonstonus 1657, 111; see also Lovell 1661, 74). This is very reminiscent of the properties ascribed to *Aetites*, the Eagle Stone (Duffin 2012). William Drage reinforces belief in this mode of action of the emerald, and adds a series of other stones (Loadstone, coral, Jasper) which were suitable for the same purpose, plus some additional items-"Garden-Tansy bruised, sprinkled with Muskadine [...] Bones of a Stags Heart worn about the Neck, or under the Arm-holes [and] a Girdle of Sea-Horse-Skin, or Wolf-Skin" (Drage 1664, 349). The list is expanded even further by James McMath (fl. late seventeenth century), who adds cornelian, azurite, sapphire and hyacinth or jacinth to the inventory of amulets supposedly effective against miscarriage (McMath 1694, 108-109).

Jane Sharp also suggests using emerald to eradicate the melancholy believed to lead to the development of cancer of the womb:

> Prepare and Purge Melancholy, from whence it proceeds: Use no sharp biting applications at first, but onely Diapompholyx, or juice of night shade, Plantane, or Purslane. Give every day three or four Grains of a Powder made of Oriental Bezoar stone, Saphyrs and Emeralds, of each one dram, in waters of Scabius, or Carduus; take also juice of Nightshade six ounces, burnt Lead washt, and Tutty, of each two drams, Camphire half a dram, put Cray-fish powder to them, and stir them well in a leaden Mortar (Sharp 1671, 282-283).

Resisting lust

Albertus Magnus recorded (see above) the experience of the King of Hungary, where the emerald in his finger ring broke whilst having sexual intercourse with his wife, indicating that this indicated that the emerald was "good and genuine". Magnus interpreted this as potentially confirming the idea that the gem "inclines the wearer towards chastity" (Wyckoff 1967, 119-120). The core of this account is often repeated in early modern texts, but the thrust of sexual probity is sometimes modified, expanded or embellished. Lovell (1661, 74) records the emerald's "antipathie to venery", while Culpeper (1649, 74) indicates that it is "called a Chast stone, because it resisteth lust, and will break (as *Cardanus* saith) if one hath it abòut him when he deflowrs a virgin" (see also Culpeper 1659, 264). Others indicate that it "loves Chastity, and is … averse to the sopperies of Venery" (Renou 1657, 413), "it cannot endure venery; for if it touch ones body in the act, it will break" (Jonstonus 1657, 413), it "represseth wanton motions of lechery" (Batman 1582, 265) and Thomas Nicols (1652, 95) records that:

> there is such an enmity betwixt it, and illegitimate venery, or the uncleannesse of the flesh, as that if it do but touch the skinne of an adulterer, it will break: and that it doth bridle the reins of lasciviousnesse, and much temper it.

Combating baldness

Lovell (1661, 74) indicates that emeralds "hinder the falling off of the hair". This appears to based on the comments of Pseudo-Aristotle and Alfonso X, detailed above, that using an emerald to treat cases of poisoning has the benefit that the patient will lose neither their hair nor their skin. The comment in Lovell seems to be entirely disassociated from a poisoning event.

Personal qualities

Many "stones" in the Western Lapidary Tradition were believed to inculcate higher personal qualities, abilities and character traits (e.g. Duffin 2007a, 2007b, 2012, 2020b). The emerald is no exception. The association of such benefits with emerald seems to date back to the writings of Albertus Magnus and Pseudo-Albertus (see above) and was sustained through various lapidaries. By no means universally promoted, notice of the supposed effect of emerald on the personal qualities of the bearer still survive in early modern texts. It was stated, for example, to eliminate folly and anger (Culpeper 1649, 74; Culpeper 1659, 264), improve eloquence and speech (Batman 1582, 265; Wirtzung 1605, 88; Culpeper 1659, 264), encourage kindness and goodness (Batman 1582, 265), and good manners (Lovell 1661, 74), stimulate prophesy when held under the tongue (Magnus 1560, unnumbered; Batman 1582, 265; Gaule 1657, 221; Culpeper 1659, 264), increase worldly riches (William of Auvergne in Thorndike 1923b, 363; Magnus 1560, unnumbered; Batman 1582, 265; Gaule 1657, 221; Culpeper 1659, 264; Lovell 1661, 74) and "facundity" (Lovell 1661, 74), calm fears (Culpeper 1649, 74; Lovell 1661, 74) and even engender a love of studying (Culpeper 1659, 264). In addition to calming tempests (Batman 1582, 265), emerald was also believed to be able to protect the bearer from enchantment (Batman 1582, 265; Culpeper 1654: 155; Culpeper 1659: 264).

Alchemy

The medical reformer and alchemist, Paracelsus proposed the idea that there were five *Ens* or entities that influenced the health of mankind: the influence of the stars (*ens astrale*), poison (*ens veneni*), the individual (*ens naturale*), actions through the spirit (*ens spirituale*) and the will of God (*ens deale*) (Paracelsus 1660, Stillman 1919). He advocated the use of *Ens* tinctures whose virtues were to rejuvenate and heal the body as well as to restore man to proper alignment with God and His purposes. He indicated that, by taking finely ground emeralds, calcining them in salt, dissolving the mixture and then placing the container in a fire, a solid could be produced-the Ens of Emerald-which contained the essence of the gem. This could then be used therapeutically to renovate and restore the body to full health (Paracelsus 1660, [A Book of Renovation and Restauration] 19), although his advice, which follows, does seem somewhat drastic. Sufficient of the material was dissolved in wine so the liquid was visibly coloured. Daily drinks of the mixture at dawn then took place "til the nails of your fingers first fall off, and then the nails on your feet, then your hair and teeth, and then lastly till your skin be dried up" (Paracelsus 1660, 20). At this point, medication should cease so that all these body parts can be renewed and regrown, "and the diseases both of the body and mind will depart away". Anyone who followed this approach to its logical conclusion must have been not only very sick, but also very disappointed.

Anonymous (1664, 239) embraced Paracelsus' teachings and commended many of his plague protections and remedies, including his "pestilential drink", "Zenecthon" amulet, and *Alexipharmacum spagiricum*. He also promoted a 'Universal Cure of the Plague' made up of "spirit of Gold, with Diaphoretical ☉ [gold] of life, the essence of Gemms, Hyacinth, Smaragdus, Saphires, Tinctures, Corals, and of Antimony with *Solificatum* and *Perlatum Laudanum*". "These mysteries of Nature", he concluded, "will expel the Plague altogether".

Goa Stones

The Lapis de Goa was the mid-seventeenth century invention of Gaspar António, a Jesuit lay brother working as an apothecary in Goa. A synthetic stone, it was produced in response to declining availability of suitable bezoar stones. The original recipe for the stones (see Barroso 2016, fig. 6; Duffin 2010a, Table 1) required seed pearl, musk, ambergris, red coral, white coral, emerald, fossil shark´s teeth, topaz, terra sigillata, ruby, Cananor stone, jacinth, deer horn tips, sapphire, and Oriental bezoar.

Subsequent recipes are similar, with some ingredients (e.g. fossil shark's teeth and Cananor Stone) omitted, but others (such as amber, spodium, garnets, Armenian earth, scrapings of unicorn horn and ivory, and crab's eyes) added. For export purposes, the stones required certification from the Jesuit pharmacies by decree of the House of India (Barroso 2016, 75). Although compounded according to a "secret" recipe, the list of ingredients entered mainstream publications and the recipe evolved over the next century and a half of its use (Duffin 2010a, 2010b). Often fashioned into balls, the product was commonly coated in gold leaf, probably partly to reduce the impact of the offensive odour they emitted, and partly to add a touch of authenticity and a sense of high value to the commodity. Indeed, their high status and expensive nature often saw them being kept in specially designed gold or silver cages (Fig. 4.20). Popular as an alexipharmic and cordial medicine, it was esteemed as a sudorific, diaphoretic and mild astringent, and commonly recommended to treat a wide variety of fevers, including those associated with plague and gout. It was also indicated in the treatment of smallpox, measles, childhood fevers, muscle spasms, and as a cardiac tonic.

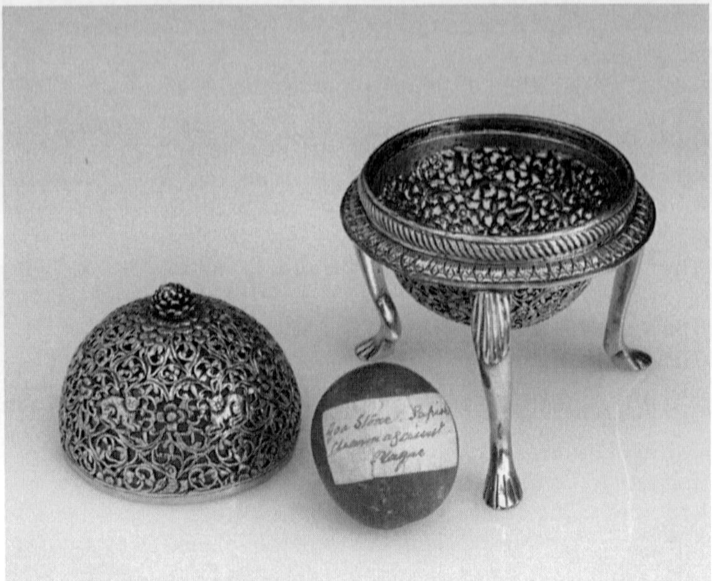

Fig. 4.20. Goa stone and holder, seventeenth century. Science Museum, CC BY 4.0

Summary and Conclusions

It is clear from the evidence presented above that the emerald held a significant place in the *materia medica* from classical times through to the mid-eighteenth century. In spite of its status and high market demand as a precious stone also sought after for inclusion in items of jewellery, and its consequent high price, it seems to have enjoyed unbroken popularity in the treatment of a wide range of diseases. Stocked in apothecary shops and featuring in *materia medica* collections, supply to the market seems to have been dominated by material won from Egyptian mines adjacent to the Red Sea up until the sixteenth century. The sixteenth century discovery of rich deposits of emeralds by Spanish conquistadors in what is now Colombia represented a new source of supply, especially via gem markets in Spain and Portugal, and thence to Goa.

Many of the medicinal uses of emerald have their roots in the magico-medical traditions established by Graeco-Roman authors in classical times, and medieval authors from both Arabic and Western traditions. The invention of printing drove early modern innovation in many areas of study, making classical and foreign texts more readily available to an increasingly educated clientele both in Latin and often in vernacular European languages. Many early modern texts repeated observations about the gem and its amuletic use from earlier authors, with occasional conflation and adaptation from the original ideas. Emerald increasingly became incorporated into compound recipes, often with alexipharmic, near wonder-drug status. These included

1. The Gem Electuary of Johannes Mesuë.
2. The Goa Stone
3. The *Aurea Hadrianea* of Adrian von Mynsicht.
4. The *Rotulae Zedoarticae pro Pueris* of Adrian von Mynsicht.
5. The *Marmelada Cephalica* of Adrian von Mynsicht.
6. The *Confectio Cephalica* of Adrian von Mynsicht.
7. The *Rotulae Smaragdinae* of Adrian von Mynsicht.
8. The *Species confectionis liberantis* of Culpeper.
9. The *Pulvis Bezoardicus Magistralis* of Culpeper.
10. The *Diamargaritum frigidum* detailed by William Bullein,

There have been several suggestions for the mode of action of the emerald in therapeutic situations:

1. The intense colour, hardness and durability of precious stones in general suggested that they possessed special healing characteristics.
2. Emeralds are examples of rare and exotic substances, many of which were ascribed special therapeutic powers (e.g. unicorn horns, glossopetrae (fossil sharks' teeth), coconut, precious red coral etc.)
3. The observation that the emerald causes the air above it to reverberate in some way implies the presence of occult or hidden powers and virtues. Culpeper (1653, 54) lists emerald as one of the stones that heals by means of a "hidden property".
4. The Biblical association of emeralds with the foundations of the New Jerusalem and the breastplates of Aaronic priests, plus the suggestion that they are washed out of the presence of God in the Garden of Eden supports the idea that their healing virtues are God-given.
5. Utilisation of the residual heat of the sun from the time of origin of the gem to stimulate a physiological response to disease (Hildegard von Bingen).
6. God uses celestial bodies as the mediums through which to work medical healing. Therapeutic gems receive their divine therapeutic powers from the stars, so that their use requires both astronomical and astrological understanding (see Pietro d'Abano).
7. According to Pietro d'Abano, anti-poison materials may act in one of three ways: one poison (such as opium) weakens the effect of another by means of its opposite qualities; expulsion of the poison by inducing sweating or vomiting; the material (e.g. emerald) causes the poison to avoid the heart and move toward the extremities, particularly the feet (Gibbs 2019, 93).
8. They could be used as *probae*-testing agents that warn of the presence of poison. In the case of emerald, this involved change (usually loss) of colour intensity.
9. Balancing the humors; Culpeper (1654) indicates that emeralds are cold in the first degree; Banister (1575, 105) agrees, stating that they are cold and dry.
10. Magnetic extraction of "virulence and malignity" (Thomson 1666, 158).

Irrespective of their perceived mode of action, emerald was ascribed various therapeutic properties, including acting as

1. An astringent.
2. An alexipharmic.
3. An exhilarant.

4. A cardiac, cephalic or general tonic.

Utilised as an amulet, emerald was believed to be an efficient prophylactic against

1. Epilepsy.
2. Hemitertian fever and ague.
3. Memory loss.
4. Poisoning.
5. Controlling the process of childbirth.

Incorporated with other geological, herbal and zoological simples into compound medicines, the therapeutic value of emerald expanded dramatically. It was used mainly in cordial and alexipharmic medicines, but also specifically in cases of:

1. Epilepsy.
2. Pleurisy.
3. Dysentery.
4. Weak sight.
5. Convulsions.
6. Plague.
7. Melancholy.
8. Apoplexy.
9. Palsy.
10. Vertigo.
11. Asthma.
12. Dropsy.
13. Leprosy.
14. Sleep disorders.
15. Smallpox.
16. Measles.
17. Excessive menstrual bleeding.
18. Swooning.
19. Palpitations.
20. Dullness (Habetation).
21. Lunacy.
22. Diarrhoea.
23. Nosebleeds.
24. Haemorrhoids.
25. Haemoptisis (spitting blood).

26. Bloody Flux.
27. Colic.
28. Sciatica.
29. Gout.
30. Fevers.

Potential tests of authenticity for the stone, for which substitutions and fakes were possible, included:

1. Bringing the stone close to a toad. If the emerald is stronger than the poisonous toad, the toad will burst (Albertus Magnus), or its eyes will liquefy (Tomassi).
2. Bringing the stone close to a snake. A genuine stone causes the eyes of the snake to pop out of their sockets (al-Biruni).
3. Bringing the stone close to a snake. The snakes' eyes bulge, the animal becomes disoriented and eventually ceases movement altogether (al-Tifachi).

Thus, emeralds enjoyed considerable respect as a geological simple, especially through early modern times. A late as the 1750s, Sir John Hill, whilst commenting that "the Virtues ascribed to this Gem by fanciful Authors are numberless", was nevertheless confident in its ability to "stop Haemorrhages and Diarrhoeas, and sweeten or obtund the too acrid Humours" (Hill 1751, 292). Noting that apothecarial stocks of the gem were generally chips of coloured Quartz, however, he remarks that the therapeutic qualities might not pertain to Emerald, but to the substituted minerals instead.

The demise of the emerald as an actively promoted medicinal simple cannot be pinpointed definitively, but by the time William Cullen (1710-1790) was writing his lectures on the Materia Medica for his students at Edinburgh University in 1761, ten years after Hill's remarks, they, together with all other precious and semi-precious stones, were no longer part of the curriculum (Cullen 1772).

Acknowledgements

I am very grateful to Maria do Sameiro Barroso (Lisbon) and Rachael Pymm (Egham) for their critical appraisal of the manuscript. Reproduction of the images used in the various figures included here has been through the kindness of the Wellcome Collection, The Arkenstone, Getty Museum

Open Content Program, The Science Museum, The University of Aberdeen and the Countway Medical Library.

References

Archival sources

Aberdeen Bestiary. Aberdeen University Library MS. 24.

De Beauvais, Vincent. 1475?. Getty Museum. Ms. Ludwig XIII 5, v1 (83.MP.148.1).

Goldsmith's Lapidary: Gamon, Hannibal. 1604. *The Gouldesmythes Storehowse. whearein is layde up manye hidden Secretes of that Ingenious Misterie. Compiled, Made, & Drawen into This Methode by H.G. Citizen And Gouldesmythe of London. Anno Salutis 1604. The Seconde Booke of this Storehowse Leadethe to the Knowledge of all sortes of Gemms or praetiose Stones: describinge the Places wheare they growe, Their Names, Coullors, Vertues, and Valewes, Accordinge as they are Bowghte from Marchaunte to Marchaunte. Worthye their studie, whiche professe them selues Iuellers: or are desirous to be made Acquaynted with these Secretes Of Nature.* Folios 34-64. MS 3181, Q1. The Worshipful Company of Goldsmiths, Goldsmiths' Hall, Foster Lane London EC2.
Le livre et la vraye hystorire du bon roy Alixandre [Royal MS 20 B XX, f. 73r]

Marra, Guglielmo di. Opusculum quod dicitur Sertum Papale de Venenis. Vatican Ms.Barb.Lat. 306. https://digi.vatlib.it/view/MSS_Barb.lat.306. Accessed 24 May 2022.

MS Worcester Cathedral F.172.

Ms. S 103 Bibliothèque Supersaxo, Bibliothèque cantonale du Valais, Sion, Switzerland; dated 1420.

Richardoune's Verses; B.M. Additional Manuscript 34360; MS. E.

Websites

https://www.thetimes.co.uk/article/bidders-fail-to-see-value-in-3m-emerald-spectacles-ws0gkdsp3 Accessed 24 May 2022.

https://www.sothebys.com/en/buy/auction/2021/arts-of-the-islamic-world-india-including-fine-rugs-and-carpets-2/a-pair-of-mughal-spectacles-set-with-emerald Accessed 24 May 2022.

Printed sources

D'Abano, Pietro. 1520. *Conciliator differentiarum philosophorum [et] medicorum*. Place of publication and publisher not indicated.

D'Abano, Pietro. 1537. *De venenis, atque eorundem commodis remediis. Liber plane aureus, per Joannem Dryandrum medicum pristino suo nitori restitutus* Marpurgi: ex officina Eucharium Ceruicorni Agrippinatis.

Agricola, Georgius. 1546. *Georgii Agricolae De ortu et causis subterraneorum, lib. V. De natura eorum quæ effluunt ex terra, lib. IV. De natura fossilium, lib. X. De ueteribus et nouis metallis, lib. II. Bermannus, siue de re metallica dialogus. Interpretatio germanica uocum rei metallicæ, addito indice foendissimo*. Basileae: Per Hieronymvm Frobenivm et Nic. Bischoff.

Ahmad, Sayeed, Rehman, Shabana, Ahmad, M. Aftab, Siddiqui, Khalid M., Shaukat, Seemin, Khan, Masood Shah, Kamal Y. T., & Jahangir, Tamanna. 2010. "Khamiras, a natural cardiac tonic: An overview". *Journal of Pharmacy and Bioallied Sciences*, 2 (2): 93-99.

Amar, Zohar & Lev, Ephraim. 2017. "Most-Cherished Gemstones in the Medieval Arab World". *Journal of the Royal Asiatic Society,* [3] 27 (3): 377-401.

Anonymous. 1528. *Here begynneth a lytell boke of the .xxiiii. stones pryncipalles / that profyteth most to mans body/ as the day & the nyght hath .xxiiii. hours/ so be there .xxiiii. stones pryncipall*. [London: R. Pynson] And be for to sell at the Sygne of seynt Iohn Euangelyst, in seynt Martyns parisshe besyde charynge Crosse.

Anonymous. 1664. *The method of chemical philosophie and physick. Being a brief introduction to the one, and a true discovery of the other. namely, of diseases, their qualities, causes, symptoms, and certain cures. The like never before extant in English*. London: printed by J.G. for Nath: Brook, at the Angel in Cornhill.

Anonymous. 1685. *The Magick of Kirani, King of Persia, and of Harpocration containing the magical and medicinal vertues of stones, herbes, fishes, beasts, and birds : a work much sought for by the learned but seen by few : said to have been in the Vatican-Library in Rome but not to be found there nor in all the famous libraries of the empire / now published and translated into English from a copy found in a private hand*. [London]: [W. Cooper].

Ardakani, Mohammad Reza Shams, Farjadmand, Fatemeh, & Rahimi, Roja. 2018. "Makhzan al Adviyeh and Pointing to the Scientific Names of Medicinal Plants for the First Time in a Persian Book". *Traditional and Integrative Medicine,* 3 (4): 186-195.

Aslam, M., Davis, S.S. & Healy, M.A. 1979. "Heavy Metals in Some Asian Medicines and Cosmetics". *Public Health,* 93 (5): 274-284.

Babb, Lawrence A. 2013. *Emerald City. The Birth and Evolution of an Indian Gemstone Industry*. New York: SUNY Press.

Bacon, Francis. 1638. *The historie of life and death With observations naturall and experimentall for the prolonging of life*. London: Printed by I. Okes, for Humphrey Mosley, at the Princes Armes in Pauls Church-Yard.

Bahler, Ingrid & Gatto, Katherine Gyékényesi. 1997. *The Lapidary of King Alfonso X The Learned*. New Orleans: University Press of the South.

Bandy, Mark Chance & Bandy, Jean A. 1955. *De Natura Fossilium (Textbook of Mineralogy) by Georgius Agricola*. The Geological Society of America, Boulder, CO, Special Papers, 63 [Dover reprint 2004].

Banister, John. 1575. *A needefull, new, and necessarie treatise of chyrurgerie briefly comprehending the generall and particuler curation of vlcers, drawen foorth of sundrie worthy wryters, but especially of Antonius Calmeteus Vergesatus, and Ioannes Tagaltius, by Iohn Banister ... Hereunto is anexed certaine experiments of mine ovvne inuention, truely tried, and daily of me practised*. London: By Thomas Marshe.

Barney, Stephen A., Lewis, W. J., Beach, J. A. & Berghof, Oliver. 2006. *The Etymologies of Isidore of Seville*. Cambridge: Cambridge University Press.

Barroso, Maria do Sameiro. 2017. "Malachite, the Healing Gem of Green Nature". *Vesalius*, 23 (1): 99-107.

Barroso, Maria do Sameiro. 2018. "Amber: Some Portuguese Artifacts and Costliest Recipes". 75-79 *In* Polyakova, Irina, Duffin, Christopher John & Suvorova, Tatiana J. (eds.) *Amber in the history of medicine: Proceedings of the International Conference*. Kaliningrad: Kaliningrad Regional Amber Museum [dated 2016].

Barroso, Maria do Sameiro. 2019. "The Touch of Health - The Lapidarius in Peter of Spain's Treasure of the Poor". *Vesalius*, 25 (2): 6-17.

Barroso, Maria do Sameiro. 2021. "The Goa Stone: Myths, Empiricism and Insights on Chemistry". Vesalius, 26 (1): 36-60 (e-supplement).

Barroso, Maria do Sameiro. 2022 (this volume). "History of Spectacles-A Collection from the Museum of Aveiro".

Batman, Stephen. 1582. *Batman Vppon Bartholome, his Booke De Proprietatibus Rerum, Newly corrected, enlarged and amended: With such Additions as are requisite, vnto euery severall Booke: Taken foorth of the most approued Authors, the like heretofore not translated in English. Profitable for all Estates, as well as for the benefit of the Mind and the Bodie*. London: Thomas East. [Georg Olms Reprint 1976].

Beauvais, Vincent de. 1478? *Speculum Naturale*. Strassburg: The R-Printer (Adolph Rusch).

Bela, Zbigniew. 2016. "The Authorship of the *Secrets of Alexis Piedmont* (Venice, 1555)". *Kwartalnik Historii Nauki i Techniki*, 61 (1): 53–73.

Bogdasarov A.A. & Bogdasarov M.A. Amber derivatives in medicine: Historical Background. In: *Amber in the History of Medicine.* Polyakova, Irina, Duffin, Christopher John, & Suvorova, T. J. (Eds). Kaliningrad: Regional Museum, 2016, 16-23.

Bowersox, Gary, Snee, Lawrence W., Foord, Eugene E. & Seal, Robert R. II. 1991. "Emeralds of the Panjshir Valley, Afghanistan". *Gems and Gemology,* Spring 1991; 26-39.

Boxer, C.R. 1963. *Two pioneers of tropical medicine: Garcia d'Orta and Nicolás Monardes*. [London]: [Hispanic & Luso-Brazilian Councils].

Brasavolus, Antonio Musa. 1536. *Examen omnium simplicium medicamentorum, quorum in officinis usus est.* Place of publication not indicated: A. Bladus de Asula.

Brigo, Francesco, Trinka, Eugen, Brigo, Bruno, Bragazzi, Nicola Luigi, Ragnedda, Giammario, Nardone, Raffaele & Mariano Martini. 2018. "Epilepsy in Hildegard of Bingen's writings: A comprehensive overview". *Epilepsy & Behavior,* 80: 135-143.

Bruce-Chwatt, Leonard Jan. 1983. "George Bate—Cromwell's Devious Physician". *Journal of the Royal College of Physicians of London*, 17 (2): 144-146.

Bullein, William. 1579. *Bulleins bulwarke of defence against all sicknesse, soarenesse, and vvoundes that doe dayly assaulte mankinde: which bulwarke is kept with Hilarius the gardener, [and] Health the phisicion, with the chirurgian, to helpe the wounded soldiours. Gathered and practised from the most worthy learned, both olde and new: to the great comfort of mankinde.* London: By Thomas Marshe, dwellinge in Fleetestreate neare vnto Saincte Dunstanes Church.

Burnet, Thomas. 1673. *Thesaurus medicinæ practicæ expræstantissimorum tum veterum tum recentiorum medicorum observationibus, consultationibus, consiliis & epistolis : summa diligentia collectus ordineq, alphabetico dispositus.* London: excudebat G. R. pro Roberto Boulter

Caley, Earle Radcliffe C. & Richards, John F.C. 1956. *Theophrastus On Stones. Introduction, Greek Text, English Translation and Commentary.* Columbus: Ohio State University.

Charas, Moyse. 1678. *The Royal Pharmacopoea, Galenical and Chymical, According to the practice of the Most Eminent and Learned Physitians of France, And Publish'd with their several Approbations. By Moses Charas, the Kings Chief Operator in his Royal Garden of Plants.* London: John Starkey.

Clément Mullet, Jean-Jacques. 1868. *Essai sur la Minéralogie Arabe*. Paris: Imprimerie Impériale.

Cohn, Ferdinand. 1891. "Scholz von Rosenau, Laurentius". *Allgemeine Deutsche Biographie,* 32: 229-230.

Croll, Oswald. 1670. *Bazilica chymica, & Praxis chymiatricæ, or, Royal and practical chymistry in three treatises : wherein all those excellent medicines and chymical preparations are fully discovered, from whence all our modern chymists have drawn their choicest remedies : being a translation of Oswald Crollius, his Royal chymistry, augmented and inlarged by John Hartman : to which is added his Treatise of signatures of internal things, or, A true and lively anatomy of the greater and lesser world : as also, The practice of chymistry of John Hartman, M.D., augmented and inlarged by his son / all faithfully Englished by a lover of chymistry.* London: Printed for John Starkey at the Mitre in Fleetstreet near Temple-Bar, and Thomas Passinger at the Three Bibles on London-Bridge.

Cuba, Johannes de. 1491. *Hortus Sanitatis.* Mainz: Jacob Meydenbach.

Cuba, Johannes de. 1536. *Hortus Sanitatis.* Strasbourg: Matthias Apiarius.

Cullen, William. 1772. *Lectures on the materia medica, / as delivered by William Cullen, M. D. Professor of Medicine in the University of Edinburgh: And now printed from a correct copy, which has been compared with others by the editors.* London: Printed for T. Lowndes, in Fleet-street.

Culpeper, Nicolas. 1649. *A physicall directory, or, A translation of the London dispensatory made by the Colledge of Physicians in London.* London: Printed for Peter Cole and are to be sold at his shop.

Culpeper, Nicolas. 1653. *Pharmacopœia Londinensis, or, The London dispensatory further adorned by the studies and collections of the Fellows, now living of the said colledg*. London: Printed for Peter Cole.

Culpeper, Nicolas. 1654. *A new method of physick: or, A short view of Paracelsus and Galen's practice; in 3. treatises. I. Opening the nature of physick and alchymy. II. Shewing what things are requisite to a physitian and alchymist. III. Containing an harmonical systeme of physick. Written in Latin by Simeon Partlicius, phylosopher, and physitian in Germany.* London: Printed by Peter Cole in Leaden-Hall, and are to be sold at his shop at the sign of the Printing-press in Cornhil neer the Royal Exchange: And by S. Howes, J. Garfield, and R. Westbrook.

Culpeper, Nicolas. 1659. *Culpeper's school of physick, or, The experimental practice of the whole art wherein are contained all inward diseases from the head to the foot, with their proper and effectuall cures, such diet set down as ought to be observed in sickness or in health: with other safe wayes for preserving of life*. London: Printed for N. Brook.

Cunha, João Teles e. 2001. "Hunting Riches: Goa's Gem Trade in the Early Modern Age". 269-304 *In* Malekandathil, Pius & Mohammed, T. Jamal (eds.), *The Portuguese, Indian Ocean and European Bridgeheads: Festschrift in Honour of Prof. K.S. Mathew.* Kannur: Institute for Research in Social Sciences and Humanities & Fundacão Oriente.

Dall, Lawrence & Stanford James F. 1990. "Fever, Chills, and Night Sweats". *In* Walker HK, Hall WD, Hurst JW (editors): *Clinical Methods: The History, Physical, and Laboratory Examinations.* 3rd edition. Boston: Butterworths.

Dirlam, Dona Mary, Rogers, Chris L., & Weldon, Robert. 2019. "Gemstones in the Era of the Taj Mahal and the Mughals." *Gems & Gemology,* 55 (3): 294-319.

Drage, William. 1664. *A physical nosonomy, or, A new and true description of the law of God (called nature) in the body of man confuting by many and undeniable experiences of many men, the rules and methods concerning sicknesses or changes in mans body, delivered by the ancient physicians and moderns that followed them ... : also, in the second part of this book is a practice of physick drawn from the best of the moderns and completely treating of those diseases specified in the table formerly, writ by the author, though added to these new scrutinies as if they were a latter work*. London: Printed by J. Dover, for the author, 1664.

Duffin, Christopher John. 2006. "Silicate Minerals. An Overview". *British Micromount Society Occasional Papers*, 1-38.

Duffin, Christopher John. 2007a. "Fish Otoliths and Folklore: A Survey".

Folklore, 118: 78-90.
Duffin, Christopher John. 2007b. "Alectorius: The Cock's Stone". *Folklore*, 118: 325-341.
Duffin, Christopher John. 2008. "Fossils as drugs: pharmaceutical palaeontology". *Ferrantia*, 54: 1-83.
Duffin, Christopher John. 2010a. "Lapis de Goa: the 'Cordial Stone'". *Pharmaceutical Historian,* 40 (2): 22-32.
Duffin, Christopher John. 2010b. "Lapis de Goa: the 'Cordial Stone'-Part Two". *Pharmaceutical Historian,* 40 (3): 42-46.
Duffin, Christopher John. 2012. "A Survey of birds and fabulous stones". *Folklore*, 123 (2): 179-197.
Duffin, Christopher John. 2013a. "Lithotherapeutical research sources from antiquity to the mid-18th century". *In* Duffin, Christopher John, Moody, Richard T.J. & Gardner-Thorpe, Christopher (eds.) *A History of Geology and Medicine.* Geological Society of London Special Publication, 375: 7-43.
Duffin, Christopher John. 2013b. "The Gem Electuary". *In* Duffin, Christopher John, Moody, Richard T.J. & Gardner-Thorpe, Christopher (eds.) *A History of Geology and Medicine.* Geological Society of London Special Publication, 375: 81-111.
Duffin, Christopher John. 2013c. "Some early Eighteenth Century geological Materia Medica". *In* Duffin, Christopher John, Moody, Richard T.J. & Gardner-Thorpe, Christopher (eds.) *A History of Geology and Medicine.* Geological Society of London Special Publication, 375: 209-233.
Duffin, Christopher John. 2013d. "Porcupine Stones". *Pharmaceutical Historian*, 43 (1): 13-22.
Duffin, Christopher John. 2013e. "History of the external pharmaceutical use of Amber". *Pharmaceutical Historian,* 43 (3): 46-53.
Duffin, Christopher John. 2014. "The pharmaceutical use of lapis lazuli in the Ancient East". *Pharmaceutical Historian*, 44 (4): 84-87.
Duffin, Christopher John. 2015a. "Pharmaceutical lore in the Lapidary of Sidrac (13th century)". *Pharmaceutical Historian,* 45 (4): 90-96.
Duffin, Christopher John. 2015b. "Historical survey of the internal use of unprocessed amber". *Acta medico-historica Adriatica*, 13 (1): 41-74.
Duffin, Christopher John. 2016. "Nathaniel Hodges (1629-1688), Plague doctor". *Journal of Medical Biography,* 24 (1): 30-35.
Duffin, Christopher John. 2017. "'Fish', fossils and fakes: medicinal unicorn horn". *In* Duffin, C.J., Gardner-Thorpe, C. & Moody, R.T.J. (eds) *Geology and Medicine: Historical Connections.* Geological Society of London Special Publication, 452: 211-259.

Duffin, Christopher John. 2018. "A Dwarf on Giant's shoulders: Sir John Hill and Geology". *In* Brant, C, & Rousseau, G. (eds.) *Fame & Fortune: Sir John Hill and London Life in the 1750s.* London: Palgrave, 2018: 243-265.

Duffin, Christopher John. 2019. "British Eighteenth Century Materia Medica Collections". 105-125 *In* Polyakova, I.A., Duffin, C.J., & Suvorova, T.J. (eds.): *Collection in the Space of Culture.* Kaliningrad, Kaliningrad Regional Amber Museum.

Duffin, Christopher John. 2020a. "Medicinal Quartz: *Crystallus* or Rock Crystal". 162-204 *In* Barroso, M. Sameiro do, Duffin, C.J. & Sousa, G. de (eds.): *Medical Heritage of the National Palace of Mafra.* Cambridge: Cambridge Scholars.

Duffin, Christopher John. 2020b. "Fifteenth century magico-medicinal minerals". *Deposits Magazine.* https://depositsmag.com/2020/05/30/fifteenth-century-magico-medicinal-minerals/

Duffin, Christopher John. 2022. "The Margrave Anti-epileptic Powder". *Pharmaceutical Historian,* **52** (1): 1-15.

Eamon, William 1994. *Science and the Secrets of Nature: Books of Secrets in Medieval and Early Modern Culture.* Princeton: Princeton University Press.

Eden, Rycharde. 1553. *A treatyse of the newe India with other new founde landes and islandes*. London: In Lombard strete, by [S. Mierdman for] Edward Sutton.

Ettmüller, Michael. 1699. *Etmullerus abridg'd: or, A compleat system of the theory and practice of physic. Being a description of all diseases incident to men, women and children. With an account of their causes, symptoms, and most approved methods of cure, physical and chirurgical. To which is prefix'd a short view of the animal and vital functions; and the several vertues and classes of med'cines. Translated from the last edition of the works of Michael Etmullerus, late professor of physic in the University of Leiptsich*. London: printed for E. Harris, at the Harrow in Little-Britain, F. Hubbard, next door to the Crown Tavern in Duck Lane, and A. Bell, at the Cross Keys and Bible in Cornhill, near Stocks-Market.

Evans, Joan & Serjeantson, Mary S. 1933. *English Medieval Lapidaries.* London: Early English Text Society, Original Text Series 190 [EETS reprint 1960].

Fèbure, Nicolas le. *A compendious body of chymistry, which will serve as a guide and introduction both for understanding the authors which have treated of the theory of this science in general and for making the way plain and easie to perform, according to art and method, all operations, which teach the practise of this art, upon animals, vegetables, and minerals, without losing any of the essential vertues contained in them.* London: printed for Tho. Davies and Theo. Sadler, and is to be sold at the sign of the Bible over against the little North-door of St. Pauls-Church, 1662.

Ficalho, Francisco Manuel de Melo Breyner, count de. 1886. *Garcia de Orta e o seu tempo.* Lisboa: Imprensa Nacional.

Führer, H. 1956. *Lithotherapie. Historische Studien über die medizinische Verwendung der Edelsteine*. Ulm: Karl F. Haug Verlag.

Gaule, John. 1657. *A collection out of the best approved authors containing histories of visions, apparitions, prophesies, spirits, divinations and other wonderful illusions of the devil wrought by magic or otherwise: also of divers astrological predictions shewing as the wickedness of the former, so the vanity of the latter, and the folly of trusting to them.* London: Printed for Joshua Kirton.

Gibbs, Frederick W. 2019. *Poison, Medicine and Disease in Late Medieval and Early Modern Europe.* London & New York: Routledge.

Giuliani, Gaston & Groat, Lee A. 2019. "Geology of Corundum and Emerald Gem Deposits: A Review". *Gems & Gemology*, Winter 2019: 464-489.

Giuliani, Gaston, Groat, Lee A., Marshall, Dan, Fallick, Anthony E. & Branquet, Yannick. 2019. "Emerald Deposits: A Review and Enhanced classification". *Minerals*, 2019 (9): 105: 1-63.

Golding, Arthur. 1587. *The excellent and pleasant worke of Iulius Solinus Polyhistor. Contayning the noble actions of humaine creatures, the secretes & prouidence of nature, the description of Countries, the maners of the people: with many meruailous things and strange antiquities, seruing for the benefitt and recreation of all sorts of persons.* London: Printed by I. Charlewoode for Thomas Hacket.

Gunnoe, Charles D. 2019. "Paracelsus, the Plague, and De Pestilitate". *Early Science and Medicine,* 24: 504-526.

Hamiduddin, Siddiqui, M.A., Ali, Waris, Jahangeer, Gazi & Akhter Al. 2019. "Unani formulations for management of diabetes: An overview". *International Journal of Green Pharmacy,* 12 (4):769-783.

Harrell, James A. 2004. "Archaeological Geology of the World's First Emerald Mine". *Geoscience Canada*, 31 (2): 69-76.

Harris, Nichola Erin. 2009. *The Idea of Lapidary Medicine: Its Circulation and Practical Applications in Medieval and Early Modern England: 1000-1750.* Unpublished Ph.D. Thesis, Rutgers, the State University of New Jersey.

Harvey, Gideon. 1689. *The art of curing diseases by expectation with remarks on a supposed great case of apoplectick fits: also most useful observations on coughs, consumptions, stone, dropsies, fevers, and small pox: with a confutation of dispensatories, and other various discourses in physick*. London: Printed for James Partridge.

Hedesan, Georgiana D. 2018. "Alchemy, Potency, imagination. Paracelsus's theories of poison". 81-202 *In* Grell, Ole Peter, Cunningham, Andrew and Arrizabalaga, Jon (eds) *"It all Depends on the Dose". Poisons and Medicines in European History.* London and New York: Routledge.

Helmont, Jean Baptist van. 1664. *Van Helmont's works containing his most excellent philosophy, physick, chirurgery, anatomy: wherein the philosophy of the schools is examined, their errors refuted, and the whole body of physick reformed and rectified: being a new rise and progresse of philosophy and medicine, for the cure of diseases, and lengthening of life*. London: Printed for Lodowick Hoyd at the Castle *in* Cornhill.

Hill, John. 1751. *A History of the Materia Medica. Containing Descriptions of all the Substances Used in Medicine, Their Origin, Their Characters When in Perfection, the Signs of Their Decay, Their Chymical Analysis and an Account of Their Virtues, and of the Several Preparations from Them Now Used in the Shops.* London: T. Longman, C. Hitch and L. Hawes.

Holland, Philemon. 1634. *The historie of the vvorld: commonly called, The naturall historie of C. Plinius Secundus*. Volume 2. London: Printed by Adam Islip.

Holmes, Urban T. 1934. "Mediaeval Gem Stones". *Isis,* 9 (2): 195-204.

Huda, Samar Najm Abul.1998. *Arab Roots of Gemmology. Ahmad ibn Yusuf Al Tifaschi's Best Thoughts on the Best of Stones*. Lanham, MD & London: The Scarecrow Press.

Jessen, Carolus. 1867. *Alberti Magni ex ordine praedicatorum De Vegetabilibus Libri VII, Historiae Naturalis pars XVIII.* Berolini: Typis et impensis Georgii Reimeri.

Jonstonus, Johannes. 1657. *An history of the wonderful things of nature set forth in ten severall classes wherein are contained I. The wonders of the heavens, II. Of the elements, III. Of meteors, IV. Of minerals, V. Of plants, VI. Of birds, VII. Of four-footed beasts, VIII. Of insects, and things wanting blood, IX. Of fishes, X. Of man / written by Johannes Jonstonus, and now rendred into English by a person of quality*. London: Printed by John Streater and are to be sold by the Booksellers of London.

Keller, Peter C. 1981. “Emeralds of Colombia”. *Gems and Gemology.* Summer 1981; 80-92.

Kemp, William. 1665. *A brief treatise of the nature, causes, signes, preservation from, and cure of the pestilence collected by W. Kemp.* London: Printed for and are to be sold by D. Kemp at his shop.

Khan, Didier. 2020. “De Pestilitate and Paracelsian Cosmology”. *Daphnis - Zeitschrift für Mittlere Deutsche Literatur und Kultur der Frühen Neuzeit*, 48 (1-2):65-86.

King, Charles William. 1860. *Antique Gems: Their Origin, Uses and Value as Interpreters of Ancient History; and as Illustrative of Ancient Art: With Hints to Gem Collectors*. London: John Murray.

Klein-Franke, Felix. 1970. “The Knowledge of Aristotle’s Lapidary during the Latin Middle Ages”. *Ambix*, 17 (3): 137-142.

Kunz, George Frederick. 1913. *The Curious Lore of Precious Stones, Being a Description of their Sentiments and Folk Lore, Superstitions, Symbolism, Mysticism, use in Medicine, Protection, Prevention, Religion, and Divination, Crystal Gazing, Birthstones, Lucky Stones and Talismans, Astral, Zodiacal and Planetary*. Philadelphia: Lippincott. [Dover reprint, 1971].

Kunz, George Frederick. 1915. *The Magic of Jewels and Charms*. Philadelphia: Lippincott. [Dover reprint, 1997].

Lecouteux, Claude. 2011. *Dictionnaire des Pierres Magiques et Médicinales*. Paris: Imago.

Leonardus, Camillus. 1502. *Speculum lapidum*. Venice: J. B. Sessa.

Leonardus, Camillus. 1750. *The Mirror of Stones; in Which the Nature, Generation, Properties, Virtues and Various Species of More Than 200 Different Jewels, are Distinctly Described. Also Certain and Infallible Rules to Know the Good from the Bad, How to Prove Their Genuineness, and to Distinguish the Real from the Couterfeit. Extracted from the works of Aristotle, Pliny, Isiodorus, Dionysius Alexandrinus, Albertus Magnus etc*. London: J. Freeman [Metatron reprint 1983].

Lier, Hermann Arthur.1898. "Wirsung, Christoph". *Allgemeine Deutsche Biographie,* 43: 521.

Lonicer, Adam. 1679. *Kreuterbuch, Kunstliche Conterfeytunge der Bäume, Stauden, Hecken, Kräuter, Getreyde, Gewürtze: Mit eigentlicher Beschreibung derselben Namen, in sechserley Spraachen, Nemblich Griechisch, Lateinisch, Italiänisch, Frantzösisch, Teutsch, und Hispanisch, und derselben Gestalt, natürlicher Krafft und Wirckung.* Ulm: Matthäus Wagner. [1962 reprint by Verlag Konrad Kölbl, München].

Loureiro, Rui Manuel. 2008. "Garcia de Orta e os Colóquios dos simples: Observações de um viajante sedentário". *In Garcia de Orta e Alexander von Humboldt: Errâncias, Investigações e Diálogo entre Culturas*, edited by Gabriela Fragoso & Anabela Mendes. Lisbon: Universidade Católica Editora, 135-145.

Loureiro, Rui Manuel. 2013. "Enter the Milanese lapidary: Precious stones in Garcia de Orta's *Coloquios dos simples e drogas he cousas medicinais da India* (Goa, 1563)". *Journal of History of Science and Technology*, 8: 29-47.

Lovell, Robert. 1661. *Panzooryktologia. Sive Panzoologicomineralogia. Or A compleat history of animals and minerals, containing the summe of all authors, both ancient and modern, Galenicall and chymicall, touching animals, viz. beasts, birds, fishes, serpents, insects, and man, as to their place, meat, name, temperature, vertues, use in meat and medicine, description, kinds, generation, sympathie, antipathie, diseases, cures, hurts, and remedies &c. With the anatomy of man, his diseases, with their definitions, causes, signes, cures, remedies: and use of the London dispensatory, with the doses and formes of all kinds of remedies: as also a history of minerals, viz. earths, mettals, semimettals, their naturall and artificiall excrements, salts, sulphurs, and stones, with their place, matter, names, kinds, temperature, vertues, use, choice, dose, danger, and antidotes. Also an [brace] introduction to zoography and mineralogy. Index of Latine names, with their English names. Universall index of the use and vertues*. Oxford: Printed by Hen: Hall, for Jos: Godwin.

Magnus, Albertus. 1476. *De Mineralibus Libri*. Petrus Maufer for Antonius de Albricis, Patavii, unpaginated.

Magnus, Albertus. 1560. *The boke of secretes of Albertus Magnus of the vertues of herbes, stones, and certayne beasts: also, a boke of the same author, of the maruaylous thinges of the world, and of certaine effectes caused of certaine beastes,* Place of publication and publisher not indicated.

Mayor, Adrienne & Heaney, Michael. 1993. "Griffins and Arimaspeans", *Folklore*, 104: 40–66.

McMath, James. 1694. *The expert mid-wife a treatise of the diseases of women with child, and in child-bed: as also, of the best ways and means of help in natural and unnatural labours. With fit remedies for the various maladies of new born babes. A work more full than any yet extant: and most necessar [sic] for all bearing women, mid-wifes, and others that practise this art.* Edinburgh: printed by George Mosman, and are to be sold at his shop in the Parliament Closs.

Meadows, J.W. 1945. "Pliny on the Smaragdus". *The Classical Review,* 59 (2): 50-51.

Mesuë, Johannes. 1497. *Canones Universales*. Venetijs: de Gregorijs.

Midgely, Robert. 1686. *A guide to the practical physician shewing, from the most approved authors, both ancient and modern, the truest and safest way of curing all diseases, internal and external, whether by medicine, surgery, or diet. Published in Latin by the learn'd Theoph. Bonet, physician at Geneva. And now rendred into English, with an addition of many considerable cases, and excellent medicines for every disease. Collected from Dr. Waltherus his Sylva medica. by one of the Colledge of Physicians, London. To which is added. The office of a physician, and perfect tables of every distemper, and of any thing else considerable.* London: printed for Thomas Flesher, at his house over against Distaff Lane in the Old Change.

Monardes, Nicolás. 1580. *Ioyfull newes out of the newfound world wherein are declared the rare and singular vertues of diuers and sundrie herbs, trees, oyles, plants, [and] stones, with their applications, aswell to the vse of phisicke, as chirurgery: which being wel applied, bring such present remedy for all diseases, as may seeme altogether incredible: notwithstanding by practize found out, to be true. Also the portrature of the sayde herbes, very aptly described: Englished by Iohn Frampton merchant. Newly corrected as by conference with the olde copies may appeare. Wherevnto are added three other bookes treating of the Bezaar stone, the herbe escuerçonera, the properties of yron and steele, in medicine and the benefite of snowe.* London: In Paules Churchyard at the signe of the Quenes Armes, by [Thomas Dawson for] William Norton.

Montaña, J. (ed.) 1881. *Lapidario del Rey. Alfonso. Códice original.* Madrid: J. Blasco.

Morales, Gaspar de. 1605. *Libro de las virtudes y propiedades marauillosas de las piedras preciosas.* Madrid: Luis Sanchez.

Münster, Sebastian. 1544. *Cosmographia: Beschreibung aller Lender durch Sebastianum Munsterum.* Basel: Getruckt durch Henrichum Petri.

Muntner, Suessman. 1966. *The Medical Writings of Moses Maimonides Volume Two. Treatise on Poisons and Their Antidotes.* Philadelphia and Montreal: J. B. Lippincott Company.

Mynsicht, Adrian von. 1682. *Thesaurus & armamentarium medico-chymicum, or, A treasury of physick with the most secret way of preparing remedies against all diseases: obtained by labour, confirmed by practice, and published out of good will to mankind: being a work of great use for the publick.* London: Printed by J.M. for Awnsham Churchill.

Newton, Thomas. 1580. *Approoved medicines and cordiall receiptes with the natures, qualities, and operations of sundry samples. Very commodious and expedient for all that are studious of such knowledge.* London: In Fleete-streete by Thomas Marsh.

Nicols, Thomas. 1652. *A lapidary, or, The history of pretious stones with cautions for the undeceiving of all those that deal with pretious stones.* Cambridge: Thomas Buck.

Orta, Garcia da. 1534. *Colóquios dos simples e drogas he cousas medicinais da Índia e assi dalgũas frutas achadas nella onde se tratam algũas cousas tocantes a medicina, pratica, e outras cousas boas pera saber.* Goa: Ioannes de Endem.

Orta, Garcia da. 1913. *Colloquies on the Simples & Drugs of India*. London: Henry Southeran & Co.

Otlewska, Magdalena. 2012. "Traktat "De lapidibus" - o kamieniach Hildegardy z Bingen". *Ogrody nauk i sztuk* nr 2012 (2): 315-323.

Paracelsus (Philippus Aureolus Theophrastus Bombastus von Hohenheim). 1660. *Paracelsus, his Archidoxis comprised in ten books: disclosing the genuine way of making quintessences, arcanums, magisteries, elixirs, &c: together with his books of renovation & restauration, of the tincture of the philsophers, of the manual of the philosophical medicinal stone, of the virtues of the members, of the three principles, and finally his seven books of the degrees and compositions, of receipts and natural things.* London: Printed for W.S. and are to be sold by Thomas Brewster.

Paré, Ambroise. 1634. *The workes of that famous chirurgion Ambrose Parey translated out of Latine and compared with the French*. London: Printed by Th: Cotes and R. Young.

Pazzini, A. 1939. *Le Pietre Preziose nella Storia della Medicina e nella Leggenda*. Roma: Casa Editrice Mediterranea.

Pechey, John. 1694. *The London dispensatory, reduced to the practice of the London physicians wherein are contain'd the medicines, both Galenical and chymical, that are now in use*. London: Printed by F. Collins for J. Lawrence.

Phayre, Thomas. 1550. *The regiment of life, whereunto is added a treatise of the pestilence, with the boke of children, newly corrected and enlarged.* London: In fletestrete at the signe of the Sunne ouer against the condite, by Edwarde Whitchurche.

Pomet, Pierre. 1748. *A complete history of Drugs, written in French by Monsieur Pomet chief druggist to the late French King Lewis XIV, to which is added what is further observable on the same subject, from*

Messrs. Lemery, and Tournefort, divided into three classes, vegetable, animal and mineral; with their use in Physic, Chemistry, pharmacy, and several other arts. London: J. & J. Bonwicke, S. Birt, W. Parker, C. Hitch, and E. Wicksteed.

Psellus, Michael. 1745. *De lapidum virtutibus Graece ac Latine / cum notis Phil. Jac. Maussaci et Joan. Steph. Bernard. Accedit fragmentum de colore sanguinis, ex doctrina medica Persarum nunc primum ex codice MS. bibliothecae Lugduno Batavae editum.* Lugduni Batavorum: Philippum Bonk.

Pymm, Rachael Jane & Duffin, Christopher John. 2020. "Dragonstones: Myth, Magic, Medicine and Material Culture". 205-256 *In* Barroso, M. Sameiro do, Duffin, C.J. & Sousa, G. de (eds.): *Medical Heritage of the National Palace of Mafra*. Cambridge: Cambridge Scholars.

Raineri, Antonio. 1818. *Fior di pensieri sulle pietre preziose di Ahmed Teifascite. Opera Stampata nel suo originale arabo, colla traduzione italiana appresso, e diverse note.* Firenze: E. R. Tipografia Orientale Mediceo-Laurenziana.

Rankin, Alisha. 2021. *The Poison Trials. Wonder Drugs, Experiment, and the Battle for Authority in Renaissance Science.* Chicago and London: The University of Chicago Press.

Rattray, Sylvester. 1658. *Aditus novus ad occultas sympathiæ et antipathiæ causas inveniendas per principia philosophiæ naturalis, ex fermentorum artificiosâ anatomia hausta, patefactus.* Glasgow: Excudebat Andreas Anderson.

Renou, Jean de. 1657. *A medicinal dispensatory, containing the vvhole body of physick discovering the natures, properties, and vertues of vegetables, minerals, & animals: the manner of compounding medicaments, and the way to administer them. Methodically digested in five books of philosophical and pharmaceutical institutions; three books of physical materials galenical and chymical. Together with a most perfect and absolute pharmacopoea or apothecaries shop.* London: printed by Jo: Streater and Ja: Cottrel; and are to be sold by Henry Fletcher at the three gilt Cups neer the west-end of Pauls.

Reys, Aurélien. 2014. "La filière brésilienne des pierres gemmes « de couleur »". *Cahiers des Amériques latines*, 77: 161-178.

Rivière, Lazare. 1685. *The secrets of the famous Lazarus Riverius, councellor & physician to the French king, and professor of physick in the University of Montpelier newly translated from the Latin by E.P., M.D.* London: Printed for Daniel Brown.

Royal College of Physicians of London. 1618. *Pharmacopoeia Londinensis : in qua medicamenta antiqua et noua vsitatissima, sedulò collecta, accuratissime examinata, quotidianâ experientia confirmata describuntur. Diligenter reuisa, denuo recusa, emendatior auctior. Opera Medicorum Collegij Londinensis. Ex serenissimi Regis mandato cum R.M. priuilegio.* London: printed for Iohn Marriott and are to be sould at his shop in Fleetstreete.

Ruscelli, Girolamo. 1562. *The thyrde and last parte of the Secrets of the reuerende Maister Alexis of Piemont, by him collected out of divers excellent authours, with a necessary table in the ende, conteyning all the matters treated of in this present worke.* London: Roulande Hall, for Nycholas Englande.

Ruska, Julius. 1912 *Steinbuch des Aristoteles mit Literartgeschichtlichen Untersuchungen nach der Arabischen Handschrift der Bibliotheque Nationale*. Heidelberg: Carl Winter's Universitätsbuchhandlung.

Said, Hakim Mohammad. 1989. *Al-Beruni's Book on Mineralogy. The Book Most Comprehensive in Knowledge on Precious Stones*. Islamabad: Pakistan Hijra Council.

Salmon, William. 1681. *Iatrica, seu, Praxis medendi, The practice of curing being a medicinal history of above three thousand famous observations in the cure of diseases, performed by the author hereof: together with several of the choicest observations of other famous men ... : wherein for the most part you will find 1. the constitution of the body of the sick, 2. the symptoms predominant, 3. the cause of the disease, what? 4. the exact method which was taken in the cure, 5. an exact account of the medicines exhibited, with the order of their exhibition, various doses and success thereupon*. London: Printed for Th. Dawks and Langley Curtiss.

Salmon, William. 1681b. *Synopsis medicinæ. A Compendium of Physick, Chirurgery and Anatomy in IV. Books*. 2nd edition. London: Printed for Thomas Dawks.

Salmon, William. 1683. *Doron medicum, or, A supplement to the new London dispensatory in III books: containing a supplement I. to the materia medica, II. to the internal compound medicaments, III. to the external compound medicaments: compleated with the art of compounding medicines.* London: Printed for T. Dawks, T. Bassett, J. Wright and R. Chiswell.

Salmon, William. 1694. *Pharmacopœia Bateana, or, Bate's dispensatory translated from the second edition of the Latin copy, published by Mr. James Shipton : containing his choice and select recipe's, their names, compositions, preparations, vertues, uses, and doses, as they are applicable to the whole practice of physick and chyrurgery : the Arcana Goddardiana, and their recipe's intersperst in their proper places, which are almost all wanting in the Latin copy: compleated with above five hundred chymical processes, and their explications at large, various observations thereon, and a rationale upon each process: to which are added in this English edition, Goddard's drops, Russel's pouder, and the Emplastrum febrifugum, those so much fam'd in the world : as also several other preparations from the Collectanea chymica, and other good authors*. London: Printed for S. Smith and B. Walford.

Scholz, Lorenz. 1610. *Epistolarum philosophicarum: medicinalium ac chymicarum a summis nostrae aetatis philosophis ac medicis exaratarum volumen*. Hanoviae: Typis Wechelianus, apud haeredes Joannis Aubrii.

Sharp, Jane. 1671. *The midwives book, or, The whole art of midwifry discovered. Directing childbearing women how to behave themselves in their conception, breeding, bearing, and nursing of children in six books.* London: Printed for Simon Miller, at the Star at the West End of St. Pauls.

Sinkankas, John. 1981. *Emerald and Other Beryls*. Radnor: Chilton Book Company: 371-377.

Stange, Emil. 1905. *Die Enzyklopädie des Arnoldus Saxo, zum ersten mal nach einen Erfurter Codex.* Erfurt: Fr. Bartholomius.

Stillman, J.M. 1919. "Paracelsus as a Reformer in Medicine". *The Monist*, 29 (4): 526-546.

Sylvio, Jacobus. 1553. *Ioannis Mesuae Damasceni, De Re Medica Libri Tres*. Paris: Publisher not indicated.

Steinschneider, Moritz. 1895. "Arabische Lapidarien". *Zeitschrift der deutschen Morgenländischen Gesellschaft,* 49: 244-278.

Tahil, Patricia P. 1989. *De Virtutibus Lapidum: The Virtues of Stones Attributed to Damigeron*. Seattle: Ars Obscura.

Tanner, John. 1659. *The hidden treasures of the art of physick; fully discovered: in four books.* London: Printed for George Sawbridge, at the sign of the Bible on Lud-gate-Hill.

Temkin, Owsei. 1994. *The Falling Sickness. A History of Epilepsy from the Greeks to the beginnings of modern Neurology.* Baltimore and London: The Johns Hopkins University Press.

Thomson, George. 1666. *Loimotomia, or, The pest anatomized in these following particulars, Viz. 1. The material cause of the pest, 2. The efficient cause of the pest, 3. The subject part of the pest, 4. The signs of the pest, 5. An historical account of the dissections of a pestilential body by the author, and the consequences thereof, 6. Reflections and observations on the fore-said dissection, 7. Directions preservative and curative against the pest: together with the authors apology against the calumnies of the Galenists, and a word to Mr. Nath. Hodges, concerning his late Vindiciae medicinae*. London: Printed for Nath. Crouch.

Thorndike, Lynn. 1923a. *A History of Magic and Experimental Science during the first Thirteen Centuries of our Era. Volume 1*. New York and London: Columbia University Press.

Thorndike, Lynn. 1923b. *A History of Magic and Experimental Science during the first Thirteen Centuries of our Era. Volume 2*. New York and London: Columbia University Press.

Throop, Priscilla. (trans.). 1998. *Hildegard von Bingen's Physica. The Complete English Translation of Her Classic Work on Health and Healing*. Rochester: Healing Arts Press.

Throop, Priscilla. 2009. *Hrabanus Maurus. De Universo. The Peculiar Properties of Words and Their Mystical Significance, The Complete English Translation. Books XII–XXII. Volume 2*. Charlotte: Lulu.com.

Tommasi, Pietro. 1968. *Pietro Tommasi. Consilium de Universali Praeservatione contra venena. Traduzione e commento di Emanuele Djalma Vitali*. Roma: Istituto di Storia della Medicina dell'Università di Roma.

Turner, Robert. 1657. *The compleat bone-setter wherein the method of curing broken bones, and strains, and dislocated joynts, together with ruptures, vulgarly called broken bellyes, is fully demonstrated. Whereunto is added The perfect oculist, and The mirrour of health, treating of the pestilence, and all other diseases incident to men, women and children. Also, the acute judgement of urines. Written originally by Friar Moulton, of the Order of St. Augustine. Now revised, Englished and enlarged by Robert Turner philomathēs*. London: Printed by J.C. for Martha Harison, at the Lamb at the east-end of Pauls.

Vitet, Louis. 1778. *Pharmacopée de Lyon, ou Exposition méthodique des médicaments simples et composés, de leurs caracteres, de leurs vertus, de leur preparation et administration, et des espèces de maladies où ils sont indiqués*. Lyon: Frères Perisse.

Willis, Thomas. 1684. *An Essay of the Pathology of the Brain and Nervous Stock: in which Convulsive Diseases are Treated of*. London: Printed by A.M. and R.R. for T. Dring, J. Leigh and C. Harper.

W.J. 1665. *A collection of seven and fifty approved receipts good against the plague Taken out of the five books of that renowned Dr. Don Alexes secrets, for the benefit of the poorer sort of people of these nations*. London: printed by Peter Lillicrap, for John Wingfield at the Bible and Anchor in Tower-street near Mark-lane end.

Wirtzung, Christopher. 1605. *The general practise of physicke conteyning all inward and outward parts of the body, with all the accidents and infirmities that are incident vnto them, euen from the crowne of the head to the sole of the foote: also by what meanes (with the help of God) they may be remedied: very meete and profitable, not only for all phisitions, chirurgions, apothecaries, and midwiues, but for all other estates whatsoeuer; the like whereof as yet in english hath not beene published. Compiled and written by the most famous and learned doctour Christopher VVirtzung, in the Germane tongue, and now translated into English, in diuers places corrected, and with many additions illustrated and augmented, by Iacob Mosan Germane, Doctor in the same facultie.* London: [Printed by Richard Field] Impensis Georg. Bishop.

Woolley, Hannah. 1670. *The queen-like closet; or, Rich cabinet stored with all manner of rare receipts for preserving, candying & cookery. Very pleasant and beneficial to all ingenious persons of the female sex.* London: printed for R. Lowndes at the White Lion in Duck-Lane, near West-Smithfield.

Wyckoff, Dorothy. 1967. *Albertus Magnus Book of Minerals*. Oxford: Clarendon Press.

Yarwood, John. 1683. *Physick refin'd, or, A little stream of medicinal marrow flowing from the bones of nature wherein several signs, particular rules, and distinct symptoms whereby the most ordinary diseases may be distinctly known, and truly judged, are perspicuously delineated : and the most proper way, safe method, and simpathetical care, whereby nature may be helped, the sick eased, and languishing patients relieved (without the use of poysonous purging potions, and venomous medicaments) is succinctly demonstrated*. London: Printed for Tho. Passinger.

Zedler, Johann Heinrich. 1741. *Grosses vollständiges Universal-Lexicon aller Wissenschafften und Künste. Volume 29, Pr-Pz.* Leipzig & Halle: Verlegts Johann Heinrich Zedler.

Zedler, Johann Heinrich. 1743. *Grosses vollständiges Universal-Lexicon aller Wissenschafften und Künste. Volume 35, Schle-Schwa.* Leipzig & Halle: Verlegts Johann Heinrich Zedler.

CHAPTER 5

MEDICAL ASPECTS FROM POUSSIN'S PLAGUE

CARLOS LEMOS AND DANIEL NUNES

Abstract
Following an outbreak of bubonic plague epidemic in northern Italy, the French painter Nicolas Poussin (1594-1665) started a composition known as *The Plague of Ashdod*. The original canvas can be found in the Louvre Museum in Paris, and the other two replicas are located, respectively, in the National Gallery, in London, and the National Museum of Ancient Art, in Lisbon. This painting has become one of the most relevant plague representations, depicting an Old Testament episode from the First Book of Samuel (4-6): after defeating the Hebrews in the battle of Ebenezer, the Philistines captured the Ark of the Covenant, which was displayed as a trophy at the temple of Dagon, in the city of Ashdod. This sacrilege was punished by Yahweh, causing the shattering of Dagon's statue, the outbreak of a widespread disease and a scourge of rodents across Ashdod. Identifying the disease as bubonic plague, Poussin suggested a new reading of this biblical episode. At the same time, the presence of several rats in this seventeenth-century painting has sparked a debate on their significance since their role as bubonic plague reservoirs was not elucidated until the nineteenth century.
Key words: Plague; bubonic plague; Poussin; *Ashdod*; rats.

Resumo
Na sequência de uma epidemia de peste bubónica no norte da Itália, o pintor francês Nicolas Poussin (1594-1665) iniciou a composição de uma pintura conhecida como *A Peste de Ashdod*. O quadro original encontra-se no Museu do Louvre, em Paris, existindo duas réplicas localizadas, respetivamente, na *National Gallery*, em Londres, e no Museu Nacional de Arte Antiga, em Lisboa. Esta pintura tornou-se uma das representações mais relevantes da peste bubónica, recorrendo a um episódio do Antigo Testamento, retirado do Primeiro Livro de Samuel (4-6): após derrotar os

hebreus na batalha de *Ebenezer*, os filisteus capturaram a Arca da Aliança, que foi exibida como um troféu no templo de *Dagon*, na cidade de *Ashdod*. O sacrilégio seria punido por Yahweh, com a destruição da estátua de Dagon, e o aparecimento de um surto epidémico, com uma invasão de ratos na cidade de *Ashdod*. Ao identificar a doença com a peste bubónica, Poussin sugeriu uma nova leitura desse episódio bíblico. Ao mesmo tempo, a representação dos ratos nesta pintura do século XVII despertou um debate sobre seu significado, uma vez que seu papel de reservatório da doença apenas foi identificado no século XIX.
Palavras-chave: Peste; peste bubónica; Nicolas Poussin; *Ashdod*; ratos.

The Plague of Ashdod

Nicolas Poussin's painting *The Plague of Ashdod* (1630-31) depicts the outcome of the Philistines after placing the Ark of the Covenant at the temple of Dagon at Ashdod.

The Philistines were an ancient people who inhabited actual Palestine between 1175 and 800 BC (Sabbatani 2010, 200). According to the biblical text of the *First Book of Samuel* (4-6), after defeating the Hebrews in the Battle of Ebenezer (around 1050 BC), the Philistines captured the Ark of the Covenant, a gold-covered wooden chest containing the Ten Commandments and placed it as a trophy in the temple of the pagan god Dagon, in the city of Ashdod. Yahweh punished this sacrilege by causing the Dagon's statue to break down.

At the same time, the Philistines were struck by widespread disease and a plague of rodents. These punishments induced the victorious Philistines to restore give back the Ark of the Covenant to the Israelites, accompanied by the guilt offering of "five gold tumours and five golden rats", models of the pestilences afflicting the city.

In 1630, when Poussin started *The Plague of Ashdod*, northern Italy was afflicted by the plague epidemic. At that time, Poussin was living in Rome, where news of "miserable events and devastation of cities by the plague, with infinite hundreds or thousands of people dying every day" arrived incessantly, causing an exodus from the cities to the villages (Barker, 2004, 671).

Intensive measures were taken to prevent an outbreak, namely the creation of the Congregazione della Sanità in 1629, a health committee of noblemen, bureaucratic officials, scientists, doctors, and public administrators headed by Cardinal Francesco Barberini (1597-1679), one of Poussin's patrons.

The congregation convened twice a week to exchange medical expertise and implement strategies to impede the spread of the epidemic in the Papal States. This institution has become of paramount relevance for epidemiological surveillance in the early modern period. Serving as a member of the congregation was another of Poussin's patrons, Cassiano dal Pozzo (1588–1657), secretary of Cardinal Francesco Barberini. Given these circumstances, it is reasonable to conclude either that Poussin began his plague canvas for one of the members of the congregation, or that he began his work without a specific commission but had this particular circle of potential buyers in mind.

However, the disease ended up reaching Rome in 1656. Although many Romans flew from the city to escape death (as many as 16,000 Romans may have fled just in the summer of 1656), pope Alexander VII (Papacy from 1655 to 1667) remained at the Quirinal Palace, along with Cassiano dal Pozzo and Francesco Barberini, among other cardinals who served in the Congregazione della Sanità (Barker 2006, 244). In the canvas of *The Plague of Ashdod,* Poussin depicted these events as one scene (Fig. 5.1).

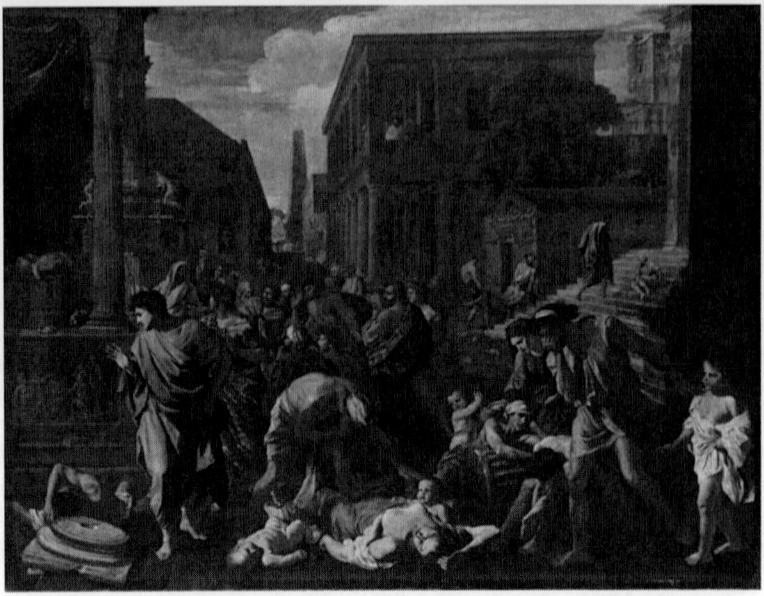

Fig. 5.1. Nicolas Poussin, The Plague of Ashdod, 1630-31, oil on canvas (148 x 198 cm). Courtesy of Louvre Museum, Paris.

The temple of Dagon is placed at the left, in the middle distance. The Ark seems suspended above its pedestal, and the Dagon statue lies on the ground with head and hands separated from the body. Rodents the size of large rats are visible on the statue's socle, in front of Dagon's temple and in the open spaces in the background. In the foreground, a boy, wearing a white tunic, advances resolutely from the far right. The figure matches Samuel's biblical description. A small figure seated on the stairs far at right must be Eli, the priest, hearing from a messenger the news of the lost battle and the capture of the Ark. A group of three men standing on the upper balcony witness the horror of the events taking place below. Actually, the painter has employed a complex use of space, combining various locations and different moments in the biblical episode. The change of space corresponds to a change in time, and each area is connected with a different event. This is partly due to the artist's experimental narrative style, which takes precedence over spatially integrated figures.

The Philistines' suffering has become one of the most appealing subjects of the painting: men, women and children lie on the ground, victims of the plague, while survivors exhibit several gestures of despair. To the left, a man regards with pity another squirming on the ground in agony. In the background, corpses of dead people are being carried away. A toddler, looking back, with his right arm upraised, cries to be carried away from the terrific scene. Broken columns everywhere heighten the atmosphere of death and destruction.

Poussin's depiction is in agreement with the biblical reference to a plague of "tumours in secret parts", since no tumours can be seen on the victims' bodies. Although the buboes of the plague are not visible in the picture, their painful presence can be intuited from the victims' postures: both the dead mother in the central foreground and the male victim to the far left have raised their right arm away from the body as if to avoid contact with the inflamed, tumescent, lymphatic axillary nodes. Artists had been using this gesture in plague imagery as a means of discreetly alluding to the presence of buboes (Barker 2004, 663). An example that confirms the association between the raised arm posture and the disease's clinical symptoms is Tintoretto's painting *Saint Roch Healing the Plague-Stricken* (Fig. 5.2).

The darkening of the victim's skin is detectable in the old woman who has collapsed against a fallen column, the deceased mother and infant in the foreground, and the male cadaver being carried away by two men in the middle ground at right. The young man in the right foreground, who feebly slumps over his knees, and the old woman slung over the broken column exhibit symptoms of exhaustion, often accompanied by fever. This old woman exhibits the so-called facies pestica, with eyes wide open and a terrified expression.

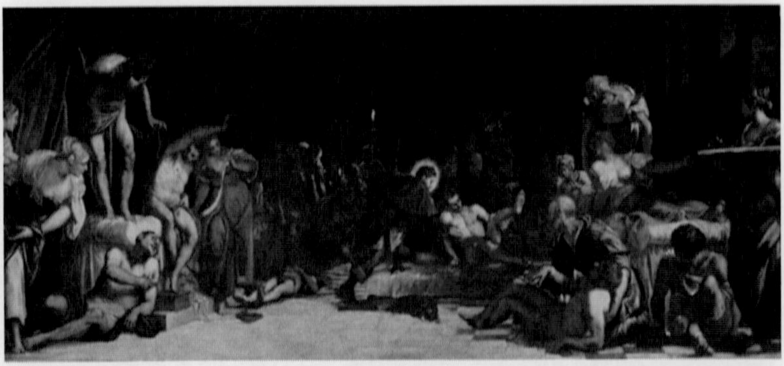

Fig. 5.2. Jacopo Tintoretto, St. Roch Healing the Plague-Stricken, 1549, oil on canvas 1549 (307 x 673 cm). Chiesa di San Rocco, Venice. Courtesy of Scuola Grande di San Rocco in Venice.

At the centre of the composition of *The Plague of Ashdod*, a dead woman lies in the foreground, with one child, also dead, at her side, and the other looking up while approaching the mother's breast. A man intervenes to save this child's life, jeopardizing his health by coming so close to the pestilential corpse of the mother. Holding his nose, he tries to protect himself from the contagion of the corpse's breath. This iconographical motif is borrowed from *The Plague of Phrygia*, known *as Il Morbetto* (c. 1512), an engraving by Marcantonio Raimondi (c.1482-c. 1534) (Fig. 5.3), following a drawing by the Italian painter Raphael Sanzio (1483-1520), illustrating a plague episode from the third book of Virgil's Aeneid (Boeckl 2000, 91-6).

This influence was highlighted by Giovanni Pietro Bellori (1613-1696), one of Poussin's first biographers, who remarked that *The Plague of Ashdod* "imitates, for the most part, Raphael's *Morbetto*, engraved by Marcantonio" (Bellori 1672, 416). This motif goes back to an ecphrasis by Pliny the Elder (c. 23-79), in his *Naturalis Historia,* describing a painting by the Greek painter Aristides of Thebes (4th century BC): he was the first of all the painters who captured and depicted the mind and expressed the feelings of a human being, what the Greeks called *ēthē,* and the emotions; he was a little too hard in his colours. His works include "on the capture of a town, showing an infant creeping to the breast of his mother who is dying of a wound; it is felt that the mother is aware of the child and is afraid that her milk is exhausted by death and it may suck blood (…)" (Pliny, *N. H.* Book 35, chapter 36, § 96 in Hendersen 1952, 333-335).

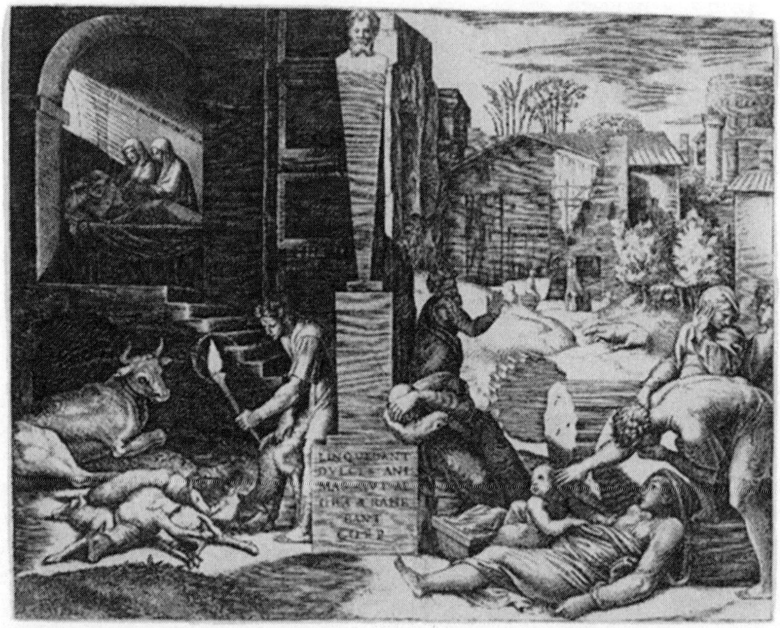

Fig. 5.3. Il Morbetto (The Plague of Phrygia), c. 1512, engraving (19.5 x 25.2cm). Courtesy of The National Gallery of Art, Washington.

Several other figures in the painting also pinch their noses or cover their faces, protecting themselves from the danger of breathing in the vicinity of putrefying corpses. Actually, the odours released were assumed to be the essence of the disease's poison and of death itself. The Florentine painter Giovanni Baldinucci (1577-1656) explained that during the Florentine plague of 1630, "the stench of the dead kills the living" (Barker 2004, 664). Pneumonic plague, or lung-based plague, may develop from inhaling infectious droplets or after untreated bubonic or septicemic plague when the bacteria spread into the lungs. The patient's condition evolves rapidly, developing pneumonia with shortness of breath, chest pain, cough, respiratory failure, and shock. It can be incredibly contagious and can trigger severe epidemics spreading from person to person through infectious droplets.

In *The Plague of Ashdod*, Poussin adds further emotional charge to this motif, placing the dead corpse of an infant that could be the living child's twin brother at the mother's other side. Poussin also depicts the mechanisms of contagion recognized by seventeenth-century physicians. Poussin draws particular attention to the physical contact between individuals by picturing several characters at the precise moment when that contact occurs. Extending from one end to the other of the canvas, there is a great concatenation of human bodies linked through their gestures, in a dangerous possibility of *contagion*. In this way, *The Plague of Ashdod* "reasserts the etymological kinship of 'contagion' and 'contact' by displaying the violence that can be hidden in the gentlest caress" (Barker 2004, 665).

The Plague of Ashdod, by Nicolas Poussin, can be placed "between the sensual colourism of the early years and the austere classicism of the middle period" of Poussin's work (Neer 2006, 299). The painting's colour scheme also helps to interpret the scene. While the plague victims in the foreground are portrayed in muted tones, conversely, the bright sky in the background promises a radiant future, suggesting duality in the themes of destruction and hope, characteristic of the seventeenth-century definition of history (Boeckl 2000, 131).

Differential Diagnosis

When Poussin executed this painting, the Philistines' disease was not interpreted as the bubonic plague in any specific medical sense. However, assembling several pictorial formulations that any viewer would recognize as bubonic plague, Poussin depicts some traits of the illness distinct from traditional exegesis of this biblical subject. The Book of Samuel does not accurately identify the plague that afflicted the Philistines at Ashdod. The disease was accompanied by the development of "tumours" ("*prominentes extales*") in "hidden regions" of the body ("*in secretiori parte*") (*Biblia Sacra Vulgatae* 1592, 206). It appeared among the army in the field and was then disseminated among the civilian population by the returning troops. After defeating the Hebrews in the battle of Ebenezer, the Philistines captured the Ark of the Covenant, which was displayed as a trophy at the temple of Dagon, in the city of Ashdod. This sacrilege was then punished by Yahweh, causing the shattering of Dagon's statue and the outbreak of a widespread disease among the Philistines.

During Antiquity, the word "pestis" referred to every disease resulting in large-scale mortality over a limited time period (Sabbatani 2010, 199). In both the Old and New Testaments of the Bible, plagues were considered to be divine punishments for some rebellious behaviour against God (Boeckl

2000, 38-9). The best known are the Ten Plagues of Egypt described in the Book of Exodus (Exodus, 7-12:36). Among these, pestilence (Exodus, 9:1-7) is one of the most serious. The Book of Isaiah mentions the appearance of a lethal disease which overnight "killed in the Assyrian camp 175,000 soldiers", forcing their King Sennacherib to withdraw his army from the Judea and preventing the conquest of Jerusalem (Isaiah, 37:36). Unfortunately, the disease features are also poor here, whereas we have the information on the number of deaths. The biblical text describing the plague striking Israel during David's reign accounts for 70,000 deaths (2 Kings 24).

The original Hebrew text of the Book of Samuel uses two words to describe the disease lesions: *"techorim"* (tumor) and *"opalim"* (boils), both appropriate for bubonic plague. The Hebrew word *"opalim"* also appears among the curses of the Law in Deuteronomy 28: 27: "The Lord will strike you with Egypt and with tumors, festering sores and itching, which cannot be cured". Nonetheless, whatever meaning is attached to the word *"opalim"*, it must have the same sense in 2 Kings 24 and Deuteronomy 28, so that in both contexts, it must mean something like swelling or protuberance, either internal or externally (Shrewsbury 1949, 249).

Bubonic plague is an infectious disease that affects humans and other mammals, caused by the Gram-negative rod-shaped bacillus *Yersinia pestis*. These bacteria maintain their existence in a cycle involving rodents and their fleas (CDC, 2019). The bacteria enter the skin through the flea bite and travel via the lymphatic vessels to a lymph node (CDC, 2018). One to seven days after exposure, patients develop fever, headaches, chills, weakness and one or more swollen, tender, and painful lymph nodes (called buboes), namely in the area where the bacteria entered the skin. Without prompt treatment, plague bacteria invade the bloodstream and spread rapidly, causing severe illness or death.

The first recorded plague pandemic was the Justinian plague (541-740 AD). Mortality rates of 15–40% were recorded, causing tens of millions of deaths throughout the Mediterranean world (Mordechai 2019, 25546-25554). In Europe, the second pandemic occurred 600 years later, from 1330 to 1346. Later known as the Black Death, it spread throughout the known world, resulting in the estimated death of 17-28 million Europeans, approximately 30-40% of the population at the time (Drancourt 2002, 105). The bubonic plague then recurred periodically until the eighteenth century. Finally, during a third plague pandemic in the 1850s, at least 10 million people died in China and India. The plague reached San Francisco in 1900 aboard rat-infested ships to make its first appearance in North America (Steensma 2020, 6). The etiological agent of the plague was discovered during this pandemic, paving the way for the modern study of the disease.

It still remains to be explained why bubonic plague should occur in an area where no previous case is known. Actually, more substantial evidence is required as to the first manifestation of the disease in a particular geographical area where the disease did not reoccur in the following centuries. Although it can be tempting to assert a direct causal connection between the swellings and the rats, their role in the transmission of the disease was unknown until the nineteenth century. On the other hand, the composition of the Books of Samuel ranged over some seven centuries, from 900-200 BC., and the rat story is believed to be a later interpolation, until now impossible to fix the date (Crawfurd 1914, 12).

Among the early modern plague treatises, there is only one reference to the Philistines' disease as the bubonic plague: this comes, in Athanasius Kircher's (1602-1680) *Scrutinium Physico-Medicum Contagiosae Luis*, a few decades after the completion of Poussin's painting (Barker 2004, 241). Though a unique case, Kircher's reference does indicate that, by the later seventeenth century at least, interpretation of the Philistines' disease as the bubonic plague -perhaps first proposed by Poussin in his painting- was both a permissible and plausible deviation from traditionally accepted views.

While recreating *The Plague of Ashdod*, it is quite possible that Poussin had consulted, besides the Vulgate, the Jewish–Roman historian Flavius Josephus (c. 37-c. 100 AD). In his work *Jewish Antiquities*, from c. 94 AD, the original Greek term *"nósos"* was translated into the Latin word *"pestis"*, which, in this context, means no more than "disease" (Josephus 1961, 164-5). As a matter of fact, another book by Josephus, *The Wars of the Jews* (written c.75 AD), had already been the artist's source for the first version of *The Sack and Destruction of the Temple at Jerusalem by Titus* (1626, The Israel Museum, Jerusalem), and the *Jewish Antiquities* were definitely a source for some of his later paintings around the figure of the prophet Moses (c. 13th century BC). Josephus translates the Hebrew word *"opalim"* as haemorrhoids, although his translation has been questioned (Asensi 2018, 166). Following this translation, Josephus states categorically that the disease was dysentery (Josephus 1961, 165). Dysentery, characterized by diarrhoea, is caused by either *Shigellae* or *Amoebas* from the consumption of contaminated water. However, the text mentions neither contaminated water nor diarrhoea and focuses on lethality and tumours.

Tularemia is another hypothesis which has been considered. Tularemia is a zoonotic disease also transmitted through rodents, and its manifestations include ulceroglandular formations, which can be misdiagnosed as bubonic plague. It is also fatal when untreated, thus fitting the episode in the text (Trevisanato 2007, 1145).

An Unsuspected Presence

When the Philistines decided to give the Ark of the Covenant back to Israel, they provided five golden tumours and five golden rats as a guilt offering. In the Hebrew text of the Old Testament, the plague of rats can only be deduced from that guilt offering. The plague of rats is only mentioned explicitly in an additional line of verse 6 of 1 Sam, included in the Greek Septuagint, the Greek translation of the Hebrew Bible dating from the third century BC, and in the post-Tridentine Vulgate, the authoritative version of the Bible in Poussin's time: "The mice went up into their land, and there was mortal panic in the city" (*Biblia Sacra Vulgatae* 1592, 206). Like the Vulgate, Flavius Josephus also includes a reference to the scourge of rats when recounting the Ashdod episode in the *Jewish Antiquities*.

Alexander Yersin (1863-1943), a bacteriologist from the Pasteur Institute, identified the etiological agent of bubonic plague in Hong Kong in 1894 for the first time (Steensma 2020, 7). Several days earlier, the Japanese physician Kitasato Shibasaburō, in Hong Kong, independently described the plague bacillus, although his initial reports were vague and somewhat contradictory. Yersin was then afforded the primary credit for discovering the bacillus, which he described as "small, stocky spindles with rounded ends" (Treille 1894, 310). First named as *Bacterium pestis* and then as *Pasteurella pestis*, in 1967, it was moved to a new genus and renamed *Yersinia pestis* in honour of Yersin. Yersin also noted that the same bacillus was present in rodents and human disease, thus underlining the possible means of transmission of the disease. Another bacteriologist from Pasteur Institute, Paul Louis Simond (1858-1947), proposed the transmission route from the black rat (*Rattus rattus*) via the flea *Xenopsylla cheopis* (Mollaret 1999, 283).

Across the centuries, when the plague was prevalent in Europe, the black rat was primarily responsible, so far as can be ascertained, for the spread of plague to man, since it is a house-haunting species (Shrewsbury 1949, 247). If the Philistines had suffered from a plague of house mice, it is conceivable that an epizootic plague among them might have given rise to a human epidemic. However, seventeenth-century writers rarely distinguished between rats and mice. The ancients did not have the Linnaean classification to name and describe their animals (McCormick 2003, 4). Even though several documents from Antiquity mention the black rat, classical Latin and Greek lacked a word for "rat" that would distinguish it from what we call "mouse". Latin "*mus*" (pl. "*mures*") and Greek may designate either rats or mice.

The biblical record of the Ashdod epidemic clearly mentions a plague of field mice: "*murium qui demoliti sunt terram*" (*Biblia Sacra Vulgatae* 1592, 206). Therefore, it is impossible to identify the exact mouse species, although it remains evident there is an allusion to some animal that devours the crops. Several studies point to the presence of *Rattus rattus* in the Mediterranean and more northern countries in Europe c. 2nd millennium BC (Toškan 2006). Although it is thought that black rats did not reach the Near East until the 1st century BC, fossilized remains of *Xenopsylla cheopis* and *Rattus rattus* have been found in the Nile Valley, dating their arrival in the Middle East to 1350 BC, well before the events reported in 1 Samuel 4-6 (Asensi 2018, 186). Nonetheless, both in the Roman and medieval world, other rodents, such as the Egyptian or African grass rat (*Arvicanthis niloticus*), might have played a role in sustaining or transmitting plague (McCormick 2003, 1).

Before *Poussin's Plague of Ashdod*, rats already figured in early pictorial representations of the Philistine's epidemic. Several textual and visual sources can be invoked to demonstrate how the connection between rats and plague originated and how it was understood (Berger, 2007). In medieval times, there was already an established tradition in book illumination for painting scourge victims together with rats. Nevertheless, this iconographical tradition does not resolve whether there was any suspicion of a correlation between rats and plague in Poussin's time. Poussin's theory that depicting the rats because he recognized an etiological link between plague and rodents has no basis in either ancient or contemporary textual sources at all (Hipp 2007, 180).

The Persian physician Avicenna (980-1037) wrote about the role of rats in plague not as vectors, but as an omen of a human epidemic: "the rats come out of their holes and stagger around as being drunken" (Köhler 2003, 338). There was the belief that rats were born of miasmas produced by stagnant water or swampy earth, as were other animals, such as dogs, cats, frogs, toads, lizards, snakes, mosquitoes, ants, snails, foxes, different species of birds, crocodiles, and dragons. The Italian Physician Hieronymus Fracastoro (c.1476-1553), known by his works on syphilis, in his *De Contagione et Contagiosis Morbis* (1546), describes how animals, normally living underground, came out of their hiding places before the outbreak of an infectious disease (Köhler, 2003, 338).

Some authors (Shrewsbury 194, 2479) argue that the two plagues were synchronous though disconnected because the Philistines made different replicas of the tumours and the mice.

Flavius Josephus also discriminates the epidemic from the scourge of mice (Josephus 1961, 165-6). However, eliminating any direct relationship between the disease and the field mice does not affect the argument that the tumours were plague buboes. On the contrary, the Clementine edition of the Vulgate states clearly that both the buboes and the mice belonged to the same plague (*"quia plaga una fuit"*) (*Biblia Sacra Vulgatae* 1592, 206). If so, the episode in the Book of Samuel could be the oldest written description of a plague epidemic that would have occurred in 1320 BC amidst the Philistines.

The sin offerings, representations in gold of the disease, were akin to the votive offerings of diseased parts dedicated to Asclepius, the god of medicine, and representations of mice associated with imitative magic (Crawfurd 1914, 11). Thus, Apollo seems to stand in the same relation to the mouse as Asclepius to the serpent. Apollo was a plague god, bringing both the disease and its cure. As a matter of fact, among Apollo's many attributes is the epithet "*Smintheus*", associated with mice and rats, both as their exterminator but also as a plague carrier. The first mention of Apollo *Smintheus* appears in Homer's Iliad when Apollo strikes the Greeks with the arrows of plague because Agamemnon has raped the daughter of Apollo's priest Chryses (Homer, *Iliad,* I:1-39). This episode from the Iliad may have inspired Poussin a quarter of a century after *The Plague of Ashdod*, following the plague of 1656, when composing a canvas with the plague arrows captured by the hands of St. Frances of Rome (1384-1440), an entirely dissimilar plague painting, without any rat depiction (*The Vision of St. Frances of Rome*, 1657-58, Louvre Museum, Paris).

Depicting a Crime Scene

The painting's origin is relatively well known, thanks to the records from a court trial involving the Sicilian art dealer Fabrizio Valguarnera (Costello 1950, 237-284). On 12 July 1631, Don Fabrizio Valguarnera had been arrested in Rome on suspicion of murdering, in Madrid, Manuel Alvares Carapeto, the Portuguese cashier of a wealthy merchant, in possession of a diamond package brought from India to Lisbon. Don Fabrizio had fled to Rome, had the diamonds cut by jewellers of the city, and used them to purchase artworks with which to launder the spoils of the robbery (Costello 1950, 255-6). When Valguanera's house was inspected, some diamond stones were found there together with 37 paintings, two authored by Poussin: *The Plague of Ashdod* and *The Realm of Flora*, both dating from the same period (1630-31). Every canvas painter that could be found was then called to testify in court to unveil the circumstances in which Valguarnera invested the diamond heist.

Poussin himself testified on July 28, establishing the date of the painting as the end of 1630, adding that, when Valguarnera visited his studio, the canvas was already underway but still incomplete (Costello 1950, 275). The circumstances that prompted Poussin to undertake this canvas remain unclear. It remains uncertain whether the artist began the painting with a specific commission which was subsequently withdrawn or whether he initiated this project without a purchaser. Probably it was not a commissioned work, since Poussin was able to sell the unfinished painting to Valguarnera, who acquired *The Plague* during February or March 1631 for the price of 110 *scudi* (Costello 1950, 275), a value that allows rating Poussin as a respected painter at the time, able to charge relatively high prices for his works.

At Valguarnera's trial, Poussin mentions the composition as "The Miracle of the Ark", revealing he was not overly concerned with the plague itself but focused instead on Samuel's text (Boeckl 1991, 129). However, since the imagery of the painting alluded to the recent outbreak of plague, this association made the work an immediate success in Italy and France. By 1670, five years after the artist's death, the painting was already called *The Plague That Struck the Philistines for Capturing the Ark of the Covenant.*

After Valguarnera was convicted a few months later, the original by Poussin was auctioned off by its creditors in 1632. André Félibien (1619-1695), a friend of Poussin and one of his biographers, mentioned that while he was in Rome, as secretary of the French Embassy, he had seen the painting at the house of Bernini's assistant, Matteo Bonarelli (died 1654), between 1647 and 1649 (Keazor 1996, 62). After his death, his wife, Constanza Piccolomini (1614-1662), maintained a thriving art dealership during the pontificate of Alexander VII (reigned 1655-1667). In 1660 she sold *The Plague of Ashdod* to the Duke of Richelieu (1585-1642) for 1000 *écus*, a price ten times higher than Poussin had received thirty years before (Rosenberg 2015, 98). In 1665, the canvas joined the royal collection of Louis XIV (1638-1715) and twelve other works by Poussin. The painting was kept in the Louvre Palace and taken to the Palace of Versailles before returning to the Louvre, where it is currently on display.

Interestingly, Valguarnera commissioned a copy of Poussin's painting from the Roman painter Angelo Caroselli (1585-1652) (Fig. 5.4), maybe with the intention of making a profitable sale. Valguarnera testified during his trial that he had paid 35 *scudi* to Caroselli, a third of the original's price (Costello 1950, 262, 272). Caroselli's painting was later owned by the Cardinal Jules Mazarin (1602-1661), prime minister of France (Rosenberg 2015, 106). In 1801, it was sold by Giovanni Gherardo De Rossi (1754-

1827) to the art dealer Alexander Day (c. 1753-1841), who, between 1804 and 1812, brought it to England. Later, it was acquired by the third Duke of Northumberland (1785-1847), who, in 1838, offered it to the National Gallery, where it can be seen nowadays.

In this version of *The Plague*, the figures are faithfully reproduced from the original painting, except for the colour of some of the garments. The differences found in the background buildings have been proposed as documenting Poussin's earlier plan for the architectural setting, suggesting that Caroselli had worked directly from it, in Poussin's studio, while the original was still unfinished (Keazor 2000, 255).

However, Carroselli's version does not correspond to the compositional changes visible in the infrared examination of Poussin's original (Thuillier, 1962, 254). Therefore, these differences seem unlikely to document an earlier state of Poussin's work and maybe just represent Caroselli's attempt to personalize his copy from Poussin's original. Since another smaller item had been faithfully copied in Caroselli's picture, it seems plausible to assume that Caroselli only had the original at his disposal for a limited time so that when he came to the background, he had to improvise (Keazor 2000, 255).

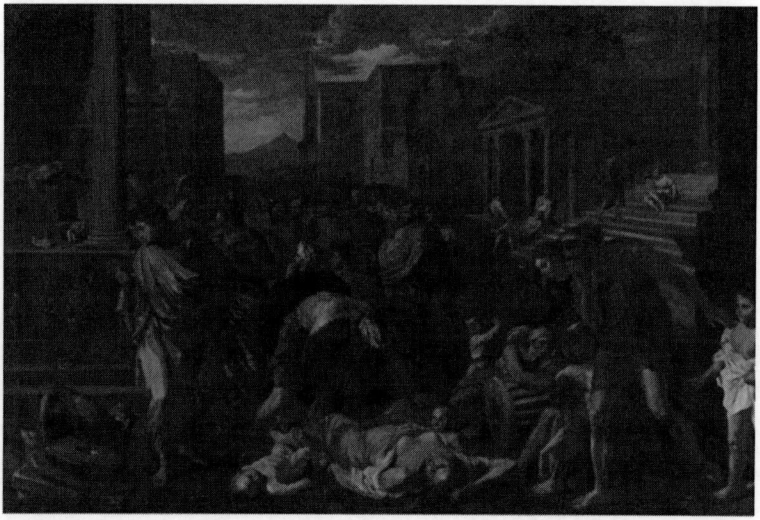

Fig. 5.4. Angelo Caroselli, The Plague at Ashdod (after Poussin), 1631, oil on canvas (148 x 198 cm), Courtesy of The National Gallery, London.

The Portuguese version of The Plague

Another version of the painting is exhibited at the National Museum of Ancient Art, in Lisbon (Fig. 5.5). This version of *The Plague* was acquired by the National Academy of Fine Arts in 1866, from the Portuguese diplomat and art collector Jorge Augusto Husson da Câmara (died 1877), along with other seventeen paintings for the amount of 20,000 réis (Portuguese currency of the time), a gift by the King D. Fernando II of Portugal (1816-1885) (Neto 2014, 54). The canvas was bought by Husson da Câmara from the Italian Prince Mario Chigi Albani Della Rovere (1832-1914), who, being in economic distress, had to sell several works of art from his family gallery. Interestingly, an ancient inventory of the art collection of the Chigi family-the 1692 inventory of the cardinal Flavio Chigi (1631-1693), nephew of the pope Alexander VII-mentioned a copy of *The Plague,* by Poussin, which we propose corresponds to the Portuguese version. This copy would have been made by Constanza Piccolomini to hang in the place of the original, sold to the Duke of Richelieu in 1660 (Yeager-Crasselt 2013, 171). Therefore, the Portuguese version would be a copy of Poussin's original and would have been painted somewhere between 1647 and 1660.

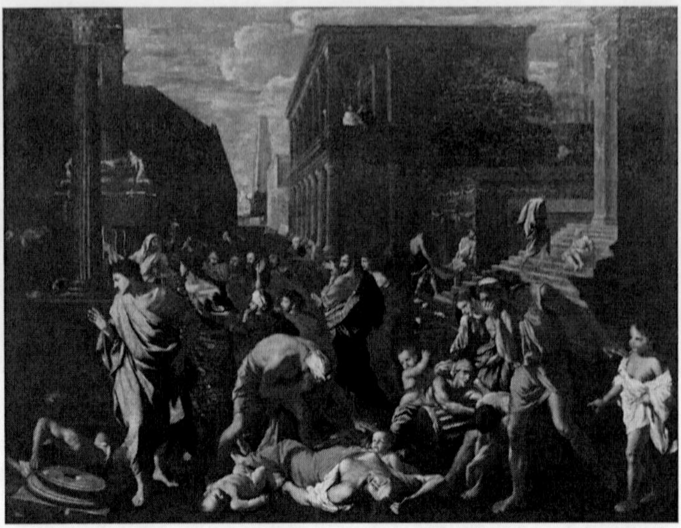

Fig. 5.5. Authored to Nicolas Poussin, The Philistines Struck by The Plague in the City of Ashdod, 1647-1660, oil on canvas (149,5 x 199 cm), Nº Invº Fotográfico 17269 a TC. Reproduced with permission.

The 1662 inventory of Constanza's collection already lists a copy of *The Plague*, whose author is not named (McPhee 2012, 92, Appendix 8, 163, fol. 652r). This copy, along with the remaining paintings from Constanza's collection, would end up in the hands of the cardinal Flavio Chigi.

The authenticity of this version was inadvisedly declared by Jean-Auguste Dominique Ingres (1780-1867) in a letter describing the painting collection of Husson da Câmara, whom he had met in Rome. In the nineteenth century, it was actually considered "a copy of *The Plague* by Poussin, with a more robust and vigorous style than that of the famous painting in the Louvre Museum since it was painted when the artist had attained the highest degree of perfection" (Biester, 1860, 485). The Portuguese version of the painting shows more similarities with the Louvre's canvas than Caroselli's copy, presenting the same architectural background and vestment colours, although in more vivid tones. However, the Portuguese version was severely damaged through the succeeding centuries and deeply retouched afterwards, hindering the recognition of the true author's style (Freire 2007, 19). Consequently, there is no certainty as to whether the Portuguese version is an original from Poussin, a studio copy or a follower's work.

Conclusion

The Plague of Ashdod, by Nicolas Poussin, with the grey-tinted bodies of the dead woman and her children, the holding of the nose from the stench of illness and the several attitudes of despair, has become an emblematic plague pattern. The French historian Jean Delumeau (1923-2020) has remarked that "these iconographic 'projections', a sort of exorcism of the plague, constituted – together with the flight from the cities and social aggression – habitual reactions in the face of a fear that grew into anguish" (Barker 2004, 681).

One of the first artists to be inspired by Poussin's *Plague* was the Flemish painter Michael Sweerts (1618- 664), in his *Plague in an Ancient City* (ca. 1652-54, Los Angeles County Museum of Art, Los Angeles). Although he also portrays a dramatic vision of the bubonic plague, encompassing a broad range of emotional and psychological states, following Poussin, he overlooked the rat's relevance.

During Poussin's lifetime, there were many outbreaks of bubonic plague in Europe, and it is therefore not surprising to find that he identified the Philistine pestilence with bubonic plague. Though his knowledge of Medicine and History was negligible, his inclusion of rats in his painting *The Plague of Ashdod* represents one of the earliest representations, in modern art, of an association between their presence and human plague. This and other depictions, far from implying an etiological link between both phenomena, suggest that such a connection was already suspected from ancient times.

References

Asensi, Victor, Fierer, Joshua. 2018. "Of Rats and Men: Poussin's Plague at Ashdod". *Emerging Infectious Diseases*, 24 (1): 186–187.

Barker, Sheila. 2004. "Poussin, Plague, and Early Modern Medicine". *The Art Bulletin,* 86 (4): 659-689.

Barker, Sheila. 2006. "Art, Architecture, and the Roman Plague of 1656". *Roma Moderna e Contemporanea,* 14 (1): 243-262.

Bellori, Giovanni. 1672. *Le vite de'pittori, scultori et architetti moderni.* Volume 1. Roma: Mascardi.

Berger, Pamela. 2007. "Mice, Arrows, and Tumors, Medieval Plague Iconography North of The Alps" 23-63. *In Piety and Plague: From Byzantium to the Baroque*. Pennsylvania: Penn State University Press.

Biblia Sacra Vulgatae Editionis Sixti V. et Clementis VIII. 1592. Roma: Typographica Apostolica Vaticana.

Biester, Ernesto. 1860. "Chronica". *Revista Contemporânea de Portugal e Brasil.* 2 (10): 484-486.

Boeckl, Christine. 1991. "A New Reading of Nicolas Poussin's The miracle of the Ark in the Temple of Dagon". *Artibus et Historiae,* 12 (24):119-145.

Boeckl, Christine. 2000. *Images of Plague and Pestilence: Iconography and Iconology*. Sixteenth Century Essays & Studies. Volume LIII. Kirksville: Truman State University Press.

Centers for Disease Control and Prevention (CDC). 2018. *Plague's Symptoms*, in https://www.cdc.gov/plague/symptoms/index.html

Centers for Disease Control and Prevention (CDC). 2019. *Plague's Ecology and Transmission,* in https://www.cdc.gov/plague/transmission/index.html accessed January 15, 2022.

Cole, Lucinda. 2016. *Imperfect Creatures Vermin, Literature, and the Sciences of Life 1600-1740*. Ann Arbor: University of Michigan Press.

Costello, Jane. 1950. "The Twelve Pictures 'Ordered by Velasquez' and the Trial of Valguarnera". *Journal of the Warburg and Courtauld Institutes.* 13: 237–84.

Crawfurd, Raymond. 1914. *Plague and Pestilence in Literature and Art*. London: Oxford University Press.

Drancourt, Michel, Raoult, Didier. 2002. "Molecular Insights into the History of Plague". *Microbes and Infection,* 4 (1): 105–109.

Freire, Luciano. 2007. "Elementos para um relatório acerca do tratamento da pintura antiga em Portugal segundo notas tomadas no período da execução desses trabalhos". *Conservar Património,* 5, November: 9-65.

Harris, James. 2006. "The Plague of Ashdod". *Archives of General Psychiatry,* 63(3): 244–45.

Josephus. 1961. *Jewish Antiquities*, edited by Heinemann, William, translated by Tackeray, Henry and Marcus, Ralph. Volume V. Book VI, Chapter 1. Cambridge: Harvard University Press.

Pliny. 1952. *Natural History*, translated by Rackam, Harris, Books 33-35. Cambridge: Harvard University Press.

Hipp, Elisabeth. 2007. "Poussin's The Plague at Ashdod. A Work of Art in Multiple Contexts". *Piety and Plague: From Byzantium to the Baroque.* Pennsylvania: Penn State University Press.

Homer. 2003. *The Iliad*, translated by Fagles, Robert. London: Penguin Classics.

Keazor, Henry. 1996. "A propos des sources litteraires et picturales de la Peste d'Asdod (1630/31)". *Revue du Louvre,* 45: 62-69.

Keazor, Henry. 2000. "Coppies Bien que Mal Fettes: Nicolas Poussin's Rinaldo and Armida Re-Examined". *Gazette des beaux-arts,* (6) 1583: 253-264.

Köhler, Werner, Köhler Michael. 2003. "Plague and rats, the 'plague of the Philistines', and: what did our ancestors know about the role of rats in plague?". *International Journal of Medical Microbiology,* 293: 333-40.

McCormick, Michael. 2003. "Rats, Communication, and Plague: Towards an Ecological History". *Journal of Interdisciplinary History.* 34: 1-25.

McPhee, Sarah. 2012. *Bernini's Beloved: A Portrait of Costanza Piccolomini.* New Haven: Yale University Press.

Mollaret, Henri. 1999. "La découverte par Paul-Louis Simond du rôle de la puce dans la transmission de la peste". *Bulletin de la Société de Pathologie Exotique,* 92: 383-7.

Mordechai, Lee, Eisenberg, Merle, Newfield, Timothy. 2019. "The Justinianic Plague: An inconsequential pandemic?". *Proceedings of the National Academy of Sciences,* 116 (51): 25546-25554.

Neer, Richard. 2006. "Poussin and the Ethics of Imitation". *Memoirs of the American Academy in Rome* Volumes 51/52, Ann Arbor: University of Michigan Press.

Neto, Maria João. 2014. "Construção e desconstrução de coleções: o Mercado da Arte em Roma no período Napoleónico aos olhos dos diplomatas portugueses". *In Coleções de Arte em Portugal e Brasil nos Séculos XIX E XX – Perfis e Trânsitos*. Casal de Cambra: Caleidoscópio.

Rosenberg, Pierre. 2015. *Nicolas Poussin – Les Tableaux du Louvre*. Paris: Louvre Editions.

Sabbatani, Sergio, Fiorino, Sirio. 2010. "The plague of the Philistines and other pestilences in the Ancient World: exploring relations between the religious-literary tradition, artistic evidence and scientific proof". *Le infezioni in medicina,* 18 (3): 199–207.

Shrewsbury, John. 1949. "The Plague of the Philistines". *The Journal of Hygiene,* 47 (3): 244-52.

Steensma, David, Kyle, Robert. 2020. "Alexandre Yersin: Discoverer of the Plague Bacillus". *Mayo Clinic Proceedings,* Jan 95 (1): 7-8.

Thucydides. 1998. *The Peloponnesian War*, Translated by Steven Lattimore Book 2: 2.47–2.54. Indianapolis: Hackett.

Toškan, Borut, Kryštufek, Boris. 2006. "Noteworthy rodent records from the Upper Pleistocene and Holocene of Slovenia", *Mammalia* 70 (1-2): 98-105.

Treille, Georges-Félix, Yersin, Alexandre.1894. "La peste bubonique à Hong Kong". *Congrès international d'hygiène et de démographie, Budapest, Hongrie*: 310-311.

Trevisanato, Siro. 2004. "Did an epidemic of tularemia in Ancient Egypt affect the course of world history?". *Medical Hypotheses,* 63 (5): 905–910.

Trevisanato, Siro. 2007. "The biblical plague of the Philistines now has a name, tularemia". *Medical Hypotheses,* 69 (5): 1144–1146.

Thuillier, Jacques. 1962. "Perspectives du XVII[e] Siecle". *Art de France,* (2) 252-54.

Yeager-Crasselt, Lara. 2013. "Michael Sweerts (1618-1664) and the Academic Tradition". Dissertation submitted for the degree of Doctor of Philosophy. College Park: University of Maryland.

CHAPTER 6

HISTORY OF SPECTACLES - PORTUGAL IN THE SIXTEENTH CENTURY

MARIA DO SAMEIRO BARROSO[1]

Abstract

Spectacles constitute one of the most remarkable and helpful inventions of the Middle Ages, first emerging as convex lenses helping to produce magnified images of objects mainly to correct presbyopia, a condition characterized by gradual loss of the ability of the eyes to focus on nearby objects in people over forty years old. Spectacles appeared mainly in monasteries and were available to members of the clergy and nobility, as well as learned and wealthy people. In the sixteenth century, these costly and valuable objects were manufactured and sold all over Europe. In this essay, I will briefly survey their invention, manufacture, trade and classification, focusing on paintings and reports about their use in Portugal, and presenting an unpublished collection of specimens from the Museum of Aveiro, former Monastary of Jesus from Aveiro (Mosteiro de Jesus de Aveiro), founded in 1458. The Monastery became illustrious when Princess Joanna (1452-1490), daughter to King D. Afonso V (reigned from 1438, being six years old up to 1477 under the regency of his oncle D. Pedro, Duke of Coimbra (1392-1499) and 1477-1481), entered the monastery in 1460, after refusing marriage proposals from European monarchs.

Key words

History of visual aids; Spectacles; History of Ophthalmology; Monastery of Jesus from Aveiro

Resumo

Os óculos constituem uma das invenções mais notáveis e úteis da Idade Média, tendo surgido primeiro como lentes convexas ajudando a produzir imagens ampliadas de objectos principalmente para corrigir a presbiopia,

[1] Unless otherwise stated, English translations are by the author.

problema ocular caracterizado pela perda gradual da capacidade dos olhos de focar objetos próximos em pessoas com mais de quarenta anos. Os óculos surgiram principalmente nos mosteiros para membros do clero e nobreza e pessoas cultas e ricas. No século XVI, eram objetos caros e valiosos, fabricados e vendidos em toda a Europa. Neste estudo, procederemos a uma breve retrospectiva da sua invenção, fabrico, comércio e tipologias, abordando pinturas e referências à sua utilização em Portugal, apresentando uma coleção inédita de exemplares do Museu de Aveiro, antigo Mosteiro de Jesus de Aveiro (Mosteiro de Jesus de Aveiro), fundado em 1458. O Mosteiro ganhou notariedade quando a princesa Joana (1452-1490), filha do rei Afonso V (reinou desde 1438, tendo seis anos até 1477 sob a regência de seu tio D. Pedro, Duque de Coimbra (1392 -1499) e 1477-1481), entrou no mosteiro em 1460, após recusar propostas de casamento de monarcas europeus.

Palavras-chave
História das ajudas visuais; Óculos; História da Oftalmologia; Mosteiro de Jesus de Aveiro

Introduction

According to Dr Plinio Prioreschi, physician and medical historian, the invention of eyeglasses stands as one of the most remarkable inventions of the Middle Ages. Most would agree that eyeglasses, the indispensable gadget used daily by untold numbers of human beings, are one of the most useful discoveries that technology has ever produced (Prioreschi 2003, 83).

The earliest eyeglasses consisted of convex lenses, which rectify presbyopia, a natural physiological change due to ageing. Presbyopia affects all types of eye in people from their early forties onwards; it is caused by the loss of elasticity of the eye lens, which reduces accommodation, resulting in focusing difficulty on nearby objects. Convex lenses also rectify farsightedness (hyperopia) a common condition caused by a refractive error in which visual images focus behind the retina, the vision being better for distant than for near objects (Allen 1972, 365 and 347).

Early evidence for the use of lenses

Reports of the use of rock crystal appear in texts as early as the Assyrian-Babylonian cuneiform tablets, whose decipherment has brought to our knowledge a surprising variety of medical and surgical instruments:

> An inventory text from third-millennium Ebla indicates that the AZU had in his toilet kit, in addition to straight and curved bronze blades each weighing 2 to 3 shekels (16 to 24 g) and bronze needles and tweezers (forceps) of similar dimensions, small bronze hammers (DUB.NAGAR), which to judge from later texts were intended for testing reflexes 'See Chapter 13'. Also available to ancient physicians were magnifying glasses made of polished rock crystal that could have been used for closer examination of skin and other tissues (Scurlock & Andersen 2005, 6).

Although the laws of optics were unknown at the time, literary and archaeological evidence points to a knowledge of magnifying lenses in the ancient cultures of the Middle East and Graeco-Roman world, which included their use for medicinal purposes[2] (Harvey 2010). Aristophanes (446-386 BC), the Greek comedy-writer, refers to magnifying glasses as igniting fire when exposed to the sun's rays (Aristophanes, *Clouds,* translated by Paul Roche, 2005, 167). Lucius Annaeus Seneca (c.4 BC-65AD), the Roman philosopher, describes how a glass globe of water magnified the letters, helping in reading:

> I have already said that there are certain mirrors that multiply every object they reflect. I may now add that every object much exceeds its natural size when seen through water. Letters, however small and dim, are comparatively large and distinct when seen through a glass globe filled with water. (Seneca, *Natural Questions,* Book I, Chapter VI, translated by Clarke 1910, 29).

In Byzantine times, Isidore of Seville (c. 650-636 AD) provided evidence for the use of gems as lenses:

> No gem or plant possesses greater intensity than *smaragdus.* It exceeds green plants and leaves, and imbues the reflected air around with its greenness. Nothing is more soothing to the eyes of gem cutters than its refreshing green. If its surface is broad, it reflects images like a mirror. Indeed the Emperor Nero used to watch gladiator matches using a *smaragdus* (Isidore of Seville translated by Barney et al. 2010, 322).

---

[2] Harvey, Anna, 2010. "The use of Magmifying lenses in the Classical World." *History of the Ancient World* https://www.historyoftheancientworld.com/2012/11/the-use-of magnifying-lenses-in-the-classical-world/ accessed 10 August 2021.

Reading magnifiers (*Lapis ad legendum*) in the Middle Ages

Roger Bacon (c. 1219/20-c. 1292), an English natural philosopher and Franciscan friar, also known as Doctor Mirabilis, gave a decisive contribution to the invention of eyeglasses by studying the laws of optics. In the fifth chapter of his work *Opus Majus,* written in 1267, he reviewed the early work on eye anatomy, physiology and optics by ancient authors like Euclid (325-265 BC), Aristotle (384-322 BC) and the Arabic mathematician, astronomer and physicist Alhazen (Ḥasan Ibn al-Haytham c. 965 – c. 1040), the author of *Kitāb al-Manāẓir* (Arabic: كتاب المناظر, "Book of Optics"), written during 1011–1021, and translated into Latin by Gerard of Cremona in the twelfth century AD (Bergholdt 1994, 111-120).

Bacon added valuable contributions to the understanding of light and vision. In the following passage, Bacon highlights his comprehension of the laws of refraction, which, in turn, led to an understanding of the functioning of lenses:

> "For we can so shape transparent bodies, and arrange them in such a way with respect to our sight and objects of vision, that the rays will be refracted and bent in any direction we desire, and under any angle, we wish we shall see the object near or at a distance. Thus, from an incredible distance, we might read the smallest letters and number grains of dust and sand ..." (Bacon translated by Burke, vol. 2. Part 5, Chapter IV, 582).

Bacon made the introductory statement that plano-convex lenses could be ideal for older people and people with weak eyes. One could see even the most miniature letters at a larger size by using them. Although Bacon was not the "inventor" of the "reading stone", he recognized the importance of this visual aid, made improvements to its design and searched for a scientific explanation of the phenomenon. The miracle of the reading stone soon caused such a sensation in the learned and educated world that even the poets proclaimed it enthusiastically (Bergholdt 1994, 111-120).

Aside from Bacon, other scholastic students like John Peckham (c. 1230 – 8 December 1292), Archbishop of Canterbury in the years 1279–1292, and Vitello (c. 1230–1280), a Polish friar, theologian and natural philosopher who wrote a book on Optics, also contributed to a better understanding of optics. Their motivation was primarily theological as part of their search for the divine *Miracle of Grace (Wunder der Gnade).*

According to Neoplatonic philosophy, light and grace are different levels of emanation of the Creator. In their view, the rays of light falling into the eye show striking parallels to the analogous stream of grace, understood purely physically (Bergholdt 1994, 111-120). Evidence of gems, namely beryls ("Berillus" from which the German word 'Brillen' for eyeglasses is derived), used as lenses, are mentioned in poetry from the second half of the thirteenth century.

Albrecht, about whom little else is known (Killy 1988, 96), is the author of the epic poem *Jüngeren Titurel* (*The Young Titurel*), written between around 1260-1275. In it he commended the magnifying properties of beryl: "As the beryl enlarges the writing when you read in it, your heart resembles it with all its virtues. It grows in height, broadness and also in length"[3].

It is not surprising that rock crystal also appears as magnifying glass material because of its transparency, purity and religious symbolism; it was one the most celebrated holy stones in ancient cultures. In Antiquity, it was believed to be frozen ice (Rätsch & Guhr 1989, 44). An ancient Greek hymn, possibly dedicated to Orfeus, translated into German by Christian Rätsch and Andreas Guhr, praises the properties of rock crystal: "rejoicing the heart of the gods":

> Take the crystal in your hands
> The incomparable, radiant stone.
> The sky rays light
> Lies in this wonder stone.
> Its unearthly transparency
> Rejoices the hearts of the gods.
> Come into the holy temple with the crystal in thy hand,
> Heaven will listen to your humble request.
> Hear now and recognize the stone's magical power. (…)[4]

Pieces of crystal were familiar to learned thirteenth century Germans, cut as magnifying lenses and provided with a handle (Bergholdt 1994, 120) as implied in the poem *The Golden Forge* (*Die Goldene Schmiede*) written

---

[3]Sam der berillus grozzet . die fchrift . in im zv lefene. Din hertze fich dem genozzet . dar inne alle tvgende mit wefende.Wehfet hoch breit wit vnd ovch die lenge (v. 1400 Albrecht translated by Hahn 1842, 140); ("Wie der Beril vergrössert die Schrift, in ihm zu lesen, dein Herz sich dem gleicht mit allen Tugenden, die darin sind. Es wächt hoch, breit und auch in die Länge" (Translated into modern German in Bergoldt 1994, 111-120).

[4] Nimm in die Hände den Kristall,/Den unvergleichlichen, strahlenden Stein./Der Himmelsstrahlen Licht/Ist in diesem Wunderstein eingeschlssen./Seine unirdische Durchsichtigkeit/Erfreut die Herzen der Götter./Kommst du in den heiligen Tempel mit dem Kristall in der Hand,/Wird der Himmel deine unterwürfige Bitte erhören./ Höre jetzt und erkenne des Steins zauberhafte Kraft.(..) (Rätsch & Guhr 1989, 44).

between 1270-1275 by the German poet Konrad von Würzburg (1220/1230-1287). Würzburg dedicated the poem to the Virgin Mary and compared her purity to that of a rock crystal lens of help in reading:

> I have compared you (i.e. the Virgin Mary)
> with a crystal stone,
> to which I want to compare you, again,
> oh, pure virgin.
> It (i.e. the crystal) has in itself the great and mighty power
> that writing would never be so small
> its appearance in it would be larger:
> If this stone is covered and overspread,
> if someone would want to cut it thin
> and hold it on the script,
> would see the small letters
> appear larger through it.
> (Greef 1923, 90-101)[5]

Semi-precious stones and rock crystal lenses, known as *Reading magnifiers (Lesensteinen* in German and *Lapis ad Legendum* in Latin writings), are the earliest known aids to vision (Greef 1923, 90-101). Albrecht mentioned using topaz as an aid when watching fights: "*Topaz, for fighting, can enlarge the sight*" (*Topasius fvr striten.hat er craft die grozzen*; v. 538 in Hahn 1842, 53). Glass was not utilized in this way at this time. According to Greeff, even in Roman times, colourless glass was difficult to obtain, being more highly appreciated and expensive than coloured glass; the same was true in the Middle Ages. Greeff cites a poetic expression: *Schwarz wie glass* ("*Black like glass*") by a German poet. Only Venetians, well versed in the characteristics of glass, could produce clear glass at this time, but they kept the production process secret. In the course

[5] Original version: "ich hân dâ vor gelìchet dich /dem kriſtallinen ſteine: /dem wil ich, vrouwe reine,/ noch zeimâl dich genôzen ./er hât an im die grozen/und die gewalteclichen art ,/ daz nie kein fchrift fo kleine wart,/ ir ſchîn enwürde breiter/ob dirre ſtein vil heiter/fi daht und übergriffe :/ fwer in ot dünne fliffe,/ und ûf die fchrift in wolde haben ,/ ern fæhe ir kleinen buochſtaben/ durch in breiter fchinen ." (Schröder 1926, 99, vv. 1766-1810). Modern German translation: Ich habe dich (d.h. die Jungfrau Maria) verglichen/mit einem kristallen Stein,/dem will ich dich, reine Jungfrau,/noch einmal vergleichen./Er (d.h.) der Kristal hat in sich die gröβe und gewältige Art,/daβ nie eine Schrift so klein wäre,/ihr Aussehen in ihm würde gröβer:/Wenn dieser Stein/sie überdachte und übergriffe,/Sofern ihn jemand dünn schliffe/und auf die Schrift halten wollte,/der sähe durch ihn die kleinen Buchstaben/gröβer erscheinen. (Greeff 1923, 98-101).

of time, Venetian glass seems to have been traded over the Alps (Greeff 1923, 98-101).

The invention of eyeglasses

The invention of eyeglasses is still shrouded in mystery, as is the case with some other innovations. We are certain that eyeglasses were unknown in Classical Antiquity, the Middle Ages, and to Arabic authors. The possibility of the Chinese having invented eyeglasses has been ruled out by Hirschberg, who thoroughly reviewed the writings of Marco Polo (1254-1324), the famous traveller who would surely have brought the innovation from China back to Europe. However, he could find nothing on that subject in Marco Polo's work (Hirschberg 1905, 265).

Although some inventions appeared in ancient China before they did in Europe, this was not the case in spectacles as visual aids. The Chinese used spectacles before 2000 BC, not to improve sight but to help weak-sighted people through the imaginary power of "Yoh Shui" supposedly existing in the spectacles. These glasses were made from mica in light and dark colours and worn as light shields (Holtmann 1978, vii-xxii).

A tradition of unknown origin attributes the invention of spectacles to Saint Jerome (also known as Jerome of Stridon; 331-420) (Bock 1903, 14-15). A spectacles vendor from Venice held the Saint as his patron and wrote in his store "S. Girolamo inventore degli occiali" (Saint Jerome, inventor of the eyeglasses).

The Saint is depicted with a pair of riveted spectacles hanging over a notebook on his work desk in a wall painting by Ghirlandaio (1449-1494) in the Church Ognisanti in Florence (Bock 1903, 15, Bild 7) (Fig. 6.1). Because he was frequently depicted with a lion, a skull and spectacles, he was credited with being the patron saint of eyeglass manufacturers (Holtmann 1978, vii-xxii).

Saint Jerome was one of the most erudite Christian scholars. One of his most outstanding achievements was translating the Bible into Latin; this is known as the *Vulgata.* He is considered the patron saint of librarians, scripture scholars, students, translators and interpreters who celebrate International Translation Day on September 30, honouring his death[6].

A plausible reason for his wearing spectacles in various representations is the fact that he spent long periods of time reading. He lived, however, long before they were available as aids to vision.

---

[6] https://www.collinsdictionary.com/dictionary/english/erudite-scholar accessed 20 June 2022.

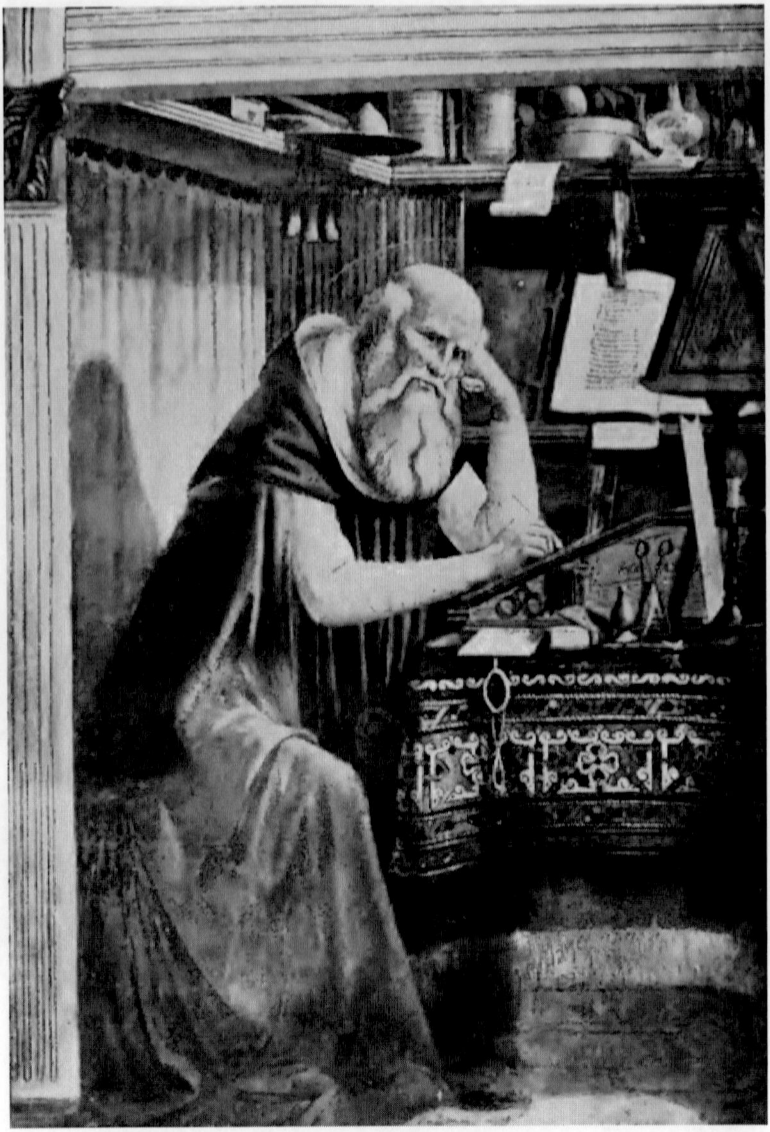

Fig. 6.1. Saint Jerome. Wall painting by Ghirlandaio (1449-1494 in the church Ognissanti in Florence, reproduced from Bock 1903, 15 fig. 7.

The possible development of two eyeglasses worn directly in front of the eyes may have taken place like this. The spherical segments of convex lenses became flatter. Instead of placing it directly over the writing, hanging the lens in front of the eyes may have taken place until, finally, the idea of connecting two such reading stones with a frame appeared (Holtmann 1978, vii-xxii). According to Bergholt:

> The inventor simply had to reduce the height radius of a flat or biconvex glass to such an extent that the magnifying effect occurred immediately in front of the eye. This and the glass no longer acted as a reading magnifier. For this, technical know-how was necessary, which at the end of the 13th century was only available in Venice, where glass production on Murano technically developed the most in Europe (Bergholdt 1994, 111-120).

Spectacles were invented around 1285, most likely by a craftsman. The date is derived from Sermon XV by the Dominican theologian Jordan of Pisa (Italian: Giordano da Pisa) or Jordan of Rivalto (c. 1255-1311) in 1305:

> It is not yet twenty years since there was found the art of making eyeglasses, which make for good vision, one of the best arts and most necessary that the world has. And it is so short a time that this new art, never before extant, was discovered. And the lecturer [Giordano] said: I saw the one who first discovered and practised it, and I talked to him[7].

The earliest visual aids were initially only spherical segments of transparent Murano glass, quartz, rock crystal or semi-precious stones such as beryls (Schmitz 1982, 67). Monocles and rivet spectacles (*Nietbrillen*), rimless eyeglasses consisting of two lenses mounted with metal rivets, appeared by the end of the thirteenth century and were manufactured until the sixteenth century. Initially, their frame was made of metal (iron, silver, gold) and, later, of bone or horn; the lenses were made of crystal or semi-precious stones, such as beryl, or Murano glass. They were manufactured in Venice and a city in the North of Europe, presumably Brabant, until 1570-80. Rivet spectacles evolved into folding glasses *(Gelenkbrillen*) that were easily doubled over each other, giving a pear-like shape and kept in a case. Folding spectacles were fabricated until the end of the eighteenth century (Hallauer 1929, 9-11).

---

[7] Non e ancora venti anni che si trovo l'arte di fare gli occhiali, che fanno vedere bene, ch'e una de le migliori arti e de le piu necessarie che '1 mondo abbia, e e cosi poco // che ssi trovo: arte novella, che mmai non fu. E disse il lettore: io vidi colui che prima la trovo e fece, e favellaigli (Delcorno, 1974, 75).

Scissor-spectacles, consisting of a double monocle which could be stowed in a fixed case, also provided an alternative means of greater comfort when reading. They were made from horn, to begin with, and later, of brass, wood or or bone. Precious metals like silver and gold were also employed, different materials sometimes being combined in the same piece. They were also called Lorgnettes, and their shape was maintained until around 1850 (Pflugk 1929, 214-215).

Since 1684, it was believed that an epitaph in the Church of Santa Maggiore in Florence belonged to the inventor of eyeglasses. The inscription "Here lies Salvino D'Armato of the Armati of Florence Inventor of Spectacles. May God forgive his sins: AD 1317 (*Quindiaci Salvino D'Armato delli Armati di Firenzi, Inventor degli ochialli; Dio gli perdoni la pecata, Anno D, MCCCXVIII*) is now known to be fraudulent and of unknown date (Goes 2013, 131).

Around 1300, the mass production of eyeglasses, involving the manufacture of cheaper glasses, regulated by standards, was established in Venice (Bergholdt 1994, 111-120). Testimonies of the use of eyeglasses appear shortly after this date in medical literature. The French physician Bernard de Gordon (c.1260-c.1318), a professor at the University of Montpellier, referred in his *Lilium Medicinae,* the earliest manuscript of which dates from 1306, to a collyrium that allows older men to read even the smallest letters without eyeglasses.[8]

In 1313, Friar Allessandro della Spina (birth and death dates unknown) also reported on the manufacture of eyeglasses in an Ancient Chronicle by Bartolomeo da San Concordio (d. 1347) of the Dominican Monastery of St. Catherine in Pisa, and whose first compiler was Friar Bartolomeo da San Concordio (d. 1347):

> Friar Alexander della Spina, a modest and good man, whatever he saw that had been made, he knew how to make it. Eyeglasses, having first been made by someone else, who was unwilling to share them, he [Spina] made them and shared them with everyone with a cheerful and willing heart. He knew how to sing, write, illuminate [manuscripts] and everything which mechanically skilful hands can do. Ingenious in corporeal things, by his ingenuity, he made himself a room in the house of the Eternal King (Ilardi 1975, 6).

---

[8] Transcribed in Hirschberg 1905, 271, note 2 and Bergholdt 1994, 111-120: "est tantae virtutis quod decrepitum faceret legere litteras minutissimas sine ocularibus". Original manuscript from 1303: Utrecht University https://www.uu.nl/en/utrecht-university-library-special-collections/collections/manuscripts/medieval-medical-manuscripts/lilium-medicinae-by-bernard-de-gordon, accessed 16 September 2021.

Spectacles appeared in public documents roughly at the same time as in medical literature (Pansier 1901, 21). As early as 1319, the Lord of Padua (Podertà of Padua), which is not far from Venice, caused surprise and all kinds of excitement and sensation when he appeared at a prince's wedding party in Vienna wearing eyeglasses (Schmitz 1982, 66-68).

Poets also conveyed testimonies of the use of eyeglasses. The most outstanding was the Italian poet Francesco Petrarca (1304-1374), who confessed in his autobiography (*Secretum Meum*), written in 1342-43, that, by that time, unfortunately, he could not read without eyeglasses (Bergholt 1992, 114).

The Minnesänger (Minstrel) in the Manessischen Liederhandschrift. ("Manessian Song Manuscript"), a late thirteenth century collection by numerous poets, mentions magnifying glasses as "*lichte Spiegel*" (light mirrors), another expression for eyeglasses. The following lines are by Mizener (Meissner):

> So, when our face ages
> everything goes so blurry
> that we no longer can see
> the noble writing,
> we must be given more,
> so, our candle for it
> is a clear mirror,
> fully illuminating the script
> providing clear vision[9].

When dealing with vision impairment, the French physician and surgeon Guy de Chauliac (c. 1300-1368) prescribed eye drops in his work *Chirurgia Magna*, published in 1363. However, if that did not work, he advised wearing glass or beryl spectacles. It seems that beryl eyeglasses were also fabricated, possibly in France or other countries in which transparent glass was not available: "And if these things do not benefit, we have to resort to glass or beryl glasses"[10].

The earliest representation of eyeglasses appeared in 1352. The Italian painter Tommaso da Modena (1325-1379) was commissioned to paint a

---

[9] Original version: "so that we can see. Svenn uns daz alter die gesicht/betimbert al ze sere,/Daz wir die edlen schrift niht/vol geschen mügen mere,/so sint unser kere/zuo z'einem lichten spiegel klar/Der uns die schrift erliuten kan/unt vol gesihtik machen/so wir si dur in sehen an." (*Hagers Minnesängern*, II, 224, transcribed in Hirschberg 1905, 272).

[10] "Et si ces choses n'y profitente, il faut auoir recours aux oculaires de verre ou de berilles" (Nicaise 1980, 491).

fresco of forty Dominican scholars in the chapter room of the former Dominican convent of San Nicolo at Treviso, portraying the Cardinal Hugo of Provence (or Hugh St. Cher) (c. 1200-1263), reading at his desk, wearing a pair of rivet spectacles placed on the nose without additional support. The Cardinal died before the invention of eyeglasses (Ilardi 1975, 19-20) (Fig. 6.2a).

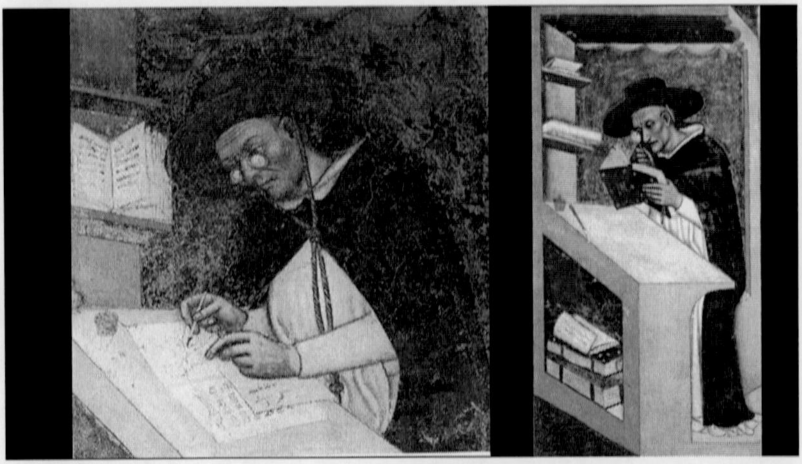

Fig. 6.2a. Detail of fresco from by Tommaso da Modena depicting Cardinal Hugo of Provence wearing glasses. Serie dei Quaranta domenicani illustri, ex convento di San Niccolò, Sala del Capitolo, Treviso, 1352. Credit: Wiki Commons.
Fig. 6.2b. Detail.Cardinal Nicholas of Rouen using a monocular lens.

Tommaso da Modena portrayed Cardinal Nicholas of Rouen (1326-1379) using a monocular lens (Ilardi 1975, 20) (Fig. 6.2b). According to Chiara Frugoni, this painting proves that the Dominicans were concerned with reading books and used eyeglasses.

Thus, this painting introduced the reproduction of earlier religious figures wearing eyeglasses, long before their actual invention:

> His seemingly capricious depiction of spectacles on the nose of a person who had died some twenty years before their invention, while withholding them from others contemporary with their first use, started a trend to anachronistically depict scholarly and saintly figures with glasses (Ilardi 1974, 21).

Representations of spectacles appear in religious communities. Around 1380, Saint Paul is depicted wearing rivet spectacles, presumably coping with the light of revelation in a manuscript of the French *Bible Historiale* (Goes 2013, 131) (Fig. 6.3).

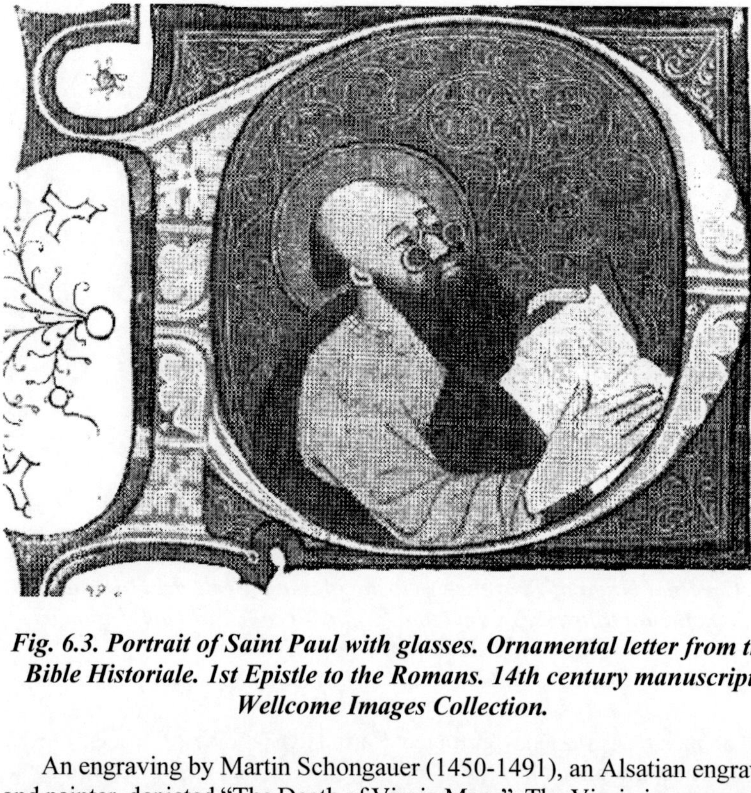

Fig. 6.3. Portrait of Saint Paul with glasses. Ornamental letter from the Bible Historiale. 1st Epistle to the Romans. 14th century manuscript. Wellcome Images Collection.

An engraving by Martin Schongauer (1450-1491), an Alsatian engraver and painter, depicted "The Death of Virgin Mary". The Virgin is surrounded by the apostles. Two are kneeling on the right, at her bedside, reading a book. One holds a pair of rivet spectacles close to the page, using it as a reading lens, according to Bock (Bock 1903, 11, fig. 5) (Fig. 6.4).

However, an alternative explanation by the Bristish ophthalmologist Carl Barck (Barck 1907, 206-226) was that this man might be nearsighted; he could be checking how the lenses worked, realising that, in his case, they they were of no help.

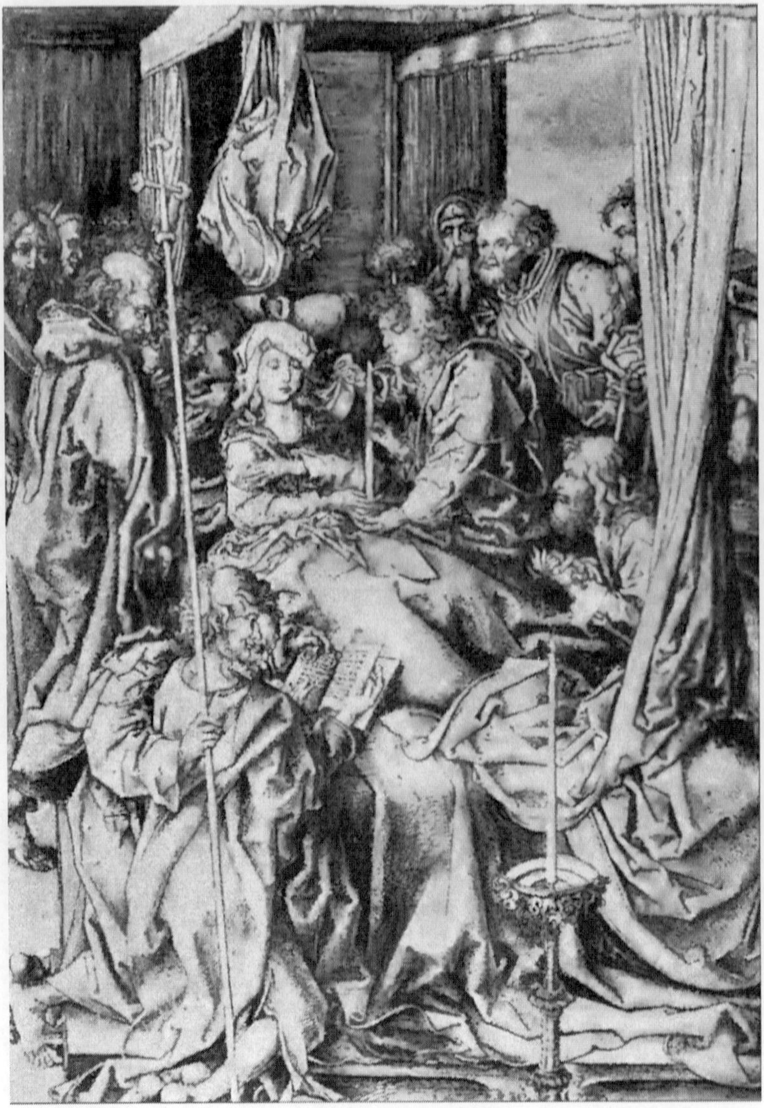

Fig. 6.4. Death of the Virgin, engraving by Martin Schongauer in Bock 1903, 11, fig.5.

Master of Heiligenkreuz, an Austrian painter who lived possibly around 1395-1430, also depicted "The Death of the Virgin" currently housed at the Cleveland Museum of Art (U.S.A.). The Apostles visit the Virgin upon her deathbed. Saint Peter performs the funerary rites, reciting prayers, wearing robes and the papal tiara, sprinkling holy water on the Virgin's body, while the angels above celebrate the assumption of the Virgin heavenward (Fig. 6.5a).

Notice that Saint Peter holds the book a long way from his eyes. His hair and beard are white. Being aged, he suffers from presbyopia. However, the open book shows an illumination on the odd page and big lettering on the even page. Two apostles are sitting on a dais at the bottom of the painting. With a long grey beard and hair, the one on the right is leafing through a book from afar. Also aged and suffering from presbyopia, he cannot thoroughly read the book. The apostle on the left, although younger, is reading the book closely, wearing a pair of rivet spectacles, holding it upwards with the hand against his forehead. This detail illustrates how uncomfortable it would have been to hold the spectacles in place when reading (Fig. 6.5b).

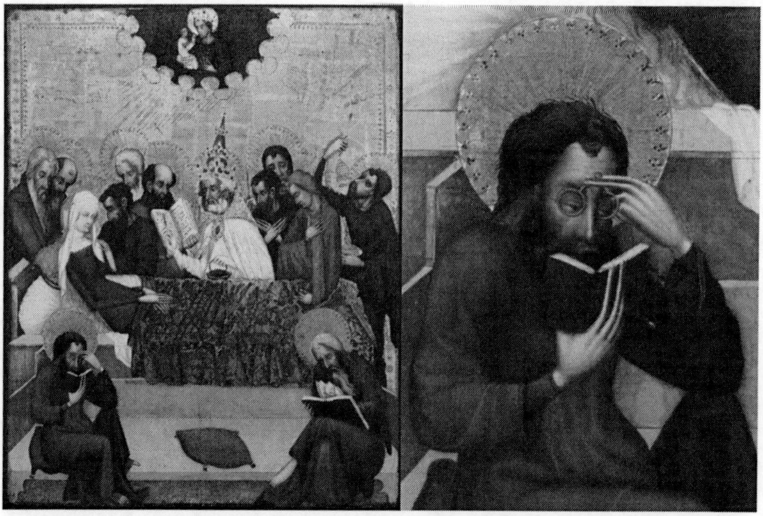

Fig. 6.5a. "The Death of the Virgin. Cleveland Museum (U.S.A.). Open Access. CC. Fig. 6.5b. Detail. Apostle wearing rivet spectacles while reading a book.

In artworks, people are depicted holding spectacles in their hands when pausing from reading as seen in "Saints Peter and Dorothy" by Master of the Saint Bartholomew Alterpiece, dating from 1505-1510, and housed at the National Gallery, London. Taking a break from reading with the help of spectacles, Saint Peter holds an open Bible with his right hand and his vision aid with his left hand (Fig. 6.6).

The Museum description of the painting reads as follows:

> Saint Peter clutches a Bible with a soft leather cover to his chest. In the same hand he holds two unwieldy keys – those to the kingdom of heaven, promised to him by Christ. Saint Dorothy holds only a tiny delicate flower to her breast, presumably plucked from the basket of blooms in her left hand. The flowers are a reference to a miracle told in her legend: at Dorothy's martyrdom, Christ delivered a basket of flowers from heaven to an unbelieving onlooker[11].

When travelling, spectacles were hung in a sheath on the belt, as in an altarpiece painted by Conrad Leib (c.1410-1460/1465) depicting Bernardine of Siena (1330-1444), a famous preacher of the Franciscan Order, with his spectacles hanging from the belt in a small pouch (Frugoni 2004, 25, fig. 7).

Wearing "pince-nez" or holding them in the hand became quite impractical. Bernardine of Sienna and, later, Girolamo Savonarola (1452-1498), a preacher friar of the Dominican Order, wore them, provided with hooks to hang on his clothes. The preachers' spectacles and cap were essential elements of their clothing, which were later considered to be valuable relics (Frugoni 2004, 31).

Anachronistic representations of ancient Christian figures wearing spectacles was a theme also extended to illustrious Graeco-Roman poets.

The German painter and engraver Ludger tom Ring the Elder (1496-1547), who spent his apprentice years in the Netherlands and later settled in Münster, Germany, painted a series of fifteen sibyls and pagan prophets for the walls of the Münster cathedral (around 1538, 7 panels, currently housed in the Westphalian State Museum of Münster)[12].

---

[11] Saints Peter and Dorothy by Master of the Saint Bartholomew Alterpiece. National Gallery, London.
https://www.nationalgallery.org.uk/paintings/master-of- the-saint bartholomew-altarpiece-saints-peter-and-dorothy accessed 10 November 2021).

[12] Lorenz, Angelika, "Ring, Ludger tom" in: Neue Deutsche Biographie 21 (2003), S. 629-630 [Online-Version]; URL: https://www.deutsche-biographie.de/pnd119485451.html#ndbcontent accessed 25 june 2022.

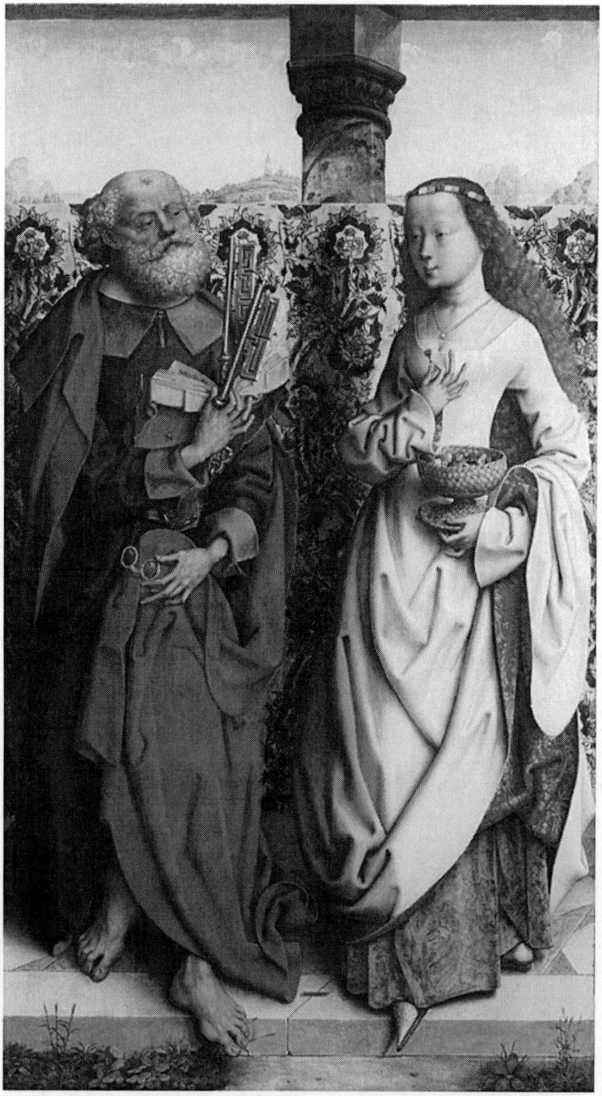

Fig. 6.6. Master of the Saint Bartholomew Altarpiece, 'Saints Peter and Dorothy', The National Gallery, London. Photo credit: Chris Duffin.

Ludger tom Ring the Elder also painted the Latin poet Virgil (70-21 BC) c. 1538. He depicted the poet with a long beard, wearing a turban and Oriental clothes, which are not typical of Roman garments. The poet holds a pair of scissor spectacles upwards with his right hand, leafing through and reading a bulky printed book (Fig. 6.7).

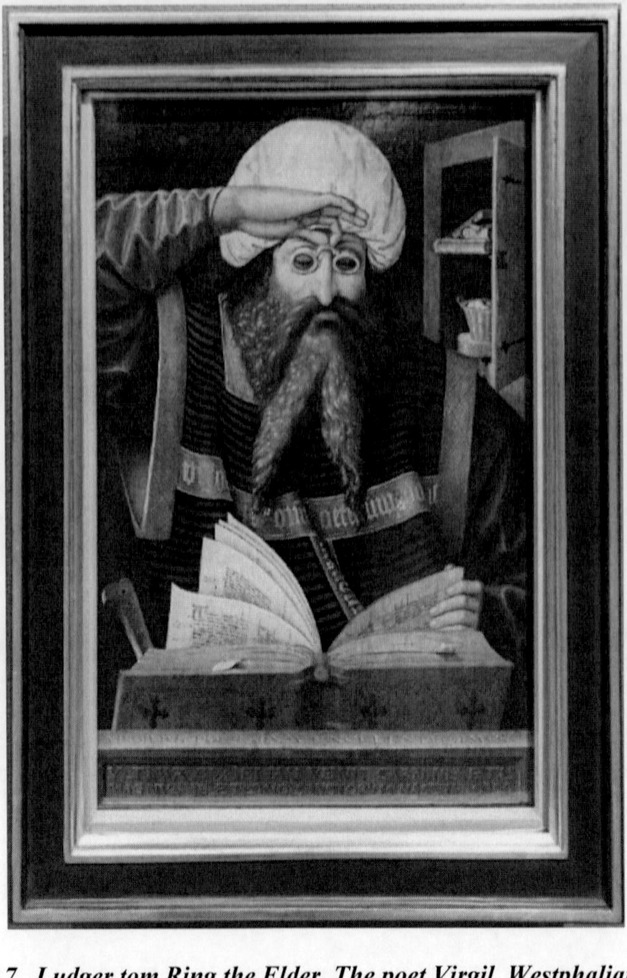

Fig. 6.7. Ludger tom Ring the Elder. The poet Virgil. Westphalian State Museum of Art and Cultural History, Münster. Public domain.

The earliest spectacles in Europe

Rivet spectacles belonging to nuns who sang in the choir have been discovered during restoration work to the choir stalls at Wienhausen Monastery. Similar spectacles were discovered at the Freiburg Augustinian monastery. All have the shape of the rivet spectacles depicted by the Italian painter Tommaso da Modena (1326-1379) (Schmitz 1982, 72).

The rivet spectacles from the Wienhausen Monastery date from the mid-fourteenth century and are made of wood. Shattered remains of a pair of scattered spectacle frames, made from the metacarpal bone of a bull, were discovered during the excavations of the Trig Lane site, by the Museum of London in 1974-75. These are also among the most ancient spectacles known, dating from the mid-fifteenth century. These spectacles have a unique feature: a row of three teeth on the sides of both handles where they widen to join the rims, and a cluster of three drilled holes in the centre of the same area, which would help to adjust contact with the nose (on this subject, see Rodes 1980, 23-25).

In the seventeenth century, quacks and market vendors also used spectacles of transparent or coloured glass to attract attention to their products. In the seventeenth century, eyeglasses were also worn in masquerades (Weve 1929, 44-48).

The benefit of wearing glasses to visual acuity is pointed out in the 1415 ballad addressed to Sir John Oldcastle (c.1378-1417) by the English poet and clerk, Thomas Hoccleve or Occleve (1368 or 1369–1426), a key figure in 15th-century Middle English literature:

> Right as a spectacle helpith feeble sighte
> Whan a man on the book redith or writ,
> And causith him to see bet than he mighte,
> In whieh spectacle his sighte nat abit
> But gooth thurgh, and on the book restith it;
> The same may men of ymages seye
> Thogh the ymage nat the seint be, yit
> The sighte vs myngith to the seint to preye.
>
> (Hoccleve, *Ballad to Sir John Oldcastle,* stanza 53 translated by Toulmin 1982, 9-42).

The ballad was written two years before the execution of Sir John Oldcastle, an English Lollard leader, hanged and burned for heresy and treason in 1417. In the ballad, Thomas Hoccleve intended to convince Sir John to give up following the movement, held as being heretic, of John

Wycliffe (1328-1384). Hoccleve uses the metaphor of spectacles as a way to make him see better.

In the sixteenth century Elizabethan play "Sir John Oldcastle", the controversial rebel was seen as a proto-Protestant martyr, inspiring William Shakespeare's character John Falstaff originally called John Oldcastle (Toulmin 1982, 9-42).

From the early fourteenth century onwards, spectacles made of convex lenses were well known but very expensive, appearing as items listed in inventories and wills.

Spectacles with lenses interconnected by means of a clip, and nose pinch glasses with no ear support ("*Bügelbrille*" in German or "*pince-nez*" in French), were developed during the late fifteenth to mid-sixteenth century. They first appeared in Germany in 1490, being adopted for everyday use throughout the country, replacing rivet spectacles which had disappeared completely from paintings of this time period (Weve 1929, 12-16).

Although spectacles provided with "temples" (the technical word used for the arms of a pair of spectacles), were fully developed in the mid-eighteenth century, pince-nez were attached to the hat or ears by wire or leather straps. This was depicted by some painters in the sixteenth century, such as Peter Bruegel the Elder (1526-1569) in the painting "Adoration of the Magi", housed at the London National Gallery (Frugoni, 2004, 31, fig. 18) (Figs 6. 8a and 8b).

A miniature from a choir book of the Monastery of Saint Mark in Florence also shows a man whose pince-nez are attached to a hat (Pansier 1901, 26).

Benito Daça de Valdes (1591-1634), known as the Father of Optometrics because he authored the first book on the subject, provided the technique for using a rudimentary ear support for pince-nez, adopted by King Filipe II (reigned 1556-1598 in Spain and 1581-1598 as Filipe I of Portugal):

> I am going to provide you with a technique that I was told King Philippe II used so that you can wear spectacles attached to a wing or stretcher so that you can hold them between the hat and the forehead so that you keep the spectacles under your eyes and can see with them, hanging from the wing, not touching the nose.[13]

---

[13] Yo os darè una traça para eso que ʃegón me dixeron la vʃava el Rey don Felipe ʃegundo,y es que pongáis los antojos afidos aun ala , ó paletilla como de calcador, y luego la encaxeis por entre el bonete y la cabeça, haʃta tanto q̃ʃe tenga y com efto vcrnã a quedar en bago los antojos, y podréis ver con ellos, eʃtando aʃsi pendiẽtes de aquel ala, ʃin que os toquen á las narizes (Valdes 1623, 85-86).

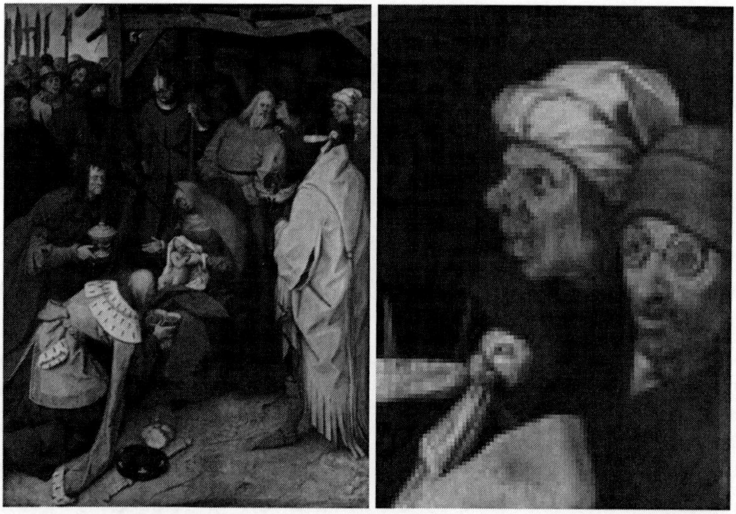

Fig. 6.8a and 8b. "Adoration of the Magi" by Peter Bruegel and detail of man wearing spectacles attached to his cap. National Gallery. Photo credit: Chris Duffin.

Sometimes, eyeglasses served purposes other than the purely optical. In Spain, spectacles were used as a symbol of status and style (Weve 1929, 44-46). By the end of the sixteenth century, spectacles were used as items of jewelry, decorated with precious stones, and kept in beautiful cases (Schmitz 1982, 195).

Following the increased accessibility of the written word following the invention of the printing press by the German goldsmith Johannes Gutenberg (1396-1469) around 1436, spectacles had started to be manufactured, becoming part of everyday life (Hirschberg 1905, 281).

The Flemish painter and engraver Jan van der Straet (Stradanus in Latin; 1523-1605), depicted the interior of a printing workshop among the great medieval and sixteenth-century discoveries in science and art. The proof reader is wearing spectacles. The explanation of the figure provides details about the printing work:

> PRINTING BOOKS – Just as one voice can be heard by a multitude of ears, so single writings cover a thousand sheets.
>
> The interior of a printing shop represents the possible appearance of Gutenberg's own shop. At the right are two screw presses. In the background a printer applies

ink with two daubers. At the left compositors set type while an apprentice gathers the sheet. The proof reader wears an early form of spectacles (Stradanus 1953, Plate 4) (Fig. 6.9).

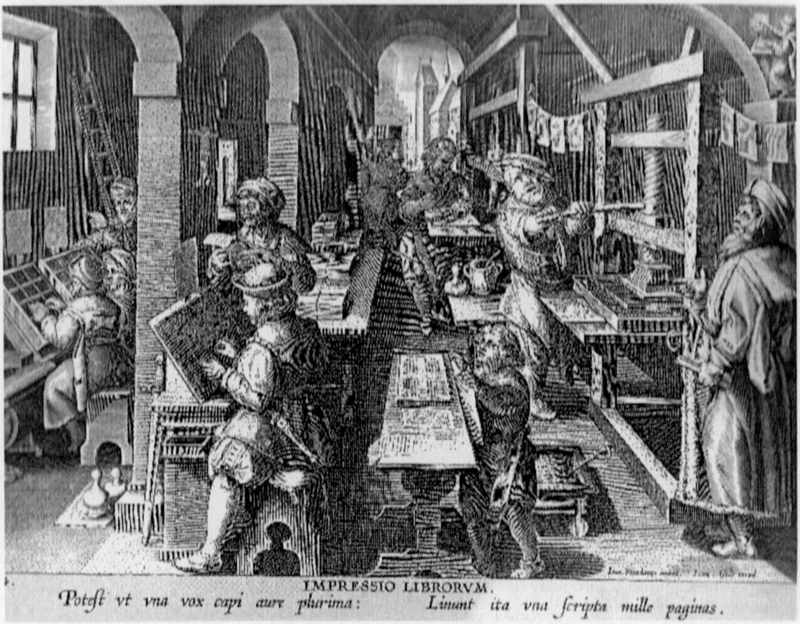

Fig. 6.9. Jan van der Straet. Impressio Librorvm. Reproduced from Stradanus 1953. Plate 4.

Engraving on copper was developed by Florentine goldmisths in the 1400s. Jan van der Straet also depicted an engraving workshop, displaying the production of engravings. On the right side, a man is composing the letters, wearing spectacles (Fig. 6. 10).

The lenses were manufactured according to empirical knowledge. According to Barck: "The earliest numbering of the lenses was crude and arbitrary. The age for which they were considered most suitable was scratched scales" (Barck 1907, 206-226). Early spectacles were supported without earpieces by pinching the bridge of the nose. A handwritten manuscript from 1600, housed in the Germanic Museum in Nuremberg, documents the first set of regulations for eyeglasses manufacturers, dating from 1483, together with images of folding spectacles, scissor spectacles, monocles and bow spectacles (Bock 1903, 29, fig.17) (Fig. 6.11).

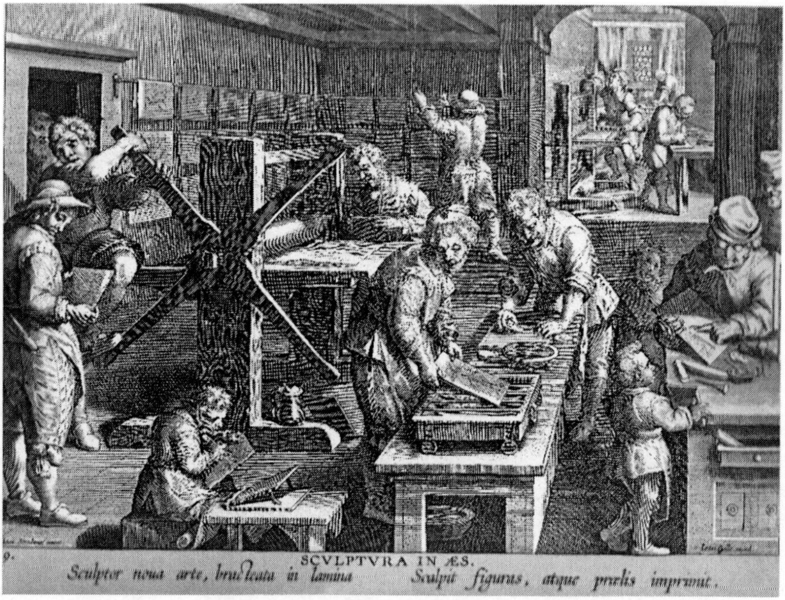

Fig. 6.10. Jan van der Straet. Engraving on copper. Reproduced from Stradanus 1953. Plate 19.

In 1482, eyeglass manufacturers from Nuremberg were mentioned. Images illustrating vendors and customers of spectacles trying them out in stores or outdoor markets frequently appear in sixteenth century books and engravings.

Another engraving by Jan van der Straet dedicated to the invention of spectacles, provides a vivid representation of the sale of spectacles. The vendors display their products on their shop counters, showing the lenses and spectacles available at the time and people trying them on, while a dog leads a less happy blind man. The subtitle and explanation of the figure read as follows:

> Also invented were eyeglasses which remove dark veils from the eyes. At the left the optician (note this trade banner) dispenses ready-made spectacles and magnifiers. These were equipped with neither temple-bars nor nose-grip. At the right their use is shown, while in the back the blind man is led by a dog (Stradanus 1953, Plate 15) (Fig. 6.12).

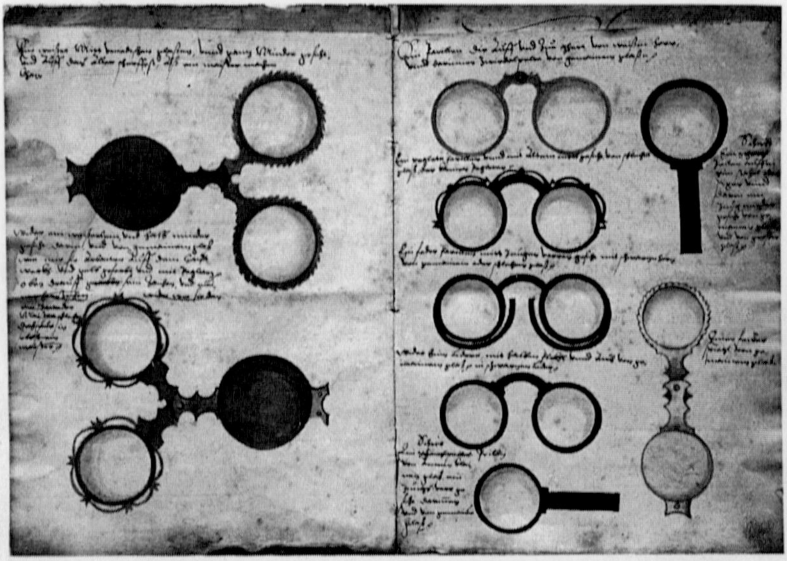

Figure 6.11. Folding spectacles (on the right); scissor spectacles and bow spectacles on the left. Germanic Museum, Nuremberg, Germany. (Bock 1903, 29, fig.17).

It should be noted that spectacles do not remove dark veils, which include anything that opacifies the ocular structures, such as cataracts that obscure the lens.

At that time, physicians had no scientific background understanding as to how spectacles worked, leaving the job to traders who could conduct some tests with clients to check out what would best suit their needs, a task shrouded in mystery (Bock 1903, 16).

The physiological events of vision, namely, refraction of light when entering the eye and focusing of the image on the retina by accommodation of the lens, were not known until the German astronomer, mathematician and natural philosopher Johannes Kepler (1571-1630) published his work *Ad Vitellionem paralipomena, quibus astronomiae pars optica traditur* in 1604. Kepler, known as the Father of Optics, was the first to understand that the image was formed on the retina and how the crystalline lens functioned (Pansier 1901, 43). His remarkable contribution marks the beginning of Medical Optics, permitting an understanding as to how lenses interact with the human eye for vision correction with spectacles.

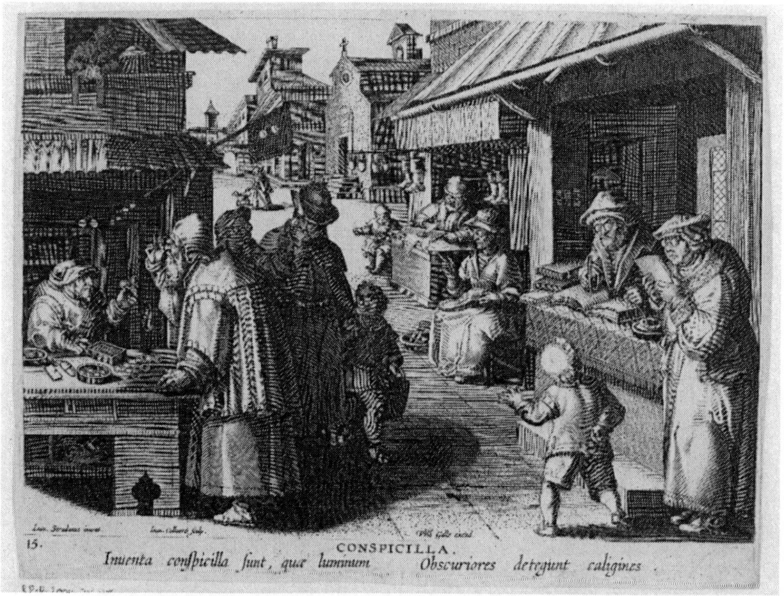
15.
CONSPICILLA.
Inuenta conſpicilla ſunt, quæ luminum Obſcuriores detegunt caligines.

Fig. 6.12. Jan van der Straet. Spectacles. Reproduced from Stradanus 1953. Plate 15.

Until that time, the "crystalline" (the lens in the eye) was considered the main organ of vision, as stated by the French physician Andre du Laurens (1558-1609), court physician of King Henry V (reigned 1589 to 1610):

> Here are all the layers; it is time to discover the most precious treasure of the eye, the rich diamond, the beautiful crystalline, which is of greater price than all the pearls of the Orient: it is this icy humour which is the principal instrument of sight, the soul of the eye, the inner lens: it is the only one which is changed by the colours, and which receives all the images from it.[14]

Despite some advances, knowledge of the anatomy of the eye and an understanding of its physiology contained significant gaps and errors from

[14] Voila toutes les enueloppes oftees, il eft temps de defcouvrir le plus précieux threfor de Il'oeil, le riche diamant, le beau cryftallin, qui eft de plus grand prix que toutes les perles d'Orient: c'eft cefte humeur glacee, qui eft le principal inftrument delà veuë, l'ame de l'oeil, la lunette intérieure: c'eft celle qui eft feule altérée des couleurs, & qui en reçoit toutes les images (Laurent 1600, 43).

Antiquity onwards (on this subject, see Retriet et al. 2008, 697-700). Physicians relied mainly on the opinions of Claudius Galen (129-c. 216 AD) (on this subject, see Pansier 1901. 34-35). The "Prince of Medicine" as he has been called, carried out relevant dissections, especially on extraocular musculature (on this subject, see Wade 2010, 33-68). However, although he described the lens, the corpus vitreous, the retina and the optic nerve in his anatomical dissections (Simon 1906, 26-33), he did not understand the physiology of vision.

Further surgical contributions to ophthalmology were carried out by Georg Bartisch (1535-c.1607), a skilled barber-surgeon born in Dresden from a poor social background, who was Court Oculist to Duke August I (Elector of Saxony from 1553 to 1586).

Bartisch authored the first ophthalmic textbook, *Ophthalmodouleia. Das ist Augendienst*, published in 1583 (Fig. 6. 13a). The work, written in German since he had no university studies and studied Latin by himself, was the first Renaissance work on eye surgery and established a new surgical ophthalmological speciality. He described new diseases and treatments and devised several surgical instruments, giving a new shape to ancient needles for cataract couching (Fig. 6.13.b).

Bartisch viewed refractive errors, which provoked blurred vision if not corrected with appropriate lenses, as part of corneal and lens opacity, along with other conditions leading to vision impairment and loss of vision. He recommended several recipes to improve eyesight, including purging pills, electuaries, powders, waters, and amulets such as a dead fox tongue and precious stones carried around the neck.

Recommending "Medo", would prevent blindness and refresh sick and weak eyes. Such amulets should be carried in beautiful earrings, rings, pendants, booklets or other lavish containers "To carry around the neck to prevent weak and dark eyesight" (*Am halse zu tragen vor ein blöde und dunckel geſichte*) or should be kept in a place where they could be beheld so that the eyes could benefit from their healing powers (Bartisch 1583, chapter III, unpaginated (Fig. 6.14). 'Medo' is the stone called "Medius" by Albertus Magnus or Saint Albert the Great, a German Dominican friar, philosopher, scientist and Catholic Saint (c.1200-1280), because it came from Media whose inhabitants are called Medes (Best & Brightman 1973). Albertus Magnus authored one of the earliest medieval lapidaries. His work *Liber secretorum Alberti Magni*, incorporated magical traditions and some mineralogical knowledge from Roman times. It circulated in manuscript copies and was published in 1502. Information drawn from these lapidaries was frequently integrated into medical prescriptions until the end of the 18th century.

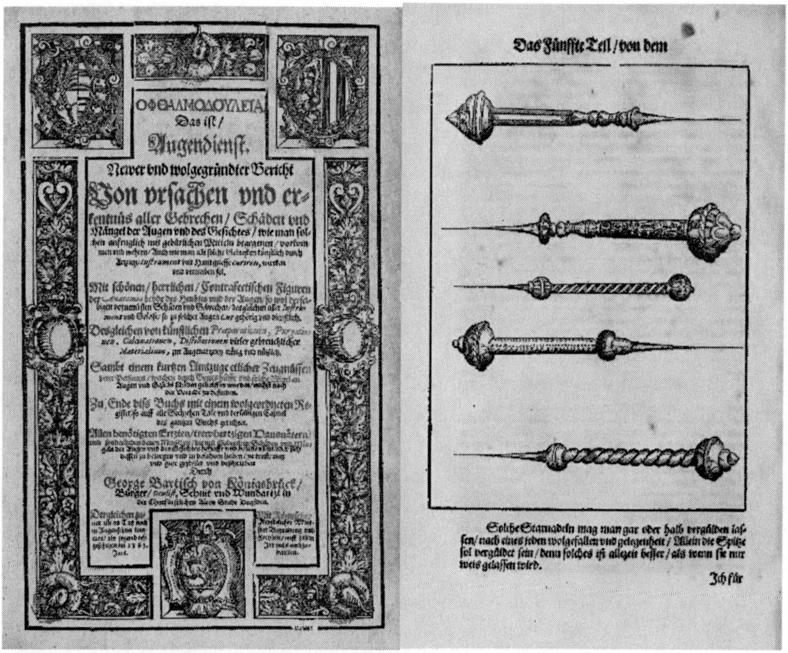

Fig. 6.13a. Georg Bartisch. 6. 13b. Title page. [Ophthalmodouleia] das ist, Augendienst, 1583. 6.13.b. Cataract needles.

The stone, probably a copper mineral, was said to be "good against the gout and blindness of the eyes, and it nourisheth hurt and weak eyes" (Best & Brightman 1973, 29-30).

Copper minerals like malachite were empirically known to be beneficial for the eyes because of the antimicrobial properties of copper (on this subject, see Barroso 2017, 99-107). However, used as an amulet, its properties relied on magic, at best acting by psychological effect or sympathetic magic, according to the principle *Similia Similibus Curantur (Like Cures Like)*. However, in this case, it should be noted that refractive errors of the eyes do not benefit from drugs, only from correction by appropriate lenses.

When addressing lenses and spectacles, it is clear that Bartisch had no scientific background on which to rely for understanding and prescriptions purposes. He insisted that, rather than wearing spectacles, it was better to strengthen the eyesight and advised lenses and spectacles only for those who thought they might benefit from using them. He provided several recipes for electuaries which included vegetable ingredients like myrrh, used to improve eyesight since Antiquity. Some recipes include comminuted minerals like jade, white coral, white agate, rubies, crabs' eyes and amethyst. He stated that sometimes it was better to wear nothing at all in front of the eyes, gave recipes based on herbal ingredients which would act better than lenses and that it was always better to be two-eyed than four-eyed.

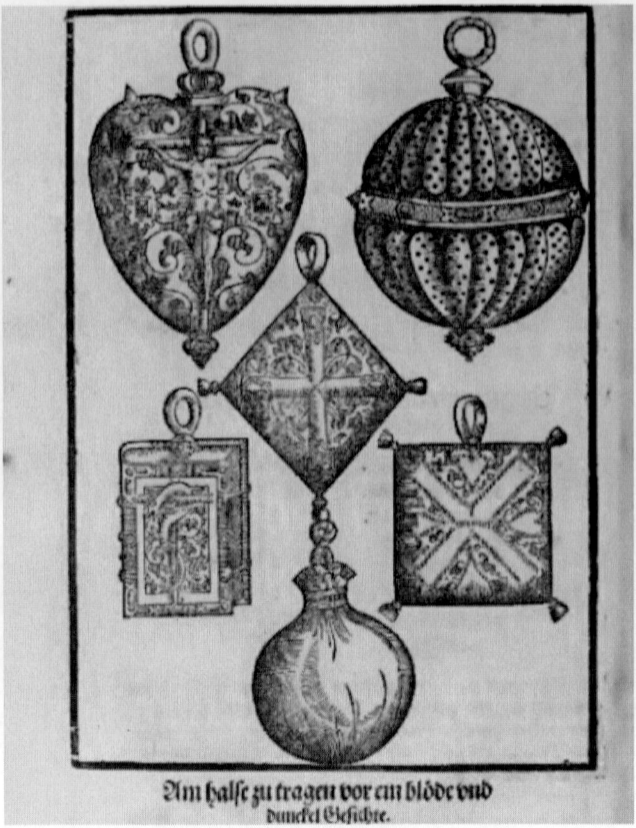
Am halse zu tragen vor ein blöde vnd
dunckel Gesichte.

Fig. 6.14. Georg Bartisch. Amulet containers. In [Ophthalmodouleia], das ist, Augendienst, 1583.

Notwithstanding, at the beginning of the chapter, he is depicted reading a book, wearing spectacles, and having what seems to be a spectacles' mould on his desk (Fig. 6.15).

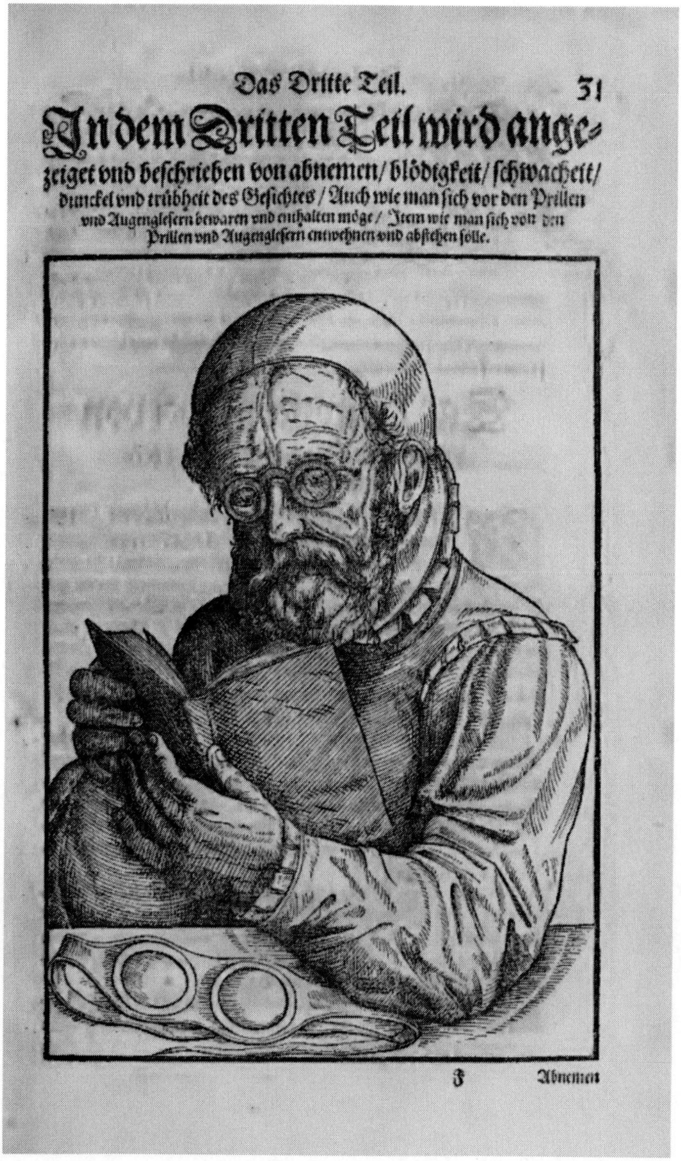

Das Dritte Teil. 31

In dem Dritten Teil wird angezeiget vnd beschrieben von abnemen / blödigkeit / schwacheit / dunckel vnd trübheit des Gesichtes / Auch wie man sich vor den Prillen vnd Augenglesern bewaren vnd enthalten möge / Item wie man sich von den Prillen vnd Augenglesern entwehnen vnd abstehen solle.

3 Abnemen

Fig. 6. 15. Bartisch. Chapter 3 in [Ophthalmodouleia], das ist, Augendienst, 1583.

Spectacles in caricatures

Although books were rare but increasingly available items after the invention of the printing press, too much reading was targeted in a satire of manners by the German humanist and theologian Sebastian Brant (1458-1521), *Das Narrenschiff (The Ship of Fools)*. A scholar is depicted with a hallucinated gaze, sitting at his lectern. He is surrounded by books that he can neither read nor understand, wearing a big pair of pince-nez, a sleeping cap, and holding another cap and a broom (Sebastian 1872, 1) (Fig. 6.16).

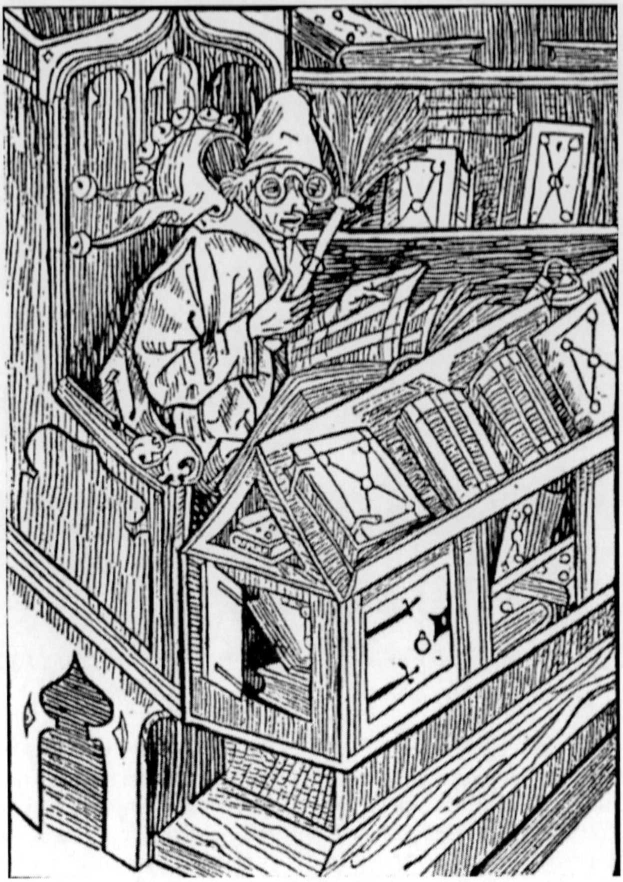

Fig. 6. 16. A scholar crazy for books in Sebastian Brant. Das Narrenschiff, 1872.

Caricatures of tooth pullers and quacks abounded, sometimes depicted wearing spectacles. A theriac[15] vendor advertises the anti-poison effect of his Theriac in a public square. Wearing a large pair of spectacles, he holds one snake while others crawl around in a box at his feet (Peters 1976, 45 fig. 47). The spectacles were meant to impress and attract customers (Fig. 6.17).

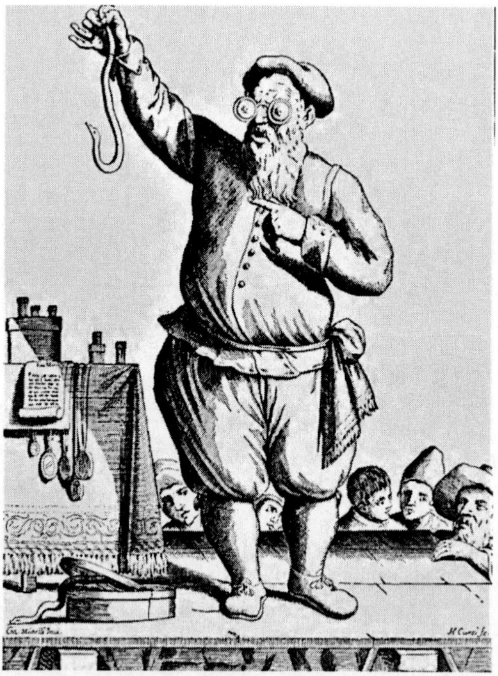

Fig. 6. 17. Theriac dealer after an engraving from Curti (1634-1718). Reproduced from Bock 1903, 21, fig 10.

[15] Theriac was an anti-poison electuary, used especially against snake toxins. It was introduced into medical practice by the Greek poet and physician Nicander of Colophon (197-170 BC). Andromachus of Crete, physician to Emperor Nero (1st century AD), reformulated the compound. The new formula contained seventy-three ingredients, one of which was the flesh of a snake, considered to be the most poisonous animal. The recipe was considered to be a cure-all remedy figuring in a poem dedicated to Emperor Nero. Theriacs by other physicians followed. Galen gave particular attention to these medicines (Drey 1978, 234).

Spectacles in representations of the devil

The reason why there should so many representations of the devil with spectacles in the Middle Ages is unclear. Perhaps people wanted to document the devil's age and preoccupation with the register of human sins (Holtmann 1978, vii-xxii). On the other hand, depicting eyeglasses in association with the devil shapes might have reflected the fact that the glasses were long considered to be a magical, deceitful tool. For that reason, spectacles were often part of the devil's costume (Reiss 1929, 107-109).

Moreover, the scientific contributions of Friar Roger Bacon were misunderstood; his works were considered to issue from witchcraft and spectacles to be things of the devil (Bock 1903, 13).

In medieval Christian iconography, representations of the devil were the ugliest imaginable. Demons took the shapes of animals like snakes, dragons, goats, pigs or boars or in the human body with animal parts (bird's feet, horns, tails, horses' feet). Ordinary people associated the spectacles with dubious decency and behaviour. In Germany, the word "Brüllenreiszer" (a gossiper with spectacles) designated a screamer or one who talked too much (Reiss 1929, 107-109). Spectacles could also denote an evil character, as seen in the poem by the German mastersinger and shoemaker Hans Sachs (1494-1576) *The devil looks for a place to rest on earth* (*Der Teufel sucht ihm ein Ruhstatt auf Erden*):

> (...) the prince looked through spectacles
> and went after the devil's passions.[16]

These infernal creatures sought to mislead mankind to embrace their most heinous and darkest works until the Final Judgement. This was represented in two trials in the late Middle Ages, in which Christ opposed the Old Testament devil Belial.

The German "Belial" is an anonymous translation of the Latin work, *Litigatio Christi cum Belial sive Consolatio peccatorum (Christ's Dispute with Belial or Consolation of Sinners*) by Jacobus Palladinus de Teramo (1349-1417), an Italian canon lawyer and bishop. This work appeared in several manuscripts with beautiful illuminations from 1461 onwards, and, later, in a series of incunabula and printed book editions. Some manuscripts are illustrated with illuminations in which devil figures are wearing spectacles. The work was very popular and was translated into other european languages. The story began when Christ entered Limbo, delivered

---

[16] (...) der Furst sah durch die Brillen/und ging nach des Teufels Willen. (Sachs 1966, 259).

the Patriarchs, led them to paradise and snatched the Old Testament from the devils. The devils felt robbed and tried to regain their possessions but, not succeeding, filed a lawsuit against Jesus for theft. Solomon was the judge and Moses defended the devils, appearing in a miniature with a Belial, wearing eyeglasses and two other devils[17] (Fig. 6.18).

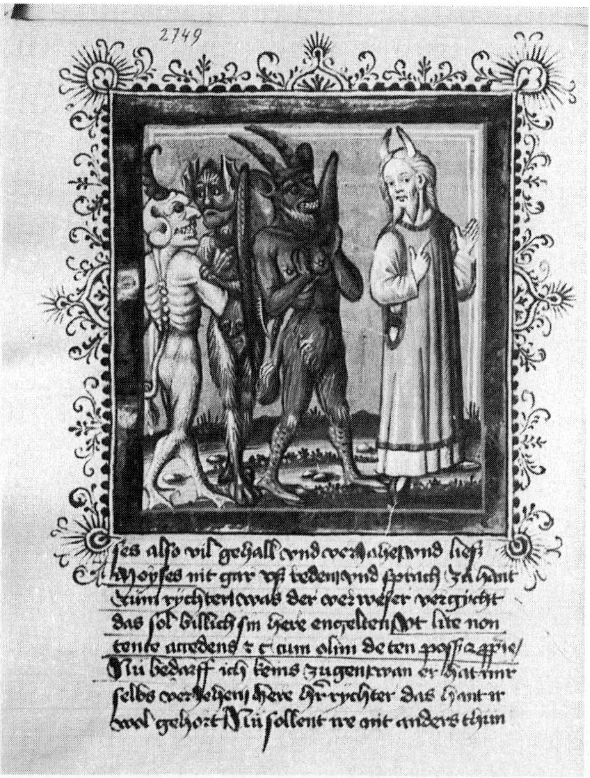

Fig. 6. 18. Belial, two other Devils and Moses. Part of Jacobus Palladino de Anacarano. Miniature. 1461. Deutsche Digitale Bibliotek.

[17] The explanation of Moses' depiction with horns would lie in a misinterpretation of Sait Jerome when translating the Hebrew word for rays of light coming from Moses' head when descending the Mount Sinai, for horns, another meaning for the word, which Saint Jerome adopted (https://blog.ititranslates.com/2014/01/17/patron-saint-of-translators/ accessed 20 June 2022).

Moses missed the date of the judgment. The story extends over two trials in which Jesus Christ is always the winner. After the resurrection, Christ, the Son of God, reigns over the whole creation. However, the devils won the right to continue persecuting and tormenting men, and dance, celebrating their triumph (Jezler 1994, 364-367). The scene is depicted in a manuscript from the State Library of Münich. In the centre, a devil reads the court's decision, wearing spectacles (Fig. 6.19).

The devils continued to pose as seductive creatures who are callous, empty and perfidious. They only emerge victorious when they manage to lead men astray.

The poet John Milton (1608-1674) characterized Belial with a fairly accurate picture of treacherous and wicked people as follows in his masterpiece *Paradise Lost:*

> (…) On th'other side up rose
> Belial, in act more graceful and humane;
> A fairer person lost not Heav'n; he seem'd
> For dignity compos'd and high exploit:
> But all was false and hollow; through his Tongue
> Dropt Manna, and could make the worse appear
> The better reason, to perplex and dash
> Maturest Counsels; for his thoughts were low,
> To vice industrious, but to noble deeds
> Timorous and slothful; yet he pleas'd the ear,
> And with persuasive accent thus began.
> (Milton, *Paradise Lost*, *Book II. Lines 98-112* (edited by Christopher Ricks) *31,*1969).

Since the interpretation of Belial's story could be misinterpreted, Pope Paulus IV (papacy 1555-1559) included the *Litigatio Christi cum Belial sive Consolatio peccatorum* in the *Index librorum proibitorum* (list of the works prohibited by the Christian Chuch), claiming the following:

> Also, no one should understand the copied book so unequivocally that he thought that he copied it correctly and understood what happened so clearly[18].

The work was included in the Index until 1981 (Degola 1841, 224).

---

[18] Auch soll niemand das nachgeschrieben bůch also einfeltiglich verstan das er geloub das das nachgeschriben recht und krieg also sichtlich geschehen sey (Jezler 1994, 364-367).

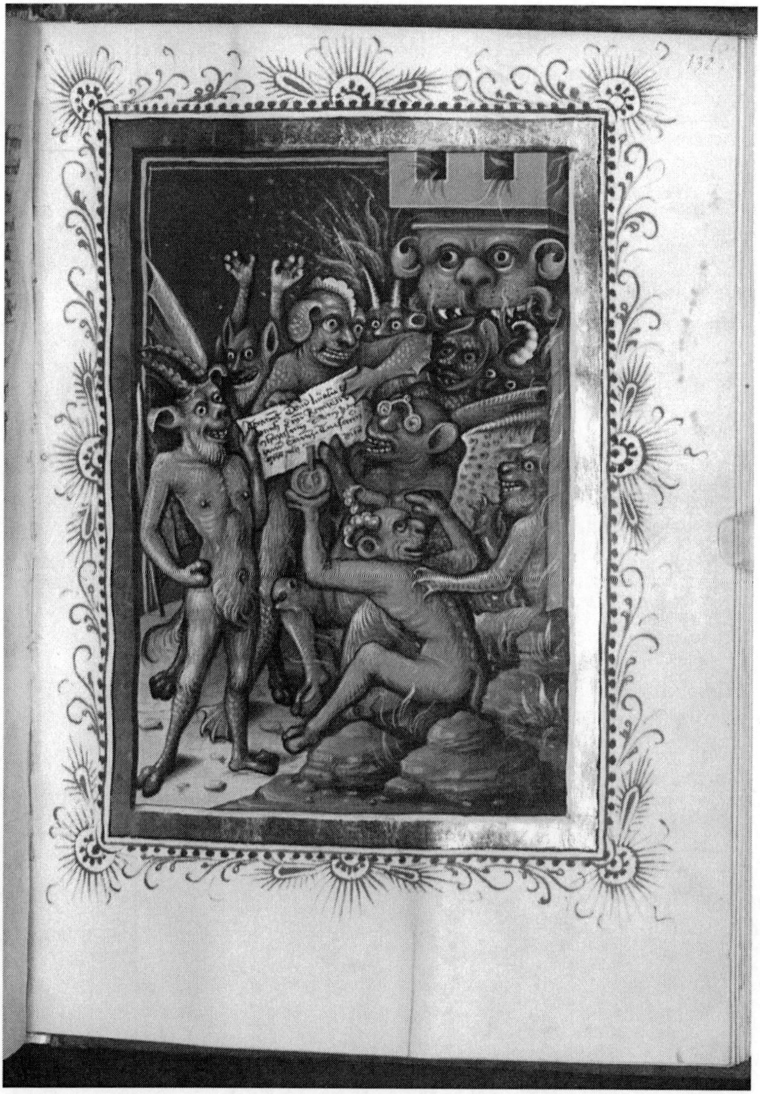

Fig. 6. 19. Devils' dance, celebrating their license to lead men to evil. Bayerische Staatsbibliothek München, Cgm 48, fol. 132r.

The torments afflicted by horrendous figures of demons and monsters on saints in isolation is one of the dominant themes of the painting "Saint John in Patmos" by Flemish painter Hieronimus Bosch (1450-1516); it is part of a series on the Saints' Triumph. In solitude on the island of Patmos, where he wrote the Book of Revelation, Saint John is not free from the devil's tricks. A little monster appears next to him in idyllic scenery (Bosing 2001, 79-81). In cases like this, Bosch's devils appear pale and pathetic, the lower body presented something like a black beetle with a reptilian tail, and he is wearing eyeglasses (Fig. 6. 20).

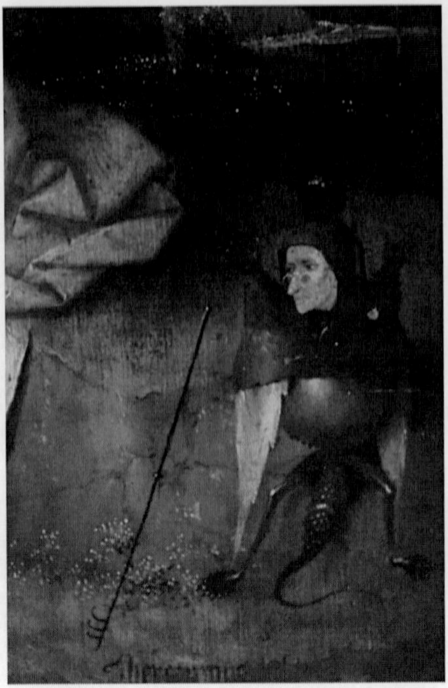

Fig. 6.20. Hieronimus Bosch. St. John on Patmos (1506). Berlin. Gemälde Galerie. Detail. Public domain.

Bosch also portrays the darkest side of humanity in several paintings where weird monsters and devils appear side by side with the pure and bright side of humanity as if the man could choose the path to follow, as expressed by the Italian Renaissance philosopher Picco della Mirandola (1463-1494):

> We have made you a creature neither of heaven nor earth, neither mortal nor immortal, in order that you may, as the free and proud shaper of your own being, fashion yourself in the form you may prefer. It will be in your power to descend to the lower, brutish forms of life; you will be able, through your own decision, to rise again to the superior orders whose life is divine (Picco della Mirandola, *Oration on the Dignity of Man,* translated by Caponigri 1956, 7-8).

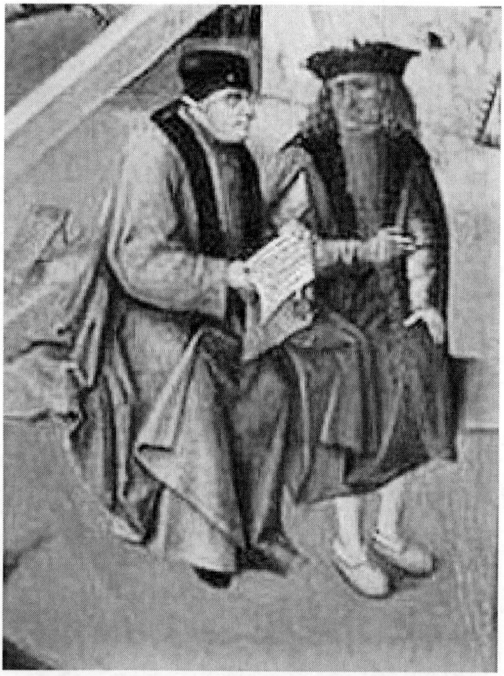

Fig. 6.21. Hieronimus Bosch. Table of the Mortal Sins. Avaritia (Greed). Museo do Prado. Madrid (Spain). Detail. Public domain.

His work "The Seven Deadly Sins and the Four Last Things", painted between 1500-1510, depicts men between Hell and Glory[19]. When portraying greed (Latin *avaritia),* a crooked judge accepts a bribe, wearing spectacles (Fig. 6.21).

[19] Hieronymus Bosch. Table of the Seven Deadly Sins. Museo del Prado (https://www.museodelprado.es/en/the-collection/art-work/table-of-the-seven-deadly-sins/3fc0a84e-d77d-4217-b960-8a34b8873b70 accessed 24 June 2022).

According to the art historian Reginal Howard Wilensky, in 1581, one year after King Filipe II of Spain was reigning in Portugal as King D. Filipe I (reigned in Spain from 1556 and Portugal 1580 until he died in 1598) whilst watching a procession in the streets of Lisbon, commented to his fifteen year-old daughter Isabella "I'm really sorry you and your brother can no longer see some devils like those painted by Bosch". Isabella's brother, Infant Philipp, later King D. Filipe III of Portugal (reigned 1598- 1621), was three years old by that time and an admirer of Bosch's depictions of the devil. He already owned twelve or more paintings of Bosch's devils, some of which can still be seen at the Palaces of Prado and Escorial. Bosch was the painter of demons and haunted creatures, as well as fantastic, satirical and didactic paintings, which were admired and disputed by other European sovereigns (Wilensky 1958, 2).

Friar José de Siguënza (1544-1606), the prior of the monastery of Escorial, also held Bosch in great esteem, stating about his paintings that:

> his paintings require care and study and should be beheld with study. The owl is a nocturnal bird, dedicated to Minerva and studying, a symbol of the Athenians, where Philosophy flourished and can be reached with the stillness and silence of the night, spending more oil than wine[20].

Paintings such as "The Seven Deadly Sins and the Four", "The temptations of Saint Anthony" and Tryptich of "The Last Judgement" are among the numerous painting by Hieronymus Bosch that he donated to the Escorial Monastery (Cuevas 1930, 545-668).

Around 1530, Damião de Góis (1502-1574), a humanist and philosopher at the court of King D. Manuel I, had acquired a horrendous triptych, "The temptations of Saint Anthony", painted c. 1505 and currently housed at the National Museum of Ancient Art in Lisbon (Wilensky 1958, 2).

In the central panel, the devils are incarnations of the sinful tendencies Antonius has to contend with in the solitude of the desert (Bosing 2001, 88); demon priests and monsters are depicted. One with a pig's head is reading a book and wearing spectacles (Bosing 2002, 93-94, figs 94-95). At the bottom of the image, a man whose face emerges from a plucked goose with open hands, seemingly trying to float on the water, is also wearing spectacles, reading a manuscript a little too far away from his eyes (Fig. 6.22).

---

[20] sus pinturas son de cuidado y estúdio y com estúdio se han de mirar. La lechuza es ave nocturna, dedicada a Minerva y al estúdio, símbolo de los atenienses, donde floresció la Filosofía, que se alcanza com la quietude y silencio de la noche, gastando más aceite que vino (Sigüenza 1963, 275).

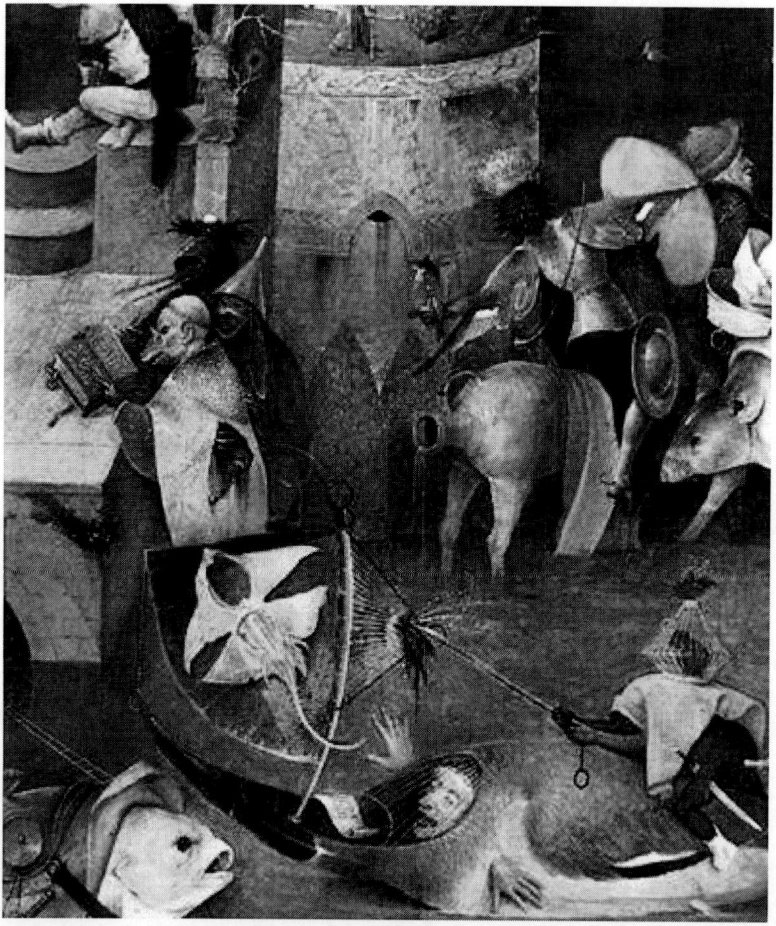

Fig. 6. 22. Hieronimus Bosch. Triptych of Temptations of St Anthony (between 1505 and 1506). National Museum of Ancient Art, Lisbon. Detail from WGA2587.jpg Wikimedia.

In the Tryptich, "The last Judgement", painted after 1482, currently housed in the Academy of Fine Arts in Vienna, Bosch dedicated the left panel to a vision of the entrance to hell. At the gate, a dark-skinned devil apprentice, wearing spectacles with white rims, reads the register of those destined to enter the hell (Fig. 6.23).

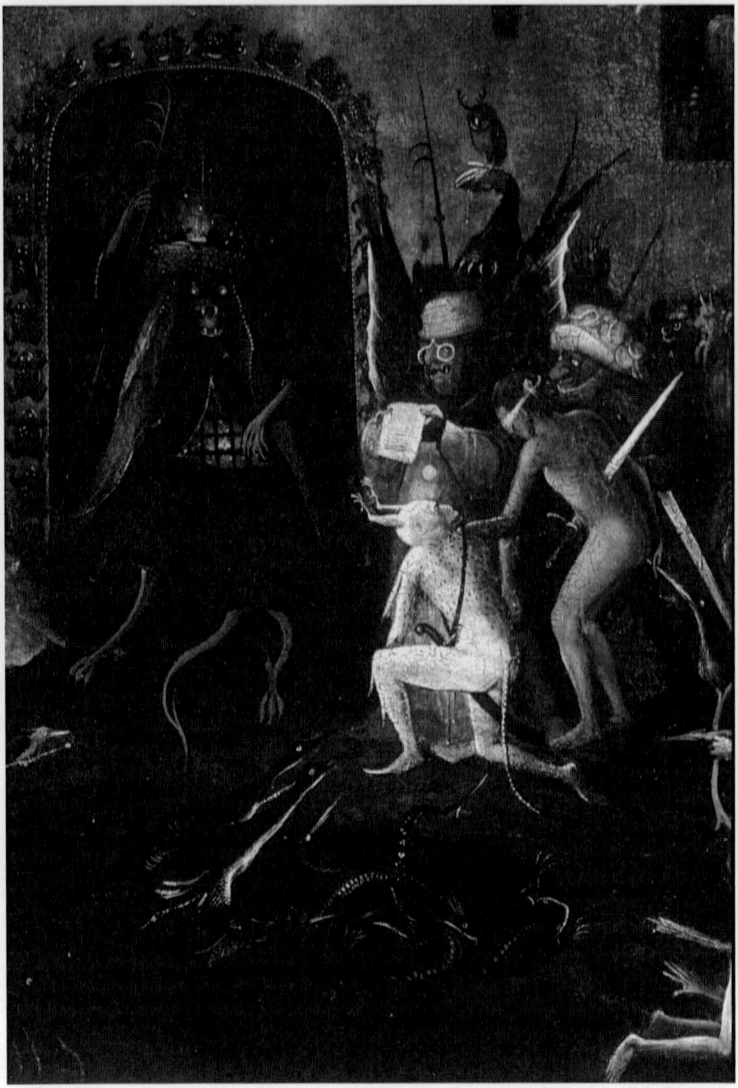

Fig. 6.23. Hieronymus Bosch. The last Jugement. Academy of Fine Arts, Vienna. Detail of the left panel. Photo credit: Nimatallah/ AKG Images/Fotobanco.pt.

Spectacles in Portugal

Reynaldo dos Santos (1880-1970), physician and pioneer of Vascular Surgery, was also a writer and one of the most eminent Portuguese art historians. He carried out a study of the earliest paintings from medieval times onwards. Many were stored in the museum's reserve collection. They were restored and studied. In a substantial number of these paintings, the authorship was unknown. In King D. Manuel's time, following the Portuguese overseas discoveries, Portuguese art stepped into a new artistic period reflecting enrichment and adopting new forms following the King's magnificence. A fruitful period of architectural initiatives followed, and commissions for altarpieces, imported from Flanders, gave Manueline painting unprecedented splendour. Some Flemish painters were hired to come to work in Portugal (Santos 1953, 20).

Thirteen panels of Flemish origin, dating from the late fifteenth century, were commissioned by the Portuguese monarchs from Flemish painters to decorate the altarpiece of the Cathedral of Évora. The Portuguese taste of the time favoured monumentality in Cathedrals dedicated to the cult of the Virgin (on this subject, see Taquenho, 2007). The Flemish painter Gerard David (c. 1460-1523), probably born in Oudwater, near Utrecht, is an artist of great value yet insufficiently appreciated (Puyvelde 1947, 17).

He also authored one of the earliest representations of spectacles in Portugal, the painting "Jesus among the Doctors", in which one of the Doctors (second from the right upper corner) is reading a book, wearing spectacles. The work is part of the panel "Polyptych of the Virgin", painted between 1495-1510, currently housed at the Evora Museum (Museu de Évora - Museu Nacional Frei Manuel do Cenáculo)[21].

In a Manueline church, Igreja Matriz de S. Miguel from Freixo de Espada à Cinta, a medieval city in Northwest Portugal near the border with Spain, a sculptural frieze of polychrome wood represents the four Evangelists with their attributes: the Angel for Saint Matthew, the Lion for Saint Mark, the Ox for Saint Luke and the Eagle for Saint John. Saint Matthew, is wearing a pair of scissor spectacles and holding a manuscript[22] (Fig. 6.24).

The provenance of the frieze is unknown. It is possibly of Flemish origin, dating from the late fifteenth century or early sixteenth century. So far, no

---

[21] Museu de Évora - Museu Nacional Frei Manuel do Cenáculo http://www.matriznet.dgpc.pt/MatrizNet/Objectos/ObjectosConsultar.aspx?IdReg 14098 accessed 10 October 2021.

[22] Igreja de S. Miguel, Matriz de Freixo de Espada-à-Cinta https://www.e-cultura.pt/patrimonio_item/6677 accessed 22 June 2022.

document has emerged to help establish the provenance and date. However, it is undoubtedly one of the earliest representations of spectacles in Portuguese art.

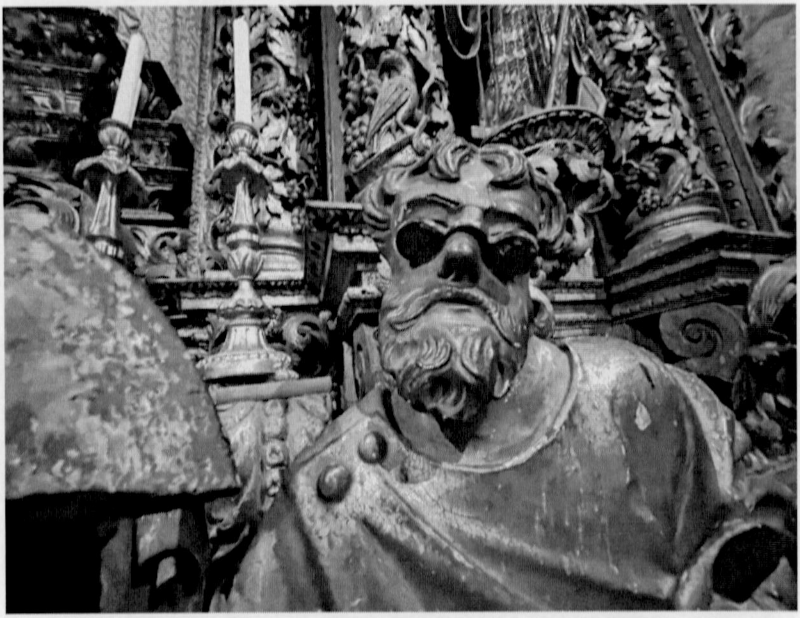

Fig. 6.24. Igreja Matriz de S. Miguel de Freixo de Espada à Cinta. Detail of the Evangelists' frieze - Saint Matthew wearing spectacles. Photo: Câmara Municipal da Câmara Municipal de Freixo de Espada à Cinta.

Scissor spectacles are also depicted in paintings from Portuguese artists from the sixteenth century. A painting housed at the National Museum of Ancient Art in Lisbon (Museu Nacional de Arte Antiga), depicts a male figure with a long white beard belonging to the Order of the Knights of Christ, as indicated by the cross on the doublet. The knight, already aged, is holding a manuscript in his left hand and a pair of spectacles in the right, meaning he wore spectacles when reading. The author is unknown. It has been attributed to Gregório Lopes (c. 1490-1550), one of Portugal's most outstanding painters of the sixteenth century. This portrait has been presumed to be of the famous explorer Vasco da Gama (1469-1524), the Portuguese explorer who discovered the sea route to India.

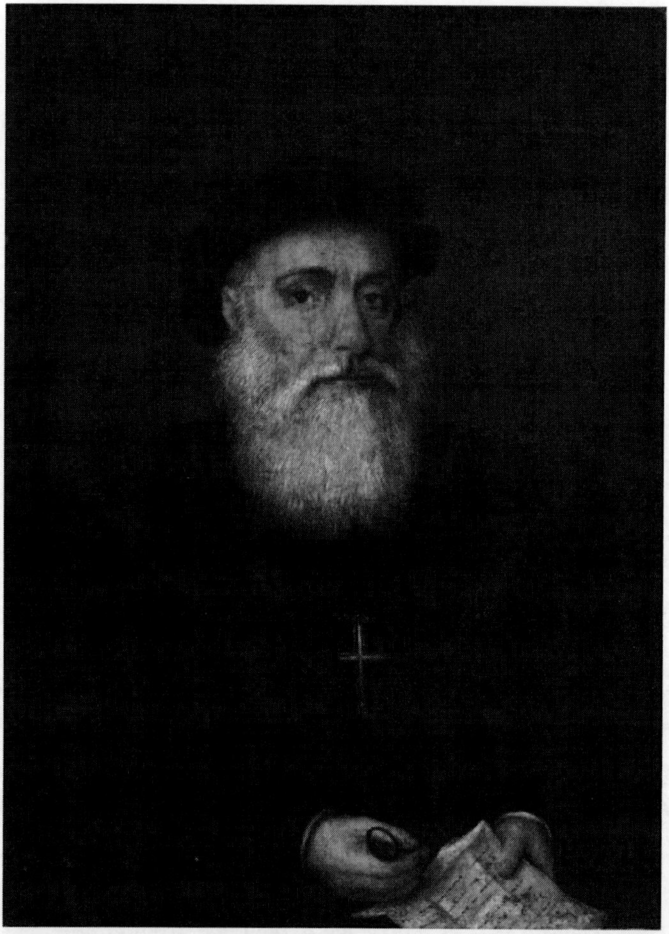

Fig. 6.25. Portrait presumed to be of Vasco da Gama (1469-1524) holding spectacles (Image reproduced from Coutinho 1946, nº 26).

Since no other portrait of Vasco da Gama, Camoens' hero in his epic poem *Lusiads,* is extant, this image was chosen to depict the explorer in a book about Camoens' iconography (Coutinho 1946, nº 26) (Fig. 6.25).

A seventeenth century oil painting of unknown authorship depicting Saint Jerome is housed at the National Palace of Mafra. Saint Jerome is depicted as an aged man, wearing a red waistcoat according to his status as cardinal on his naked breast, and holding a stone he used for self-flagellation. He is sitting at his working desk. At the centre, a skull, a pair of spectacles and manuscripts of his notes for the Bible translation, commissioned by Pope Damasus I (papacy 366-384), and a book illustrate the main characteristics for which he became known[23] (Fig. 6. 26).

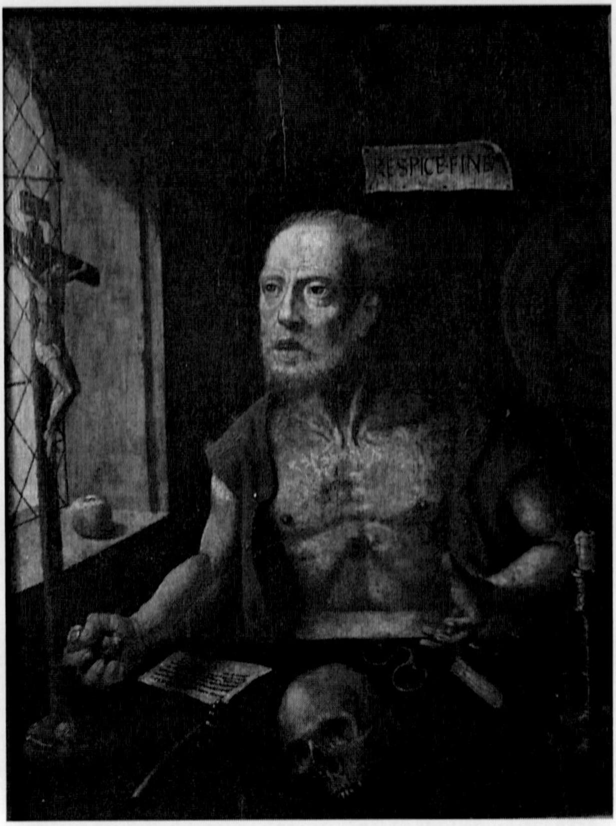

Fig. 6.26. Oil painting. Saint Jerome. Unknown author. 17th century. National Palace of Mafra. Photo credit: National Palace of Mafra.

---

[23] S. Jerónimo PNM 1925 http://www.matriznet.dgpc.pt/MatrizNet/Objectos/ObjectosConsultar.aspx?IdReg=992536 accessed 30 June 2022.

During the sixteenth and seventeenth centuries, we find people using reading eyeglasses in literary and artistic sources before they came into general use, with the exception of Portugal and Spain (Weve 1929, 44-46).

Sometimes, spectacles were used metaphorically, symbolically or allegorically implying an opposite meaning or appearing as an expression of light, clairvoyance, knowledge, or precaution (Greef 1929, 80). Luis de Camoens (c.1524-c.1580) employed the word *antolhos,* which means "eyeglasses" in sixteenth century Portuguese, and used metaphorically to indicate limited vision, limited understanding or delusions[24].

In the Elegy *(O Poeta Simónides, falando,* line 79) he writes: "*Eu, trazendo lembranças por antolhos"* (Saraiva 2002, 154-161), "while I, blinkered by my memories" (translated into English by White 2008, 148-154).[25]

A special report on spectacles comes from the Portuguese Royal family. In 1553, Queen Catherine of Habsburg (1507-1578) married King D. João III (reigned 1521-1557), an exceptional collector of exotic and luxury goods from all over the world. She offered his brother, Charles V (1500-1558), Holy Roman Emperor, King of Germany and Italy, eyeglasses made from Indian rock crystal and a tortoiseshell case, among other rarities:

> To please and delight her elder brother, Charles V, Catherine sent him bezoar stones in 1553, which he brought with him from Brussels to Yuste (Extremadura) when he retired there in 1556, while other gifts (among them an ebony box containing a tortoiseshell case and eyeglasses made from Indian rock crystal) were sent to him from Portugal two years before he died (Trnek Haag 2000, 6).

Queen Catherine developed the refined taste for collecting typical of other Renaissance monarchs and members of the nobility, especially the Habsburg family. She was queen of an overseas empire, a unique position in which she took great pride. Her collection was the first significant Renaissance *Kunstkammer* in Iberia (Gschwend 1995, 1-8). Gift-giving secured her position as Queen of Portugal, using her financial resources for special patronage, confirming and strengthening her dominant position as a ruler of the vast Portuguese empire (Gschwend & Beltz 2010, 34).

---

[24] OsDicionarios.com
http://www.osdicionarios.com/c/significado/antolhos accessed 10 October 2021

[25] *Gafas* and *Anteojos* are the Spanish word for spectaclas; *Doblos ojos* (Double eyes) is a popular expression (Hirschberg 1903, 283). *Óculos* and *anteolhos* in Portuguese.

Spectacles from the Museum of Aveiro

An unpublished collection of four pairs of pince-nez glasses without earpieces, housed at the Museum of Aveiro, contains three of the oldest spectacles discovered in Portugal. The Museum was a former monastery for Dominican nuns of the Preachers Order. The Monastery of Jesus from Aveiro (Mosteiro de Jesus de Aveiro) was founded in 1458, and became illustrious when Princess Joana (1452-1490) entered it in 1460 after refusing several marriage proposals from various European monarchs.

Princess Joana was the daughter of King D. Afonso V (reigned from 1438, being six years old, to 1477, under the regency of his uncle D. Pedro, Duke of Coimbra (1392-1499), and 1477-1481). The Princess, the sworn heir to the Crown of Portugal, kept her title until the birth of her brother, the future King D. João II (1455-1495). She was regent of the Kingdom in 1471, during the expedition of D. Afonso V to Arzila. She had always been prone to a religious vocation (Paula 2018, 19) and was later beatified by Pope Innocent XII (papacy 1691-1700) in Rome in 1693 (Braga 2020, 14).

In 1834, within the "General Ecclesiastical Reform" undertaken by the Minister and Secretary of State, Joaquim António de Aguiar (1792-1884), and carried out by the Commission for the General Reform of the Clergy (1833-1837), by Decree of May 30, all convents, monasteries, colleges, hospices and houses of all religious orders were closed. The county bishops ran the nuns' institutions until the death of the last nun, which marked the date of definitive closing. All assets were incorporated into the goods of the National Treasury. In 1874, on March 2, the Monastery of Aveiro became defunct at the death of the last nun (Braga 2020, 8). In 1911, the assets were taken to the Museum of Aveiro.

These items included reading spectacles used by the nuns over forty years old. The shape of each of the four items is similar. All are pince-nez (or scissor-spectacles) with round lenses of transparent glass. Three items have a very close parallel in a pair of leather spectacles, presumably from 1500, housed at the Nurnberg Museum in Germany (Pflugk 1929, 17-18). They also match the leather pince-nez from the catalogue of the Zeiss Museum (Poulet 1978, Z3) (fourteenth-fifteenth century) (Fig. 6.27 a-d). All have a similar shape, the lenses are transparent glass, and the frame front and bridges are made of leather. Therefore, the Aveiro specimens might also date from around 1500.

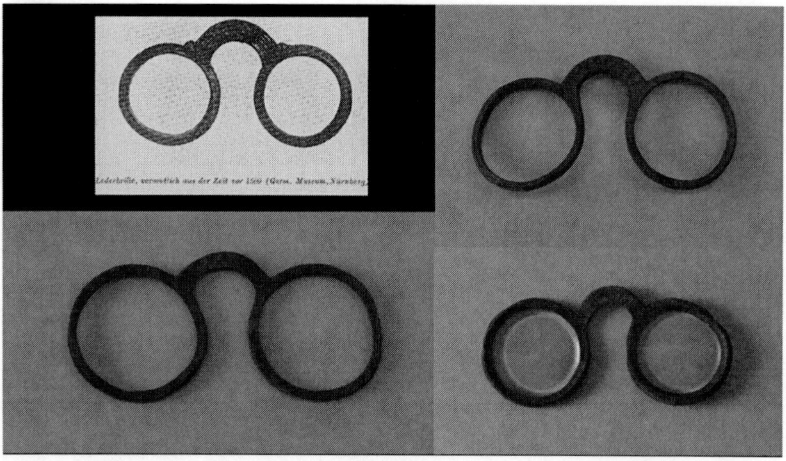

Fig. 6.27a. Leather scissor spectacles from the Nurnberg Museum (Presumably 1500) reproduced from Pflugk 1929, 17).
Fig. 6.27b. Scissor spectacles from the Museu of Aveiro / Saint Joana. From up right to left: Inv. Nr. 55/L. Lenses: Transparent glass; frame front and bridge: leather. H: 4,6 cm, W: 9,2 cm.
Fig. 6.27c. Inv. Nr. 56/L. Lenses: Transparent glass; frame front and bridge: leather. H: 5 cm, W: 10 cm.
Fig. 6.27d. Inv. Nr. 57/L. Lenses: Transparent glass, frame front and bridge: leather. H: 4,6 cm, W: 10 cm.
Copyright: © Museu de Aveiro / Santa Joana - Câmara Municipal de Aveiro. Reproduced with permission.

A pair of frame spectacles of silver-plated copper from the seventeenth to mid-nineteenth century from Greeff's catalogue (Fig. 6.28a) is a close parallel to Inv. Nr. 54/L from Museu de Aveiro. The right lens is broken (Fig. 6.28b). Therefore, this pair of spectacles, probably also dates from the seventeenth century.

A leaflet from the monastery, currently housed at the Museum of Aveiro, refers to the *lunettes* (eyeglasses) and glasses of the nuns from the convent, among other items. The date is unknown. It gives notice:

> "Curiosities of convent life: Lunettes - coin - bezel rings - and glass of nuns from the Jesus convent" (Fig. 6.28c).

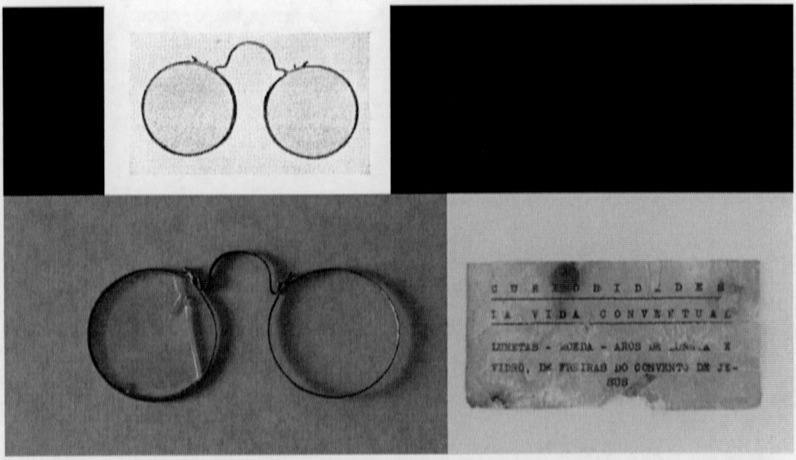

Fig. 6.28a. Wire frame spectacles from the 17th to mid-nineteenth century. In Greeff 1929, 24-26. Fig. 6.28b – Inv. Nr. 54/L. Wire frame pair of spectacles from Museu de Aveiro, Lenses: transparent glass, the right lens is broken; frame front and bridge: silver plated copper. Fig. 6.28c –Curiosidades da vida conventual. Leaflet from the inventory of the monastary, housed at the Museu de Aveiro.

Concave lenses

Concave lenses or plano-concave lenses (lenses with one concave surface and one flat surface) to rectify myopia were mentioned by the end of the fifteenth century, although this condition was only fully understood after the work of Kepler. Pope Leo X (1475-1521) (Papacy 1513- 1521) was myopic. Being a great lover of hunting, he used concave glass, which increased his visual power, making him see distant objects (Pansier 1901, 29). A portrait by the Italian painter Raphael (1483-1520) depicts Pope Leo X holding his monocle (Fig. 6.29).

The Flemish painter Jan van der Straet, known in Italy as Giovanni Stradano, was a painter at the court of Francesco I, Grand Duke of Tuscany (1541-1587), a patron of the arts between 1574-1587. His father, Cosimo I (1519-1574), was a great alchemy enthusiast. One of the paintings by van der Straet for Franco's studiolo depicts the Renaissance prince in his alchemical laboratory at the Palazzo Vecchio (Fig. 6.30).

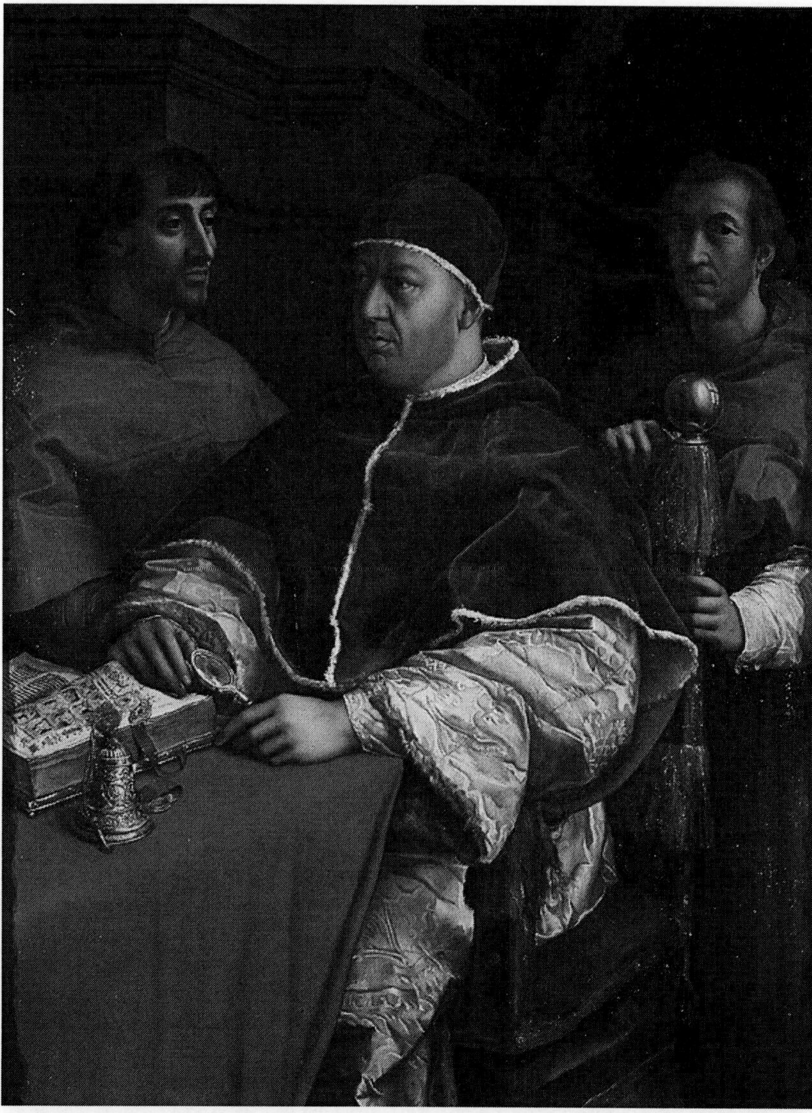

Fig. 6.29. Portrait of Pope Leo X with Cardinals Giulio de Medici and Luigi de Rossi. Raphael, 1518. Uffizi, Florence. Public domain.

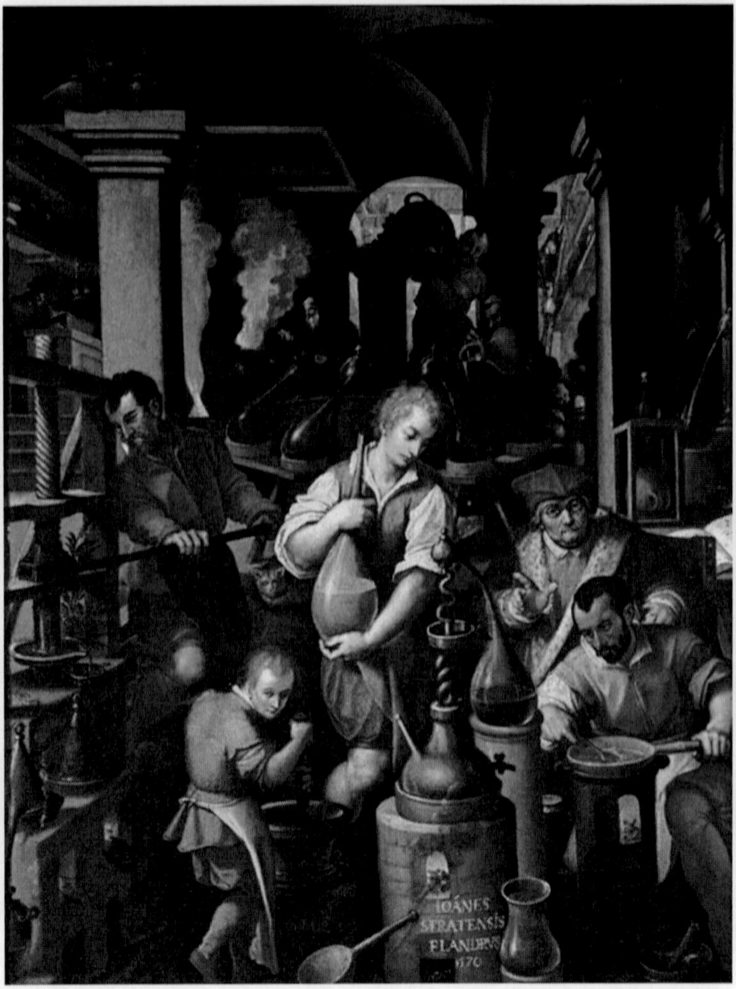

Fig. 6.30. Jan van der Straet 'The Alchemist's Laboratory' (1570). Museo di Palazzo Vecchio. Public domain.

An alchemist identified as Sisto de Bonsisti from Norsia is wearing spectacles on the bridge of his nose. This alchemist was employed in early 1560 because of his skill in counterfeiting precious stones. Francesco also employed his son Nicoló to produce crystal glass (Beretta 2014, 129-156). Sisto de Bonsisti is neither reading nor holding any books. Therefore, it is likely he is wearing concave lenses for the correction of myopia. The painting also provides insights into the close relationship between alchemy and the production of crystal glass.

A physician wearing a stalked monocle occurs in the title page of *De humani corpora fabrica libri septem*, written by the great anatomist Andreas Vesalius (1514-1564) and published in 1543. This illustration does depict a myopic scholar (Weve 1929, 44-48) (Fig. 6.31a and detail 6.31b).

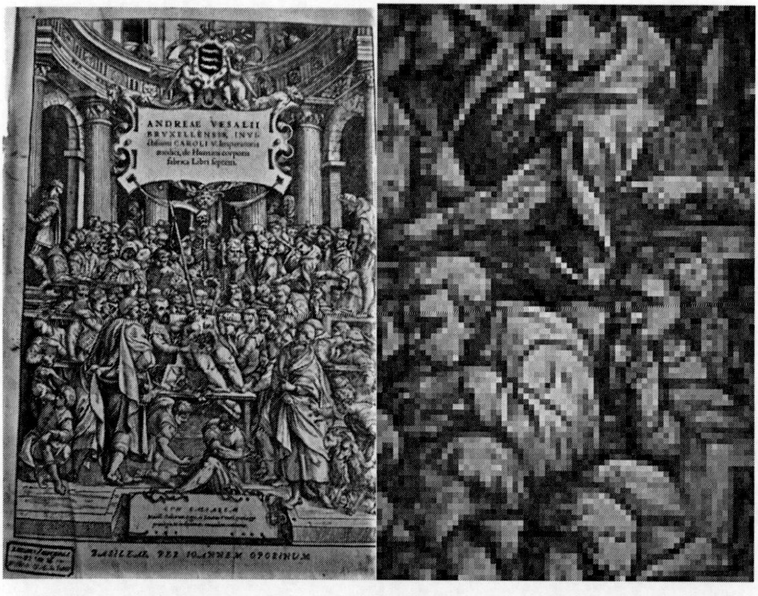

Fig. 6.31a. Title page of Vesalius' De humani corporis fabrica, 1543. Courtesy of the Library from Faculty of Medicine, University of Lisbon. Fig. 6.31b. Detail. Myopic physician with a stalked monocle.

Another physician near him is wearing a pair of scissor-spectacles, more clearly visible in a copy from the facsimile edition produced by the Mexican Academy of Surgery (2011). (Fig. 6.32a and detail 6.32b).

Cylindrical lenses to rectify astigmatism were developed in the early nineteenth century (Hirschberg 1905, 281). When one finds distance spectacles depicted in an ancient artwork, it cannot be inferred that this represents correction for myopia; on the contrary, presbyopic hypermetropics may have had a need for this intervention, as well as those suffering from aphakia a condition characterized by congenital absence of the lens, or following cataract surgery or due to an injury (Allen 1972, 235 and 249).

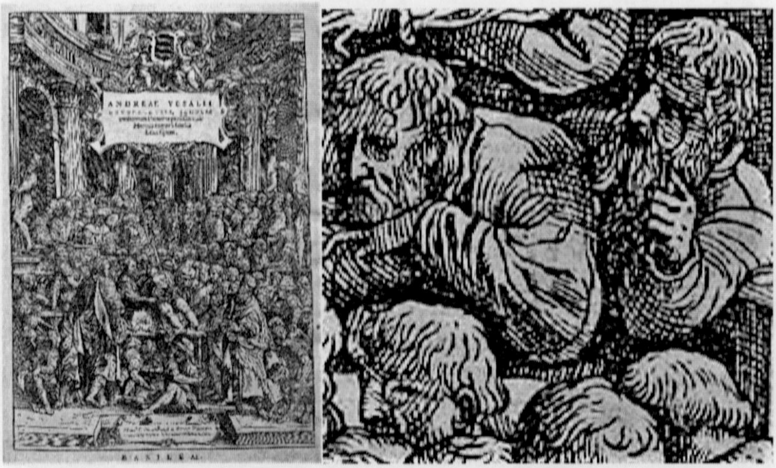

Fig. 6.32a. Title page of Vesalius' De humani corporis fabrica, 1543. Facsimile. Mexican Academy of Surgery, 2011.
Fig. 6.32b. Detail of scholar wearing scissor-spectacles.

Spectacles as protective equipment

Daza de Valdes (1591-1634) advised wearing protective eyeglasses with plain lenses, neither convex nor concave, to maintain healthy sight (Valdes 1623, 10-11). Valdes considered rock crystal the best material from which to fashion eyeglasses, but specimens should be carefully selected to avoid impurities harmful to the eyes, making them less effective than those made from glass. Quartz or rock crystal is well known for a wide range of impurities, including colour gradations caused by the presence of chemical substitutions and trace elements, and inclusions of small vesicles and inclusions of other phases including fluid vesicles and minerals.

The finest glass from Murano was also good for eyeglasses since they were light and more adaptable than rock crystal. Spectacles from average glass, lacking purity and perfection, were the poorest because they damaged the eyes rather than enhancing vision (Valdes 1623, 17-18).

Valdes understood the dangers of sudden changes from darkness to light and also advised protection from extreme cold and bright sunshine. Lenses of all colours could provide protection, such as citrine (from citrine quartz) or turquoise because it was the colour of the sky. Green was also recommended (Valdes 1623, 89-90).

Eye protection to keep dirt and debris from entering the eyes is detailed in the German translation of the philosophical work by the Italian poet Francesco Petrarca (1304-1374), *Von der Artzney bayder Glück, des gutes and widerwertigen (De Remedis Utriusque Fortunae),* meaning *On remedies for Good and Bad Luck;* this work was very popular long after his death.

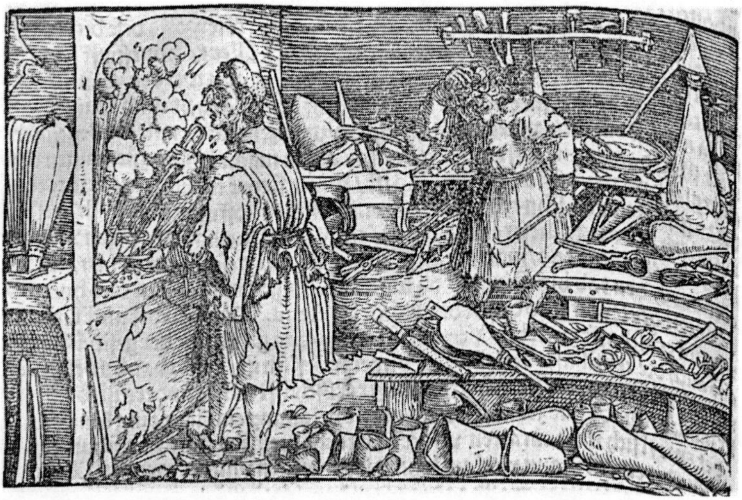

Fig. 6.33. Alchemists' workshop. Woodcut by Hans Weiditz (1495-1537). Petrarca 1532, CXI Capitel, unpaginated.

A woodcut by Hans Weiditz (1495-1537), also known as the Petrarch Master for his woodcuts illustrating Petraca's writings, depicts a caricatured scene of two alchemists at work. One alchemist stands near a stove, mixing a melting pot wearing protective spectacles (Schmitz 1982, 194; Petrarca 1532, CXI Capitel, unpaginated) (Fig. 6.33).

Furthermore, drawings by Leonardo da Vinci (1452-1519) depict coral and pearl divers wearing protecting glasses (Schmitz 1982, 194).

Ambroise Paré (1510-1590), the great French surgeon of the Renaissance, when giving advice to cataract patients concerning post-operative protection from the light, recommended that they should avoid excessive clarity and use green taffeta or spectacles to diffuse the light until they could tolerate it without pain (Paré, 1840-1841, 441).

Sunglasses have long been known to protect the eyes from harmful wavelenghts of light. In Antiquity, green gems were used to protect the eyes of gemstone cutters. From this tradition, green was deemed the most suitable colour for sunglasses appearing from the end of the fifteenth century onwards. Reports on the use of protective eye glasses date from the early sixteenth century (Schmitz 1982, 194).

Georg Bartisch also advises wearing a visor to protect the eyes from flames, light and the sun's radiation (Fig.6.34).

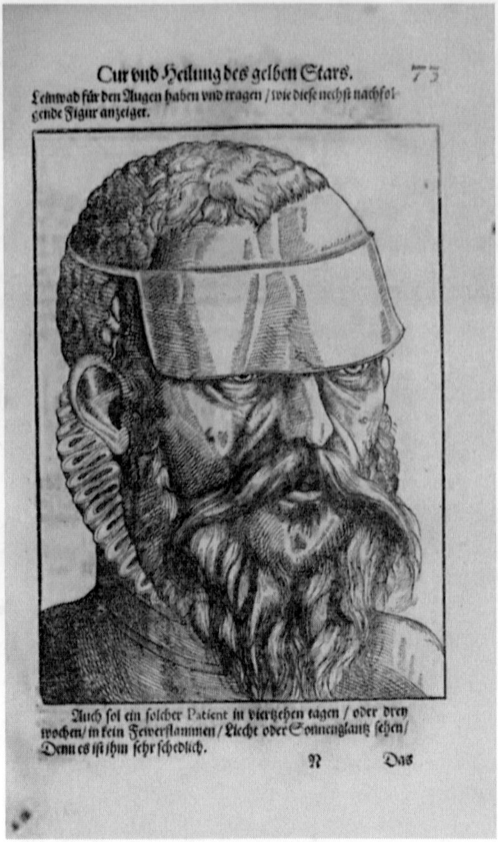
Cur vnd Heilung des gelben Stars. 73
Leinwad für den Augen haben vnd tragen / wie diese nechst nachfol-
gende Figur anzeiget.
Auch sol ein solcher Patient in viertzehen tagen / oder drey
wochen / in kein Fewerflammen / Liecht oder Sonnenglantz sehen /
Denn es ist jhm sehr schedlich.
N Das

Fig. 6.34. Georg Bartisch. Protective visor. In [Ophthalmodouleia], das ist, Augendienst, 1583.

In the mid-seventeenth century, spectacles appear as part of the personal protective equipment of physicians working with plague victims.

During the epidemics which hit Europe from the fourteenth through to the eighteenth century, physicians tried to protect themselves from contagion when approaching patients affected with plague (Peters 1969, 58, fig. 63). A copper engraving of *Doctor Schnabel, von Rom* ("Dr Beak from Rome"), a plague doctor in seventeenth-century Rome dating from after 1656, has a satyrical poem in German and some Latin words in bold:

Vos creditis als eine fabel **quod scribitur** vom Doctor Schnabel, **der fugit die contagion** **et autert** seinen Lohn darvon **Cadavera** ſucht er zu ſristen gleich wie der **Corvus** auf der Miſten . **Ah credite** , zihet nicht dort hin, dann **Romae** regnat die Pestin . **Quis non deberet** sehr erſchrecken für seiner **Virgul** oder ſtecken , **qua loquitur,** als wäre er ſtumm , und deutet sein conſilium. Wir mancher **Credit** ohne zweifel, dass ihn **tentir** ein schwarzer Teufel. **Marſupium** heisst seine Höll , und **aurum** die geholte ſeel .	Do you believe, like in a fable, on what is written about Doctor Beak, who runs away from contagion and from it earns his salary. He tries to extend cadavers' life just like the crow on the dung. Oh, believe me, do not go there For the plague is queen in Rome. You should not be so frightened for his rod or disposition, because he speaks as if he were dumb, interpreting his *Concilium.* Some of us believe, not doubting that a black devil is tempting him. His purse is his hell, and gold is his procured soul.

At the bottom of the engraving, is a description of the physician's costume in German: *Kleidung wider den Tod zü Rom Anno 1656.* At the bottom of the engraving, the clothing is described:

> Also gehen die Doctores medici daher zü Rom, wann ſie die an der Pest erkrankte Perſonen beſuchen, ſie zü curiren und tragen, sich vor dem Gift zu ſichern, ein langes Kleid von gewäxtem Tuch. Ihr Angeſicht iſt verlarvt, für den Augen haben ſie grosse crystalline Brillen, vor den Naſen einen langen Schnabel voll wohlriechender Specereÿ, in der Hände, welche mit

Handʃchʃhen wohl versehen ist, eine lange Rütje und damit deüten ʃie, was man thün und gebraüchen ʃoll. (Fig. 6.35)

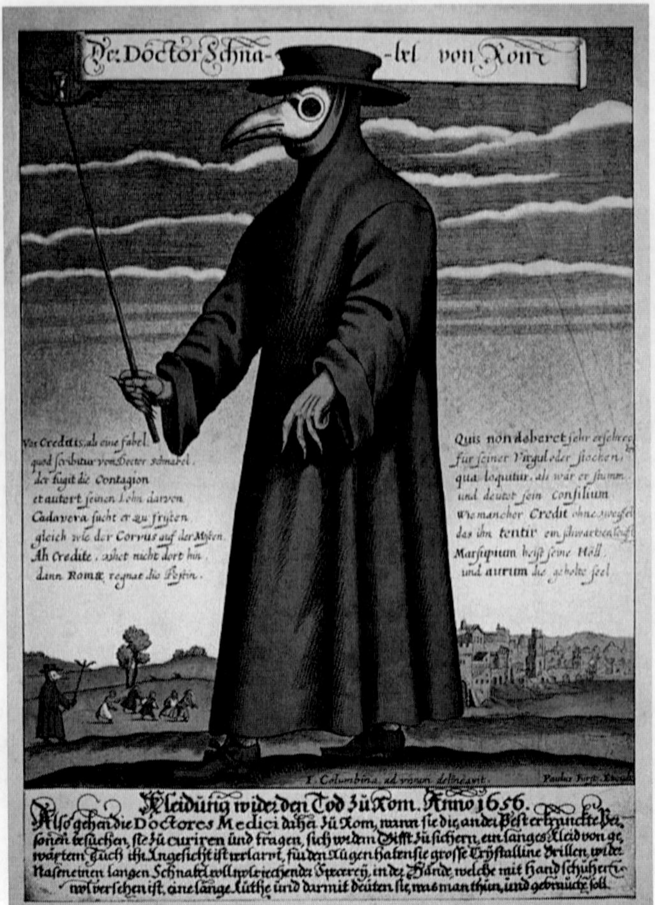

Fig.6.35. Copper engraving of Doctor Schnabel, a plague doctor in seventeenth-century Rome. Date: after 1656. Wikimedia Commons. The bottom caption describes "Clothing against death in Rome in 1656".

This is how the Medical Doctors go from here to Rome, when they visit people who are sick of plague to treat them, to protect themselves from the poison, wearing a long dress of waxed cloth. Their face is hidden, for their eyes, they have large crystalline glasses, in front of their noses a long beak full of fragrant spices, in their hands, which are well equipped with gloves, a long rod, and with this they indicate what one should do and use.

The rock crystal from Dr Beak's eyeglasses was supposed to have the virtue of purifying the rays entering the eye and, through their purity, avert the contaminated air, dangerous to the eye (Pansier 1901, 76).

Conclusion

Investigating the history of spectacles is a challenging but fascinating task, intimately linked to the development of the history of discoveries about optics and the application of optics to telescopes, microscopes and the visual arts, which are beyond the scope of this essay. Although spectacles stand among the most valuable discoveries for humanity, they frequently go unnoticed, mainly in their early history. As Dr Wolfgang Pfeiffer mentioned in his introduction to Poulet's Atlas, it is not easy to understand why such a small number of museums of optics exist (Pfeiffer 1978, iii-v). From the eighteenth century onwards, optical material and medical literature abound. It is somctimes difficult to disentangle the story from legends or forgeries until then. For our part, we have sought to add some insights into the earliest spectacles known from Portugal, presenting an almost unknown sculpture, some paintings and a hitherto unpublished collection.

Acknowledgements

I thank Professor Alfredo Rasteiro, Professor of Ophthalmology of the University of Coimbra, for the opthalmological supervision of this essay and Dr Christopher J. Duffin for his critical reading of the manuscript and to reproduce his images. I am grateful to Dr Miguel Capão Filipe, Councillor of the Aveiro City Council and Dr José António Cristo, Director of the Museum of Aveiro, for their kind permission to study and reproduce the unpublished collection of spectacles from the Museum of Aveiro. I thank the permission to reproduce images The National Gallery, London, Deutsche Digitale Bibliotek, Bayerische Staatsbibliothek München, and Dr Susana Henriques, Librarian of the Faculty of Medicine of the University of Lisbon and Professor Victor Oliveira, Director of the Library of the Lisbon Faculty of Medicine for their permission to reproduce the cover of Vesalius' *De humanis corporis fabrica*. I am very grateful to Professor Maria Teresa Dias Furtado and Dr. Ana de Sousa Dias for bringing the sculpture frieze of Freixo de Espada à Cinta to my knowledge and Dr. Jorge Duarte for the available information on the sculpture. I also thank Dr. Sérgio

Gorjão, Director of the National Palace of Mafra and Dr. Teresa Amaral for kind permission to reproduce the painting of Saint Jerome with spectacles.

References

Albrecht. 1842. *Der Jüngere Titurel.* Übersetzung von Karl August Hahn. Quedlingburg Leipzig: Druck und Verlag von Gottfried Basse.

Aristophanes. 2005. *Aristophanes. The Complete Plays.* Translated by Paul Roche. New York, USA: New American Library.

Allen, James. 1972. *Manual de las Enfermidades de los Ojos.* Spanish version by Palomar-Petit. Reprint of the 16th Edition. Barcelona: Salvat Editores S. A.

Bacon, Roger. 1962. *The Opus Majus of Roger Bacon.*Translated by Robert Belle Burke. New York: Russell & Russell, Inc.

Barck, *Carl*. 1907. "The *History of Spectacles*. (Illustrated)." The *Open Court,* (4) 4: 206-226. Available at: https://opensiuc.lib.siu.edu/ocj/vol1907/iss4/4 accessed 5 June 2022.

Barroso, Maria Do Sameiro. 2017. "Malachite, the healing gem of Green Nature." *Vesalius*, (23) 1, June: 99-107 www.vesalius.org.uk

Bartisch, George. 1583. *[Ophthalmodouleia], das ist, Augendienst : Newer und wolgegründter Bericht von Ursachen und Erkentnüs aller Gebrechen, Schäden und Mängel der Augen und des Gesichtes, wie man solchen anfenglich mit geburlichen Mitteln begegnen, vorkommen und wehren, auch wie man solche Gebresten künstlich durch Arzney, Instrument und Handgriffe curiren, wirken und verreiben sol ....* [Dreszden]:[Matthes Stöckel].

Beretta, Marco. 2014. "Material and Temporal Powers at the Casino di San Marco." 136-156 *In* Dupre, S. (ed.): *Laboratories of Art: Alchemy and Art Technology from Antiquity to the 18th Century*. Berlin: Freie Universität, Max Plank Institute for History of Science.

Bergholt, Klaus. 1992. *Artz, Krankheit und Therapie bei Petrarca. Die Kritik an Medizin und Naturwissenschsft im italienischen Frühhumanismus.* Weinheim: VCH Verlagsgeselschaft mbH.

Bergholdt, Klaus. 1994. "Die Erfindung und Verbreitung der Brille im Spätmittelalter." *Medizinhistorisches Journal,* 29 (2): 111-120.

Best, Michael & Brightman, Frank (eds). 1973. *The Book of Secrets of Albertus Magnus.* Boston, M/Ayork Beach, ME: Weiser Books.

Bock, Emil. 1913. *Die Brille und ihre Geschichte.* Wien: Verlag von Josef Safr.

Bosing, Walter. 2001. *Alle Schilderijen.* Vertaling door Klaas de Graaf. Köln: Taschen Verlag.

Braga, Joana. 2020. *Ordem dos Pregadores. Mosteiro de Jesus de Aveiro. Instrumento de descrição arquivística L 756.* Lisboa: Torre do Tombo.

Coutinho, Xavier. 1946. *Camões e as Artes Plásticas.* Porto: Livraria Figueirinhas.

Brant, Sebastian. 1872. *Das Narrenschiff* (erneut von Kark Simrock). Berlin: Franz Lipperheide.

Cuevas. Julián Zarco.1930. "Inventario de las alhajas, relicarios, estatuas, pinturas, tapices, y otros objetos de valor y curiosidad donado por el rey don Felipe II al Monasterio de El Escorial. Años de 1571 a 1598." *Boletín de la Real Academia de la Historia,* 96: 545-668.

Delcorno, Carlo (ed.). 1974. *Giordano da Rivalto. Quaresimale fiorentino, 1305-1306.* Firenze: G. C. Sansoni.

Degola, Friar Thomas Antoninus (ed.). 1841. *Index Librorum Prohibitorum Sanctissimi Domini Nostri Gregorii XVI Pontificis Maximi.* Roma: Ex Typographia Camertae Apostolica.

Drey, Rudolf. 1978. *Apothecary Jars. Pharmaceutical Pottery and Porcelain in Europe and the East 1150-1850. With a Glossary of Terms used in Inscriptions.* London: Faber and Faber Limited.

Frugoni, Chiara. 2004. *Das Mittelalter auf der Nase. Brillen, Bücher, Bankgeschäfte und andere Erfindungen des Millelalters.* 2. Auflage. München: C.H. Beck Verlag.

Goes, Frank Joseph. 2013. *The Eye in History.* New Delhi, London: Jaypee Brothers Medical Publishers (P) Ltd.

Gschwend, Annemarie Jordan. 1995. "In the Tradition of Princely Collections: Curiosities and Exotica in the *Kunstkammer* of Catherine of Austria." *Bulletin of the Society of Renaissancs Studies,* 8 (1): 1-8.

Gschwend, Annemarie Jordan & Beltz, Johannes. 2010. *Elfenbeine aus Ceylon. Luxusgüter für Katarina von Habsburg (1507-1578).* Zurich: Museum Rietberg.

Greeff, Karl Richard. 1923. "Der vergrößernde Krystal des Konrad von Würzburg (c. 1275)." *Zeitung Ophthalmologie,* Optik 8: 98-101.

Greeff, Karl Richard; Hallauer, Otto; Lundsgaard, Konrad; Reiss, Wiktor; Weve, Henricus Jacobus & Simón, Jose Maria (hrg). 1929. *Katalog einer Ausstellung zur Geschichte der Brille. Im Auftrag des Vorsstandes des XIII Internationalen Ophthalmologischen Kongresses zu Amsterdam.* Amsterdam: Verlag A. E. d' Oliveira.

Greeff, Karl Richard. 1929. "Klemm, klamm – oder Federbrilles." 24-26 *In* Greeff, K. R. ; Hallauer, O.; Lundsgaard, K.; Reiss, W,; Weve, H. J. & Simón, J. M. (hrg). *Katalog einer Ausstellung zur Geschichte der Brille. Im Auftrag des Vorsstandes des XIII Internationalen Ophthalmologischen Kongresses zu Amsterdam.* Amsterdam: Verlag A. E. d' Oliveira.

Hirschberg, Julius. 1905. *Geschichte der Augenheilkunde bei den Arabern* Band 2 Leipzig: Verlag Engelmann.

Hollauer, Otto. 1929. "Nietbrillen." 9-11 *In* Greeff, K. R.; Hallauer, O.; Lundsgaard, K.; Reiss, W.; Weve, H. J. & Simón, J. M. (hrg). *Katalog einer Ausstellung zur Geschichte der Brille. Im Auftrag des Vorsstandes des XIII Internationalen Ophthalmologischen Kongresses zu Amsterdam.* Amsterdam: Verlag A.E. d' Oliveira.

Holtmann, Horst. 1978. "Abriß zur Brillengeschichte." vii-xxii, Band I. *In* Poulet, W. *Atlas zur Geschichte der Brille mit Einschluss der Contactlinse.* Bonn: Wayenborgh.

Ilardi, Vincent. 2007. *Renaissance vision from spectacles to telescopes.* Philadelphia: American Philosophical Society.

Isidore of Seville. 2010. *The Etymologies of Isidore of Seville*. Edited and translated by Stephen A. Barney, W. J. Lewis, J. A. Beach & Berghof, O. Cambridge: Cambridge University Press.

Jetzler, Peter. 1994. *Himmel, Hölle, Fegefeuer. Das Jenseits im Mittelalter. Eine Ausstellung des Schweizerischen Landesmuseums in Zusamenarbeit mit dem Schnütgen-Museum und der Mittelalterarbeit des Wallraf-Richartz-Museums der Stadt Köln*. Zürig: Verlag Neue Zürcher Zeitung.

Kepler, Johannes.1604. *Ad Vitellionem paralipomena, quibus astronomiae pars optica traditur*. Francofurti: apud Claudium Marnium & haeredes Ioannis Aubrii.

Killy, Walther (hrg.). 1988. *Literatur lexikon. Autoren und Werke deutscher Sprache.* Band I. München: Bertelsmann Lexikon Verlag.

Laurens, André du. 1600. *Discours de la conservation de la veue: des maladies melancoliques des catarrhes, & de la vieillesse.* Rouen: Claude Le Villain.

Laufer, Berthold. 1913. "Zur Geschichte der Brille." *Mitteilungen zur Geschichte der Medizin und der Naturwissenschaften.* Deutsche Gesellschaft für Geschichte der Medizin und für Naturwissenschaften 6: 379-385.

Milton, John. 1968. *Paradise Lost* (Ricks, Christopher (ed.). London: Penguin Books.

Nicaise, Edouard. 1890. *La grande Chirurgie de Guy de Chauliac composée en l'an 1363.* Paris: Félix Alcun Éditeur.

Paré, Ambroise. 1840-1841. Malgaigne, Joseph-François (ed.) *Oeuvres complètes d'Ambroise Paré*. Paris: Balllière.

Paula, Gonçalo Rebelo da. 2018. *O culto a Santa Joana Princesa em Aveiro – memórias e percursos.*Thesis. Porto: Faculdade de Letras.

Pansier, Pierre. 1901. *Histoire des Lunnetes.* Paris: Éditeur A. Maloine.

Peters, Hermann. 1976. *Der Arzt und die Heilkunst in alten Zeiten.* Düsseldorf, Köln: Eugen Diederichs Verlag.

Petrarca, Francesco. 1532. *Von der Artzney bayder Glück, des guten und widerwertigen.* Augsburg: Heynrich Steyner.

Picco della Mirandola, Giovanni. 1956. *Oration On The Dignity Of Man.* Translated by A. Robert Caponigri. Introduction by Russell Kirk. Chicago: Henry Regnery Company.

Pflugk, Albert Otto von. 1929. "Lederbrillen." 17-18 *In* Greeff, K. R.; Hallauer, O.; Lundsgaard, K.; Reiss, W.; Weve, H. J. & Simón, J. M. (hrg). *Katalog einer Ausstellung zur Geschichte der Brille. Im Auftrag des Vorsstandes des XIII Internationalen Ophthalmologischen Kongresses zu Amsterdam.* Amsterdam: Verlag A. E. d' Oliveira.

Pflugk, Albert Otto von. 1929. "Scissor spectacles." 214-215 *In* Greeff, K. R.; Hallauer, O.; Lundsgaard, K.; Reiss, W.; Weve, H. J. & Simón, J. M. (hrg). *Katalog einer Ausstellung zur Geschichte der Brille. Im Auftrag des Vorsstandes des XIII Internationalen Ophthalmologischen Kongresses zu Amsterdam.* Amsterdam: Verlag A. E. d' Oliveira

Poulet, William. 1987. *Atlas zur Geschichte der Brille mit Einschluss der Contactlinse.* Band I. Bonn: Wayenborgh.

Prioreschi, Plinio. 2003. *A History of Medicine.* Volume V. Medieval Medicine. Ornaba: Horatius Press.

Puyvelde, Leo van. 1947. *Les Primitifs Flamandes. Catalogue.* Paris: Musée de l'Orangerie.

Rätsch, Christian & Guhr, Andreas. 1989. *Lexikon der Zaubersteine aus ethnologischer Sicht.* Wiesbaden: VMA-Verlag.

Reiss, Henricus Jacobus. 1929. "Teufel mit Brille." 107-109 *In* Greeff, K. R.; Hallauer, O.; Lundsgaard, K.; Reiss, W.; Weve, H. J. & Simón, J. M. (hrg). *Katalog einer Ausstellung zur Geschichte der Brille. Im Auftrag des Vorsstandes des XIII Internationalen Ophthalmologischen Kongresses zu Amsterdam.* Amsterdam: Verlag A. E. d' Oliveira.

Retief, François Pieter; Stulting, Andries & Cilliers Louise. 2008. "The eye in antiquity". *South African medical jornal/Suid-Afrikanaase tydskrit vir Geneeskunde,* 98 (9): 697-700.

Rodes, Michael. 1980. "A pair of late medieval spectacles from the Trig Lane site." *The London Archaeologist,* 4: 23-24.

Rosenthal, Jonas William. 1996. *Spectacles and other Vision Aids. A History and Guide to Collecting.* San Francisco (USA): Norman Publishing.

Sachs, Hans. 1966. *Werke in zwei Bände.* Berlin und Weimar: Aufbau-Verlag.

Santos, Reynaldo. 1957. *Os Primitivos Portugueses.* 2ª edição, corrigida e aumentada. Lisboa: Academia Nacional de Belas Artes.

Saraiva, Maria de Lurdes. 2002. (2ª edição). *Luís de Camões – Lírica Completa III*. Lisboa: Imprensa Nacional – Casa da Moeda.

Schmitz, E. H. 1982. *Handbuch zur Geschichte der Optik.* Bd 1 (Von der Antike bis Newton). Bonn: Wayenborgh Verlag.

Schröder, Edward (hrg.). 1926. *Die Goldene Schmiede des Konrad von Würzburg*. Göttingen: Vandenhoeck & Ruprecht.

Scurlock, Jo Ann & Burton R. Andersen. 2005. *Diagnosis in Assyrian and Babylonian Medicine*. Urbana and Chicago: University of Illinois.

Seneca. 1910. *Physical Science in the time of Nero; being a translation of the Questiones naturales of Seneca.* Translation by John Clarke. Bombay. Calcutta, Melbourne: Macmillian and CO, Limited. Sigënza, Fray José de. 1963. *La Fundación del Monasterio de el Escorial.* Aguilar: Madrid.

Simon, Max.1906. *Anatomie des Galens. Zum ersten mal veröffentlicht ins Deutsche übertragen und kommentiert.* II Band. Leipzig: J. C. Hinrichs'sche Buchhandlung.

Smith, Lucy Toulmin. 1982. "Ballad by Thomas Occleve Addressed to Sir John Oldcastle, A. D. 1415". *Anglia,* 5: 9-42.

Stradanus. 1953. *New Discoveries: The Science, Inventions and Discoveries of the Middle Ages and the Renaissance as Represented in 24 Engravings Issued in the Early 1580 by Stadanus.* Dibner, Bern: Burndy Library.

Tacanho, Maria das Mercês de Carvalho Daun e Lorena. 2007. *Um particular olhar no Políptico da Virgem da Sé de Évora* (Thesis). Évora: Universidade de Évora.

Trnek, Helmut & Haag, Sabine (hrg.). 2000. *Exotica. Portugals Entdeckung im Spiegel fürstlicher Kunst-und Wunderkammern der Renaissansce. Die Beiträge des am 19. und 20. Mai 2000 vom Kunshistorisches Museum Wien veranstalteten Symposiums.* Wien: Kunshistorisches Museum.

Valdes, Benito Daça de. 1623. *Vso de los antoios para todo genero de vistas: en que se enseña a conocer los grados que a cada vno le faltan de su vista y los que tienen qualesquier antojos*. Seuilla: Diego Perez.

Vesalius, Andreas Bruxellensis. 1543. *De humanis corporis fabricamlibri septem.* Basilea: ex oficina ioannis Oporinis.

Vesalius, Andreas Bruxellensis. 2011. *De humanis corporis fabricamlibri septem.* Basilea: ex oficina ioannis Oporinis. Facsimile 1543. Candida Fernández de Calderon. Mexico: Academia Mexicana de Cirurgia.

Wade, Nicholas. 2010. "Pioneers of eye movement research." *i-Perception*, (1) 2: 33-68. doi:10.1068/i0389.

Weve, Henricus Jacobus. 1929. "Brille für die Ferne." 44-48 *In* Greeff, K. R.; Hallauer, O.; Lundsgaard, K.; Reiss, W.; Weve, H. J. & Simón, J. M. (hrg). *Katalog einer Ausstellung zur Geschichte der Brille. Im Auftrag des Vorsstandes des XIII Internationalen Ophthalmologischen Kongresses zu Amsterdam.* Amsterdam: Verlag A. E. d' Oliveira.

Weve, Henricus Jacobus. 1929. "Die Bügenbrille." 12-16 *In* Greeff, K. R.; Hallauer, O.; Lundsgaard, K.; Reiss, W.; Weve, H. J. & Simón, J. M. (hrg). *Katalog einer Ausstellung zur Geschichte der Brille. Im Auftrag des Vorsstandes des XIII Internationalen Ophthalmologischen Kongresses zu Amsterdam.* Amsterdam: Verlag A. E. d' Oliveira.

White, Landeg. 2008. *The Collected Lyric Poems of Luís de Camões.* Princeton, New Jersey: Princeton University Press.

Wilensky, Reginald Howard. 1958. *Bosch Hieronymus.* Berlin: Kunstreihe des Safari-Verlags.

Websites

Collins Dicionary https://www.collinsdictionary.com/dictionary/english/erudite-scholar accessed 20 June 2022.

Harvey, Anna, 2010. "The use of Magnifying lenses in the Classical World." *History of the Ancient World* https://www.historyoftheancientworld.com/2012/11/the-use-of magnifying-lenses-in-the-classical-world/ accessed 10 August 2021.

Hieronymus Bosch. Table of the Seven Deadly Sins. Museo del Prado https://www.museodelprado.es/en/the-collection/art-work/table-of-the-seven-deadly-sins/3fc0a84e-d77d-4217-b960-8a34b8873b70 accessed 24 June 2022.

Igreja de S. Miguel, Matriz de Freixo de Espada-à-Cinta https://www.e-cultura.pt/patrimonio_item/6677 accessed 22 June 2022.

Interpreters and Translators INC Blog https://blog.ititranslates.com/2014/01/17/patron-saint-of-translators/ accessed 20 June 2022.

Lorenz, Angelika, "Ring, Ludger tom" in: Neue Deutsche Biographie 21 (2003), S. 629-630 [Online-Version]; URL: https://www.deutsche-biographie.de/pnd119485451.html#ndbcontent accessed 25 june 2022.

Museu de Évora - Museu Nacional Frei Manuel do Cenáculo http://www.matriznet.dgpc.pt/MatrizNet/Objectos/ObjectosConsultar.aspx?IdReg 14098 accessed 10 October 2021.

OsDicionarios.com http://www.osdicionarios.com/c/significado/antolhos accessed 10 October 2021.

Saints Peter and Dorothy by Master of the Saint Bartholomew Masterpiece. National Gallery, London https://www.nationalgallery.org.uk/paintings/master-of-the-saint-bartholomew-altarpiece-saints-peter-and-dorothy accessed 10 November 2021.

Utrecht University https://www.uu.nl/en/utrecht-university-library-special-collections/collections/manuscripts/medieval-medical-manuscripts/lilium-medicinae-by-bernard-de-gordon, accessed 16 September 2021.

CHAPTER 7

SANITARY PRECAUTIONS AGAINST THE PLAGUE IN PORTUGUESE PORTS (14TH-19TH CENTURIES)

JOÃO MARTINS E SILVA

Abstract
The human plague is an epidemic disease of great lethality, caused by the bacterium *Yersinia pestis* which was identified in 1884. From Antiquity onwards, the disease was recognized by large ganglionic engorgements that, when appearing in affected individuals, characterized bubonic plague. The development of commercial exchange, wars and human migrations, among other factors, boosted the development of the three pandemics that affected humanity between 540/541 and the 1960s. The second plague pandemic, which started with the devastating Black Death (between 1347 and 1351) and continued with recurrent outbreaks in Europe, the Near and Middle East, North Africa and Asia up until the beginning of the 19th century, caused serious demographic, socio-economic and political consequences on the populations of the most affected regions. In a bid to spare the Kingdom from the contagion and damage caused by *Yersinia pestis*, Portuguese monarchs sought information about possible plague epidemics in the countries from which the ships heading for Lisbon and other coastal ports of the Kingdom had come. Based on the health situation in the places of origin of these ships, Portuguese governments were empowered to authorize the docking and unloading of goods, as well as the free passage ashore of the crew and passengers or, alternatively, when infected or suspected of being infected, imposing on them a mandatory ban on entry into the ports or compliance with regulated sanitary measures.

Key words: Plague; Ports; Provenance; Prevention; Sanitary Measures

Resumo:
A peste humana é uma doença epidémica de grande letalidade, causada pela bactéria *Yersinia pestis*, identificada em 1884. Anteriormente, deste a Antiguidade, a doença era sinalizada por ingurgitamentos ganglionares volumosos que, ao surgirem nos indivíduos afectados, caracterizavam a peste bubónica. O desenvolvimento das trocas comerciais, guerras e migrações humanas, entre outros factores, potenciaram o desenvolvimento das três pandemias que afectaram a Humanidade entre 540/541 e os anos 60 do século XX. A segunda pandemia de peste, iniciada com a devastadora Peste Negra (entre1347 e 1351) e continuada por surtos recorrentes na Europa, Próximo e Médio Oriente, norte de África e Ásia até ao início do século XIX, trouxe graves consequências demográficas, socioeconómicas, políticas, entre outras, às populações das regiões mais atingidas. De modo a poupar o Reino ao contágio e estragos causados pela *Yersinia pestis*, os monarcas Portugueses procuraram informar-se da existência de eventuais epidemias de peste nos países donde provinham as embarcações que se dirigiam para Lisboa e outros portos costeiros do Reino. Com base na situação de saúde vigente nos locais de procedência desses navios, os governos Portugueses ficavam habilitados a autorizar a atracação e descarga das mercadorias dos navios, assim como o livre-trânsito em terra às tripulações e passageiros ou, em alternativa, quando infectados ou suspeitos de o estarem, a impor-lhes a proibição de entrada nos portos ou ao cumprimento de medidas sanitárias regulamentadas.
Palavras-chave: Peste; Portos; Procedências; Prevenção; Medidas Sanitárias

Introduction

The many contagious pestilences that have affected humans from time immemorial, especially those which were the most serious, prolonged and/or accompanied by very high levels of mortality, were called (amongst other things) “plagues”.

Some of these infectious pestilences probably included smallpox, typhoid fever, exanthematic typhus, malaria and cholera, among other bacterial, parasitic and viral agents, all of which were only recognised from the 19th century onwards as a consequence of advances in the development of microbiology (Pye 1721, 3-4; Marks 1975, 6). Differentiating itself from these various pestilences, what came to be called bubonic plague was characterized by very painful ganglionic engorgements in buboes (which appeared, in particular, in the groin, armpits, neck, and even more rarely in other ganglionic tracts), and which, after the onset of fever, could break resulting in exudation of pus. The designation of the adjective "bubonic", derives from the pre-Greek *βουβών* (swelling in the groin) and Medieval Latin *būbō* (groin).

Contagious diseases were the first to require community preventive measures. In this essay, the discovery of the causative bacterium of plague and the dissemination of the disease will be briefly reviewed.

The cause of plague was only clarified in 1894 by Alexandre Yersin[1], who was assigned to the Pasteur Institute in Hong Kong, where a serious plague had broken out. Yersin found that plague was an infection of the human body caused by a gram-negative bacterium present in the blood and pulp of the buboes of the infected individuals (Yersin 1894, 664-667). This bacterium was first called *Bacterium pestis* until 1900, then *Bacillum pestis* until 1923, when it was changed to *Pasteurella pestis*, until eventually being renamed *Yersinia pestis* in 1944; the generic name was constructed to honour its discoverer. However, this designation only became widespread approximately twenty-five years later.

Yersinia pestis has also been detected in rats that, before or at the beginning of the human epidemic, were found dead in large numbers in the streets and homes of the sick and those who died from the plague. Like humans, infected animals often showed the presence of bulky bubo-like ganglia filled with specific bacilli on autopsy. Yersin was able to develop plague in healthy rats, mice and/or guinea pigs by inoculating them with bubo pulp, by making them ingest fragments of liver, spleen, or pure bacterial cultures from dead animals, or by placing infected animals in contact with healthy ones, which quickly became sick. In each case, the induced infection was quickly lethal, with characteristic lesions and numerous bacilli in the blood, ganglia and spleen showing at autopsy. From these observations, Yersin drew the following conclusions: (a) plague was a contagious and inoculable bacterial disease; (b) there was a causal relationship between the outbreak of a human epidemic and a nearby epizootic[2] disease of rats; (c) In this cause-effect relationship, infected rats were likely to be the main vehicle of transmission of plague to humans and healthy rats or other rodents (Yersin 1894, 665-667; Yersin 1897, 82).

---

[1] Alexandre Yersin (1863-1943) was Swiss doctor and bacteriologist who became a naturalised Frenchman.

[2] An epizootic defines an infectious disease arising at a given period in the human population (local, general or universal), in which the number of new cases of those infected and dead increases considerably. Term corresponding to epidemic in human medicine.

Four years later, Paul-Louis Simond,[3] Yersin's compatriot and colleague at the Pasteur Institute in Bombay, found that human deaths followed a trail parallel to the emigration and place of death of the pestiferous rats, on which the spread of the plague by land or sea depended in large part (Simond 1898, 640-642, 650). Although *Yersinia pestis* caused similar epidemic diseases in humans and rats, their interdependence remained to be confirmed. Through successive observations and laboratory experiments, Simond demonstrated that the link between healthy humans and infected rats was established by the fleas that parasitized the rodents. These animals, once contaminated, acted as hosts and propagating vehicles for *Yersinia pestis*, which was transmitted to healthy humans or rats through the bite of infected fleas (or bedbugs). Thus, the entry point for the infection was the skin where, in the liquid of the (rare) blisters remaining from the flea bite, Simond found the presence of *Yersinia pestis* (Simond 1898, 671-677).

Simond's seminal conclusions, especially regarding the transmission of plague by flea bites, were not immediately accepted by the contemporary medical community which still adhered to miasmatic theory and other hypotheses, now obsolete, as explanations for the transmission of infectious diseases. Even though the results were confirmed by other researchers (Thompson 1901, 164-165; Gauthier 1903, 426), it was not until 1907 that Simond's observations on the fundamental role of fleas in the plague transmissibility cycle was verified by the Advisory Committee Appointed by the secretary of state for India, the Royal Society and the Lister Institute (Lamb 1907, 156-157). Finally, three years later, the same organisation established Simond's discovery as a scientific principle (Greenwood 1910, 566-568).

At the beginning of the 20th century a degree thesis presented to the University of Edinburgh argued that "the plague was primarily a disease of rats and only secondarily a disease of men", so that "without rats there was no plague epidemic" (Blackmore 1906, 4-14). This conclusion was reiterated about a century later by Michel McCormick (2003, 1), when he asserted that "plague is a rodent disease; in man it is overwhelmingly a by-product of the infection of rodents by an insect bite". In other words, bubonic plague is a zoonotic[4] disease of rodents, dependent on *Yersinia pestis*, in a flea-rodent-flea life cycle that, only by coincidence or particular circumstance, affects humans (Gage 2005, 506-509). On this basis, it was possible to understand the cause, development and consequences of the three bubonic plague pandemics that emerged in the 6th, 14th and 19th

---

[3] Paul-Louis Simond (1858-1947), physician, biologist and French naval officer.

[4] Infectious disease of animals, potentially transmissible to humans.

centuries, as well as subsequent outbreaks that have continued to manifest themselves until the present in different regions of the world.

However, in addition to bubonic plague (predominantly, making up 80 to 85% of all cases), there are other clinical forms of plague caused by *Yersinia pestis*, namely pneumonic plague (rare, more virulent and with a high rate of mortality). The bubonic and pneumonic forms correspond to the two main gateways of infection into the organism, the first through the skin or mucous membranes, and the second through the airways. Other rarer or clinically minimal instances of the infection caused in humans by the same bacteria have been identified, especially the septic (or systemic) plague, which is virtually fatal. The latter two has one of two origins, either primary or secondary (Poland 1999, 43-46).

Most likely originating in Central or East Asia, the second pandemic plague reached the Crimea in 1343, following the Silk Road and other routes. Three years later the epidemic entered the Genoese city and trading port of Kaffa, on the Black Sea coast, which had been under siege for a year by Khan Janibeg's Tartar army. Suddenly, the soldiers besieging the city began to die very quickly from a devastating pestilence. Before ending the siege and retreating with the rest of his army, Janibeg decided, frustrated and out of revenge, to catapult their dead into the besieged city, while the defenders sought to avoid the disease by sending the bodies of the dead attackers into the sea. However, the year-long siege had created serious limitations regarding resources for the Genoese, both in terms of supplies and elementary hygiene care, so that it was only a matter of time before they too became contaminated and died just as quickly. Those who were still apparently healthy boarded ships and sailed from Kaffa back to their own lands. However, the rats and fleas that transmitted the bubonic plague to Europe followed with them, after disembarking in November 1347 in the port of Messina, followed by those of Genoa and Marseille (Marks 1970, 1-2). As such, the second plague pandemic was under way which, after a devastating initial period in the 14th century (1347-1353), commonly known as the Black Death, continued through repeated outbreaks until the middle of the 19th century (Benedictow 2004,380-382). Changes recently observed in traces of *Yersinia pestis* DNA and proteins collected from human skeletons at the time, found in mass graves in northern, central and southern Europe, suggest that the Black Death reached this continent on two or more occasions by different routes (Haensch 2010, 3-4).

The third pandemic began around 1855 in southwest China, in the province of Yunnan, and from there it slowly progressed to the cities of Guangzhou and Hong-Kong. In 1894, it spread throughout southern China and, by sea, reached Singapore and India (Yersin 1894, 664-667; Simpson

1905, 50-65). Up to the point when it was considered to be extinct in 1959 (when there was a total of 200 fatalities in the world), it spread to every continent (except Antarctica), having claimed about fifteen million victims, mostly inhabitants of India, China and Indonesia (Tikhomirov 1999, 11; Echenberg 2007, 5). In the two previous pandemics, apart from some correct preventive recommendations, the cause and treatment of the plague were little more than a set of imaginative proposals without scientific foundation. However, the one of 1855 brought the answer that was then necessary but which, even today, continues to be meticulously strengthened.

In 1899, the city of Oporto was the last in nineteenth century Europe to be infected with bubonic plague. The outbreak diagnosed by Ricardo Jorge (1858-1939), (1899, xiii, 44, 46, 47), remained active for about half a year, resulting in between 109 to 132 deaths (Souza Júnior 1902, 115; Silva Correia 1937, 476; Férran and Clua 1907, 103, 110). The application of appropriate sanitary measures and less bacterial virulence must have contributed to such a reduced number of victims in that city, compared to those registered in previous catastrophic pandemics.

From antiquity to the discovery of *Yersinia pestis*, the presumptive diagnosis of human bubonic plague was signalled by buboes that developed in infected humans, generally starting days after episodes of murine epizootics. When in June of that year the first patients appeared in Oporto, the infecting bacteria already had an identity, its propagation by vector insects and small mammals was known, and the first antibacterial serums were being tested.

This work aims to review the most critical moments from the fourteenth to the nineteenth century, when Portugal, including adjacent islands, were at risk, or were contaminated, by bubonic plague, through vessels from infected regions in Europe, North Africa and Asia, generally from mercantile ships arriving by sea in Lisbon and other port cities of the country. In the text which follows, the term "plague" covers the designation which, throughout the period covered here, was given to any pestilence with the characteristic signs of the bubonic type and, more rarely, pneumonic or septicaemic variants.

Most of the references used, regarding more explicit examples of protective measures and other measures relating to maritime traffic that could potentially call at Portuguese ports, especially Lisbon, were collected through the Municipal Archive of Lisbon-Historical Archive and denoted by the acronym AML-AH.

Earliest alerts and protecting measures at the 15th century

In 1421, the still *Infante*[5] D. Duarte (1391-1438) criticized the district of Lisbon for having authorised the mooring of an unattended British ship that carried several crew members with plague on board; this had resulted in an outbreak of this disease in Lisbon (Fig.7.1).[6] To avoid future similar occurrences, the (now) King) D. Duarte I - who reigned

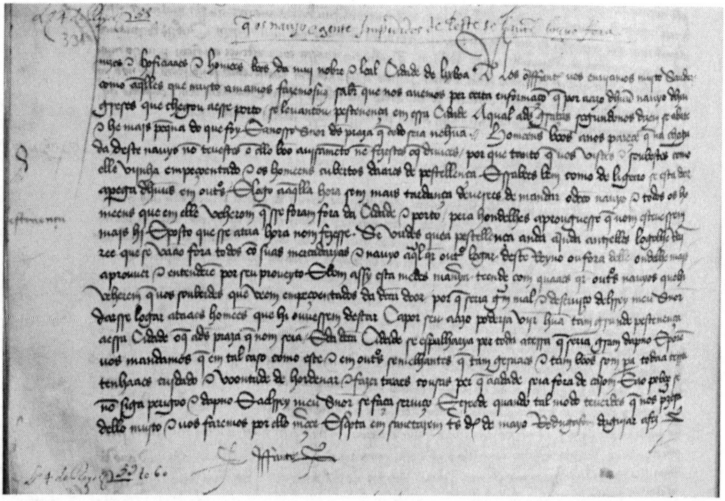

Fig. 7.1. Reproduction of the letter of May 3, [1421-1433], written in Santarém, in which Prince D. Duarte orders the judges, officials and good men of the council of Lisbon "to fulfil and enforce all the measures stipulated for prevent outbreaks of plague in the capital of the Kingdom", besides criticizing them for the council of Lisbon having allowed an English ship with plague patients on board to dock in Lisbon. Photo: Arquivo Municipal de Lisboa.

from 1433 to 1438 - and who was already experienced in matters of governance, together with his father, King D. João I (who reigned from 1385 to 1433), ordered the reinforcement of preventive measures against the plague (Fig. 7.1). These provisions included the institution of a period

---

5 Prince and heir.

6 AML-AH. 3 de Maio [1421-1433], Chancelaria Régia, Livro dos Pregos, doc. 331, f. 258v.

of quarantine off Lisbon for ships suspected of carrying pest-infected crew members.

Irony of ironies, the disease D. Duarte had wanted to protect the Kingdom from, took his own life on 9 September 1438, on a day marked by a "major eclipse of the sun". It is said that the monarch had been infected by a letter from Santarém, which he received in Ponte de Sor (Oliveira 1882, 458).

In that same year there was a great shortage of cereals and bread in Lisbon, such that in a royal charter of 23 September 1438, ships from Brittany were allowed to come "continuously to the port of Lisbon with cereals and other goods" for a year; the cereals and vegetables that they brought were exempted from paying the tithe (Oliveira 1882, 319).

Sanitary measures from the 15th to the 16th century

Following those precautions, King D. João II (his first reign in November 1477 lasted four days; his second was from 1481 to 1495) warned the council, in 1486, about the presence of a French privateer in the port of Lisbon; he decided to send ships to capture it if it did not obey their orders.[7]

Six years later, he instructed the Lisbon council on the procedures to be taken concerning a ship anchored off the city, and then extended this to all vessels coming from affected places. For this purpose, he ordered that a shelter be built in Belém to house goods and men arriving in Lisbon on ships suspected of being contaminated with the plague. In addition, he ordered the placing of two mainstays with flags in the riverside area, above which no ships from places affected by the plague could pass[8]. Apparently, this last recommendation was not fulfilled to his liking, so he reiterated it in 1494.[9] Previously, he had already ordered the council to take measures to prevent the entry of ships from Andalusia, especially Seville, because they were infected with the plague.[10] The following year, that monarch ordered

[7] AML-AH. 16 de Março de 1486, Chancelaria Régia, Livro 2º de D. João II, f. 87 - 87v.

[8] AML-AH.28 de Agosto de 1492, Provimento da Saúde, Livro 1º do provimento da saúde, f. 10 -10v. AML-AH. 5-7 de Setembro de 1492, Provimento da Saúde, Livro 1º do provimento da saúde, f. 11- 11v. AML-AH. 16-17 de Outubro de 1692, Provimento da Saúde, Livro 1º do provimento da saúde, f. 13 -13v.

[9] AML-AH. 29 de Maio-18 de Junho de 1494, Provimento da Saúde, Livro 1º do provimento da saúde, f. 25 - 25v.

[10] AML-AH. 29 de Maio-4 de Junho de 1494, Provimento da Saúde, Livro 1º do provimento da saúde, f. 24 -24v.

the expulsion of some French ships from the port of Lisbon, where cases of this disease had been detected.[11]

However, despite all these precautions, plague broke out in Lisbon in 1505 and spread throughout the Kingdom, "a plague so fierce" that it came on the ship, "touching without him knowing it", from where the bishop of Oporto, D. Diogo de Sousa disembarked. The seriousness of the situation was such that "the king went with all his court to Almeirim" (Damião de Goes 1926, I-208).

At the end of 1513 and beginning of 1514, the Lisbon council informed King D. Manuel I (reigned from 1495 to 1521) of the measures taken regarding a vessel coming from Bristol in which crew members were sick with the plague. It was immediately forbidden for ships from England (where, at the time, many cases of plague were known to exist) to come into Lisbon and Cascais.[12] He then ordered the council to appoint two members to obtain information about foreign ships arriving in Lisbon coming from countries afflicted by the plague.[13] At the end of that year, he issued an order prohibiting the entry of two ships from Genoa, where the plague had been recorded, and, once again, from England, for the same reason.[14] In 1517, the actions of the Lisbon council merited the congratulations of that monarch regarding a ship from Galicia, suspected of carrying patients with plague on board. The ban on ships from that region entering the port of Lisbon was extended until 1 January 1518.[15] The following year, King D. Manuel I expressed satisfaction with the improvement of sanitary conditions in Lisbon.[16]

In 1534, King D. João III (who reigned from 1521 to 1557), upon learning of the existence of cases of plague on the island of Madeira, ordered

---

[11] AML-AH. 29 de Abril de 1495- Provimento da Saúde, Livro 1° do provimento da saúde, f. 27-27v.

[12] AML-AH. 29 de Dezembro de 1513- 3 de Janeiro de 1514, Provimento da Saúde, Livro 1° do provimento da saúde, f. 42 - 43v. AML-AH. 15 de Janeiro de 1514, Provimento da Saúde, Livro 1° do provimento da saúde, f. 44 - 44v. AML-AH. 16 de Janeiro de 1514, Provimento da Saúde, Livro 1° do provimento da saúde, f. 45 - 45v.

[13] AML-AH. 25 de Janeiro de 1514, Provimento da Saúde, Livro 1° do provimento da saúde, f. 48 - 48v.

[14] AML-AH. 12 de Dezembro de 1514, Provimento da Saúde, Cópia do Livro 1° do provimento da saúde, f. 34. AML-AH. 18 de Dezembro de 1514, Provimento da Saúde, Livro 1° do provimento da saúde, f. 50 - 50v.

[15] AML-AH. 9 de Novembro de 1517, Provimento da Saúde, Livro 1° do provimento da saúde, f. 56 -57v.

[16] AML-AH.23 de Maio de 1519, Provimento da Saúde, Livro 1° do provimento da saúde, f. 58 e 58v

the Lisbon council to pay attention to the ships arriving from the island.[17] Two years later, he issued the same order to the council, but now in relation to ships coming from England, where several outbreaks of plague had been announced, and once again for the same reason, in 1541 and 1544, for ships coming from London.[18] The following year, that monarch ordered Lisbon council to find out whether the fleet from Flanders heading for Lisbon contained ships from England and other countries infected with plague that were forbidden from docking in the Kingdom.[19] In the same year, he thanked the Lisbon council for the sanitary measures taken against the plague concerning two French ships that had entered the port of Belém (Fig. 7.2), repeated for all ships of that origin, allegedly due to the plague outbreaks verified there. The monarch also wanted to know detailed information about a Biscay ship moored in Belém, which had come from Bristol, where there were plague cases.[20] In 1546, royal concerns turned to outbreaks of plague in Bordeaux and Brittany and ships from there, so he instructed the Lisbon council regarding the measures to be taken[21].

Another dispatch of that monarch applied to a control post in Belém, which included a health provider *(provedor de Saúde*), a clerk, a bailiff and two other men, as guards, to attend to the ships that arrived in Lisbon. None of these ships were authorized to anchor upstream of the tower of Belém (Fig. 7.3a, 7.3b) without first receiving an order from the captain of the tower, after which the master of the vessel had to disembark to show its passport to the health provider so that it was known, under oath, where he came from, how long ago he had left his land, and if he had dropped anchor in a contaminated port. Next, two sailors from the same ship were summoned, who, also under oath, had to answer the same questions; if the answers were in agreement, the crew obtained entry permission and

---

[17] AML-AH. 6 de Março de 1534, Provimento da Saúde, Livro 1º do provimento da saúde, f. 119- 120v.

[18] AML-AH. 27 de Outubro de 1536, Provimento da Saúde, Livro 1º do provimento da saúde, f. 121- 122v.AML-AH. 15 de Fevereiro de 1541, Provimento da Saúde, Livro 1º do provimento da saúde, f. 125- 126v. AML-AH. 12 de Janeiro de 1544, Provimento da Saúde, Livro 1º do provimento da saúde, f. 127 - 127v.

[19] AML-AH. 20 de Abril de 1545, Provimento da Saúde, Livro 1º do provimento da saúde, f. 134 - 135v.

[20] AML-AH. 8 de Outubro de 1545, Provimento da Saúde, Livro 1º do provimento da saúde, f. 143- 143v.

AML-AH. 28 de Outubro de 1545, Provimento da Saúde, Cópia do Livro 1º do provimento da saúde, f. 6.

[21] AML-AH. 28 de Abril-7 de Maio de 1546, Provimento da Saúde, Livro 1º do provimento da saúde, f. 146-147v. AML-AH. 29 de Outubro de 1546, Provimento da Saúde, Livro 1º do provimento da saúde, f. 148-149v.

authorisation to circulate. If any ship entered and the previous requirements were not met, the master of the vessel was found guilty, with the sentence being handed down by the city's inspectors. If the ship came from an uninfected land, two guards were sent to authorize the merchandise unloading and mooring the ship at Trafaria for thirty days; if any member of the crew wanted to go into the town, they could disembark after changing the attire for another, presumably clean (Oliveira 1903, 140).

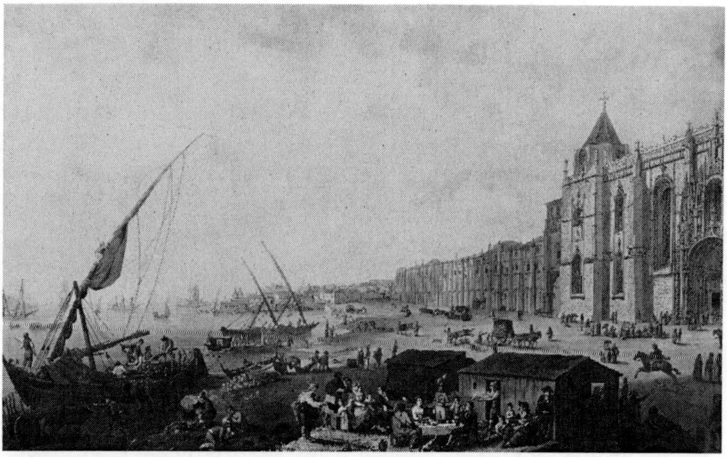

Fig. 7.2. Port of Belém and Jerónimos Monastery. Engraving- Old jurisdiction, Lisbon, Portugal. Photo: Arquivo Municipal de Lisboa.

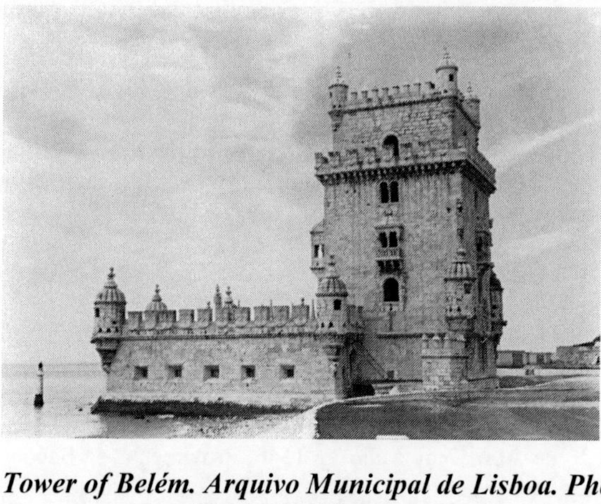

Fig. 7.3a. Tower of Belém. Arquivo Municipal de Lisboa. Photo credit: Mário de Oliveira.

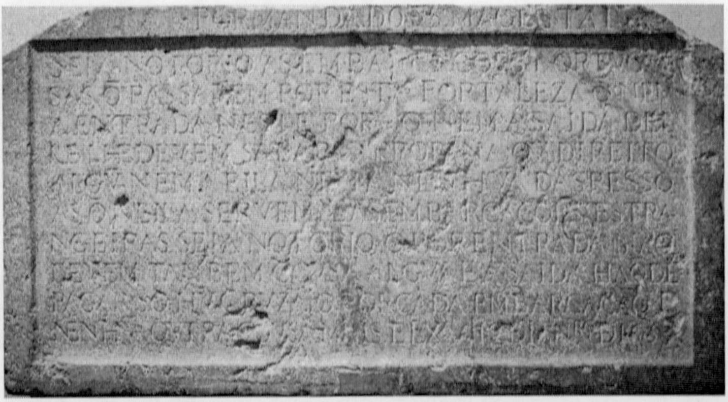

Figure 7.3b Plaque from the Tower of Belém. "It should be noted that, by order of His Majesty, the Portuguese vessels passing along this fortress are not entitled to a fee or right, neither when entering nor leaving this port nor those who utilize them. It should be noted that foreign vessels are not entitled to any payment when entering; each vessel should pay one cruzado, when leaving, and nothing more". Lisbon, April 19, 1655. Arquivo Municipal de Lisboa. Photo credit: José Vicente.

King D. João III, very attentive to the sanitary conditions of the capital of the Kingdom—which was potentially at risk of being infected by epidemics that, at the time, were devastating distant lands, through the hundreds of ships that docked in Lisbon for commercial exchanges—promoted the creation of a private health house in the centre of the city, "with officials who provided whatever was necessary for the health of the city". Twenty-nine men were also appointed to this structure, designated as "heads of health", in principle one for each parish. Their main function was to collect the death certificates issued by the *físico* [22]of the respective parish, and every day, after attending mass, to deliver them to the inspectors' *menza*, [23] which was affiliated to the church of S. Sebastião da Padaria. In this way, the number of deaths that had occurred the day before in each parish could be known. (Oliveira 1903, 139).

---

[22] Term which, in medieval times, designated those who legally practised medical functions.

[23] Term derived from Latin, equivalent to the round table (e.g. of inspectors) of a medieval organisation with charitable purposes, affiliated to a Catholic church.

In 1577, King Sebastião (reigned from 1557-1578) ordered preventive measures to be carried out against ships that docked in the ports of the Kingdom, especially Lisbon, in order to prevent their crews, if infected, from contaminating the city. Anyone who did not comply with those dictates was sentenced to certain punishment. King D. Sebastião congratulated the way in which Lisbon council had fulfilled its orders, thereby avoiding the contamination of the city, as well as the rigid implementation of dispatches concerning the departure of those infected from the city.[24]

Sanitary measures in the seventeenth century

In 1625, the city of Lisbon asked the governors to order the captains of the Towers of Belém, St. Julião, St. António of Cascais, and the entire Kingdom, to prohibit the entry of soldiers on ships from England, moored in the Tagus river bar (*barra*) due to the risk of being infected by plague (Fig. 7.4). On the other hand, contagion did not seem to be the main concern of the English merchants residing in Lisbon, because, from their point of view, they complained about the impossibility of ships from England coming into port and obtaining the respective municipal orders.[25]In 1636, the inspection of foreign ships was ordered before entering Portuguese ports, to avoid contagion from plague in England. Weeks later, the sailors of an English ship that had been detained in Lisbon due to plague and had not disembarked, were sent to quarantine in Trafaria. [26]

When the existence of plague in Catalonia and Denmark was known in 1654, the council was advised to take the usual measures in the ports of the Kingdom.[27]

In April 1656, the council informed the monarch that it was its opinion, and for the convenience of public health, that preventive norms against the plague should be maintained, despite the displeasure of certain merchants,

---

[24] AML-AH. 12 de Julho de 1577, Provimento da Saúde, Cópia do Livro 1º do provimento da saúde, f. 79. AML-AH. 3 de Dezembro de 1577, Provimento da Saúde, Livro 1º do provimento da saúde, f. 194- 195v.

[25] AML-AH. 19 de Julho-3 de Outubro de 1625, Provimento da Saúde, Cópia do Livro 2º do provimento da saúde, f. 68v - 70v.

[26] AML-AH. 17 de Novembro de 1636, Chancelaria Régia, Livro 2º de consultas e decretos de Filipe III f. 46- 47v. AML-AH. 10 de Dezembro de 1636, Chancelaria Régia, Livro 2º de consultas e decretos de Filipe III, f. 45 - 45v.

[27] AML-AH. 3 de Fevereiro de 1654,Chancelaria Régia, Livro 3º de consultas e decretos de D. João IV, f. 100 - 101v; AML-AH. 16 de Setembro de 1654, Chancelaria Régia, Livro 3º de consultas e decretos de D. João IV, f. 119 - 120v.

who were indifferent to the reasons for this precaution and because they thought only of profit and who wanted their goods to be quickly unloaded without being quarantined at Trafaria.[28]

By order of the secretary of state, on 13 July 1657, the Lisbon council learned of the devastation caused by the plague in Genoa (where around two hundred people were dying each day), along with the recommendation of taking the "care that is appropriate in safeguarding from that". Ten days later, in a consultation by the council with the king, all the care and attention concerning that issue was reaffirmed.

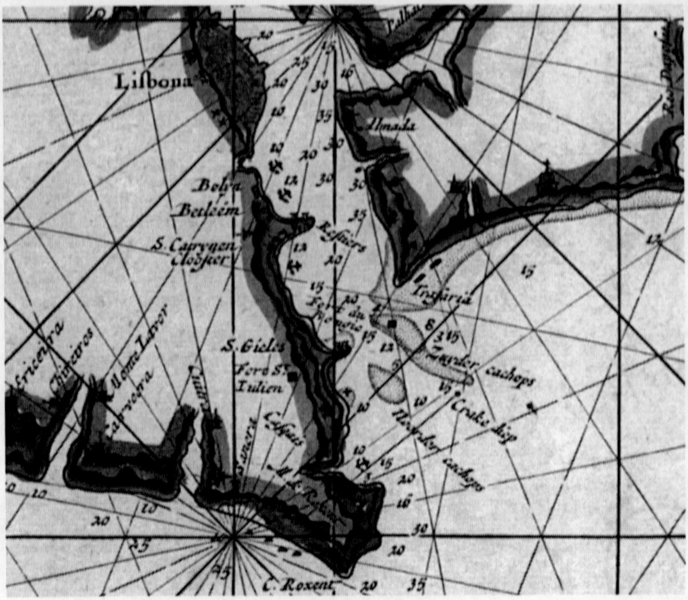

Fig. 7.4 - Map of the Tagus estuary up to the city of Lisbon, displaying the area bordering the barra, between the fortress of St. Julião da Barra and the tip of the Trafaria Cape, passing by the Tower of Bugio, in the middle of a sandy beach. In: VOOGHT, Claes Jansz, fl. ca 1680-1696 (Cutting from Nieuwe paskaart van de kust van Portugal Beginnend 3 a 4 Myl Benoorde C. Roxent. tot aen C. d S. Vincente, met al zyn Diepte, en Drooghre, des ver naaukeurigh Opgesogrt). Public copy. Biblioteca Nacional de Portugal.

---

[28] AML-AH. 26 - 28 de Abril de 1656- Chancelaria Régia, Livro 3º de consultas e decretos de D. João IV, f. 159- 160v.

It was warned, however, that such surveillance would be impossible if letters, bulls and other documentation from France, Italy (mainly Rome), England and Holland continued to arrive on land as, since they came in unopened bundles, it was feared that plague could be transmitted through the mail. Thus, it was essential that the council be authorised to open those packets, without which, upon entering Lisbon in that state, they could cause "very serious damage". Equal danger came from people on boats collecting correspondence for the monarch from ships, which should not be allowed. By royal resolution, the council received authorisation to resolve the matter as proposed (Oliveira1893, lxxvi-lxxvii).

In an order of 5 November 1662, the secretary of state gave an account of the warning sent by the governor and captain-general of the Algarve, and other entities, of the existence of plague, "from which God deliver us",[29] in Algiers, Tetouan and Tangier. Given that English ships frequently traded with those locals, it advised, by order of King D. Afonso VI (who reigned from 1656 to 1683)[30] that, "for health, they should be as vigilant as possible, warning that the seaports have also been warned" (Oliveira 1891, 377-378). The next day, that secretary of state communicated in an order that the monarch had warned him about an English ship that had arrived from Tangier, where there was plague, and "from which people had disembarked without wishing to obey the health officials" so that he ordered everyone to be collected from the ship, that note be taken of the houses into which they had entered, in addition to "not a single thing" from the ship being allowed to leave (Oliveira 1891, 378). In response, the mayor of Lisbon council informed the secretary of state on 14 November that all the necessary steps had been taken, although he noted that the crew of a British warship that had passed through Tangier had refused to obey, claiming that it was a military vessel. Subsequently, the monarch ordered the council to "pass on orders to the ambassador and consul of England to oblige the warships of his nation to obey health officials". In the steps taken at that time, it became known that a Hebrew merchant had been transported on that frigate "with

[29] At that time, it was customary to follow the term "plague" with a short invocation of faith and appeal to God in difficult situations ("may God deliver us"), which is, after all, identical to the phrase still in use today ("God deliver us"), either by believers in a kingdom with divine sovereignty in difficult situations or simply due to social habit.

[30] The kingdom of King D. Afonso VII was ruled during his childhood by his mother, Dona Luisa de Gusmão. Because of alleged mental incapacity, following an infectious illness (meningoencephalitis is suggested, which was contracted during childhood), his Kingdom was ruled from 1668 by his younger brother, Peter, until the latter succeeded him on the throne.

merchandise he had brought from Tetouan" and that other passengers had disembarked in Lisbon. Given this, the council had sent all the merchandise and people remaining in Lisbon to quarantine in Trafaria, while the ship was "impounded", as well as the communication "of its people" with the city, until the days of quarantine were over (Oliveira 1891, 384).

In 1663, by signed notice of the former secretary of state, the council was ordered by the health services to inspect a vessel coming from Amsterdam that was infected with plague.[31] Curiously and contradictorily, on the same day and signed by the same member of the government, an opinion was required from the council senate on the measures to be taken for a ship arriving at Belém from Hamburg, loaded with fabrics, with it being known that there was plague in that city.[32] To reinforce the paradox, the following day, people and goods were authorized to disembark from a vessel coming from Rotterdam that had moored at Belém, saying that there was no danger of contagion from the plague.[33] However, on that same day, contradicting the previous decision, the secretary of state issued a warning to the council that did not authorize the disembarkation of people and goods from vessels coming from Amsterdam and Hamburg because there was indeed a danger of contagion.[34] Two weeks later, in view of the news that the presence of plague in Madeira had been confirmed, the council was, along with the health services, ordered to prevent the spread of that disease.[35]

At the beginning of the following year, another incomprehensible decision authorised the mooring of a ship (which had previously been prohibited) from the Netherlands, which at the time was infected with plague.[36] Although the situation in that country remained unchanged, great care and preventive measures were, a few months later, ordered for ships arriving at the port of Lisbon.[37] On 16 July 1664, the warning was reiterated

---

[31] AML-AH. 10 de Dezembro de 1663, Chancelaria Régia, Livro 2º de consultas e decretos de D. Afonso VI, f. 290 -291v.

[32] AML-AH. 10 de Dezembro de 1663, Chancelaria Régia, Livro 2º de consultas e decretos de D. Afonso VI, f. 292 - 293v.

[33] AML-AH. 11 de Dezembro de 1663, Chancelaria Régia, Livro 2º de consultas e decretos de D. Afonso VI, f. 294-295v.

[34] AML-AH. 11 de Dezembro de 1663, Chancelaria Régia, Livro 2º de consultas e decretos de D. Afonso VI, f. 296 -297v.

[35] AML-AH. 27 de Dezembro de 1663, Chancelaria Régia, Livro 2º de consultas e decretos de D. Afonso VI, f. 298 - 299v.

[36] AML-AH. 6 de Janeiro de 1664, Chancelaria Régia, Livro 2º de consultas e decretos de D. Afonso VI, f. 335 - 335v.

[37] AML-AH. 16 de Junho de 1664,Chancelaria Régia, Livro 2º de registo de consultas e decretos de D. Pedro II, doc. 471, f. 259.

that in Holland "the evil of the plague continues with great force, may God protect us", and the order was given to "serve orders more strictly and to fully cautious and watchful over ships entering this port, originating from where there might be suspicions" (Oliveira 1891, 506). This type of recommendation was still in force a year later.[38]

The Lisbon council informed the king, on 9 September 1665, of the strengthening of surveillance in Belém, in particular for ships arriving from London, where there had been an outbreak of plague. Furthermore, it instructed that for ships coming from there or from neighbouring ports, "even if they are carrying bread and other types of cargo that do not carry contagion, in no way should they be admitted into our ports, nor allowed to dock or be given assistance". However, those coming from other parts of England that were not infected were allowed to dock, although they were forced to quarantine at Trafaria, where they could unload. Precautions covered correspondence, as was the case with a French ship that had brought letters from London to private individuals. Letters were to be collected and "benefited" (as the regulatory disinfection process was called) in the health centre. The population was warned that in the future, those receiving letters from England should take them to health inspectors to be opened and ventilated, under penalty of the offenders spending "forty days at Trafaria and for however long seemed right, because any rigour is fair in such a case". The monarch was asked to find out what the French were doing to protect their ports from contamination from the English, even though it was said that "they did so with cannons, and if this is not the case or not practised with rigour, it will be necessary to pay more attention to the ships that come from there". In this event, it would be necessary to reinforce the surveillance personnel on the coast near the Belém and S. Julião Towers, as well as in Cascais, in order to prevent crews and others from disembarking in the sands from ships originating from there. It was also requested that the governors and lieutenants of the towers be instructed to help the health personnel and to comply with all such orders communicated to them by the main inspector (Oliveira 1891, 570-572).

The extreme caution contained in those messages was justified, since on 1 September 1666, the secretary of state sent a new notice to the head of the senate of Lisbon council to comply with the regulations and royal orders as news had arrived from England of a "furious plague" in all that territory, though London was the least affected (Oliveira 1891, 603).

[38] AML-AH. 7 de Janeiro de 1665, Chancelaria Régia, Livro 2º de consultas e decretos de D. Afonso VI, f. 336- 338v.

During the reign of King D. Pedro II (reigned from 1668 to 1671), preventive measures were ordered against a possible spread of the plague brought on ships from Rouen and Normandy, with those measures ceasing in 1670, once that danger no longer existed. Lisbon council was told to ask health officials to find out if the ships from Holland were carrying crews with plague, in order to prevent the contagion from spreading to Lisbon. A few days later, the council was advised that ships from northern Europe would be allowed to dock, as there was no longer any danger of contagion from the plague. The following year, the English consul guaranteed that there was no longer any danger of contagion from plague coming from England.[39]

In 1676, two British ships were not allowed to dock, as it was alleged that they had come from places where there was plague.[40] The same happened to a French vessel, suspected of having been in contact with outbreaks of plague.[41] During this period, there were consular complaints against impediments to ships concerning entry to the port of Lisbon or being held in quarantine. This was the case of the English consul, who complained that there was no reason to detain a ship from his country, suspected of plague, and which had been quarantined in Trafaria,[42] while the French consul accused the council of ignoring the bills of health he had presented as proof that the ships had not been in contact with the plague, and the fact that by keeping the goods in quarantine, his merchants were being disadvantaged.[43] In the same year, a blockade of the port of Lisbon had been proposed, using more vessels that would effectively avoid the entry of ships

[39] AML-AH. 25 de Setembro de 1668, Chancelaria Régia, Livro 1º de consultas e decretos de D. Pedro II, f. 55 - 56v. AML-AH. 3-6 de Agosto de 1669, Chancelaria Régia, Livros 1º e 5º de consultas e decretos de D. Pedro II, f. 169 -172v e f. 19 - 22v. AML-AH. 10 de Maio de 1670, Chancelaria Régia, Livro 1º de consultas e decretos de D. Pedro II, f. 288 - 289v. AML-AH. 29 de Maio de 1670, Chancelaria Régia, Livro 1º de consultas e decretos de D. Pedro II, f. 296 - 297v. AML-AH. 26 de Julho de 1671, Chancelaria Régia, Livro 1º de consultas e decretos de D. Pedro II, f. 482 - 483v.

[40] AML-AH. 27 de Julho de 1676, Chancelaria Régia, Livro 4º de consultas e decretos de D. Pedro II, f. 296 - 297v.

[41] AML-AH. 4 de Agosto de 1676, Chancelaria Régia, Livro 4º de consultas e decretos de D. Pedro II, f. 298 - 299v.

[42]AML-AH.28-31 de Agosto de 1676, Chancelaria Régia, Livro 4º de consultas e decretos de D. Pedro II, f. 302 - 304v.

[43]AML-AH. 11-21 de Setembro de 1676, Chancelaria Régia, Livro 4º de consultas e decretos de D. Pedro II, f. 325-326v.

suspected of having been in contact with places infected with that disease,[44] and for which an advisory document on the prevention of contagion from the plague that had spread throughout several ports in the Levant and Africa, had been issued in the senate.[45]

On 3 October of that year, the Lisbon council consulted the king about the English war frigate "Assistance" which had arrived in the port of Lisbon from near Turkey and was *in transit* to London. The ship's captain did not want his statements to be witnessed by members of the crew, or allow guards aboard because it was a warship, and he was not carrying a certificate of health from the country of origin as it was not required from the ports of that country for those of England. On the way, the ship had stopped for water provisions and repairs in Malta (which had come down with the plague months before), Liorne, Tangier and Cádiz, where it was neither allowed to dock nor given assistance. At the port of Lisbon, it intended to take on water provisions once more and undertake some repairs. The signs of suspicion of contagion in the said frigate were very strong, either because of those ports it went through, or because of the state of the individuals on board. Accordingly, the council was of the opinion that the frigate should immediately leave the harbour, leaving the final decision in the hands of the monarch. The king ordered the frigate to be sent away within twenty-four hours (Oliveira 1894, 167-168).

Three days later, the monarch was once again consulted by the Lisbon council regarding the petition presented by the English consul, in which it was alleged that that war frigate had taken shelter in Lisbon "to be fixed and repair the damage caused by storms and during the voyage", and had only passed through the ports of Liorne, Cadiz, and Tangier, "where they had not entered or been granted permission to dock and receive assistance" because they only wanted to hear news about the English navy. Thus, that royal decision was equivalent to "the same as sinking, because so much water is entering that "two hundred sailors… are not enough to work the pump". Continuing, the consul alleged that with so much work nobody could be dispensed with to disembark on land, in addition to the good disposition of the crew to "remove all suspicion of contagious disease", offering to go on board with the health officials for the necessary examinations, and concluding by stating that "without repairing the damage, it would not be just for this ship to leave this port". In view of these statements, the council concluded that the consul's petition contradicted the oath made by the ship's

[44]AML-AH.28-31 de Agosto de 1676, Chancelaria Régia, Livro 4º de consultas e decretos de D. Pedro II, f. 305 - 312v.
[45]AML-AH. 7-9 de Setembro de 1676, Chancelaria Régia, Livro 4º de consultas e decretos de D. Pedro II, f. 318 - 319v.

captain on several carefully detailed points. For these reasons, the council sent its opinion to the monarch: "that the resolution be carried out, that this ship should immediately leave the harbour, without any delay". The royal resolution granted eight days to the captain to undertake repairs, for which he had to ground the ship in Trafaria, where guards would be placed to prevent any communication with the population (Oliveira 1894, 167-170).

In 1677, the council inquired from the governor of arms of Cascais whether orders were being carried out for soldiers not to board vessels calling at that port before they were inspected by health personnel.[46]

The following year the council was advised to take all measures to prevent the plague, including the quarantining of ships coming from the Mediterranean, due to the epidemic that was raging in Constantinople.[47]

In 1679, the council issued several advisory documents. The first referred to a ship anchored in the port of Cascais, coming from Salé and Tangier, from which a passenger who had not been inspected by the health service had disembarked, endangering the population that could have been infected by the plague.[48] The second culminated in a ban on unloading merchandise of ships coming from Tangier and Andalusia and the unloading of wax and hides from the Santa Ana ship, at the port of Trafaria, as there was a danger of contagion from the plague, given that the vessel had embarked from Tangier, where there was an outbreak of the epidemic.[49] In the third, regarding the plague that was growing in Andalusia, the council was consulted on the measures to be taken to prevent contagion[50]; it was ordered to place two feluccas (*faluas*) [51] so as to spend day and night in front of the beaches and another in front of the port of Belém near the tower, each with a trusted person appointed by the council plus six musketeers, to inspect the beaches and boats which fish on the high seas and those coming from Setúbal and Alcácer do Sal and other sea ports, "because these often take passengers from ships and bring them to this city (Lisbon)" (Oliveira

---

[46] AML-AH. 23 de Julho - 6 de Setembro de 1677, Chancelaria Régia, Livro 5º de consultas e decretos de D. Pedro II, f. 62 - 63v.

[47] AML-AH. 6 de Agosto de 1778, Chancelaria Régia, Livro 2º de consultas e decretos de D. Maria I, f. 200 - 200v.

[48] AML-AH. 2 de Junho de 1679, Chancelaria Régia, Livro 6º de consultas e decretos de D. Pedro II, f. 77 a 78v

[49] AML-AH. 21-27 de Junho de 1679, Chancelaria Régia, Livro 6º de consultas e decretos de D. Pedro II, f. 102 a 103v.

[50] AML-AH. 16 de Junho de 1679, Chancelaria Régia, Livro 6º de consultas e decretos de D. Pedro II, f. 75 -76v

[51] A *falua* was a small vessel, with two triangular lateen sails, used to transport cargo and passengers between the two banks of the Tagus River.

1894, 347). This decision was reinforced by the decree on the following 17 August, which established a ban, in Lisbon and all the other ports of the Kingdom, on the activity of vessels bringing passengers from ships or giving them pilots (except for Portuguese ships that had come from their conquests), under penalty of being flogged and exiled in the galleys for five years, and their boat being burned. In the event of a passenger being deposited at any seaport via a boat, the health inspector was immediately to be notified by the health guards about the identity of the passenger, the ship's master and its place of origin, and to be publicly disclosed by the authorities in their areas of jurisdiction (Oliveira 1894, 357-358).

The following year, the entry of ships coming from Malaga was banned, in order to avoid contagion from the plague that was raging in that city, and such measures were insisted on for that disease in Andalusia. In September of that year, the senate advised the monarch, considering that "the contagion of Castile, by the mercy of God, "has ceased"; and as this was the cause of the precautions and caution, with which this Kingdom has defended itself up to the present", in the sense of "suspending the health guards in those parts where there was less fear of danger", while still maintaining some vigilance. Given the proximity of Andalusia and Malaga, the parts referred to include the provinces of the Alentejo and the Algarve and the seaports of the latter (Oliveira 1882, 484-485).

In 1681, the entry into the port of Belém of a Portuguese ship from Cádiz that had to quarantine was noted, to avoid the city from being contaminated with the plague which had been detected in Castile.[52] Meanwhile, as there was no longer any suspicion of plague in northern Europe, the consuls of the countries whose vessels used the port of Lisbon signed a petition that their ships be authorised to go up the river and pass beyond the tower of Belém.[53]

In 1683, the Lisbon council was advised that the goods transported on ships coming from Maranhão (Brazil) could be unloaded with an exemption from quarantine, as there was no plague in the Portuguese dominions.[54]

For the prevention of the plague and the safeguarding of public health, in 1687, it was decreed that no crew member of ships at anchor was authorised to disembark before being inspected by health officials; failure

[52] AML-AH. 27 e 28 de Abril de 1681, Chancelaria Régia, Livro 6º de consultas e decretos de D. Pedro II, f. 467- 468v.

[53] AML-AH. 19 de Setembro de 1681, Chancelaria Régia, Livro 7º de consultas e decretos de D. Pedro II, f. 15- 17v

[54] AML-AH. 28 de Março de 1683, Chancelaria Régia, Livro 9º de consultas e decretos de D. Pedro II, f. 56 -57v.

to comply with this provision was punishable by a sentence of exile in Angola.[55]

Three years later, an advisory document was issued about an English ship suspected of being infected with the plague, which Lisbon council intended not to allow to dock and unload its goods in any port in the Kingdom.[56] Concerns about the entry of plague through foreign ships led to an advisory document issued by the head of the Lisbon council, signed by other individuals in the city, about the health measures to be taken to avoid contagion in the city.[57] The matter had been raised by a letter from a Portuguese representative sent to London, in which he reported "diseases of the plague" at Plymouth. As a result, the council advised the monarch suggesting that "an order be sent" to the governors of the towers not to allow any ship above their respective position to pass by on the Tagus, nor to have any type of communication without them "being visited and cleared by health officials". As for vessels coming from England, regardless of the country of origin, including Portuguese ships, they should not be admitted or allowed to moor nor should they be given assistance in any of the seaports of the Kingdom, "rather they must immediately leave, as it is not fair to admit them with the danger and harm to the public health of this court and Kingdom". And if sailors or other persons were discovered, who had come from those impeded ships, the king should order that any official of justice or guard "may freely kill him, without further commotion or act of judgment". And if the ships not authorized to enter continued not to leave, they would "feel the bite of the cannons of the towers". However, if any of the captains and masters of non-English ships that sailed the English Channel showed that they had neither been in nor communicated with English ports, they were required to comply with a strict quarantine on their ships, while their merchandise (on suspicion of being infected) went to the Trafaria quarantine station to "be washed and purified".[58] By royal decree, the proposals were generally approved, albeit with reservations. Thus, the deaths of those restricted would only be in the event of resisting the order, while the restriction on entry and allowing mooring and receiving assistance was limited to ships coming from Plymouth (Oliveira 1896, 168-171).

---

[55] AML-AH. 17 de Novembro de 1687, Chancelaria Régia, Livro 9º de Consultas e Decretos de D. Pedro II, f. 280 - 281v.

[56] AML-AH. 10 de Abril a 6 de Maio de 1690, Chancelaria Régia, Livro 11º de consultas e decretos de D. Pedro II, f. 171 -176v.

[57] AML-AH. 22-24 de Abril de 1690, Chancelaria Régia, Livro 11º de consultas e decretos de D. Pedro II, f. 156 -157v

[58] Isolated facility where carriers of contagious or suspected diseases were confined under quarantine.

In 1694, a French consul once again filed a complaint regarding five ships from his country not being allowed entry into the port of Belém, as they did not have a clean bill of health.[59] The same happened for the same reason to an English ship coming from England and another, Dutch vessel, arriving from Amsterdam, which also caused complaints from their respective consuls. These events could almost be superimposed on each other.[60]

Sanitary measures in the eighteenth century

Government concerns about improving surveillance conditions at national maritime borders were justified. One of the measures consisted in establishing a health inspection regime and a health regime for the port of Belém, started in the reign of King D. Pedro II, which was reconfirmed on 7 February 1695 and 26 March 1696, and once again applied through the order of his son, King João V (who reigned from 1706 to 1750). These regimes[61] were utilised when there was plague in some Kingdom or province bordering Portugal.[62]

On August 1720, João V was informed, through the ambassador in Madrid that plague had broken out in the quarantine hospital of Marseille, from where it had spread to the city. As a result, all the Portuguese councils were advised to activate the measures that had been regulated. By royal deliberation it was ordered not to allow any ship coming from the French Mediterranean ports to moor or receive assistance, as well as not to allow the entry into the Kingdom of any fugitives originating from there who might come by land (Oliveira 1901, 428-429).

---

[59] AML-AH. 13 de Fevereiro-3 de Março de 1694, Chancelaria Régia, Livro 13º de consultas e decretos de D. Pedro II, f. 386 - 391v.

[60] AML-AH. 19 de Fevereiro-3 de Março de 1694, Chancelaria Régia, Livro 13º de consultas e decretos de D. Pedro II, f. 392 -395v. AML-AH. 10 de Fevereiro-3 de Março de 1694, Chancelaria Régia, Livro 13º de consultas e decretos de D. Pedro II, f. 382 - 385v.

[61] The oldest known codified and systematised health regime dates from 27 September 1526. It was drawn up because of an outbreak of plague in Lisbon and included in the report of a voyage as the "Regime followed by Pedro Vaz concerning the good of the health of Lisbon in 1526". (Oliveira 1906, p. 327) However, we cannot ignore the first draft of a health regulation, which dates back to 1481, drawn up by King João II for the city of Beja, and later extended to Lisbon, which included essential rules for protection against the plague: isolation of the city, quarantine of the sick and disinfection of dwellings.

[62] AML-AH. 20 de Dezembro de 1693-1708, Chancelaria Régia, Livro 2º de Consultas e Decretos de D. João V, do senado oriental, f. 1 - 14v.

In next September, measures had already been taken against the plague coming from the Mediterranean by not allowing the unloading of goods from Spain, where the plague was raging. These measures, including reinforcing the surveillance of vessels entering the harbour, were extended to all vessels coming from ports where there were outbreaks of that disease,[63] while the chief guard (*guarda-mor*) at Paço de Arcos was ordered, along with his personnel, to visit all the ships that had entered Tagus Bay (Fig. 7.5).[64]

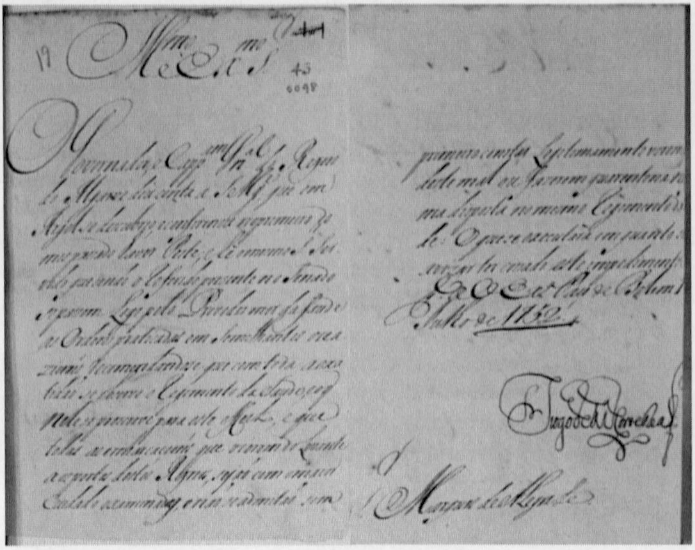

Fig. 7.5. Reproduction of the announcement of 7th July 1752 on the existence of plague in Algiers. Photo: Arquivo Municipal de Lisboa.

On 3 November, the clerk of the council was told by the secretary of state to keep a watch on ships arriving from France and the Levant (Oliveira 1901, 445). At the end of the following month, precautions were also extended to ships, silks, cottons and other merchandise coming by sea from

[63]AML-AH. 23 de Setembro de 1720, Chancelaria Régia, Livro 8º de Consultas e Decretos de D. João V, do senado oriental, f. 119- 121. AML-AH. 3 de Novembro de 1720, Chancelaria Régia, Livro 8º de Consultas e Decretos de D. João V, do senado oriental, f. 71.

[64] AML-AH. 3 de Outubro de 1720, Chancelaria Régia, Livro 8º de Consultas e Decretos de D. João V, do senado oriental, f. 118.

the "Turks and Moors", whatever their origin was. When it became known, through a warning stemming from Sicily, that two (unidentified) English ships coming from the Levant with most of their crews sick with plague and which had been refused entry by all the ports on that island, the monarch determined to ban entry to the ports and beaches of the Kingdom to all English vessels coming from the Levant (Oliveira 1901, 462). However, it turned out that the news was false, as these ships had arrived at their ports and destination, London and Hamburg "without any harm, so the previous royal determination was revoked only for those ships that had been supposed to be carrying the plague, while keeping all the other prohibitions in force" (Oliveira 1901, 482-483).

The ban ended in 1721 for ships coming from Spain, while entering into force for those originating from Italy and Turkey.[65] In fact, throughout that year, government authorities remained particularly vigilant to the entry of the plague through national ports, reinforcing security measures,[66] preventing ships from the Levant (where there were outbreaks of contagion) from entering the ports of the Kingdom. This also applied to French vessels and those of other nationalities suspected of having been in contact with the plague,[67] and the unloading in ports of the Kingdom of goods from the Mediterranean in ships that had been in the vicinity of that disease.[68] Meanwhile, the main health inspector provided information about a situation in which an English ship was found carrying a number of goods from Genoa and five passengers, none of whom had a passport and, through fear of having been in contact with the origins of the plague, were

---

[65] AML-AH. 19 de Junho-8 de Julho de 1721, Chancelaria Régia, Livro 2º de consultas e decretos de D. João V, do senado ocidental, f. 93 - 94.

[66] AML-AH. 18 de Março de 1721, Chancelaria Régia, Livro 8º de Consultas e Decretos de D. João V, do senado oriental, f. 156. AML-AH. 24 de Maio de 1721, Chancelaria Régia, Livro 8º de Consultas e Decretos de D. João V, do senado oriental, f. 155. AML-AH. 21 de Novembro de 1721, Chancelaria Régia, Livro 8º de Consultas e Decretos de D. João V do senado oriental, f. 157.

[67] AML-AH. 16 de Maio de 1721, Chancelaria Régia, Livro 8º de Consultas e Decretos de D. João V do senado oriental, f. 165. AML-AH. 23 de Setembro de 1721, Chancelaria Régia, Livro 8º de Consultas e Decretos de D. João V, do senado oriental, f. 45. AML-AH. 19 de Setembro de 1721, Chancelaria Régia, Livro 8º de Consultas e Decretos de D. João V, do senado oriental, f. 46. AML-AH. 8 de Dezembro de 1722, Chancelaria Régia, Livro 4º de consultas e decretos de D. João V, do senado ocidental, f. 130 – 131.

[68] AML-AH. 22 de Dezembro de 1721, Chancelaria Régia, Livro 8º de Consultas e Decretos de D. João V, do senado oriental, f. 42.

quarantined and prevented from disembarking.[69] However, these impositions were not always fulfilled.[70]

Due to the resurgence of the plague in Marseilles, on 30 June 1722, an order was issued for all seaports in the Kingdom to take the precautions established at the time of the first such news. As Castile was taking precautions concerning all the Barbary ports, some of which were believed to have plague, the king ordered that no vessel originating from there be admitted (Oliveira 1901, 564). Months later, the council received the order to prohibit the entry of ships from Constantinople, where there was a serious plague epidemic.[71]

In 1726, with the continuation of the plague in some European cities, the council was advised to deny entry to ships without a prior sanitary inspection by health officials.[72] On 8 November that year, information was received that in Constantinople and in Grand Cairo "there was a plague so violent that six to seven thousand people died every day". It was also reported that two ships had arrived in Marseilles loaded with wheat from the Levant, where some sailors and a captain had died during the voyage and in the quarantine station. Under these circumstances, King D. João V ordered the national councils to carry out rigorous examinations of the crews of vessels arriving from those ports, in order to exclude any suspicious contamination or, as an alternative, quarantine was imposed, as established in the health regime (Oliveira 1903, 109).

Upon learning that Italy, Spain and northern European countries were taking precautions concerning commerce that came from various places bordering the Turkish dominion, where there was a "contagious mal", the monarch ordered all the councils to issue instructions provided for in the health regime, in terms of guarding against everything stemming from those parts, not admitting vessels or anything that carried, in particular, people, clothing, barley and other grains (Oliveira 1903, 153).

In 1728, the ban on entry into national ports was extended to all vessels coming from the vicinity of the Turkish dominion, on suspicion of being

---

[69] AML-AH. 31 de Maio-7 de Junho de 1721, Chancelaria Régia, Livro 8º de Consultas e Decretos de D. João V, do senado oriental, f. 286 - 288.

[70] AML-AH. 28 de Setembro de 1722, Chancelaria Régia, Livro 4º de consultas e decretos de D. João V do senado ocidental, f. 148 - 149.

[71] AML-AH. 1 de Setembro de 1722, Chancelaria Régia, Livro 4º de consultas e decretos de D. João V, do senado ocidental, f. 214- 215.

[72] AML-AH. 18 de Julho de 1726, Chancelaria Régia, Livro 4º de consultas e decretos de D. João V, do senado ocidental, f. 334 - 335.

infected with the plague.[73] However, the end of the restriction on ships coming from Marseilles was announced, as it was no longer suspected there was plague in this city.[74]

In 1733, the public attorney for the city of Lisbon was notified, through a letter from a cleric, of the arrival of a ship from England, in which there were deaths and possible sources of plague, and for which public protection measures were requested; the arrangements decided on by the medical board for that ship were communicated to the council by the health inspector.[75] In the same year, the council senate received orders to activate the provisions set out in the health regime against a possible contagion of plague brought by ships from the Mediterranean, apparently associated with the outbreaks of that disease recorded in Tripoli.[76] Ships arriving from that port were to be inspected, and not admitted before it was confirmed that they were free of this problem or else they had to quarantine (Oliveira 1903, 499)

Two years later, the council was alerted to the threat of plague coming from Smyrna, Alexandria and neighbouring ports, which involved the sending of prevention letters to the chief guards of the ports of the Kingdom.[77] In the same year, the secretary of state sent a notice to the head of the council senate to carry out the strict quarantining of all ships coming from the ports of the city of Danzig, Royal and Ducal Prussia, Pomerania, Semigallia, Courland, Livonia and Poland. [78]

In 1741, a new alert was given to all the chief guards of the seaports of the Kingdom regarding the plague that was sweeping over the southern coast of the Mediterranean, in Barbary, [79] especially in Algiers, Tétouan and

---

[73] AML-AH. 19 de Junho de 1728, Chancelaria Régia, Livro 5.º de Consultas e Decretos de D. João V, do senado ocidental, doc. 95, f. 132 - 132v.

[74] AML-AH. 27 de Dezembro de 1728, Chancelaria Régia, Livro 5.º de consultas e decretos de D. João V, do senado ocidental, doc. 11, f. 21 - 21v.

[75] AML-AH. 10 de Junho de 1733, Chancelaria Régia, Livro 8º de consultas e decretos de D. João V, do senado ocidental, doc. 88, f. 132 - 132v. AML-AH. 12 de Junho de 1733, Chancelaria Régia, Livro 8º de consultas e decretos de D. João V, do senado ocidental, doc. 89, f. 133 - 134v.

[76] AML-AH. 23 de Junho de 1733, Chancelaria Régia, Livro 8º de consultas e decretos de D. João V, do senado ocidental, doc. 96, f. 141 -141v.

[77] AML-AH. 27 de Julho de 1735-17 de Outubro de 1740, Chancelaria Régia, Livro 10º de consultas e decretos de D. João V, do senado ocidental, f. 137. AML-AH. 15 de Setembro de 1741, Provimento da Saúde, Livro de registo de expediente do provedor-mor da saúde sobre a peste, f. 2 -3v.

[78] AML-AH. 6-7 de Novembro de 1770. Provimento da Saúde, Livro de registo de expediente do provedor-mor da saúde sobre a peste, f. 34v - 35v.

[79] Berberia or Barbaria was the term used from the 16th to the 19th century to refer to the coastal regions of the present-day Maghreb.

Tunis, as well as in the Levant, [80] and the contagious diseases that were plaguing Malaga.[81]

Two years later, the council was ordered not to authorise the entry of ships from Sicily due to plague in the ports of Messina and Trapani, and to quarantine those coming from the Mediterranean, which was followed by the decision not to allow communication with ships, people or goods suspected of plague, coming from Sicily and Ceuta.[82] Following on from the information that the plague in Sicily and the coast of Calabria had died out, on 8 November 1745, the precautions and extraordinary measures in force for vessels from that origin were suspended, while keeping in force those provided for in the health regime and other laws established for any ship entering the ports of the Kingdom (Oliveira 1904, 469). In 1750, the council was advised to avoid contagion entering the Kingdom from the plague that was continuing in North Africa. [83]

In 1752, in the reign of King D. José I (who reigned from 1750-1777), a new outbreak of plague occurred in Algiers, requiring identical preventive measures in the ports of the Kingdom, [84]which were repeated the following year for all vessels coming from that city and the Levant, which were requesting entry to national ports.[85] Through having prevented the application of those measures in the harbour and on the coasts, the chief guard of Cascais received a reprimand. [86]

In 1754, the secretary of state issued a warning to undertake all protective measures and gave orders to the chief health inspector to prevent

[80] AML-AH. 15 de Setembro de 1741, Provimento da Saúde, Livro de registo de expediente do provedor-mor da saúde sobre a peste, f. 5.

[81] AML-AH. 28-28 de Dezembro de 1741, Provimento da Saúde, Livro de registo de expediente do provedor-mor da saúde sobre a peste, f. 5v – 6.

[82] AML-AH. 14 de Julho de 1743, Chancelaria Régia, Livro 15° de consultas e decretos de D. João V, do senado ocidental, doc. 1, f. 4 - 4v. AML-AH. 14-15 de Julho de 1743, Provimento da Saúde, Livro de registo de expediente do provedor-mor da saúde sobre a peste, f. 6v. AML-AH. 29 de Julho de 1743, Chancelaria Régia, Livro 15° de consultas e decretos de D. João V, do senado ocidental, doc. 30, f. 60 - 60v.

[83] AML-AH. 23 de Julho de 1750, Chancelaria Régia, Livro 27° de consultas e decretos de D. João V, do senado ocidental, f. 308 - 309v.

[84] AML-AH. 7 de Julho de 1752, Chancelaria Régia, Livro 3° de consultas, decretos e avisos de D. José I, f. 51 - 52v.

[85] AML-AH. 20 de Junho de 1753, Chancelaria Régia, Livro 4° de consultas, decretos e avisos de D. José I, f. 40 - 41v.

[86] AML-AH. 11 de Outubro de 1753, Cascais, Chancelaria Régia, Livro 4° de consultas, decretos e avisos de D. José I, f. 196 - 197v.

the plague coming from the Mediterranean from spreading within the Portuguese Kingdom. [87]

In 1756, the Lisbon council was advised to take measures to avoid the consequences of infection by plague, such as those cases which had occurred in Genoa and on the island of Corsica.[88] At the end of that year, the secretary of state ordered that all sanitary measures be taken upon the arrival of a ship from Martinique, because its sailors would be contaminated with the plague.[89] Two days later, as a precaution against the plague, the council was instructed to order the health officials of all the ports in the Kingdom to quarantine ships from the ports of France, except that of Le Havre. [90]

In 1759, it was learned that Alexandria and the surrounding regions, as well as other areas involving Turkish commerce, were infested with the plague, which had spread to four ships then sailing in the Mediterranean. By royal order, communicated by the secretary of state to the Lisbon council, the chief health inspector and his team were immediately sent to Paço de Arcos, so that, from that place, they could organize the appropriate measures for that situation (Oliveira 1908, 418-419). However, the Government instructed that, after disembarking, the bales of silk ordered for the royal silk factory should not be kept in the quarantine station due to possible contamination by the plague, given that they came from Piedmont, which was not under suspicion, and not from the Levant. [91]

In 1761, Lisbon council was ordered to impose strict quarantine on all vessels coming from the Adriatic Sea.[92]

Three years later, the council was advised to issue quarantining instructions and the full range of preventive measures against the plague for ships arriving from Italy at the ports of the Kingdom.[93] A few days later, it became known, through the commissioner and inspector of the council, that

---

[87] AML-AH. 19 de Dezembro de 1754, Chancelaria Régia, Livro 6º de consultas, decretos e avisos de D. José I, f. 398 - 399v.

[88] AML-AH. 21 de Maio de 1756, Chancelaria Régia, Livro 9º de consultas, decretos e avisos de D. José I, f. 330 - 331v.

[89] AML-AH. 13 de Novembro de 1756, Chancelaria Régia, Livro 10º de consultas, decretos e avisos de D. José I, f. 355 - 356v

[90] AML-AH. 30 de Janeiro de 1758, Chancelaria Régia, Livro 11º de consultas, decretos e avisos de D. José I, f. 147 - 148v.

[91] AML-AH. 15 de Fevereiro de 1760-29 de Maio de 1765, Chancelaria Régia, Livro 14º de consultas, decretos e avisos de D. José I, f. 87 - 89v.

[92] AML-AH. 6 de Outubro de 1761,", Chancelaria Régia, Livro 12º de consultas, decretos e avisos de D. José I, f. 228 a 229v

[93] AML-AH. 28 de Julho de 1764, Chancelaria Régia, Livro 13º de consultas, decretos e avisos de D. José I, f. 192 - 193v.

there was plague in Naples so that, by royal command, the secretary of state ordered that that responsible individual issue instructions to the health officials that, as an alternative to the previous quarantine, they should rather suspend entry into the port of Lisbon originating from that region, and reserve quarantine to ships those coming from Sicily (Oliveira 1908, 567).

In 1767, two three-masted English galleys, had been driven out of Gibraltar on account of their ongoing reputation of being infected with the plague. Given this fact, regulatory measures were ordered, preventing the entry of these vessels into the Portuguese ports.[94]

The information about the contamination of the Gibraltar ships by plague was confirmed on the same date by the English vice-consul.[95]Other ships that had approached them would be admitted, although with the necessary precautions and only after confirming that there had been no direct communication with the galleys (Oliveira 1911, 168-169). A few days later, quarantine was lifted for ships coming from Ragusa, as fears of plague had proven unfounded; however, surveillance for health purposes continued for ships arriving from the Levant.[96] At the end of September, the head of the Lisbon council received a new warning from the secretary of state indicating the measures to be taken for all ships arriving in the Kingdom with suspected plague.[97] The next year, the consul in Genoa informed the secretary of state, and the latter the leaders of Lisbon council, of a French ship infected with plague.[98]

In 1770, the secretary of state sent a warning to the head of Lisbon council, through which strict quarantine was imposed on ships coming from the Mediterranean, due to plague in Alexandria, Smyrna and other ports under Turkish dominion, as well as those coming from the Baltic Sea, because there was also plague in the Kingdom of Poland.[99] The alert was repeated the following year for maritime traffic in the Baltic, when the

---

[94]AML-AH. 1 de Setembro de 1767, Chancelaria Régia, Livro 15º de consultas, decretos e avisos de D. José I, f. 243 - 244v.

[95] AML-AH. 1 de Setembro de 1767. Chancelaria Régia, Livro 15º de consultas, decretos e avisos de D. José I, f. 245 a 250v.

[96]AML-AH. 12 de Setembro de 1767, Chancelaria Régia, Livro 15º de consultas, decretos e avisos de D. José I, f. 253 -254v.

[97]AML-AH. 27 de Setembro de 1767, Chancelaria Régia, Livro 15º de consultas, decretos e avisos de D. José I, f. 259 -262v.

[98] AML-AH. 11-12 de Junho de 1768, Provimento da Saúde, Livro de registo de expediente do provedor-mor da saúde sobre a peste, f. 26- 27.

[99]AML-AH. 12-!3 de Julho de 1770, Chancelaria Régia, Livro 17º de consultas, decretos e avisos de D. José I, f. 46 - 47v. AML-AH. 12 de Novembro de 1771, Chancelaria Régia, Livro 17º de consultas, decretos e avisos de D. José I, f. 228 - 229v.

existence of plague in Moscow became known, where, in a month, it had caused four thousand deaths (Oliveira 1911, 567, 351).

The head of Lisbon council, instructed to order a rigorous inspection of ships from Sweden and Denmark,[100] was informed by his superiors in 1772 of the end of the plague in the Baltic ports.[101]

It should be noted, that there were strange exceptions to the strict sanitary standards established, as was the case with an Irish bishop and his family who, coming from Italy, were allowed to disembark (Fig.7.6), despite the fact that the ship that carried them had been placed under quarantine.[102]

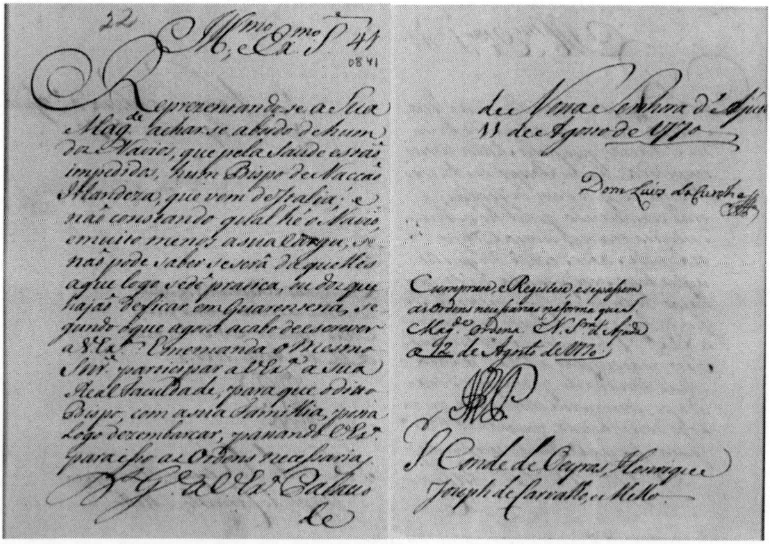

Ill.mo e Ex.mo S.r

Representando-se a Sua Mag.de acharse abordo de hum dos Navios, que pela Saude estaõ impedidos, hum Bispo de Naccaõ Irlandeza, que vem de Italia; e naõ constando qual hé o Navio, e muito menos a sua Carga, se naõ pode saber se será daquelles a que logo se dê pratica, ou dos que hajaõ de ficar em Quarentena, segundo o que agora acabo de escrever a V. Ex.a Ordena o Mesmo Snr. participar a V. Ex.a a sua Real Faculdade, para que o dito Bispo, com a sua Familia, possa logo dezembarcar, passando V. Ex.a para esse as Ordens necessarias. D.s G.e a V. Ex.a Palacio de N. Snra. d'Ajuda 11 de Agosto de 1770

Dom Luiz da Cunha

Cumprase, e Registese, e expeçaõ-se as Ordens necessarias na forma que S. Mag.de Ordena. N. Snra. d'Ajuda a 12 de Agosto de 1770

S. Conde de Oeyras, Henrique Joseph de Carvalho e Mello

Fig. 7.6. Reproduction of the document granting authorization to disembark in Lisbon in August 1770 to an Irish bishop travelling with relatives, although the ship was held in quarantine. Photo: Arquivo Municipal de Lisboa.

[100] AML-AH. 2-3 Janeiro de 1771, Provimento da Saúde, Livro de registo de expediente do provedor-mor da saúde sobre a peste, f. 35v – 36.

[101] AML-AH. 30-31 de Outubro de 1772, Provimento da Saúde, Livro de registo de expediente do provedor-mor da saúde sobre a peste, f. 37.

[102] AML-AH. 11-12 de Agosto de 1770, Chancelaria Régia, Livro 17º de consultas, decretos e avisos de D. José I, f. 50 - 51v.

During the reign of Queen Dona Maria I (from 1777 to 1816)[103], the head of Lisbon council was responsible for ordering the necessary measures to avoid the contamination of the Kingdom by the plague that was raging in Algiers by vessels from here and from the Mediterranean. For this reason, and as a preventive measure against contagion by the plague, the main health inspector had been ordered to take up residence in Paço de Arcos, in order to better coordinate his efforts with those of the governor of the court of arms of the province of Extremadura.[104]

Sanitary measures in the nineteenth century

There is a record from the Portuguese secretary of state, in 1804, about the news of vessels arriving from ports in Spain, because they were contaminated with plague.[105] Two months later, Lisbon council was advised to send documentation on the plague in Spain to the Health Inspection Board, so that this entity could promote measures to avoid contagion in the Kingdom.[106] In addition to this prevention, the council was informed that two brigantines had been deployed to guard the Atlantic coast, one between Caminha and Figueira da Foz and the other between this location and Cabo de S. Vicente,[107] while two sanitary cordons were being established along the borders of Minho and the Beiras provinces for protection against the plague in Spain.[108] The Board's deliberations for the prevention of contagion from the plague were approved, [109]and the secretary of state

[103] Due to alleged dementia, the Kingdom was ruled by his son, Prince João, from 1792 to 1816.

[104] AML-AH. 30 de Abril-2 de Maio de 1787, Chancelaria Régia, Livro 1º de avisos de D. Maria I, f. 105 - 106v; AML-AH. 2 -26 de Maio de 1787, Provimento da Saúde, Livro de registo de decretos, alvarás e ordens da casa da saúde, docs. 36 - 37, f. 39 - 43v; AML-AH. 24 de Maio-30 de Maio de 1787; Chancelaria Régia, Livro 1º de avisos de D. Maria I, f. 111 - 112v.

[105] AML-AH. 1-23 de Setembro de 1791. Provimento da Saúde, Livro de Registo de Avisos da Secretaria de Estado à Provedoria-Mor da Saúde, doc. 132, f. 63 - 63v.

[106] AML-AH. 17-21 de Novembro de 1804, Provimento da Saúde, Pasta n.º 2 de reais avisos expedidos das Secretarias de Estado, doc. 24, f. 48 - 49v.

[107] AML-AH. 27-28 de Novembro de 1804, Provimento da Saúde, Pasta n.º 2 de reais avisos expedidos das Secretarias de Estado, doc. 31, f. 62 - 63v.

[108] AML-AH. 8-14 de Dezembro de 1804, Provimento da Saúde, Pasta n.º 2 de reais avisos expedidos das Secretarias de Estado, doc. 35, f. 70 - 71v.

[109] AML-AH. 22-23 de Novembro de 1804, Provimento da Saúde, Pasta n.º 2 de reais avisos expedidos das Secretarias de Estado, doc. 28, f. 56 - 57v.

advised the council to commend the effectiveness of the Health Inspection Board in protecting the Kingdom. [110]

At the beginning of 1805, together with the news of the existence of a person sick with the plague at Oporto General Hospital, a statement was issued that all matters relating to public health should be referred to the Health Inspection Board.[111] Outbreaks of plague near the Portuguese border, namely in Cádiz, Gibraltar and Cartagena were recorded, of which the head of Lisbon council was informed, so that the Health Inspection Board could implement the regulatory measures. [112] Shortly thereafter, those entities were informed that the outbreak of plague in Spain was over. [113]

The surveillance of the dangers of contagion led the government to specify how and when it would be necessary to implement preventive measures. Therefore, a public notice was published in July 1813 regulating that the fishing boat skippers (*arrais*) who wanted to fish beyond the Tower of Belém should place a banner with the image of St. Sebastian (*S. Sebastião*) on the boat.[114] In addition, all the crew should carry health passports to present to the chief guard of the Belém port when leaving for registration. In this way, it was possible to control the number of returning workers. If an unregistered crew member happened to show up at the exit, the boat master would incur the punishment foreseen in the 1695 health regiment.[115]

In subsequent years, during the government of King D. João VI (reigned from 1816 to 1826), successive legislation was issued to prevent the approach of ships from "infected" or "suspicious" countries, with those prevented from docking and subject to strict quarantining at the port of Lisbon. Vessels calling at this port were given a pilot belonging to one of the six fishing boats nominated for this service. Seafarers who transgressed

---

[110] AML-AH 1-3 de Dezembro de 1804, Provimento da Saúde, Pasta n.º 2 de reais avisos expedidos das Secretarias de Estado, doc. 33, f. 66 - 67v.

[111] AML-AH. 11 de Janeiro de 1805, Provimento da Saúde, Pasta n.º 3 de papéis remetidos das Secretarias de Estado, f. 81- 84v.

[112] AML-AH. 11-22 de Março de 1805, Provimento da Saúde, Pasta n.º 2 de reais avisos expedidos das Secretarias de Estado, doc. 62, f. 126 - 127v. AML-AH. 24 de Abril de 1805, Provimento da Saúde, Pasta n.º 2 de reais avisos expedidos das Secretarias de Estado, doc. 65, f. 132 - 133v. AML-AH. 12-13 de Maio de 1805, Provimento da Saúde, Pasta n.º 2 de reais avisos expedidos das Secretarias de Estado, doc. 68, f. 138- 139v.

[113] AML-AH. 26-27 de Junho de 1805, Provimento da Saúde, Pasta n.º 2 de reais avisos expedidos das Secretarias de Estado, doc. 74, f. 150 -151v.

[114] St Sebastian is sometimes known as the "plague saint" because of his supposed intercession during a plague outbreak in 7th century Pavia.

[115] Edital de 3 de Julho de 1813, 212-213.

this service were severely punished with imprisonment and ten years of exile in Africa.[116] Also as a precaution against contagion by the plague, the crew and masters of all fishing boats that went out below Belém Tower, or Paço de Arcos or Cascais, were required to meet a detailed list of obligations (which included the marking of the boats with a triangular banner of the same colour and predetermined size, and the identification of their equipment in a health passport), to be checked by the authorities of the respective Health Court every time they left and returned, in addition to being prohibited from entering into any contact with other vessels. The transgression of any of the established rules resulted in quarantining in the quarantine station, and the stranding or loss of their boat and cargo.[117] In the same year, a total ban from entry into the ports of the Kingdom was ordered for all ships from Norway, where it was said that "a dangerous and contagious disease" had broken out, attacking people, leading to death in less than twelve hours. Moreover, it was reported that it had originated in the relics from a shipwreck that had come ashore".[118]

Precautions against contagions from countries infected with contagious or suspected diseases were extended to the Azores archipelago, where Boards of Health were created. Before mooring ships from suspected ports, the respective bill of health would have to be verified, as well as the undertaking of the remaining regulatory procedures provided for in the health regulations of Belém, by employees of the "health longboat"; as a precaution, the ships would be fumigated and would wait three days, with a yellow flag hoisted on the large mast, before being allowed to anchor and before any individual on board being allowed to communicate with land. In the event they were ships without a bill of health, or that had sick people on board who might have suspected illnesses, they had to hoist a yellow flag and all their passengers and crew were sent to quarantine in a lazaretto, and their goods were disinfected. [119] It was not explained, however, where the quarantine would take place, given that in Portugal there was, at that time, only one provisional lazaretto, located in Porto Brandão.

In 1837, during the reign of Queen Dona Maria II (who reigned from 1826 to 1828 and from 1834 to 1853) several captains of English ships coming from Bristol to Madeira and the Azores did not request

[116] Edital de 30 de Março de 1816a, 127. Edital de 30 de Março de 1816b, p.128. Edital, 19 de Junho de 1816, 195-196.

[117] Edital de 30 de Março de 1816c, 129-130.

[118] Edital de 19 de Junho de 1816, 222-223.

[119] Portaria de 20 de Março de 1832, pp.12-13.

authorization in the health cards, and some passengers did not carry a passport, which resulted in the sanctioning of those offenders.[120]

An alert by the Naval Command against the risk of contagion by cholera and plague, coming from Mediterranean ports and some European cities (Danzig, Berlin and Hamburg), led to strict sanitary surveillance or, in suspected or confirmed cases of infection, the prohibiting of all ships from Norway from entering the ports of the Kingdom. All ports in Denmark were also considered very suspicious. Only those which had obtained entry permits could dock at the port of Lisbon, where they would be quarantined for ten days.[121]

Attesting to these precautions, the text of a royal statement is transcribed:[122]

> Having already been instructed by an order issued to the Public Health Council, dated 29 September 1838, which, as the health visit to the ships at the Belém station cannot be verified, but from sunrise to sunset, in accordance with the respective regulation, if this was undertaken with respect to the English steamships of the peninsular shipping company, when they arrive in Belém after sunset, and only while on a health visit, in the same way as always practised with ocean liners and other special vessels, in this case, the naval officer who carries the bags is obliged to deliver to the commanding officer of the port registry a certificate of health, vouchsafing the good state of health of all the individuals on board; and Her Majesty the QUEEN, considering that the same, or more powerful reasons are given to grant the same concession to the Portuguese steamships *Porto* and *Quinta do Vesúvio* coming from a port in the Kingdom, with voyages of twenty-four hours, there can be very little suspicion about their health status; it is hereby ordered, through the Secretary of state for Affairs of the Kingdom, that the aforementioned Portuguese steamships the *Porto* and *Quinta do Vesúvio* proceed in the same way, as by the aforementioned Order of 29 September 1838 it was ordered to proceed with respect to the steamships of the Peninsular shipping company, with the health visit only, when they arrive in Belém after sunset, forcing the respective captains to deliver to the commanding officer of harbour the certificate that is referred to in the said Order. Which is shared with the Public Health Council for its awareness and undertaking.
> *Palácio das Necessidades, 26 March 1840. Rodrigo da Fonseca Magalhães.*

Ten years later, at the behest of the Lisbon Health Council, a notice was posted which, among other matters, determined that ships of any origin that

---

[120] Portaria de 3 de Março de 1837, p. 192.
[121] Portaria de 16 de Setembro de 1837, pp. 111-112.
[122] Portaria de 26 de Março de 1840, p. 45.

arrived at any port in the Kingdom, carrying such patients on board or where deaths had occurred, had to comply with quarantine, which was necessary for public health safety. This was further reinforced by the requirement of bills of health or personal certificates issued by doctors in the area who were local, authenticated by the Portuguese consulate or any other nation that had a commercial relationship with Portugal.[123]

In the reign of King D. Pedro V (reigned from 1853 to 1861), health certificates were required to fully mention the number of passengers and crew being carried, and without this information the ship's crew, passengers and cargo were subject to quarantine and the envisaged sanitary measures.[124] As the health certificates continued to be the subject of frequent infringements, it was decided to apply the same penalty to all ships which landed under those conditions.[125] However, the Public Health Council, as soon as it classified a certain European port as suspect or "dirty", was obliged to inform the national consuls in service in the respective countries by telegraph, in order to know of the commercial aspects.[126]

Vessels from "suspicious provenances" that arrived at ports in the Kingdom, having travelled at least eight days (from the port departure date), were authorized for free local mooring and assistance, while those who did not yet have that travel time could do so at the port of arrival, during "observed quarantine".[127] This requirement assumed that, within eight days, the first manifestations of the more dangerous and frequent infectious-contagious diseases of the time, such as the plague, cholera and yellow fever, would have appeared.

In the event that the unseaworthiness of vessels from suspicious sources arriving at Portuguese ports was invoked, and in order to avoid abuses and serious inconveniences, it was determined that repairable damages were authorized under a strict ban on communications and a ban on the disembarkation of people, wares and goods, after which they would have to leave that port for the accredited lazaretto. If, by chance, there was no possible repair of the ships, their owners or representatives would have to undertake transhipment, under quarantine, to a chartered vessel with the same destination. [128]

Ships that had had yellow fever patients on board were prevented from entering national ports, while they were unable to show documentation of

---

123 Edital de 24 de Outubro de 1850, 841-842.
124 Edital de 9 de Junho de 1855, 121-122.
125 Edital de 12 de Outubro de 1860, 722.
126 Portaria de 18 de Setembro de 1861, 345.
127 Edital de 29 de Setembro de 1853, 610-611.
128 Ofício de 24 de Outubro de 1853, 667.

this having been purged.[129] Those who came from ports suspected of, or "dirty" with cholera, were subject to observation quarantine for, respectively, 3 or 5 days, or more, if this was advisable. [130]

A few months earlier, the Royal Public Health Council had informed the ship owners, consignees and captains meeting the quarantine deadline that they should pay for ship whitewashing (in areas that could not be washed) and the disinfectant drugs to be used. The Belém chief guard would indicate the quality and quantity for washing furniture, clothes and utensils and everything coming from these ships. The chief should verify the required work after the quarantine ended, which could be extended for the time necessary until those improvements were completed to guarantee public health.[131]

To carry out the works and other improvements that were taking place at the lazaretto, and to ensure compliance with the regulatory standards for the quarantine of susceptible goods or coming from "dirty" ports, that department decided to keep the lazaretto closed only for these materials in January 1859. Surprisingly, that department claimed that "dirty" ports had decreased "a lot". The unloading of ships from those origins in national ports was also prohibited unless they had already undergone purges and quarantine in lazarettos of nearby countries. Meanwhile, the lazaretto remained open to passengers arriving from those "dirty" ports.[132]

In view of the conclusions of the international conferences held in Paris in 1851 and 1859 (Howard-Jones 1975, 15, 31-34), the Government decided to unite the quarantine measures established for yellow fever, cholera and plague under one meticulous regulation; the following stood out: (a) no ship could enter the Kingdom ports without being scrupulously visited by personnel from the respective health station; (b) ships coming from clean ports with a clean and regular health pass, without any suspicious occurrences on board during the travel, and in good hygienic conditions, were immediately admitted to free circulation; (c) ships arriving from ports declared suspect were subject to an observation quarantine of three days if the ports of origin were declared suspect of cholera, of five days if it was yellow fever, and of eight days in the case of plague; quarantines for yellow fever and plague would only take place in the port of Lisbon; (d) if casualties occurred during the trip or at the port of origin due to that kind of disease, they had to comply with those quarantine periods, which could be extended if the circumstances of the ship and public safety so required, (and) if

[129] Edital de 7 de Abril de 1858, 104-105.
[130].Edital de 27 de Setembro de 1858, 378-379.
[131] Edital de 2 de Abril de 1858,103.
[132] Edital de 26 de Janeiro de 1859, 21.

quarantine was refused, the ship would have to leave the port along with its passengers and goods. [133]

Observation quarantine was also applied, in the reign of King D. Luis I (1861 to 1889), to passengers, crew, cargo, baggage and ships arriving from ports considered "clean", but which did not show a bill of health or one which did not have consular validation. [134]

In 1897, during King D. Carlos I's reign (from October 19, 1889 to February 1, 1908), the Consultative Board of Public Health considered it convenient to eliminate or reduce some regulatory provisions on maritime health that, at that time, were excessive, replacing them with less rigorous and more adequate measures to insure the progress of science and the preservation of public health. The new and detailed general regulation of maritime health, approved by the monarch, consisted of a detailed set of rules under the responsibility of the government, civil governors, or those responsible for ships and other vessels; the following functionalities were also defined: (a) organization, staff and functions of the health stations; (b) health letters, visas and expeditions; (c) free circulation, impediments and disinfection; (d) lazarettos; (e) disinfectants and their application; (f) staff from health stations and lazarettos; (g) complaints against the application of sanitary measures; (h) customs; (i) duties and taxes; (j) the services of the public disinfection post in Lisbon; (k) criminal sanctions.[135] Months later, a doubt in general regulation of maritime health was clarified, regarding the medical examination of passengers carried to the lazaretto. According to the opinion of the Consultative Board of Public Health, it was determined that the medical examination would just be carried out at the lazaretto since, by *force majeure*, it could not be carried out on board.[136]

Conclusion

The socioeconomic disruption and, above all, the high mortality rate caused by the second pandemic of bubonic plague, from the fourth century through to the mid-nineteenth century, were a constant source of concern for the Portuguese monarchs reigning at that time. Since Lisbon was, throughout these times, a centre with a large flow of maritime trade from the most distant ports in the world, the arriving crews, passengers and goods from ships that headed for the capital posed a constant threat of possible

[133] Edital de 8 de Março de 1860, 87-92.
[134] Portaria de 26 de Fevereiro de 1875, 482.
[135] Decreto de 21 de Janeiro de 1897, 7-34.
[136] Portaria de 2 de Abril de 1898, 103.

contamination. These threats were confirmed by news about the existence of pestiferous outbreaks or suspected lethal contagious diseases in distant places.

Based on these data, the Kingdom rulers from the fifteenth to the nineteenth century took steps to prevent the spread of the plague or other suspicious diseases in the national territory, carrying out a concerted and continuous health prevention strategy. In framing these dictates, initial norms were created, which evolved into a detailed sanitary regulation, put into practice by a hierarchy of zealous employees. Secretaries of state, city councils, medical entities, and a group of other workers with specified assignments intervened in this process. Failure to comply with superiorly established measures was grounds for punishing offenders with a court sentence to the galleys or exile in overseas territories.

As measures to assure naval circulation free of dangerous contagion, impediment of entry into the port and immediate removal order for vessels suspected or known to be infected would be issued, or a mandate to confinement and quarantine of persons and goods in the lazaretto, proved to be effective.

Acknowledgments

My gratitude to colleague Dr. Maria do Sameiro Barroso for clarifying textual details. My thanks to Arch. António Duarte Correia,-for the technical improvement in the images presented.

Arquival Sources and References

Arquivo histórico da câmara municipal de lisboa
Chancelaria Régia, Livro dos Pregos.
Chancelaria Régia, Livro 2º de D. João II.
Provimento da Saúde, Livro 1º do provimento da saúde.
Provimento da Saúde, Cópia do Livro 1º do provimento da saúde.
Provimento da Saúde, Cópia do Livro 2º do provimento da saúde.
Chancelaria Régia, Livro 2º de consultas e decretos de Filipe III.
Chancelaria Régia, Livro 3º de consultas e decretos de D. João IV.
Chancelaria Régia, Livro 2º de consultas e decretos de D. Afonso VI.
Chancelaria Régia, Livro 2º de registo de consultas e decretos de D. Pedro II.
Chancelaria Régia, Livro 1º de consultas e decretos de D. Pedro II.
Chancelaria Régia, Livros 1º e 5º de consultas e decretos de D. Pedro II.
Chancelaria Régia, Livro 4º de consultas e decretos de D. Pedro II.

Chancelaria Régia, Livro 5º de consultas e decretos de D. Pedro II.
Chancelaria Régia, Livro 2º de consultas e decretos de D. Maria I.
Chancelaria Régia, Livro 6º de consultas e decretos de D. Pedro II.
Chancelaria Régia, Livro 7º de consultas e decretos de D. Pedro II.
Chancelaria Régia, Livro 9º de consultas e decretos de D. Pedro II.
Chancelaria Régia, Livro 11º de consultas e decretos de D. Pedro II.
Chancelaria Régia, Livro 13º de consultas e decretos de D. Pedro II.
Chancelaria Régia, Livro 2º de Consultas e Decretos de D. João V, do Chancelaria Régia, Livro 2º de consultas e decretos de D. João V do Senado Oriental.
Chancelaria Régia, Livro 4º de consultas e decretos de D. João V do Senado Ocidental.
Chancelaria Régia, Livro 5.º de Consultas e Decretos de D. João V, do Senado Ocidental
Chancelaria Régia, Livro 8º de Consultas e Decretos de D. João V, do Senado Oriental.
Chancelaria Régia, Livro 8º de consultas e decretos de D. João V, do Senado Ocidental.
Chancelaria Régia, Livro 10º de consultas e decretos de D. João V, do Senado Ocidental.
Chancelaria Régia, Livro 15º de consultas e decretos de D. João V, do Senado Ocidental.
Chancelaria Régia, Livro 27º de consultas e decretos de D. João V, do Senado Ocidental.
Provimento da Saúde, Livro de registo de expediente do provedor-mor da saúde sobre a peste.
Chancelaria Régia, Livro 3º de consultas, decretos e avisos de D. José.
Chancelaria Régia, Livro 4º de consultas, decretos e avisos de D. José.
Chancelaria Régia, Livro 6º de consultas, decretos e avisos de D. José I
Chancelaria Régia, Livro 9º de consultas, decretos e avisos de D. José I.
Chancelaria Régia, Livro 10º de consultas, decretos e avisos de D. José I.
Chancelaria Régia, Livro 11º de consultas, decretos e avisos de D. José I.
Chancelaria Régia, Livro 12º de consultas, decretos e avisos de D. José I.
Chancelaria Régia, Livro 13º de consultas, decretos e avisos de D. José I.
Chancelaria Régia, Livro 14º de consultas, decretos e avisos de D. José I.
Chancelaria Régia, Livro 15º de consultas, decretos e avisos de D. José I.
Chancelaria Régia, Livro 16º de consultas, decretos e avisos de D. José I.
Chancelaria Régia, Livro 17º de consultas, decretos e avisos de D. José I.
Chancelaria Régia, Livro 1º de avisos de D. Maria I.
Provimento da Saúde, Livro de registo de decretos, alvarás e ordens da casa da saúde.

Provimento da Saúde, Livro de Registo de Avisos da Secretaria de Estado à Provedoria-Mor da Saúde.
Provimento da Saúde, Pasta n.º 2 de reais avisos expedidos das Secretarias de Estado.
Provimento da Saúde, Pasta n.º 3 de papéis remetidos das Secretarias de Estado.

Legislação Régia
Decreto de 18 de Setembro de 1844, sem entidade, Livro 1844.
Decreto de 26 de Novembro de 1845, D. Maria II (1826-1827; 1834-1853), Livro 1845.
Decreto de 21 de Maio de 1846, sem entidade, Livro 1846.
Decreto de 3 de Dezembro de 1868, Ministério do Reino, Livro 1868.
Decreto de 12 de Novembro de 1874, Ministério do Reino, Livro 1874.
Decreto de 4 de Outubro de 1889, Ministério do Reino, Livro 1889.
Decreto de 21 de Janeiro de 1897,Ministério do Reino, Livro 1897.
Edital de 3 de Julho de 1813, Governo do Reino, Livro 1812-1814.
Edital de 30 de Março de 1816ª, Junta da Saúde, Livro 1815-1816.
Edital de 30 de Março de 1816b, Junta da Saúde, Livro 1815-1816.
Edital de 30 de Março de 1816c, 1815-1816.
Edital de 19 de Junho de 1816, Junta da Saúde, Livro 1815-1816.
Edital de 24de Outubro de 1850, Conselho de Saúde Pública, Livro 1850.
Edital de 29 de Setembro de 1853, Conselho de Saúde Pública, Livro 1853.
Ofício de 24 de Outubro de 1853, Conselho de Saúde Pública, Livro 1853.
Edital de 9 de Junho de 1855, Conselho de Saúde Pública, Livro 1855.
Edital de 2 de Abril de 1858, Conselho de Saúde Pública, Livro 1858.
Edital de 7 de Abril de 1858, Conselho de Saúde Pública, Livro 1858.
Edital de 27 de Setembro de 1858, Conselho de Saúde Pública, Livro 1858.
Edital de 26 de Janeiro de 1859, Conselho de Saúde Pública, Livro 1859.
Edital de 8 de Março de 1860, Conselho de Saúde Pública, Livro 1860.
Edital de 12 de Outubro de 1860, Conselho de Saúde Pública, Livro 1860.
Portaria de 3 de Março de 1837, Secretaria de Estado dos Negócios do Reino, Livro 1837 - 1º semestre.
Portaria de 20 de Março de 1832, Junta da Saúde, Livro 1832.
Portaria de 16 de Junho de 1837, Secretaria de Estado dos Negócios do Reino, Livro 1837 - 2º Semestre.
Portaria de 16 de Setembro de 1837, Secretaria de Estado dos Negócios do Reino, Livro 1837 - 2º Semestre.
Portaria de 26 de Março de 1840, Secretaria de Estado dos Negócios do Reino, Livro 1840.
Portaria de 5 de Maio de 1850, Ministério do Reino, Livro 1850.

Portaria de 14 de Julho de 1859, Ministério do Reino, Livro 1859.
Portaria de 18 de Setembro de 1861, Ministério do Reino, Livro 1861.
Portaria de 26 de Fevereiro de 1875, Ministério do Reino, Livro 1876.
Portaria de 1 de Fevereiro de 1876, Ministério do Reino, Livro 1876.
Portaria de 2 de Abril de 1897, Ministério do Reino, Livro 1897.

References

Benedictow, Ole Jørgen. 2004. *The Black Death 1346-1353: The Complete History*. Woodbridge: The Boydell Press.

Blackmore, George John.1906. *Rats, fleas, and plague*, Thesis for the degree of M.D. University of Edinburgh.

Echenberg, Myrin. 2007. *Plague Ports: The global urban impact of Bubonic Plague, 1884-1901*. New York: New York University Press.

Férran y Clúa, Jaime; Viñas y Cusí, Federico; Grau, Rosendo de.1907. *La Peste Bubónica: memoria sobre la epidemia ocurrida en Porto en 1899*. Barcelona: Tipografia Sucesor F. Sánchez.

Gage, Kenneth L; Kosoy, Michael Y.2005. "Natural history of plague: perspectives from more than a century of research". *Annual Review of Entomology,* 50 (1):505-528.

Gauthier, J., Constantin, & Raybaud, Antoine. 1903. "Recherches expérimentales sur le rôle des parasites des rats dans la transmission de la peste". *Revue d'Hygiène et Police Sanitaire,* 25: 426-438

Goes, Damião. 1926. *Crónica do Felicíssimo Rei D. Manuel*. Parte I. Coimbra: Imprensa da Universidade.

Greenwood Jr, Major. 1910. "Reports on plague investigations in India. I issued by the Advisory Committee appointed by the Secretary of state for India". *The Journal of Hygiene*, 10 (3): 313-568.

Haensch, Stephanie; Bianucci, Raffaella & Signoli, Michel. 2010. "Distinct clones of Yersinia pestis caused the Black Death". *PLOS. Pathogens* 6 (10): e1001134.

Howard-Jones, Norman. 1975. *The Scientific Background of the International Sanitary Conferences 1851-1938*. Geneva: World Health Organization.

Lamb, George; Liston, William Glen; Petrie, George Ford; et al. 1907. "Reports on plague investigations in India. Advisory Committee Appointed by the Secretary of state for India, the Royal Society and the Lister Institute". *The British Medical Journal* 2 (2429):155-157.

Marks, Geoffrey. 1971. *The Medieval Plague: The Dark Death of the Middle Ages*. Garden City, New York: Doubleday & Company.

McCormick, Michael. 2003. "Rats, communications, and plagues: toward an ecological history. *Journal of Interdisciplinary History,* 34 (1):1-25.1-3, 22-24.

Oliveira, Eduardo Freire de.1882. *Elementos para a História do Município de Lisboa.* 1ª Parte, Tomo I. Lisboa: Typographia Universal.

Oliveira, Eduardo Freire. 1891. *Elementos para a História do Município de Lisboa.* 1ª Parte, Tomo VI. Lisboa: Typographia Universal.

Oliveira, Eduardo Freire de.1893. *Elementos para a História do Município de Lisboa.* 1ª Parte, Tomo VII. Lisboa: Typographia Universal.

Oliveira, Eduardo Freire de.1894. *Elementos para a História do Município de Lisboa.* 1ª Parte, Tomo VIII. Lisboa: Typographia Universal.

Oliveira, Eduardo Freire de.1896. *Elementos para a História do Município de Lisboa.* 1ª Parte, Tomo IX. Lisboa: Typographia Universal.

Oliveira, Eduardo Freire de.1901. *Elementos para a História do Município de Lisboa.* 1ª Parte, Tomo XI. Lisboa: Typographia Universal.

Oliveira, Eduardo Freire de.1903. *Elementos para a História do Município de Lisboa.* 1ª Parte, Tomo XII. Lisboa: Typographia Universal.

Oliveira, Eduardo Freire de.1904. *Elementos para a História do Município de Lisboa.* 1ª Parte, Tomo XIV. Lisboa: Typographia Universal.

Oliveira, Eduardo Freire de.1906. *Elementos para a História do Município de Lisboa.* 1ª Parte, Tomo XV. Lisboa: Typographia Universal.

Oliveira, Eduardo Freire de.1908. *Elementos para a História do Município de Lisboa.* 1ª Parte, Tomo XVI. Lisboa: Typographia Universal.

Oliveira, Eduardo Freire de.1911. *Elementos para a História do Município de Lisboa.* 1ª Parte, Tomo XVII. Lisboa: Typographia Universal.

Poland, Jack; Dennis, David. 1999. "Diagnosis and clinical manifestations". In: David Dennis et al, *Plague Manual: epidemiology, distribution, surveillance and control.* Geneva: 43-53.

Pye, George.1721. *A discourse of the plague; wherein Dr Mead's notions are consider'd and refuted.* London: J. Darby.

Jorge, Ricardo. 1899. A *Peste Bubónica no Porto-1899. Seu Descobrimento—primeiros trabalhos.* Porto: Repartição de Saúde e Higiene da Camara do Porto.

Silva Correia, Fernando da. 1937. *Portugal Sanitário: subsídios para o seu estudo.* Dissertação de doutoramento apresentada à Faculdade de Medicina de Coimbra. Coimbra: Biblioteca da Universidade.

Simond, Paul-Louis. 1898. "La propagation de la peste". *Annales de l'Institut Pasteur,* 12: 625-687.

Simpson, William John. 1905. *A Treatise of Plague Dealing with the Historical, Epidemiological, Clinical, Therapeutic and Preventive Aspects of the Disease.* Cambridge: University Press.

Souza Júnior, António Joaquim de. 1902. *Peste Bubónica (Estudos da epidemia do Porto)*. Porto: Tipografia a vapor de Artur José de Souza & Irmão.

Tikhomirov, Eugene. 1999. "Epidemiology and distribution of plague". *In Plague Manual: epidemiology, distribution, surveillance and control*. Geneva: World Health Organization, 11-41.

Thompson John Ashburton. 1901. "A contribution to the aetiology of plague". *The Journal of Hygiene,* 1 (2):153–167.

Yersin, Alexandre. 1894. "La peste bubonique à Hong-Kong". *Annales de l'Institut Pasteur,* 8 : 662–667.

Yersin, Alexandre. 1897. "Sur la peste bubonique (sérothérapie) ". *Annales de l'Institut Pasteur,* 11: 81-93.

CHAPTER 8

THE LAZARETTO MARITIME OF LISBON AND OTHER HEALTH STRUCTURES AND PROCEDURES

JOÃO MARTINS E SILVA

Abstract

Between the 14th century and the early 20th century, to avoid the devastating consequences of the second plague pandemic, the Portuguese monarchs started to develop structures and procedures to reinforce health precautions in the ports and land borders of the Kingdom. The port of Lisbon, the capital of the Kingdom and the principal place of sea routes with the Portuguese Atlantic islands and empire in Africa, Asia, Brazil, and other countries, received particular attention. To achieve this purpose, the Portuguese monarchs set up a project of building health stations in the main ports of the Kingdom and a lazaretto to ensure the quarantining and disinfection of passengers, crews, luggage and merchandise from potentially infected ships, especially when arriving from regions actively hit by plague and other epidemic diseases. At the end of the 19th century, most functions of the lazaretto were transferred to the new Maritime Disinfection Station in Lisbon. From the beginning of the 20th century, all the procedures had been assigned to the Public Disinfection Post of Lisbon.

Key words: Health station; Lazaretto; Quarantine; Disinfection stations; Sanitary regulations.

Resumo

De modo a evitar as consequências arrasadoras da segunda pandemia de peste, os monarcas Portugueses procuraram desenvolver, entre o século XIV e o início do século XX, estruturas e procedimentos que reforçassem as precauções sanitárias investidas nos portos e fronteiras terrestres do Reino. Foi dada particular atenção ao porto de Lisboa, por esta cidade ser a capital do Reino e pelo que representava como principal lugar de

intercomunicação marítima com as ilhas adjacentes e possessões ultramarinas Portuguesas em África, Ásia e Brasil, e o relevante intercâmbio comercial com outros países. Para o efeito, foi apresentada a estrutura e funcionamento das estações de saúde nos principais portos do Reino, a par da instalação de um lazareto que assegurasse o confinamento e a desinfecção de passageiros, tripulações, bagagens, mercadorias de navios potencialmente infectados ou provenientes de regiões com peste activa e outras doenças epidémicas. No termo do século XIX, grande parte das funções do lazareto transitaram para o novo Posto Marítimo de Desinfecção de Lisboa, sendo completadas, desde o início do século XX, com as atribuições conferidas ao Posto de Desinfecção Pública de Lisboa.
Palavras-chave: Estação de saúde, Lazareto, Quarentena, Postos de desinfecção, Regulamentos sanitários.

Introduction

This essay reviews the construction of strategic buildings, mainly from the seventeenth century onwards, and the procedures for preventing the outbreaks of plague and other epidemic diseases from infecting Portuguese territory. We focused mainly on the facilities established in the port of Lisbon for the sanitary inspection of ships, crews and passengers arriving by sea.

The Lisbon Lazaretto, located on the left bank of the Tagus River, deserves particular mention since a quarantine facility was indispensable for the sick and suspected of being infected with plague or other epidemic diseases. At the lazaretto, individual baggage and goods transported on ships arriving from infected ports, infected or suspected of being infected, were disinfected. The lazaretto and the health station (the latter located on the right bank of the same river) ensured the sanitary services of the port of Lisbon at the end of the nineteenth century when a Maritime Disinfection Post in Lisbon was constructed. The Public Disinfection Post in Lisbon was completed at the beginning of the following century.

Origin of lazarettos and quarantine periods

When the Black Death broke out in southern Europe in 1347, there were still those who believed that evil had spread through the air or was the result of divine retribution for human sins, plagues, planetary conjugations, cataclysms, or poisonous miasmas, among other mysticisms and superstitions (Isidore of Seville 1857, 47; Stathakopoulos 2005, 5-8; Jouanna 2012, 119-120; Gimbel 2012, 35-37, 41-42). In fact, it took until the 16th century for

Fracastoro, a brilliant Italian physician from Verona, to propose the first ideas about the propagation of infectious particles by person-to-person contact. The term 'infection' emerged as a synonym for 'contagion' (Fracastoro, 1546, 1-7).

Faced with a lack of knowledge of the nature of that plague and the inexistence of effective treatments, the populations and governments of the European regions most affected by the plague sought to avoid, prevent or cancel its spread with haphazard measures. Besides processions, pilgrimages to shrines, prayers, pious self-flagellation and other religious practices to assuage divine displeasure (Ziegler 2009, 86-88; Benedictow 2004, 104; Cirus 2021, 2-4), incense or sulfur dioxide fumigations, incineration of houses and objects, or sprinkling quicklime on the tombs of those who had died from the plague were carried out to purify the ambient air and neutralize miasmas (Franco 1569, 22-23, 25-27; Alvarez 1598, 4; Byrne 2008, 64, 75-76, 507).

Meanwhile, part of the panicking crowd was trying to survive the plague by fleeing from the infected and leaving their belongings behind (Benedictow 2004, 104). The situation was nothing new since it was known in pre-modern societies when faced with critical situations. In Hippocratic times, when a prevalent disease appeared and because it was believed to have originated in the air, people were advised to leave that place and go as far away as quickly as possible (Hippocrates 1959, 29) in order to breathe safely, which was also the meaning of an aphorism attributed to Galen (AD 129- AD 199 or AD 217), "*Cito, longe fugas, et tarde redeas*" (Stathakopoulos 2007, 111)[1]. Unknowingly, however, these fugitives spread the epidemic throughout the populations in the places where they settled.

During the repeated epidemic crises of the Middle Ages and early Modern times, the authorities of the various regions tried to prevent outsiders, mainly merchants and undesirable groups, from entering their lands, either by imposing *cordons sanitaires* or other measures that aimed to isolate the sick from the rest of the supposedly uncontaminated population.

Isolation could result from the expulsion of plague patients from the cities (which entailed the risk of contagion in the places where they settled) or by locking them down in their own homes or adapted community facilities (known as "*plague houses* or *lazarettos*"[2] where those infected

[1] The phrase in Latin means: "Run fast, run far away and come back slowly".

[2] The Italian word Lazzaretto (*Lazareto* in Portuguese) probably originates in the Military Order of St Lazarus of Jerusalem, founded by the Crusaders in a leper hospital in the late twelfth century. Lazarus would be the leper in Jesus' parable,

would often die and rarely recovered) or even in hospitals, the latter two supported by public finances. During severe epidemic outbreaks with insufficient hospital support being available, there was an anarchic installation in the vicinity of all kinds of tents and shelters to safeguard the sick (Byrne 2008, 468).

Italian cities, such as Venice, Milan and Florence, were early to utilize critical public health solutions involving cleaning, garbage removal and care for the atmosphere. At the same time, Venice and Ragusa[3], important seaports in the Mediterranean, prevented passengers, crew, and goods arriving by sea or land from contacting the local population (Byrne 2008, 468, 482). The public health systems enacted in these towns, followed later by Genoa, reached their most refined levels in the sixteenth and seventeenth centuries, taking inspiration from the public health systems in the cities of Northern Italy (and other European countries, North Africa and the Middle East), and modified by frequent updates in the main cities. When a notifiable disease was identified, long term distancing measures were undertaken. If the disease was not confirmed, short-term contact was suspended. A complex *cordon sanitaire*, consisting of forts, towers, outposts, and surveillance boats under military control, was launched to ensure territorial confinement among the various countries in the Mediterranean and the Adriatic Sea (Cliff 2009, 200, 201, 204-208).

In 1374, the Venetian authorities issued a legal provision requiring ships heading to the port to remain at anchor near the small island of San Lazzaro until the Health Council authorized docking and access to the city (Bakija-Konsuo 2018, 76). The waiting time could be forty days, '*quarantine*' in Italian, deriving from the number '*Quaranta*' (forty). This referred to the retention period of forty days for each docked ship, during which time they were not permitted to disembark people, goods or merchandise. However, this means of trying to avoid infecting the cities caused considerable damage to trade and the livelihoods of the members of the population.

In 1377, the Grand Council of Ragusa opted for a more selective measure which did not involve blocking of mercantile traffic, instead imposing thirty days (*trentine*) of isolation and disinfection of people, animals and luggage arriving by sea or land from actually or potentially infected places of origin, prohibiting entry into the city and its surroundings by those who came from places where the plague was rampant (Milosević 2018, 169). Those who

---

recorded by Luke (Luke 16:19-31), whom Christianity celebrates as the patron saint of Hansen's disease patients. That designation would also apply to places of confinement for patients with plague.

[3] Ragusa, a city and seaport in southern Croatia on the Adriatic Sea coast, was under the rule of Venice between 1205 and 1358. It has been called Dubrovnik since 1929.

appeared to be infected in the city also had to isolate themselves (Bakija-Konsuo 2018, 65, 71, 72). This period was later extended to 40 days, as in Venice (Milosević 2018, 169-170). Although various explanations have been proposed, the justification for the forty days allocated to quarantine remains unclear (Sehdev 2002, 1072).

The Italian maritime lazarettos could be temporary or permanent. In 1397, the abandoned Benedictine monastery, which occupied almost the entire island of Mljet, was adapted as one of the first temporary lazarettos for plague patients, and this continued to operate, with some gaps, until 1527. In 1419, confinement began in buildings surrounded by high walls, with hospital features and governmental support. However, because these places of confinement were scattered on islands far from the port and land routes, the government decided to join them in a large hospital building on the island of Lokrum, opposite Ragusa. In 1590 it was decided to replace this with another building in Plŏce[4] (a neighbourhood of the city close to the old port), which was decisive in controlling and ending the local plague. In fact, this lazaretto (serving, like the others, for the unloading and loading of goods transported in caravans and ships) ceased to function as an institution of the health services of Ragusa around 1872 (Bakija-Konsuo 2018, 65, 72, 77; Milosević 2018, 168).

The Venetians adapted an initial temporary structure on the island of Santa Maria di Nazareth in 1403, replacing it with a permanent lazaretto built on one of the islands in the Gulf of Venice in 1424. As it quickly filled up (it was designed for 300 passengers), in 1468, another lazaretto was built on a nearby island (for 200 passengers but which, on one critical occasion, contained 8,000 isolated detainees), known as the new lazaretto (*Lazaretto Nuovo*), to distinguish it from the previous one, the old lazaretto (*Lazaretto Vecchio*) (Cliff 2009, 212).

Those who did not comply with the quarantine conditions in Ragusa or Venice were fined and sentenced to severe punishments, including death (Cliff 2009, 204). It should be noted that quarantine, meaning isolation or confinement of infected people or suspected of being infected, was nothing new, as it had already been practised thousands of years before to protect healthy communities from the emergence of lethal or harmful agents spreading rapidly throughout most of these populations. Among other examples, there are well-known Old Testament references to patients struck by leprosy (Hansen's disease) being considered "unclean", and forced to live far away from the rest of the community (Leviticus, 13:46), as were

[4] The lazaretto began to be built in 1627 and was completed around twenty years later.

those who presented bodily "discharges" of purulent origin (Numbers, 5:2; Deuteronomy, 23:10). Before the 14th century, lepers were isolated in the Middle Ages, usually until they died in monastic facilities, generally known as *leprosarium* or *lazarettos*.

Lisbon Health Station

The preamble to the regulation[5] decreed in 1693 by King Pedro II (reigned from 1683 to 1706) laid out its key aspects:

> The port of the City of Lisbon is one of the busiest commercial harbours; therefore, it is frequently used by domestic and foreign vessels. Since everyone can find easy and comfortable places to land safely on the beaches from both banks, disembarking, warning business-people to arrange their needs in advance, taking merchandise off the ships, avoiding expenses of compulsory duties — one must fear that people may become infected in some contagious manner, as so often has happened in the world. From these situations, regrettable damage resulted not just to the Cities, Provinces and Kingdoms. All care is needed to avoid a similar calamity. There can be no caution which is not essential in such a matter. A new Regime is needed to apply the available means to obviate the dangers to which public health is exposed. Consequently, the Town Hall Senate has determined that such should be done when this city is suffering from the ravaging curse of plague, to manage the cure of this pernicious disease. Lacking the means to preserve health in this port and all the others in the Kingdom, in Algarve,[6] and the lands bordering the dominion of the King of Castile, lacking instructions for protective means, Laws, means that punishment is needed and deserved for those who transgress. Consequently, it is urged to provide the ports and routes of the Kingdom with the required vigilance and precautions that most political Nations use. For this purpose, this Regime was ordained.

This diploma was the first in Portugal to detail the measures required to protect national ports (particularly the port of Belém) as gateways to the Kingdom from epidemics originating from abroad. It is worth considering the details of its articles to a certain extent, as these constituted the inspiration for later regulations.

---

[5] Regimento de 20 de Dezembro de 1693a, 333-340.

[6] Until the establishment of the Republic, the province of Algarve was honorifically designated as a second Kingdom of the Portuguese Crown (with no autonomy, institutions or privileges of its own), by right of its conquest from the Almohad Caliphate in 1189 and the reconquest of some Muslim enclaves in 1249.

Among the issues covered, particular importance was given to the required health cards and visits to all the ships from infected regions or suspected of being infected. These tasks were assigned to the health station in Belém. Disinfection and quarantine of passengers, crew and goods transported, to be performed in a demanding and thorough manner, was the full responsibility of the Lazaretto of Lisbon. When behaving with malfeasance, the responsible personnel were subject to severe pecuniary penalties or exile.

The staff at that port consisted of a chief guard (*guarda-mor*), a health provider (*provedor da saúde*), a clerk, a flag guard (*guarda-bandeira*), and an interpreter. This staff lived in the health station.

It was up to the Chief Health Provider to watch over the health of the Kingdom, as established by the regimes and dictates of the monarchs, and to be well informed about the appearance of plague or any other contagious disease in other foreign ports. Chapter I of the regiment indicated the path to achieving such knowledge:

> (…) must have correspondence with the ministers that his Majesty has in foreign Courts; with Portuguese intelligence individuals who are serving in mercantile parts; and, where there are none, with the health magistrates of the maritime cities and towns with whom we have peace, to know, through more credible notices, whether in those parts there is cause to fear their communication; and even if in places where there is contagion care is taken to cover it up, so that the news of what they are suffering does not make it impossible for them to trade, with the hope of our finding in such cases the same correspondence that may oblige them not to hide the truth from us; and those that reach him will be communicated to all the ports of this Kingdom, so that the health officials of each one of them take all necessary precautions; and if he learns that there is plague in any part, or any other contagion, he will report this to the Town Hall Senate, so that his Majesty may be asked to send a letter to all the places that must be guarded, that they try to do so with great care and attention.

The chief guard who supervised the station was responsible for carrying out various tasks, especially carefully examining the "health cards" of the ships which had docked. These printed or manuscript documents were not very trustworthy and often had to be compared with previous ones issued by the same port to check their veracity.

When suspicious cases came forth, the chief guard was to summon the authorities to take the appropriate steps or arrest the suspects by order of the Chief Town Hall Senate. Likewise, vessels carrying no health card were expected to quarantine for forty days or longer. However, vessels arriving from Newfoundland (Norway and Canada at the time), if carrying nothing apart from cod, brine fish or wood, could benefit from a health card waiver in national ports. Several "cargoes" were subject to impediment or mandatory cleaning at the lazaretto. This legislation was applied to those arriving from the Levant and Maghreb (carrying cotton and derivatives, raw silk, leather, wax and copper), Turkey (carpets and rugs), and Persia (gold and silver canvases, feathers, apothecary drugs, indigo, and similar commodities). Wheat and all kinds of grains, vegetables and rice from suspicious places were baked, while halfah grass (*Stipa tenacíssima*) was unloaded in the lazaretto for the treatment of patients.

The clerk was responsible for overseeing all the administrative procedures relating to the docked vessels, the type and quantity of goods that were received from the ships and which went to the lazaretto, recording the money collected, convictions and other details.

The flag guard was attentive to the arrival of ships and closely monitored all approach manoeuvres, not allowing prior contact between crew and staff on land, and he also guarded the money for fines for possible malfeasance.

The interpreter was expected to master all European languages, particularly from countries with more frequent trade relations with the port of Lisbon. He was told to observe, carefully noting any hesitancy, equivocation or possible errors in the answers provided to official questions. On arrival, the skippers of the vessels were questioned when disembarking and presenting themselves at the health department, and were led by the flag guard to the chief guard and his officers who awaited them.

Kept in seclusion so that no others could listen during the (thorough and suspicious) questioning by the interpreter, the questioned individual and two further witnesses signed the final statement. The health cards, passengers and crew passports were attached to the record by the notary. This documentation was subjected to supposed disinfection, which included application of a vinegar solution, which did not destroy the documents, followed by smoking over a brazier and drying, for which "a long cane or stick opened at the end" was used.

The remaining fifteen chapters of the regulations provided detailed instructions, among other strict rules, concerning the anchoring place for caravels, ships or any other vessel that could not go beyond the Tower of Belém. Descriptions of various types of health cards followed with instructions as to what to do in the event that ships lacked them. The procedures for ships arriving from potentially infected places were detailed. They covered quarantining people and merchandise, the duties of the guards boarding the ships, entry restrictions for certain people into the ships, and impediments to entry or mandatory measures before listing the products from Asia or North Africa were imposed. Restrictions and health care measures to be carried out with people, food, or other assets carried on ships that docked were also considered, and convictions for breaching the law were also compulsory.

The penalties imposed for non-compliance were stringent. Two-thirds of the value of the fines applied to the offenders went to the Public Health Expenditure Fund. The remaining part was given to the complainant or the accuser. Any captain or other crew members who let ashore "any person, merchandise, clothing, letters, or any other papers, or animals with hair or feathers, without first being processed by the Health service would", in addition to being fined twenty-five cruzados, be sent to the lazaretto to undertake "a rigorous quarantine". Penalties were applied to anyone who removed people or goods from ships not yet cleared (authorised, after inspection by health officials), received them in their homes, or who, coming from infected sites, disembarked anywhere in the Kingdom. In addition to a fine, they were sentenced to the galleys or exile in Brazil, Angola or Castro Marim (in Algarve). Finally, the regulation established that quarantines were only to be carried out at the Lisbon Lazaretto, given that "(…) in none of the other ports of this Kingdom, and of the Algarve, is there a lazaretto, nor the convenience and safety conditions to accept suspicious vessels for quarantine, and it is convenient to do this in the port of Lisbon; and all ports are prohibited from accepting them into quarantine" (Oliveira 1911, 39-46).

To ensure that the stipulated regulations were intended for everybody, King D. Pedro V (reigned from 1853-1861), and his brother and successor, Prince Luís (reigned 1861-1889), undertook an observation quarantine on the ship *Mindello*, which transported them from a visit to England in 1854.

Attached to this regime were rules to be complied with in the event of plague in Spain, with the following title: "Regime to be observed if there is a plague (and God forbid) in any kingdom or province bordering Portugal".[7] Amongst the articles, the following were noteworthy: (a) It was the responsibility of the Chief Health Provider to communicate with all the councils of the cities and towns of the Kingdom, especially those closest to the places in Spain most affected by the plague, such that their guards remained vigilant, ensuring that no person from that country could travel to Portugal; he had to regularly inform the Chief Health Provider of the state of health in the area under his jurisdiction as to whether there were any diseases, and if so what type they were and their possible transmissibility, together with the certificate issued by the local doctor; (b) All citizens or residents of those cities and towns near the border or neighbouring areas

[7] Regimento de 20 de Dezembro de 1693b, 340-342.

who wished to travel to any part of the Kingdom safely and without impediments had to have passports issued by the clerk from their respective area; (c) Entry into Lisbon by vessels from both banks of the Tagus required, in addition to their passport, inspection of travellers by a local authority, before being allowed to disembark; (d) If any of the travellers on those vessels were not carrying a passport, all those on board were immediately taken to the lazaretto in Trafaria, where they remained until the decision of the mayor was made public, while the ship's captain was punished with a fine and sent into exile in Brazil for five years; (e) Mail coming from Madrid was brought to the Badajoz bridge by a local courier, where he removed the correspondence from the bags in which he had transported it, to "purify" it with vinegar and fire, exchanging it with the correspondence brought there weekly by the Portuguese courier, who was returning to Lisbon with an escort.

The far-sighted set of rules established by D. Pedro II proved to be particularly useful in subsequent occurrences. Thus, when an alert of a (presumed) epidemic plague epidemic raging in Andalusia and Cádiz of neighbouring Spain was sounded in 1800, the Chief Health Provider ordered posting copies of public notices at all the beaches of Lisbon and in the ports on both banks of the Tagus river bar (*barra*) up to the Spanish border. According to this edict, no one from that area could enter Lisbon, by land or sea, or in transit from one to another, without carrying a passport as provided for in the health regulations, presumably attesting that the bearer was not suffering from any contagious disease. Ships arriving at the Port of Lisbon were required to dock at pre-designated moorings. However, transported people were not allowed to dock or disembark without being observed by personnel specially assigned to this task. Those transgressing this rule were subject to the sanctions mentioned in the said regulation[8].

Four years later, due to a great pestilence in Spain, the Chief Health Provider reiterated the previous warnings concerning incidents of foreigners and the local population entering Lisbon without a passport or health certificating their state of good health. These people were to be called out and taken to the lazaretto together with their luggage. If those who let them free were nobles, they were sentenced to five years of exile in Africa, while commoners served the same length of time in the galleys.[9] At the time, measures were also taken, with a cordon and lazarettos along the Alentejan

[8] Edital de 22 de Outubro de 1800, 651-652.
[9] Edital de 8 de Outubro de 1804, pp. 282-283.

land border with Spain, in order to prevent the plague from entering the Kingdom.[10]

Apparently, the measures implemented failed to ensure proper security. By a decree dated 1804, an internal Board was created to take all the necessary measures to protect the Kingdom from all communication, "both by sea and by the land route" (*tanto por mar como pela raia seca*) against the plague which was ravaging Spain. The Board was authorized to transmit all orders to the province generals and magistrates, obliging them to give an account of these orders, punishing any misdemeanour.[11]

Believing that contagion of plague and other pestilences arriving from seaports hit by overall extinct epidemics and, therefore, posing no disturbances to the public health of the Kingdom, the so-called Board of Inspectorate of Provisions against the Plague (*Junta de Inspecção de Providências contra a Peste*) decided, through the provision of the 27 July 1807, to prevent future contamination, supported by the regulation of 18 July.[12]

Among the measures provided, the observation of the quarantine map deserves to be noted: (a) Six days for all ships arriving from the Levant or other places of origin that they contacted, including those practicing privateering; (b) Five days without a health certificate for vessels arriving from any port, including military ships or corsairs, commanded by navy personnel; however, if the commanding officers attested on their honour that they had come from ports over which there were no suspicions, which had not been in contact with other vessels and their crew was in good health, they were exempt from quarantining; (c) Three days for ships arriving directly from calling at Morocco and from the United Provinces of America; if any national or foreign ship had entered one of those contaminated ports, the measures provided in this regulation would be immediately suspended,

[10] AML-AH. 25 de Outubro-26 de Novembro de 1804, Provimento da Saúde, Pasta n.º 8 de Papéis Pertencentes à Província do Alentejo, f. 91 - 146v. AML-AH.4 de Novembro-3 de Dezembro de 1804, Provimento da Saúde, Pasta n.º 8 de Papéis Pertencentes à Província do Alentejo, f. 221 - 266v. AML-AH. 25 de Novembro-7 de Dezembro, 9 -19 e Dezembro de 1804, Provimento da Saúde, Pasta n.º 8 de Papéis Pertencentes à Província do Alentejo, f. 274 -289v, 295 a 298v. AML-AH. 13-19 de Dezembro de 1804, Provimento da Saúde, Pasta n.º 8 de Papéis Pertencentes à Província do Alentejo, f. 302 - 307v. AML-AH.22 de Março-3 de Abril de 1805, Provimento da Saúde, Pasta n.º 8 de Papéis Pertencentes à Província do Alentejo, f. 387- 390v.

[11] Decreto de 21 de Outubro de 1804, 284.

[12] Regulamento de 18 de Julho de 1807 (Provisional das Quarentenas, e outras providências relativas a Cautelas para evitar comunicação de Contágio), 452-455: Provisão de 27 de Julho de 1807, 451-452.

replaced by the rules established (in the previous health regime) for contagion in the ship and port(s) from which it had come or at which it had stopped over; it was up to the chief guard at the arrival port to inform the superior authorities of the situation.

The final decision on the measures to be implemented in preventing the spread of diseases depended on the navy seaport governors, the legitimate inspectors, and the magistrates of the respective territories, guardians of civil interests related to Public Welfare.

Notwithstanding, the reactivation of the feared epidemics a few years later frustrated the optimistic desires for permanent protection. The New Board of Health (*Nova Junta da Saúde*) was established in 1813 to manage these new threats and declared the aim of promoting "all the indispensable precautions to preserve the Kingdoms of Portugal and the Algarve from the terrible scourge of the plague" occurring in Alexandria, Malta and other Mediterranean ports at the time. It was up to the Chief Health Provider of the Court and the Kingdom to deal exclusively with the activities provided in the regime laid down in the order,[13] with the collaboration of further nominated members of the organism, [14] for which it had available funds, subject to the rigorous scrutiny of income and expenses.[15] Everything indicates that the Prince Regent D. João wanted to ensure that the Medical Board took "the most energetic and prompt measures to prevent the communication of the contagious diseases that rage in some countries", for which he placed it under the jurisdiction of the Medical Board inspector, temporarily combining it with his effective activities, ensuring the "first place in the Medical mentioned above Board". When it could not meet, it could issue orders relating to Health, taking all necessary measures in extraordinary situations. [16]

On 9 October of that year, the health official of Almada residing in Trafaria, and the health official of Paço de Arcos, were instructed not to authorize the vessels that had entered the Tagus harbour to dock on the beaches of their respective districts without first obtaining approval through a health visit. The Royal Navy ensured compliance with this rule for the first time. From that time onwards, the health authorities had the help of "the troops or military forces from their districts" to maintain and enforce

---

[13] Portaria de 28 de Agosto de 1813a, Ilegível.

[14] Portaria de 28 de Agosto de 1813b, page unreadable. Members: besides the Chief Health Provider of the Court and Kingdom, a natural member, two military officers, six physicians, the interim inspector of the Royal Navy Arsenal, a judge and a politician who acted as secretary were appointed.

[15] Portaria de 28 de Agosto de 1813c., 254.

[16] Decreto de 20 de Outubro de 1813,-275.

their deliberations. Those instructions also included the obligation for the senior guards to issue health certificates to those who wanted to cross from one bank of the Tagus to the other, in addition to the police passport required from passengers, as ruled out in 1693 (Oliveira 1911, 46-47).

In the 1814, the maritime and terrestrial *cordon sanitaire* was renewed to prevent the entry of plague into the Kingdom. A warship was anchored in the Tagus, below Belém Tower, and military detachments were present on both sides. The governors and commanders of the remaining troops stationed in the ports of the Kingdom had to request the military staffing that was needed for this purpose (Oliveira 1911, 47).

However, the functioning of the port of Lisbon showed problems requiring full clarification. In 1819, the central Town Hall Senate of the Crown and the Kingdom became aware of a complaint addressed to the monarch by many Austrian captains of ships moored in the port of Belém, based on "inattention, injustice and vexations" by the chief guard and other health officers of the port. Subsequently, the Chief Health Provider opened a public inquiry seeking to call other complainants and witnesses about equivalent abuses carried out by those officials. [17] Initially, it was unclear whether the participants had to do with a specific group of complainants of people of the same nationality who did not accept the conditions of personal reception or considered the health standards imposed by the national authorities to be excessive, refusing to comply with them. The solution to this matter is not known.

In 1839, there was also news that seven applicants from the Lisbon customs office refused to inspect the English schooner *Spy*, which the Belém health station had placed in strict quarantine as it had come from the Black Sea. Their disobedience was punished with the suspension of their duties. They appealed because the refusal was not out of disobedience or insubordination but love for their lives and families. This declaration was complied with, with subsequent abolition of the initial order but on unintelligible grounds. As if on the other hand, it was determined that, except for ships coming from infected ports which, prevented from doing practice, were inspected outside the port, customs aspirants were obliged to enter all others, even if infected and obliged to quarantine.[18]

Physicians from the Belém health station carried out health surveillance on ships that arrived in Lisbon. The health services provided to ships docked in Belém were limited to the period between sunrise and sunset. There were exceptions: regulation of ships of the peninsular shipping company when

[17] Edital de 8 de Fevereiro de 1819, 230.
[18] Portaria de 2 de Outubro de 1839, 404-405.

arriving after sunset, and privileged vessels like Queen Maria II. The same procedure was justified for the Portuguese ships *Porto* and *Quinta do Vesuvius* for the same reasons. In any case, the inboard doctor had to issue a medical certificate, delivered to the port authorities, in which he was designated as being responsible for the health status of all individuals on board.[19]

In 1844, the liberal government of the Duke of Terceira updated the offices and health stations in the Kingdom[20] upon prior approval through a Legal Charter. Essentially, thirty-two health stations were established in the ports of the mainland coast and the islands, spread over four categories, of which Lisbon was (the only one) of the 1st order, while those from Oorto, Setúbal, Funchal and Ponta Delgada were of the 2nd order. This classification corresponded to differences in staffing. Referring only to these two categories, the Lisbon station (in Belém) was assigned two chief guards physicians, two interpreter clerks and an administrator for proceedings or agents, while the second category had a single member of each category.

The only lazaretto established in the Kingdom was located in the port of Lisbon, in the Tower of S. Sebastião da Caparica. The staff included a medical inspector (who also worked at the Belém station), a sub-inspector of quarantines, a surgeon, an apothecary, a nurse, a chaplain, an inspector of improvements, warehouse guards and other general employees. When necessary, up to two temporary lazarettos could be established in Oporto and adjacent islands. It was the duty of the chief guard of each port to visit all ships arriving there for medical inspection and to order the required sanitary measures. It was up to the lazaretto inspector to order and supervise undertaking (by the sub-inspector) measures determined by the Health Council "for the purification and improvement of the people and merchandise held in quarantine in the lazaretto".

Ships with a "dirty" or "suspicious" bill of health were subject to quarantine for a variable duration depending on the severity of the contagious situation detected; if it put public health at risk, they were prevented from entering any domestic port. No merchant or warship, national or foreign, that arrived at national ports from the mainland or adjacent islands were allowed to dock or establish contact with another docked ship unless authorized by the health visiting staff (the doctor and the interpreter).[21] However, six years later, instead of the rules established for

[19] Portaria de 26 de Março de 1840, 45.
[20] Decreto de 18 de Setembro de 1844, 230-270.
[21] Carta de Lei de 10 de Fevereiro de 1844.

merchant ships, it was determined that the chief guard in Belém would issue health cards to all foreign warships that entered the port of Lisbon.[22]

In 1845, the government of the Marshal Duke of Saldanha oversaw the reorganization of the health departments.[23] Thirty-seven health stations existed at the time, distributed along the mainland and islands' coasts; the port of Figueira da Foz was transferred to a 2nd order port, and the islands of Flores and Graciosa to the 3rd order. If physicians at the Belém station were simultaneously prevented from providing service due to illness, resignation or death, they were replaced, on an extraordinary basis, by any graduate with the same scientific level of expertise. The same provision applied to health stations in all the ports in the Kingdom. [24]

With the change of government, headed by the Duke of Palmela, the previous diploma was suspended, allegedly due to the prevailing financial crisis; this was not unexpected given the rivalry maintained with the Duke of Saldanha. Consequently, the health service system in the interior and Kingdom seaports was restored, governed by the provisions of the decree of 3 January 1837[25]and other rules preceding the decree of 18 September 1844.[26] This confirmed that health policy continued to be a plaything of partisan interests, re-established by a government that did not last more than six months.

In 1860, the Public Health Council of the Kingdom (*Conselho de Saúde Pública do Reino*) brought together all the quarantine regulations applied to the three most frequent contemporary epidemics (cholera, yellow fever and plague) threatening the health of the Kingdom seaports, in a single regulation.[27] Eight years later, however, the much contested reorganization of the health services in the Kingdom did not hesitate to extinguish that health council, replacing it with a political secretariat, intended to manage the entire health service from above, besides being concerned with reducing public expenditure and increasing revenue.[28] Given such a wide range of bureaucratic intervention, the effectiveness of the system in terms of offering protection against epidemic diseases arriving by sea, previously

---

[22] Portaria de 5 de Maio de 1850, 188.
[23] Decreto de 26 de Novembro de 1845, 783-822.
[24] Portaria de 15 de Julho de 1847, p.2.
[25] Decreto de 3 de Janeiro de 1837, p.34.
[26] Decreto de 18 de Setembro de 1844, pp.230-270. Lei de 7 de Abril de 1845, p.847, to autorize.
[27] Edital de 8 de Março de 1860, pp.87-92.
[28] Decreto de 3 de Dezembro de 1868, pp.431-440.

under the sanitary guidance of the former, now defunct health council, was in serious doubt.

The maritime health regulation enacted in 1874 aiming to ensure the inviolability of maritime borders for epidemic diseases (which, otherwise, would tend to spread in the national territory) was an important step, in particular by systematising the arrangements, duties and responsibilities of all the parties involved, including; health stations or similar facilities available at ports along with their personnel; classification and observance of health cards; classification of the possible level of infection based on the ports of origin; types of transported materials susceptible to contamination; types of quarantines and periods and places where they would be carried out; lazaretto (of Lisbon) and its personnel, customs, auxiliary military force, disinfectants; complaints; duties and taxes; criminal provisions. The standard template for miscellaneous documentation (clinical bulletin, health card) was also included. [29] The post of inspector of the lazaretto (filled by Dr. Homem de Vasconcelos) was reinstated.[30] This regulation was subject to certain amendments and clarifications[31] until being replaced by two later updated versions.[32]

In 1881, the Government was given permission to raise funds to acquire or construct a building for the health station at the port of Lisbon on one of the banks of the Tagus River. The cost was amortised through a house sale where the service was located by that time.[33]

The Lisbon Lazaretto

Early 16th-18th centuries

When travellers and merchandise arriving by sea were suspected of being infected with a contagious disease, requiring isolation in quarantine before entering the city of Lisbon, Cardinal Dom Henrique (regent of Dom Sebastião), in 1565, ordered the construction of a house in an inhospitable and isolated place, almost entirely sandy, on the left bank next to the mouth of the Tagus River to provide facilities for quarantining (Fig.8.1).[34] That

[29] Decreto de 12 de Novembro de 1874,-180-216.

[30] Lei de 10 de Abril de 1874, 271-272.

[31] Portaria de 1 de Fevereiro de 1876,-493-494.

[32] Decreto de 4 de Outubro de 1889, -411-438. Decreto de 21 de Janeiro de 1897,-7-34.

[33] Lei de 27 de Junho de 1881,-120.

[34] AML_AH. 7 de Agosto de 1585, Provimento da Saúde, Cópia do Livro 1º do provimento da saúde, f. 65v- 66.

accommodation, which was of dubious quality, became the first (provisional) lazaretto in Lisbon. The village of Trafaria developed around it. More than a century later, in the reign of King Pedro II, the Chief Health Provider requested a lazaretto be built in that place, submitting a plan for it. According to the Town Hall Senate, the construction was not approved because of other priorities. [35]

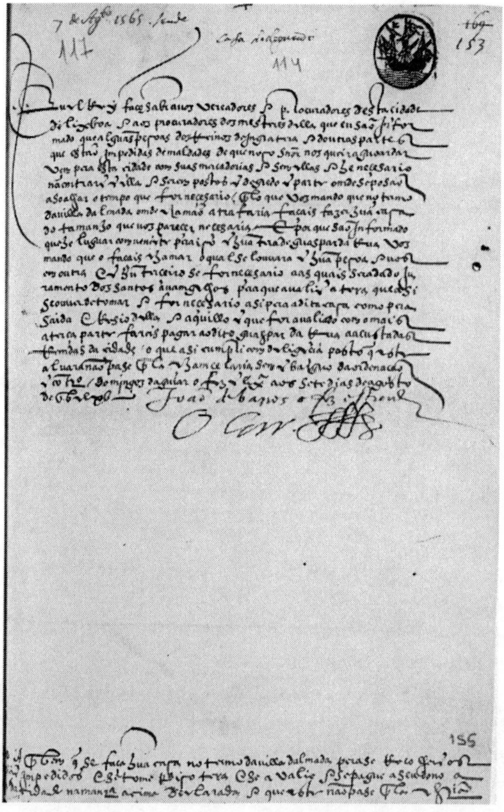

Fig.8.1. "In the name of King Sebastião, Cardinal D. Henrique, decreeted on 5 August 1565, the construction of a house where the ship crews arriving from places affected by the plague were quarantined". Photo: Arquivo Municipal de Lisboa.

[35] AML-AH. 21 de Agosto de 1682, Chancelaria Régia, Livro 5º de registo de consultas e decretos de D. Pedro II, doc. 261, f. 231v. -233.

Almost three decades later, the matter was taken up again with better knowledge and receptivity when it became evident that the temporary lazaretto was not equipped to host such quarantine demands and was unable to ensure the antiseptic cleaning of contaminated people or people suspected of contagion arriving in the port of Lisbon in ships from countries infected with the plague (Oliveira 1896,170). The sanitary service, re-established in the former Trafaria prison, also did not meet the appropriate requirements for a lazaretto, even provisionally, having only little space "just for the goods to be soaked and purified". It soon became clear that the precariousness of those facilities resulted in the loss of stored merchandise and subsequent damage, which justified a complaint from the merchants who had suffered damages, as well as the chief guard of the port of Belém.[36]

Warehouse phase with infirmary - 18th century

Finally, in 1711, King João V (reigned 1706 - 31 July 1750) ordered the construction of a lazaretto according to the plan submitted at the beginning of his reign. (Fig.8.2a).[37] The costs were supported by the council Town Hall Senate. [38] The project consisted of a chapel and warehouses for the expurgation of the goods. An infirmary was added in 1743 (Oliveira, 1911, 839).

To comply with this order, the Lisbon council informed the monarch that he should use the budget for the expansion of Rua dos Douradores. Otherwise, this improvement could not continue, despite the funds having already been spent on the demolition of annexed houses, plus the interest and compensation granted to their owners, thereby representing a "fruitless" loss to the public accounts. By royal order, it was determined that either the two works should be carried out if there were means available or, if not, the lazaretto should be built (Oliveira, 1901a, 39, 44-46).[39] And so this was the case. The lazaretto was built in 1713 by order of the Lisbon council Town Hall Senate (Fig.8.2b), royal approval followed almost a year later, and the work began in 1714 (with an estimated cost of more than seventy thousand

[36] AML-AH. 8 de Novembro- 9 de Dezembro de 1709, Chancelaria Régia, Livro 3° de Consultas e Decretos de D. João V, do Senado Oriental, f. 256 - 259.

[37] AML-AH. 19 de Novembro de 1711, Chancelaria Régia, Livro 5° de Consultas e Decretos de D. João V, do Senado Oriental, f. 150 - 155. The engineer sergeant-major Manuel do Couto was the author of the construction plan.

[38] AML-AH. 9 de Dezembro de 1713, Chancelaria Régia, Livro 5° de Consultas e Decretos de D. João V, do Senado Oriental, f. 269.

[39] AML-AH. 29 de Janeiro e 10 de Outubro de 1714, Chancelaria Régia, Livro 6° de Consultas e Decretos de D. João V, do Senado Oriental, f. 98 - 99.

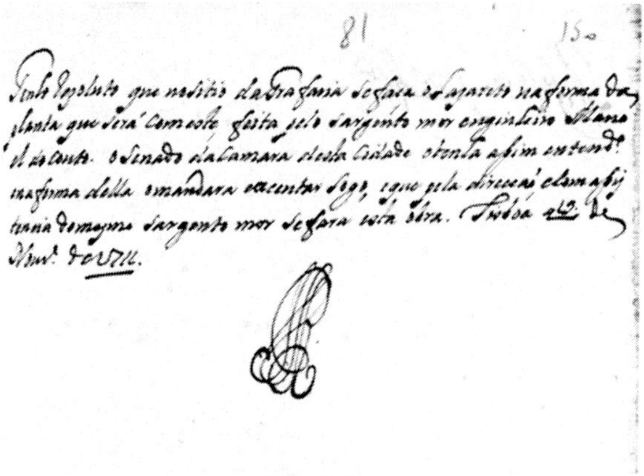

Fig. 8.2a.

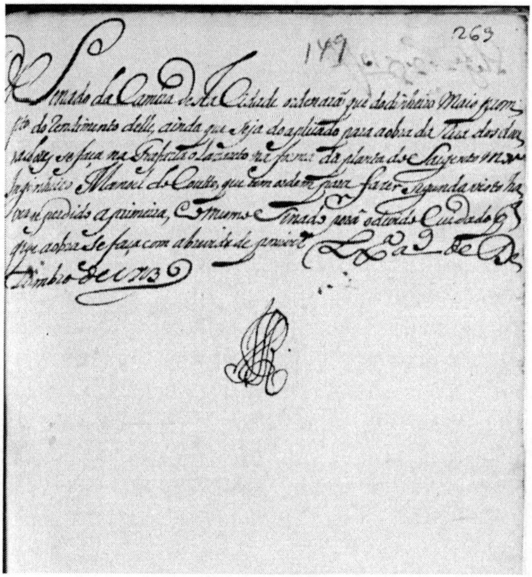

Fig. 8.2b.

Fig.8. 2a - Decree of 9 November 1711 ordering the construction of the temporary lazaretto in Trafaria, according to the plan and direction of the engineer sergeant-major Manuel do Couto.
Fig.8. 2b - On decree 19 December 1713, the Town Hall Senate of the city council of Lisbon was instructed to order the construction of the temporary lazaretto in Trafaria. Photos: Arquivo Municipal de Lisboa.

cruzados). It included a chapel, warehouses and other facilities which are not described, but it is doubtful that it had any facilities suitable to accommodate patients. However, the council later requested support from the monarch to carry out the works on that street in Lisbon but the petition was rejected (Oliveira, 1901a, 122, 125-126, 188-189).

In 1720, following the outbreak of a plague epidemic in the Lazaretto of Marseilles, all ships coming from French Mediterranean ports and fugitives seeking to cross land borders were denied entry. In that year, the delimitation of the Trafaria lazaretto was also drawn up, a wall isolating it from the village. However, before the works began, a recommendation was made concerning relocating it "further down, towards the head" of the river estuary (Oliveira, 1901a, 428-429). Apparently, no alternative location for the lazaretto was found.

Responding to a request from the chief guard of the port of Belém in 1721, attention was paid to the lack of repair of the lazaretto walls and a warehouse to store "impeded" merchandise and luggage. After that, the council consulted the monarch to authorise the works, involving the removal of the houses adjacent to the lazaretto wall and proposing instead the acquisition of nearby buildings for adaptation as warehouses to house merchandise and the men who transported them, plus two houses, one for the health officers carrying out their job in the place, and another for the guards of the warehouses containing contaminated and decontaminated merchandise. Better salaries were also proposed to award the staff and pay the village parish priest who administered the sacraments in the chapel of the lazaretto. Finally, the request pointed out that the lazaretto was located in the most convenient place: "it had been located there for so many centuries because it was the best. It was next to the beach, with the seabed for unloading merchandise, next to the mountain that covers it from the land" (Oliveira, 1901a, 497-499).

However, the works were still not satisfactory. In January of the following year, repairs were needed to the lazaretto and the pavement of the Paço de Arcos.[40] Some days later, conservation works on the lazaretto wall and warehouse, still in a deplorable condition, were urgent.[41]

---

[40] AML-AH. 26 de Janeiro de 1722-10 de Agosto de 1722, Chancelaria Régia, Livro 4º de consultas e decretos de D. João V do Senado Ocidental, f. 136 - 147.

[41] AML-AH. 30 de Janeiro de 1722, Chancelaria Régia, Livro 2º de consultas e decretos de D. João V do Senado Ocidental, f. 96.

Lack of funding to continue the works forced the Town Hall Senate to lift the pledges on incomes in 1723,[42] urging that the work be completed that year.[43] Following the rigorous accounting of public expenses imposed by D. João V, the extraordinary expenses required by the Trafaria lazaretto, and to defend public health when the plague epidemic occurred in France, totalled more than eleven "*contos de réis*" (Oliveira, 1901b, 94).

It should be noted that, through the policy of strict control of expenses, in 1728, the Government discovered an undue overlapping of salaries charged by health officers and other agents in their visits to the ships arriving at Lisbon and carried out in the lazaretto, related to persons or goods sent from these ships. This illegality also included "kickbacks" received in-kind brought by personnel from foreign ships, without the required infection control, or through bribes in money received venally, confirming the 'safety' of these vessels. This action resulted in a regrettable situation and required the necessary correction, which immediately obtained royal approval (Oliveira, 1901b, 159-170).

Given that the poor structural conditions of the lazaretto in Trafaria continued in 1743, either because there was no suitable place for an infirmary, or because of the badly ruined roofs, warehouses, walls and gates around the fencing, in a council session held on 19 August, the decision was taken urgently to initiate repair works (Fig. 8.3a). The works should ensure safety and, in particular, the construction of a house with suitable accommodation for the infirmary service. When the sick arrived, the Chief Health Provider was responsible for assigning the necessary people to administer healthcare and assistance (Oliveira, 1904, 170).

Although the Town Hall treasurer stated that he had no more money than that provided by order of the monarch for cleaning the sidewalks of Lisbon and that which belonged to creditors for pledges and auctions, it was determined by a royal resolution of 20 August to immediately move the matter forward, "paying through money received from the treasurer that will be refunded later". In compliance with that Royal determination, the Town Hall Senate ordered the delivery of the first payment "of any money it has in its possession", and when this was lacking, it would take this from the budget allocated to repair of the pavements (Oliveira 1904, 172-173). It was a courageous decision in the face of a petty and impracticable dictate since it also involved the impossibility of suspending the cleaning of pavements for a fixed period. This task was understood as public hygiene, which the

---

[42] AML-AH. 30 de Janeiro de 1722, Chancelaria Régia, Livro 2º de consultas e decretos de D. João V do Senado Ocidental, f. 96.

[43] AML-AH.15 de Outubro de 1723, Chancelaria Régia, Livro 3º de consultas e decretos de D. João V do Senado Ocidental, f. 344 - 345.

monarch particularly endorsed. Such was also the value of the pledges to be paid by the contracted party. As the council did not believe that this amount would be refunded, it proposed to the monarch that he authorize the suspension of the pledges for three months, which was granted (Oliveira, 1904, 175-178). However, as the money was insufficient to complete the task, in November 1743 the council requested another three months for the suspension of the pledges, authorized by King D. João V "only to the extent that is needed to finish the work of the lazaretto" (Oliveira, 1904, 195-196).

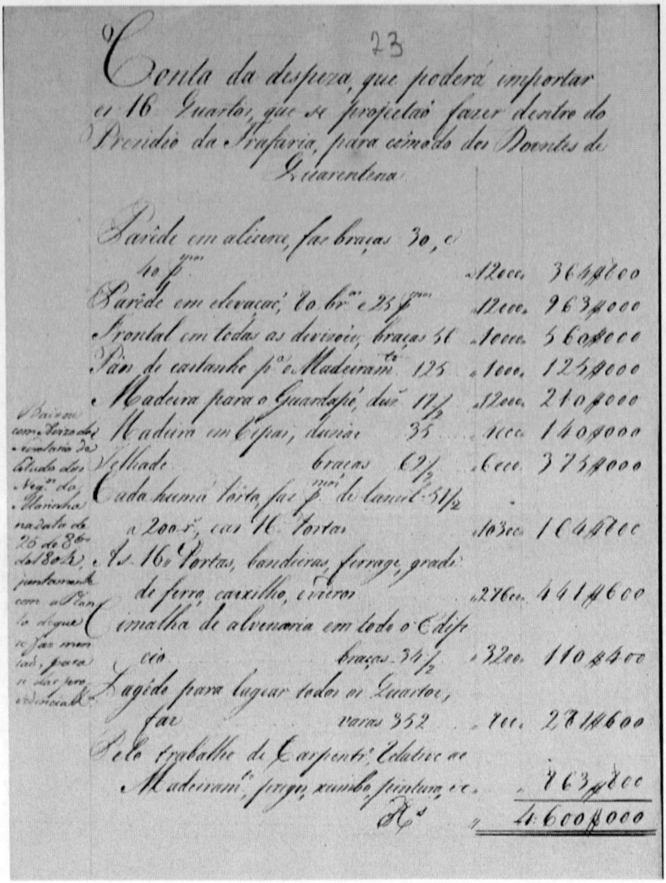

23

Conta da despeza, que poderá importar os 16 Quartos, que se projectaõ fazer dentro do Presidio da Trafaria, para comodo dos Doentes de Quarentena

Parede em alicerce, faz braças 30, e 40 p.		1200	364$800
Parede em elevaçaõ, 60 br. e 25 p.		1200	963$000
Frontal em todas as devizoens, braças 56		1000	560$000
Paõ de castanho p.ª o Madeiramento	125	1000	125$000
Madeira para o Guardapó, duz.	17½	12000	210$000
Madeira em Caços, duzias	35	4000	140$000
Telhado braças	62½	6000	375$000
Cada huma Porta, faz p. de tanoel 5½ a 200 r., nas 16 Portas		1032	164$800
As 16 Portas, bandeiras, ferrage, grades de ferro, caixilho, e vidros		2760	441$600
Cimalha de alvenaria em todo o Edificio braças	34½	3200	110$400
Lagêdo para lagear todos os Quartos, faz varas	352	800	281$600
Pelo trabalho de Carpenteiro relativo ao Madeiramento, pregos, xumbo, pintura, etc.			763$200
Rs			4:600$000

Fig. 8.3a.

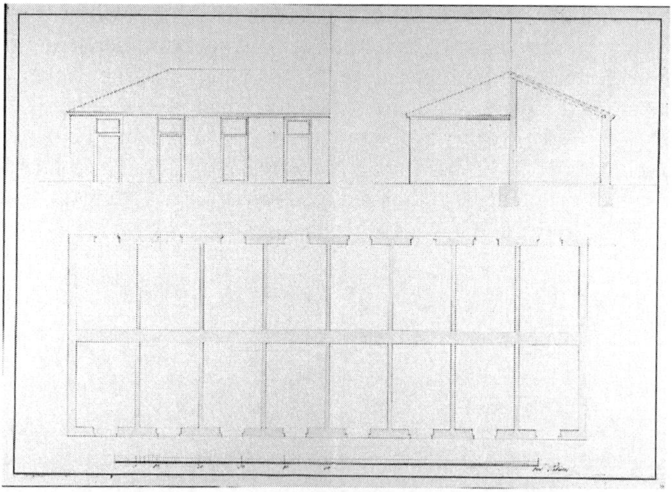

Fig. 8.3b.

Fig. 8.3a. Official letter with the expenses of the expansion works of the temporary lazaretto in Trafaria.
Fig. 8.3b. Elevation and floor plan of the ward with sixteen rooms.
Photo: Arquivo Municipal de Lisboa.

Then, the engineer in charge of the works[44] was expected to present his account and repair the doors and roof of the Trafaria lazaretto, and later on, the construction of a house for the infirmary[45] (Fig.3b). In the statement sent to the monarch in the laudatory approving words of a town councillor, the engineer stated that he “made the grandiose work of the lazaretto useful for everybody, when carrying out the mandate of His Majesty” (Oliveira 1904, 239). The petition received a favourable decision.[46]

In 1745, the houses close to the lazaretto, taken away from their occupants twenty-four years earlier, allegedly because they were too close to the lazaretto, were returned to them. The “impeded” farm goods were collected in new warehouses built on that occasion (Oliveira 1904, 471).

[44] The sergeant-major, infantry engineer and architect Carlos Mardel was the author of the works.

[45] AML-AH. 19 de-20 de Agosto de1743, Chancelaria Régia, Livro 15º de consultas e decretos de D. João V do Senado Ocidental, docs. 44 e 45, f. 95 a 98v.

[46] AML-AH. 6 e 11 de Março de 1744, Chancelaria Régia, Livro 18º de consultas e decretos de D. João V do Senado Ocidental, doc. 22, f. 68 - 69v.

Erratic lazaretto stage

Ten years later, during the reign of King José, prisoners sentenced to exile in Portuguese India were ordered to convalesce in the lazaretto before embarking. However, instead of the lazaretto, they were given the facilities of the nearby fort (Forte da Trafaria),[47] where there was only a small warehouse to store all the quarantined material. Thus, as stated by the Chief Health Provider, besides the risk of deterioration by rain, the space did not offer any suitable accommodation conditions for the sick. Therefore, the President of Town Hall Senate was assigned to prepare the facilities, ensuring that "the goods are well housed, and the sick are comfortable". Additionally, as ordered, the Treasury inspector for the division of the warehouses was to supervise the facilities designated as a lazaretto (Oliveira 1908, 128-130).

This type of letter, a Governmental initiative, signalled the intention to fully transfer policy control of the responsibilities hitherto carried out in the lazaretto by the Chief Health Provider within the scope of the Lisbon council.[48] This task was confirmed by the instruction sent to the President of the Town Hall Senate so that the keys to the lazaretto could be handed over to the inspector responsible for the Casa da India and State warehouses.[49] However, the council did not take the necessary measures, perhaps due to the earthquake of the following November that devastated the fort's installations and caused destruction in the lazaretto.

On 8 February 1756, the head of the council Town Hall Senate received a notice to vacate the lazaretto and transfer the guards and merchandise to the fort of Trafaria which was to receive prisoners, condemned to exile in Portuguese India, where there were no chains (Oliveira, 1908, 207). Two

---

[47] The fort of Trafaria, also called Fort of Nossa Senhora da Saúde da Trafaria, was built in 1683 by order of D. Pedro II to strengthen the defence against unauthorized intrusions on the Tagus bar.

[48] The Lisbon City Council, by royal delegation since the end of the 15th century, was responsible for managing some public health matters. On 27 September 1526, the post of Chief Health Provider of the Court and Kingdom was created, with attributions in the management of sanitary matters, such as food supply, city surveillance and prevention and combat of epidemics (especially the plague) and associated responsibilities such as quarantines and port surveillance; a few months later, these last competences also extended to land borders and overseas territories, from the beginning of 1580. In the two following centuries, up to 1813, most matters related to health institutions fell within the scope of the Chief Health Provider, the councillor responsible for Health at the Lisbon City Council.

[49] AML-AH. 26 de Setembro de 1755, Chancelaria Régia, Livro 8º de consultas, decretos e avisos de D. José I, f. 292 - 293v.

weeks later, the mayor was informed that having no time to carry out the works before the arrival of the prisoners, and the Chief Health Provider warning about the damage that would occur in guarding the merchandise of the fort warehouse, which was ruined by the earthquake, cells would be made ready in the fort. The merchandise would continue to be deposited in the lazaretto, although it was in ruins (Oliveira, 1908, 213). It is unknown what the solution was to be if, on that date, there were patients in the lazaretto. However, the guards also had to be resettled in the fort in order to supervise the prisoners heading Portuguese India. [50]

In April 1756, the Town Hall Senate was instructed to prepare two jails in the "lazaretto" to house prisoners who had fallen ill on the ship *Cabria*. Once again, the deteriorated merchandise had to be removed to "another part of the same lazaretto".[51] However, the lack of jails to house prisoners forced a new modification to the plans. This time, the goods were relocated to the fort of Trafaria, and the guards, while prisoners who "would come in waves to be transported to Portuguese India", should stay in the lazaretto. The Town Hall Senate should make the necessary repairs (Oliveira 1908, 294-295), isolating the wing reserved for quarantining people. A few days later, the Town Hall Senate was urged to undertake what had been determined, despite the possible damage that the ruinous state of the fort warehouse would cause to the transferred merchandise (Oliveira, 1908, 295).

The following month, the monarch ordered the Town Hall Senate to repair the damage to the lazaretto warehouses "without delay" and build a house to serve as an infirmary larger than the building of 1743. While the construction was in progress, in the cases of patients subject to confinement, the council was ordered to provide accommodation in houses close to the lazaretto. People from the houses had been previously evicted in order to prevent them from becoming infected. Measures would also be taken to prevent the lazaretto from communicating with the outside world (Oliveira, 1908, 239).

Again, in 1759, the Town Hall Senate was urged to have the lazaretto facilities and the house serving as an infirmary repaired. If more space was needed to accommodate the sick, it was authorized to "take over the houses closer to the so-called infirmary and everything needed to avoid transmitting the plague to these Kingdoms", as reported in the ports of Alexandria and Levant.

---

[50] AML- AH.8 de Fevereiro de 1756, Chancelaria Régia, Livro 9º de consultas, decretos e avisos de D. José I, f. 102 a 103v.

[51] AML-AH. 1 de Abril de 1756, Chancelaria Régia, Livro 9º de consultas, decretos e avisos de D. José I, f. 206 - 207v.

The sequence of notices sent by the Government to the Lisbon City Council between 1755 and 1759, with apparently no assistance from this institution, is still surprising. The delay in implementing the recommended measures suggests different interpretations of the concept of urgency on the part of the entities involved and the lax obedience to orders received along the chain of command, particularly under the authoritarian regime in force. The mighty Marquis of Pombal and Secretary of State (from 1750 to 1777), Sebastião José de Carvalho e Melo is said to have used the Kingdom's health defence as part of his project for political survival (Laurinda Abreu, 2018, 96-97). It could be speculated that, among other actions, this intention would benefit from the demonstration of ineffectiveness and the reduction in respect by the Lisbon Council and the Chief Health Provider for the government was an argument for taking control of the situation.

The protection system of the port of Lisbon remained alert and functional in the face of epidemic threats from the sea, for example, by forcing the quarantine of contaminated vessels, as was the case with the Dutch ship *Huys Om*.[52] Paradoxically, merchandise originating from Germany, Sweden and Denmark that was in quarantine was allowed to be unloaded.[53] In the meantime, a notice had been sent to the Chief Health Provider informing him of the appointment of a doctor and a captain for service at the lazaretto. [54]

Attention should be drawn to a substantial set of exceptions granted between the end of 1789 and 1792. Some merchants requested the immediate unloading of their goods, without their passing through the lazaretto. The merchandises were barrels of liqueur from Genoa, bales of silk and other products (some from an unknown source), only a few being identified.[55] To confirm these errors, in 1754, the chief guard of the port of Belém denounced the customs Town Hall Senate for ordering the arrest of two guards that he had sent to two ships coming from the Italian ports of Livorno and Venice. As a justification, the chief officer said he had deemed that the transported merchandise had been left unattended, resulting in a

[52] AML-AH. 6 -11 de Dezembro de1770, Chancelaria Régia, Livro 17º de consultas, decretos e avisos de D. José I, f. 64 - 65v.

[53] AML-AH. 10 - 11 de Abril de 1772, Chancelaria Régia, Livro 18º de consultas, decretos e avisos de D. José I, f. 19 - 20v.

[54] AML-AH.25 de Agosto de 1787- 5 de Junho de 1789, Provimento da Saúde, Livro de registo de decretos, alvarás e ordens da casa da saúde, f. 52 - 52v.

[55] AML-AH.10-12 de Novembro de 1789, Provimento da Saúde, Livro de registo dos avisos da secretaria de estado à provedoria-mor da saúde, doc. 1, f. 2. AML-AH. 18-20 Novembro de 1789, Provimento da Saúde, cód. n.º 8, f. 1v. AML-AH. 24-26 de Novembro de 1789AML-AH, Provimento da Saúde, cód. n.º 8, f. 2.

potential risk to public health since vessels from trade routes from Turkey and the Barbary Coast frequently arrived, requiring the most extraordinary precautions because some were not disinfected. Continuing, the chief officer gave the example of unloading from 1722. Two people unloading the goods collapsed immediately due to inhaling the vapours released when some bales were opened. The chief officers also mentioned that the epidemics in Messina and Marseille resulted from bales not being disinfected in the lazarettos (Oliveira 1906, 540-541).

In 1797, the facilities of the fort of Trafaria again required repairing. The Town Hall Senate was ordered to transfer the guards of the lazaretto and the merchandise to nearby houses and warehouses.[56]

Public loan and setbacks

Considering the urgent need for comfortable facilities that would make up for the lack of a definitive lazaretto in the port of Lisbon, Prince Regent João, under the guarantee and on behalf of his Royal Treasury, in 1800, granted a public loan of forty *contos de réis* at 5% interest, [57] for the construction of the building next to Trafaria between the prison and the Torre do Bugio (Silva 1828, 654-655). The loan was quickly provided by thirteen merchants and Lisbon, earning the gratitude of the Prince Regent (Silva, 1828, 657).

However, four years later, the choice of a construction site was still undecided. Meanwhile, the government advised the council Town Hall Senate to carry out new repairs and expand the lazaretto's structure, adding an estimated cost and floor plans for the works.[58] The Chief Health Provider of the Court and the Kingdom, after visiting the lazaretto and the fort of Trafaria, found it necessary to build a shed outside the facilities to store contaminated goods.[59]

[56] AML-AH. 18 -19 de Agosto de 1797, Chancelaria Régia, Livro de consultas de 1795-1797 de D. João VI, f. 196 - 200v.

[57] Alvará de 4 de Novembro de 1800, 664-665.

[58] AML-AH. 25-26 de Outubro de 1804, Provimento da Saúde, Pasta n.º 2 de reais avisos expedidos das Secretarias de Estado, doc. 4, f. 8 -9v. AML-AH. 25 de Outubro de 1804, Provimento da Saúde, Pasta n.º 3 de papéis remetidos das Secretarias de Estado, f. 47 - 49v. AML-AH.29 de Outubro-2 de Novembro de 1804, Provimento da Saúde, Pasta n.º 6 da Intendência-Geral da Polícia da Corte e Reino, f. 80 - 83v.

[59] AML-AH. 29 de Outubro de 1804, Provimento da Saúde, Pasta n.º 5 da Provedoria-Mor da Saúde da Corte e Reino, f. 18 a 19v. (The fort of Trafaria was

In another medical visit to the patients hospitalized in the lazaretto, the lack of an authority established in the same place that could immediately carry out the necessary measures was mentioned.[60] In fact, the Chief Health Provider was forced to provide information about the existence of competency conflicts among the health officers of the Trafaria lazaretto. [61] In addition, the mayor of Lisbon was advised about the obligation for visitors of hospitalized people in the lazaretto to be quarantined,[62] and the indispensability of military deployment to guard the facility.[63]

It is also worth noting that, from the end of 1804 through the following years, a large number of petitions was presented for payment of works, food, materials, and wages for the health personnel of the lazaretto. The delays were undoubtedly related to financial shortages or management deficiencies. Information sent by the Chief Health officer supports evidence requiring financial support for the sustenance of twenty six Spaniards and a Portuguese interned in the lazaretto.[64]

Frequent disturbances in Trafaria between civilians and soldiers of the headquarters followed, forcing the lazarettos inspector to request a magistrate who would enforce the order made by the delegation of the chief Town Hall Senate.[65]

Months earlier, upon hearing about the riots in Lisbon caused by the crew of the English frigate *Esmeralda*, the Government ordered the council Town Hall Senate that the Health Inspection Board should prevent the vessel from leaving until the time to prevent contagion from outbreaks of the plague had passed, in accordance with the health regulations.[66] According to later information sent to the council Town Hall Senate by the lazarettos' inspector, English sailors quarantined at the lazaretto had also caused

---

delivered unarmed, in 1836, at the disposal of the Companhia das Pescarias Lisbonense (Portaria de 18 Maio de 1836, 106).

60 AML-AH. 1-2 de Novembro de 1804, Provimento da Saúde, Pasta n.º 5 da Provedoria-Mor da Saúde da Corte e Reino, f. 20 -39v.

61 AML-AH. 11-12 de Novembro de 1804, Provimento da Saúde, Pasta n.º 5 da Provedoria-Mor da Saúde da Corte e Reino, f. 74 - 75v.

62 AML-AH. 18-19 de Novembro de 1804, Provimento da Saúde, Pasta n.º 5 da Provedoria-Mor da Saúde da Corte e Reino, f. 98 - 101v.

63 AML-AH. 21 de Novembro de 1804-29 de Março de 1805, Provimento da Saúde, Pasta n.º 5 da Provedoria-Mor da Saúde da Corte e Reino, f. 116 a 117v.

64 AML-AH. 18-24 de Dezembro de 1804, Provimento da Saúde, Pasta n.º 5 da Provedoria-Mor da Saúde da Corte e Reino, f. 198 - 205v.

65 AML-AH. 6 de Dezembro de 1804-7 de Janeiro de 1805, Provimento da Saúde, Pasta n.º 5 da Provedoria-Mor da Saúde da Corte e Reino, f. 214 - 217v.

66 AML-AH. 1-2 de Março de 1804, Provimento da Saúde, Pasta n.º 2 de reais avisos expedidos das Secretarias de Estado, doc. 60, f. 122 - 123v.

further disturbances.[67]

During the inquiry, it came to light that sixty-five crew members of the English frigate *Esmeralda* quarantined at the lazaretto had unleashed riots under the influence of alcoholic beverages. The incidents calmed down only after the arrival of military reinforcement, locking the mariners in their rooms with two sentries stationed in the courtyard overnight.[68] This outcome justified a new request for the construction of warehouses for the quarantined merchandise and facilities for the military detachment serving there.[69]

In the same year, crew members were infected with a suspicious disease in the vicinity of Gibraltar picked up from the Brazilian frigate *Princesa do Brasil*. The crew of the vessel was also infected. Therefore, one hundred and thirty-four patients were hospitalized in the lazaretto for about a month. After that, the ship was allowed to set sail from Lisbon. A few days later, three captains of ships from Brazil were held at Belém jail, one for falsifying the travel diary and two others for not providing reliable statements in their health inquiry.[70]

The delay in the construction of new facilities for the lazaretto, constantly requiring repairs, may explain why, in 1806, merchants from Lisbon requested moving the lazaretto from Trafaria to the Treasury customs house in Setúbal. They argued that it would avoid greater damage to trade.[71] In the same year, the interim commander of the Setúbal taskforce requested the installation of a lazaretto between Tróia and Ponta do Adoxo and accommodation for the health guards in a letter addressed to Marquis of Pombal, asking for protection against plague contagion.[72]

In 1809, and exacerbating the controversy over the Trafaria lazaretto, the council Town Hall Senate received an order from the Prince Regent João to vacate it and hand over the respective keys, so that the prisoners who were waiting to be sent to prison could be housed there. It was up to the Chief

---

[67] AML-AH.4 de Março de 1805, Provimento da Saúde, Pasta n.º 5 da Provedoria-Mor da Saúde da Corte e Reino, f. 304 a 307v.

[68] AML-AH. 3 de Dezembro de 1805, Provimento da Saúde, Pasta n.º 5 da Provedoria-Mor da Saúde da Corte e Reino, f. 217 - 220v.

[69] AML-AH. 1 de Junho- 11 de Julho de 1805, Provimento da Saúde, Pasta n.º 5 da Provedoria-Mor da Saúde da Corte e Reino, f. 342 - 397v

[70] AML-AH.10 de Julho-1 de Agosto de 1805, Provimento da Saúde, Pasta n.º 5 da Provedoria-Mor da Saúde da Corte e Reino, f. 490 - 509v.

[71] AML-AH.22 de Julho- 2 de Agosto de 1805, Provimento da Saúde, Pasta n.º 7 da Corte e Província da Estremadura, f. 141 -142v.

[72] AML-AH.23 de Junho e 18 de Setembro de 1806, Provimento da Saúde, Pasta n.º 7 da Corte e Província da Estremadura, f. 189 -190v.

Health Provider to comply with that decision.[73] Two years previously, that prince regent had ordered the handing over of the Fort of Trafaria to the General of Arms of the Court and Province of Estremadura.[74]

Transfer of a temporary lazaretto to Torre Velha

The severity of the plague outbreak in Mediterranean ports was a primary concern for the public health of the Kingdom. In 1813 it became necessary to build a temporary lazaretto for quarantining. In the same year, to "preserve these Kingdoms from the terrible scourge of the plague", Prince Regent João appointed the Public Health Board, assisted by the Chief Health Provider of the Court and Kingdom. According to the regulation, the Board was responsible for drawing up the project for the "immediate" construction of a permanent lazaretto (probably in Lisbon), taking measures to prevent the spread of the plague that was raging in Spain (and already affecting Portuguese provinces). The Board gathered information about the status of health within the Kingdom, especially in the city of Lisbon, seaports and borders, and boosted the public cleaning of cities, towns and main places of the Kingdom, establishing a cleanliness and police task force where it did not exist, improving the salubrity of the air in prisons, civil hospitals and similar buildings; cemeteries were located outside the churches, in their proper place.[75] Given the urgency of the measures taken to avoid the Kingdom from being contaminated by contagious diseases from other countries, the Prince Regent appointed the inspector of the public health area also to enact the extraordinary measures required, whenever the Public Health Board was unable to meet.[76]

---

[73] AML-AH. 18-21 de Janeiro de 1809, Chancelaria Régia, Livro 5º de registo de avisos de D. Maria I, f. 121 - 121v.

[74] AML-AH. 17 de Outubro de 1807, Chancelaria Régia, Livro 5º de registo de avisos de D. Maria I, f. 96v

[75] The Health Board included, in addition to the Chief Health Provider of the Court and the Kingdom (born member), two military officers, an interim inspector of the Royal Navy Arsenal, Judge Bartolomeu José Nunes Giraldes, and Drs Ignacio Xavier da Silva, Chief Physician of the Royal Navy, Bernardino António Gomes, Francisco José de Almeida, Francisco de Mello Franco, Henrique Xavier Baeta, José Pinheiro de Freitas, bachelor Luiz António Rebello da Silva being the secretary (Portaria de 28 de Agosto de 1813b, 232).

[76] Decreto de 20 de Outubro de 1813, 275.

Redistribution of services

At that time, it was impossible simultaneously to service the lazaretto and the Belém health station with the same staff because of their wide geographical separation. Thus, the separation of functions and employees was regulated in 1815.[77] Before and after unloading, the port entry of vessels, and onboard visits, the supervision of watching, guarding and application of security measures were carried out by the health station's personnel. The lazaretto was mainly responsible for the quarantining disinfection and the storage of foodstuff; carried out by an inspector, a clerk and several employees with specific duties (one for disinfection, a warehouse guard, another for the infirmary and a taskmaster supervising the loading and unloading). When necessary, a doctor, a surgeon, an apothecary, and a chaplain were also part of the lazaretto staff.

Following a reformist policy, the temporary lazaretto at the port of Lisbon, with its health service and new regulations, was transferred from Trafaria prison to *Torre Velha*.[78] The health department was temporarily disconnected from the Belém post. It had little function since the same health officials served both facilities.[79] On the other hand, part of the facilities of the *Torre Velha*, an old military fortification dating from 1490, was used as a temporary lazaretto (Fig. 8.4a) in a "simple and economical way".[80] It was located on a cliff on the left bank of the Tagus, between the beach at Porto Brandão and the Paulina inlet (Fig.8.4b). Until 1820, these temporary facilities presumably still benefited from the sanitary support of the prior ones in the fort of Trafaria (Sousa 1997, 101).

---

[77] Regimento de 22 de Outubro de 1815, 67-68. Edital de 10 de Maio de 1816, 137. Due to economic restrictions, the position of surgeon for visits under the responsibility of Belém port was extinct. In its place, a supplementary physician was hired, providing services just by hindrances of the resident physician paid by the general emolument division (Portaria de 29 de Julho de 1834, 332-333).

[78] Edital de 5 de Abril de 1816, 131. Edital de 10 de Maio de 1816.

[79] Decreto de 22 de Outubro de 1815, 66-67.

[80] Built on the site of an old artillery battery from the reign of King João I and enlarged in 1490 by order of King João II for the defence of the port of Lisbon (with the designation of Castle or Tower of S. Sebastião da Caparica, or the Old Tower Fortress), it was rebuilt in 1570 by order of King Sebastião, and called Tower of São Sebastião da Caparica. Being located opposite the Tower (of São Vicente) de Belém and the Bom Sucesso dock, it became known as the Torre Velha (Old Tower), as it is older than the Torre de Belém.

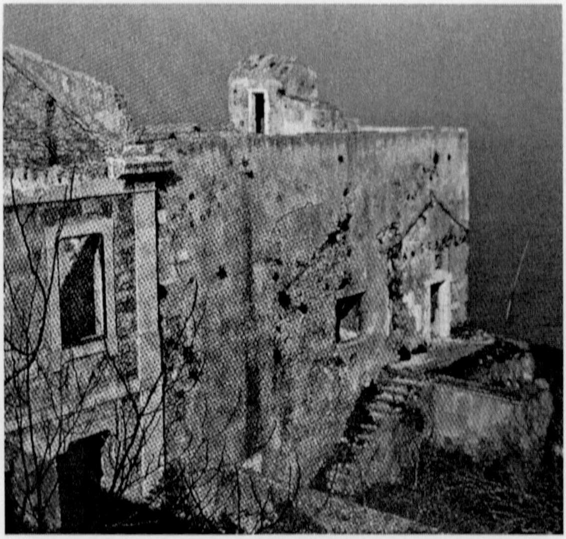

Fig. 8.4a.

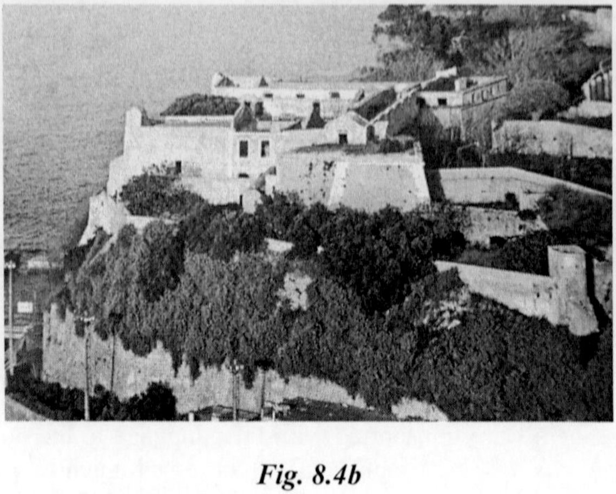

Fig. 8.4b

Fig. 8.4a. Ruins of the "summit tower" and part of the Torre Velha that temporarily housed the lazaretto in the mid-19th century.
Fig. 8.4b. Ruins of the Torre Velha. Author: Francisco Silva. Reproduced from Pedro Cid's A Torre de S. Sebastião da Caparica, figs 71 and 79, 2007. Francisco Silva. In Livro de Pedro Cid "A Torre de S. Sebastião da Caparica", 2007.

Six tents were installed next to the Tower to complement this insufficient sanitary solution. Three were used as farm warehouses, one for weighing farms goods (from which the percentage of the emoluments for the employees was calculated). The last one was used to store small boats. Around 1844, two masonry warehouses were built to protect the farms and a wall was constructed to assist with the process of unloading and landing (Fig.8.5).

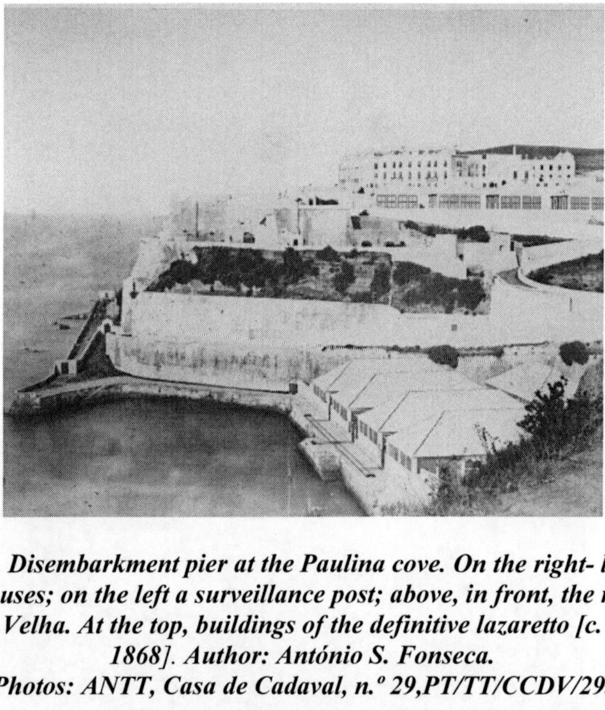

Fig. 8.5. Disembarkment pier at the Paulina cove. On the right- lazaretto warehouses; on the left a surveillance post; above, in front, the ruins of Torre Velha. At the top, buildings of the definitive lazaretto [c. 1865-1868]. Author: António S. Fonseca.
Photos: ANTT, Casa de Cadaval, n.º 29,PT/TT/CCDV/29.

However, the quarantines at the Torre Velha lazaretto only started in 1853. Passengers were transported with their luggage to the pontoons, in frigates (*fragatas do Tejo*)[81] (Fig.8. 6) which owed much to cleaning. In reality, the temporary lazaretto also suffered from a dreadful lack of privacy and unhygienic facilities, lacking adequate isolation or minimal amenities (Oliveira, 1911, 83-84).

[81]Sailing vessels with keel and smooth planking used on the Tagus River to load and unload ships and transport various goods between all the ports of the estuary.

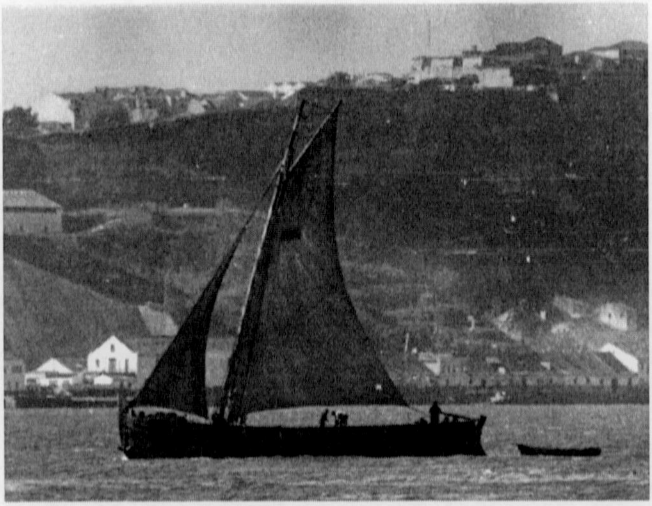

Fig. 8.6. Traditional boat on the Tagus River. Unidentified author. Photo: Arquivo Municipal de Lisboa.

Definitive lazaretto

To resolve the reported deficiencies and shortages once and for all, King João VI ordered the renting at public auction of the warehouses that had previously served as a lazaretto and had remained unoccupied in Trafaria, in order to raise the necessary funds for the construction of the new lazaretto. However, as before, there was no progress.[82]

In 1837, the Government was again alerted by the Health Council to the urgency of modifying the unsatisfactory sanitary conditions of the lazaretto, which served no contemporary practical purpose (Oliveira 1911, 84). Fourteen more years later, when Queen Maria II was aware of the "varied and repeated complaints against the same establishment… and lately repeated by the Civil Government of Lisbon", the monarch decided to pay attention to the situation and improve the conditions. He appointed a commission to properly propose the necessary reforms.[83] Following the

[82] AML-AH. 26-30 de Março de 1819, Chancelaria Régia, Livro 1° de registo de decretos de D. João VI, f. 48 a 48v.

[83] Decreto de 28 de Junho de 1851, 217-218. The commission was made up of five individuals from national civic life: Drs. Ernesto Adolfo de Freitas, Ignacio Pedro

commission's proposals at the end of 1851,[84] it was determined that special care should be taken regarding customs inspection of luggage belonging to quarantined persons, and other materials susceptible to the spread of an epidemic. [85] They would be "ventilated" and would receive other sanitary "benefits."[86]

Great care was required concerning the handling of luggage and other assets of the quarantined persons who perished in the lazaretto. These goods were the responsibility of the inspector until they were claimed by people entitled to do so. [87] It was essential to harmonize the functions of the military garrison in the lazaretto with those of the staff and sanitary surveillance.[88] It was incumbent upon the Portuguese Army Ministry to provide requisitions for goods which were indispensable for the garrison. [89] Two years later, a small armed boat was deployed to ensure the complete isolation of the lazaretto. [90]

The 1850s were worrisome. The Government was urged to strengthen health measures, in particular in defending the Kingdom from epidemics arriving from the sea. As early warnings of risk to public health started to circulate, epidemics emerged: cholera from 1853-1856. Still barely finished, it was closely followed by an outbreak of yellow fever in Lisbon, which lasted until 1857 (Gomes 1858, 85). As stated (Barbosa 1864, 210), if the "invasion of yellow fever in 1857" had not occurred, some works "highly demanded to improve public hygiene, and the decorum of the capital" would not have been carried out, nor others planned.

Finally, in 1858, the Government decided to build a new lazaretto by expropriating a site next to the *Torre Velha*.[91] Meanwhile, the project was approved, along with the construction of a wall high enough to resist the tides, and six new warehouses to store materials under quarantine at the

---

Quintella Emaus, José Vicente Barbosa du Bocage, Thomaz de Carvalho, e José Francisco de Sant'Anna e Vasconcellos.

[84] Decreto de 15 de Dezembro de 1851, 538.

[85] The following matters were included in the previous edicts on the subject: coarse or manufactured cotton; hair manufactured or in any other state; coarse or manufactured hemp; letters, newspapers and correspondence papers; fresh, dry or manufactured leather; manufactured horsehair, or in any other state; fresh animal remains, or fragments; wool, coarse or manufactured linen; manufactured skins and feathers or in any other state; coarse or manufactured silk.

[86] Edital de 9 de Setembro de 1853, 471-472.

[87] Edital de 16 de Julho de 1853,195-197.

[88] Portaria de 6 de Fevereiro de 1854,18-19

[89] Portaria de 28 de Novembro de 1856, 74.

[90] Ofício de 3 de Abril de 1858, 104.

[91] Portaria de 12 de Maio de 1858, 49.

service of the *Torre Velha* lazaretto.[92]

A preliminary project was presented to replace the precarious facilities of *Torre Velha*, where the quarantine facilities were installed, in 1860. It would be "the first work to establish a building that would meet the complex needs of the service, regarding public health requirements, without sacrificing the comfort of quarantined people". The proposal, approved the following year, included the construction of independent blocks (each with services for first, second and third-class passengers). Among other facilities, a guest house, laundry, hospital service, staff facilities and military barracks were part of the plan (Oliveira 1911, 84-85).

After the partial demolition of the Tower and almost all of the annexed fortifications, the new facilities (distributed over approximately three floors: (a) At the base (next to the quay and the mooring dock for the boats transporting quarantined people), there was a surveillance tent (with a permanent guardianship), and a little further up, the customs warehouses, including the warehouses for the collection of merchandise and luggage, the disinfection service (involving air ventilation using mechanical fans, hot air from Geneste & Herscher ovens or devices employing sulphurous acid), and the vaccination station.

When a ship arrived at the Lisbon port, sick or possibly infected passengers and crew disembarked at the Porto Brandão pier and were taken to the lazaretto for quarantine and possible treatment. Luggage and other personal belongings were sent for disinfection in steam-heated ovens or, in the most serious cases, with acid vapours; (b) On the second floor, the infirmary (also called the hospital) was utterly separated from all other buildings. It was a two-storey structure for the isolation of sick patients. The buildings of the old lazaretto (wooden and mortar tents for quarantining crews) were somewhat further away, and the new facilities for the accommodation of quarantining passengers. It was a large building composed of six blocks (*quarantines*) of four floors arranged in a semicircle in a fan-shaped structure surrounded by a courtyard (known as a *ronda*, as it provided the surveillance route of the complex, and for transporting foodstuffs, clothes and other materials).

The construction of the building, begun in 1867, was completed two years later (Sousa 1981, 102) although, in 1883, embankments and wall coatings were still being completed (Oliveira, 1911, 85). Each block looked like a hotel, provided with accommodation and catering facilities (with three pricing levels, according to the travel classes of the quarantined individuals), with garden courtyards. A kitchen (equipped to serve about a

---

[92] Portaria de 28 de Outubro de 1858, 411.

thousand people a day) was at the centre. On the upper floor, an area for visitors and a parlour (with a chapel for religious services) formed a symmetrical parallel semicircle, from where visitors could communicate through around twenty windows with the facing blocks housing the quarantined persons. Laundry, barracks for the military detachment, and a henhouse were outdoors. (c) The cemetery (with an autopsy room and chapel) and the fire station stood at the top of the property (Fig. 8.7).[93] In various places, the structure also contained the health station (for patient observation), the residences of the inspector and staff, personal disinfection house, engine room, utility room, telegraph-postal station and the office (Frazão 1897, 112-118; Oliveira 1811, 85-88).

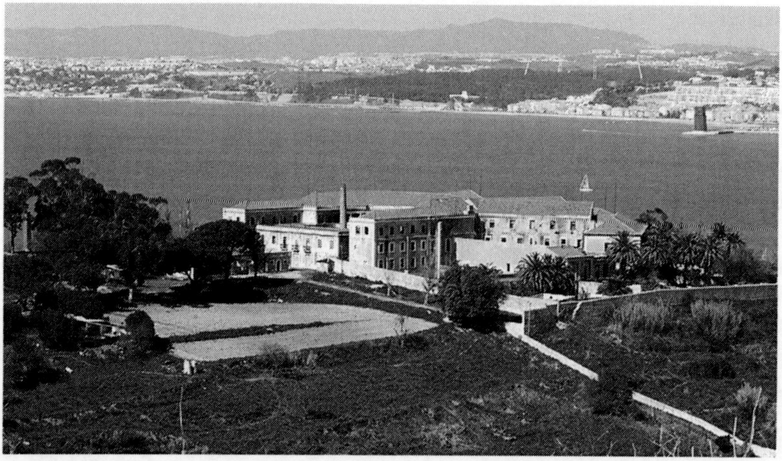

Fig. 8.7. Ruins of the definitive Lazareto in Lisbon, view from the top of the hill. In the background - the Tagus and the north bank. Unidentified author. Courtesy of the Centro de Documentação do Centro de Arqueologia de Almada.

Quarantine at the lazaretto would have been a torment for any traveller, not only because of the forced isolation under permanent surveillance by the security service, but, in particular, because of the daily expenses of a prolonged stay, paying for accommodation, catering, medicines, laundry,

[93] From here, a superb panoramic view of the Tagus is viewed: on the right, a wide river basin about 23 kilometres wide, is known as "the straw sea", and on the left, Cascais in the Atlantic Ocean. Almost the entire city extends on the north bank and outskirts, in an arc to the west, the Sintra mountain range standing out in the distance.

plus expenditure in luggage and merchandise landing fees, in addition to "the listed health taxes, broken down into a thousand and one little taxes" (Bivar 1945, 133). According to a provision of 1858, the quarantined also paid for the disinfectants used on their luggage. However, it was up to the owners or consignees of the ships to supply the drugs required for disinfection. [94] In order to guarantee the quality of those substances, in 1871, it was decided that the chief guard of the Belém health station would be responsible for their acquisition. Their distribution was assigned to the customs service.[95]

In January 1859, to finish the works and improvements of the building, the Government kept the "new lazaretto" closed for four months to the entry of merchandise, goods or other cargo from "dirty" ports every time ships and passengers had not satisfactorily passed the regulated quarantining criteria. Vessels and passengers arriving from the Vigo harbour or other regulated ports were allowed to enter.[96] In April, due to the progress of the works, passengers from those points of origin were authorized to disembark in order to quarantine in the new facilities. [97]

When the lazaretto was moved to the new health complex, the *Torre Velha,* it no longer kept its previous functions, although it did maintain a military garrison to ensure the isolation of the quarantine facilities installed at the new lazaretto. Two years later, the Government appointed a commission to check whether the state and quality of the planned works were made according to prevailing health requirements, trade interests and traveller's comfort.[98] It was also expected that this commission would point out any repairs or proposals that would benefit that project.

A floating breakwater was built to protect the boarding and disembarking of quarantined passengers, luggage, and merchandise sixteen years later.[99] Two motor speed boats (Fig.8.8) were purchased to transport the quarantined people and health and customs visitors to the lazaretto, along with a steamboat for towing them; in addition, the government announced its intention to have a dock built next to the lazaretto to facilitate loading

[94] Edital, 8 de Abril de 1858, 106.
[95] Portaria de 10 de Fevereiro de 1871, 359.
[96] Edital de 26 de Janeiro de 1859, 21.
[97] Edital de 25 de Abril de 1859, 132. Portaria de 28 de Outubro de 1858, 411.
[98] Portaria de 28 de Setembro de 1860, 636-637. The commission was constituted by the president of the Council of Public Health of the Kingdom Dr. Guilherme da Silva Abranches, and Engineers José Diogo Mascarenhas Mouzinho de Albuquerque e José Anselmo Gromicho Couceiro.
[99] Lei de 6 de Abril de 1876, 74.

and unloading of people and merchandise to and from the lazaretto.[100]

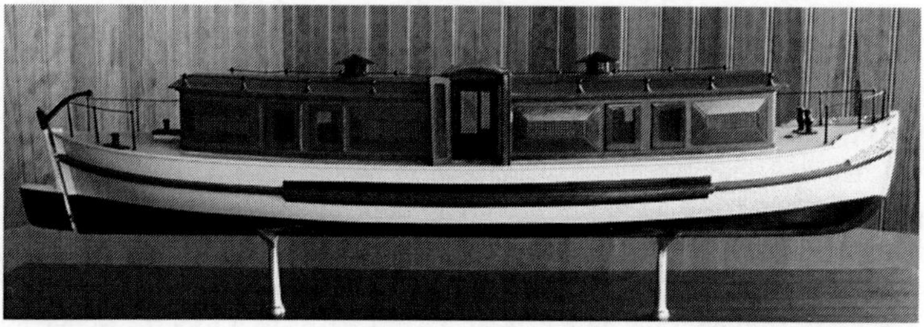

Fig. 8.8. Model of a speedboat ("Barca do Lazareto") for passengers' transport from transoceanic ships to the Lazaretto pier. Author: Lenine Rodrigues. Photo: Coleção de Museu Naval de Câmara Municipal de Almada.

Considering that the quarantined passengers and sick employees of the lazaretto made excessive claims, causing damage and exaggerated expenses that led to a higher and undue increase in public expenditure, protected by a previous provision granting free medical consultation and medication, the Government decided to revoke those rights. Indigent quarantined people were exempted from this provision. [101]

The medical staff of the lazaretto was reinforced in 1880. Additional posts were created for male and female nurses, inspectors and administrators who were mandated to reside in the building.[102] In addition, a tender was opened for the acquisition of a ventilation device and two ovens for that institution.[103] Despite these apparent improvements, the quality of the facilities at the Lisbon lazaretto was pinpointed by the sharp irony of the Portuguese artist and caricaturist Rafael Bordalo Pinheiro (1846-1905), when in 1880, returning from Brazil, he had to quarantine to prevent the dissemination of a possible yellow fever infection (Pinheiro 1881, 31-55).[104]

---

[100] Lei de 9 de Fevereiro de 1876, 31-32.

[101] Decreto de 27 de Junho de 1879, 136.

[102] Lei de 21 de Junho de 1880, 110-111.

[103] Decreto de 17 de Outubro de 1891, 635.

[104] While at the lazaretto, R.B.P. (Rafael Bordalo Pinheiro, "No Lazareto de Lisboa", 1881, 31-55) commented concerning the place on the court "These arcades are black, This slab is sepulchral, These stairs are dismal, These walls are frightening" ("*São negras estas arcadas, Sepulcral este lajedo, Lúgubres estas escadas, Estas paredes metem medo*"). A series of comments about the lazaretto and the renewed Lisbon followed. Two years later, the lazaretto seems to have improved under the direction

The distance of the lazaretto from Lisbon, forcing the sick with plague and quarantined people to move from the north bank to cross the Tagus River, was a significant inconvenience that could only be resolved by building a maritime post in Lisbon. This difficulty was particularly noteworthy during the second half of 1899 when bubonic plague broke out in Oporto. To prevent the epidemic from spreading throughout the Kingdom, the Government ordered a set of measures to prevent people from leaving the city (Martins e Silva, 2020, 12-123, 127-129). One of these provisions authorized passengers who needed to travel to Lisbon (exclusively by rail) after medical inspection, their luggage having been disinfected, and having been certified by a health passport valid for that trip. Upon arrival, passengers underwent medical inspection for nine days. They were locked down in the lazaretto, crossing the Tagus River to Port Brandão whenever suspected signs of illness became apparent.[105] When, on the advice of the Public Health Advisory Board, a sanitary cordon was established around the city of Oporto,[106] preventing travel to Lisbon by any means other than by sea, passengers were still compelled to "purge, quarantining at the Lisbon lazaretto" (Martins e Silva, 2020, 12-123,127-129).[107]

The lazaretto was also used in surveilling the inhabitants of Lisbon, whether infected with *Yersinia pestis* or not. By that time, Professor Câmara Pestana (1863-1899), moving from Oporto, had arrived in Lisbon and was asymptomatic. On the following night he was struck with the high fever and buboes characteristic of bubonic plague. As soon as the health authorities were aware, he was transferred to a hospital for isolation and quarantine. Visits from his family members with whom he had direct contact were prohibited. The other tenants of his residence were also prohibited from entering or leaving the building. They had to lock down on their residence floors as a party had occurred on another floor, attended by residents and guests. The guests were kept in the building. That night, all the residents and guests were inoculated with the Plague vaccine. On the following day, they were transported to the lazaretto for quarantining. Residents of the neighbouring buildings were mandated to undergo medical inspection for

---

of Dr. Homem de Vasconcelos. However, a final ironic assessment inevitably asserted that: "The lazaretto continues to be a penitentiary, holding everything except for yellow fever".

[105] Decreto de 23 de Agosto de 1899, 353

[106] Anais de Saúde Pública do Reino, 1904, 163.

[107] Anais de Saúde Pública do Reino, 1904, 163.

nine days.[108]

Reorganization of the health services

The days of the Lisbon lazaretto were numbered. Despite the improvements alluded to above, the structures remained unsatisfactory as did the inconvenience of crossing the River Tagus. The restructuring of the health services implemented in 1901 strongly boosted the structural and functional changes in the health services of the ports of the Kingdom. This effort, supported by the legislation of 1892, authorized the urgent expropriation of land and properties (involving compensation) for the "establishment of lazarettos, disinfection stations, hospitals and, overall, for whatever facilities funded by the State for the sanitary defense of the Kingdom against the invasion or spread of epidemics".[109]

Based on the experience acquired fighting the bubonic plague in Oporto between June and September 1899, Professor Ricardo Jorge, General Health Inspector (1899-1903), framed the regulation of national defences to manage epidemics entering from abroad with a credited level of sanitary success. The General Inspector was responsible for supervising the technical service of sections, stations and other health institutions of the Ministry of the Kingdom, among other duties. His assistants were the inspector of the Lisbon lazaretto (for maritime health matters), the director of the Royal Bacteriological Institute (bacteriological services), the Lisbon health delegate (municipal and district health), and the director of the Lisbon Public Disinfection Station (disinfection service). It was up to the health stations to carry out the sanitary services in the ports of the mainland and archipelagos of the Kingdom (including visits to vessels, under the competence of the chief guards,[110] and imposing quarantine when needed). The health services of the Lisbon port, headed by the lazaretto inspector (who also directed and administered the lazaretto and the station) were held by the health station (commanded by the chief guard) and the lazaretto. The maritime disinfection station (to be located on the right bank of the Tagus River) functioned as an annex.

---

[108] Peste bubónica- um caso de peste em Lisboa", Diário de Notícias, 11 de Novembro de 1899. "O Dr. Câmara Pestana", "Os prédios contíguos", Jornal de Notícias, 12 de Novembro de 1899.

[109] Decreto de 24 de Setembro de 1892, 716.

[110] The chief guards and the inspector of the lazaretto had medical or medico-surgical qualifications.

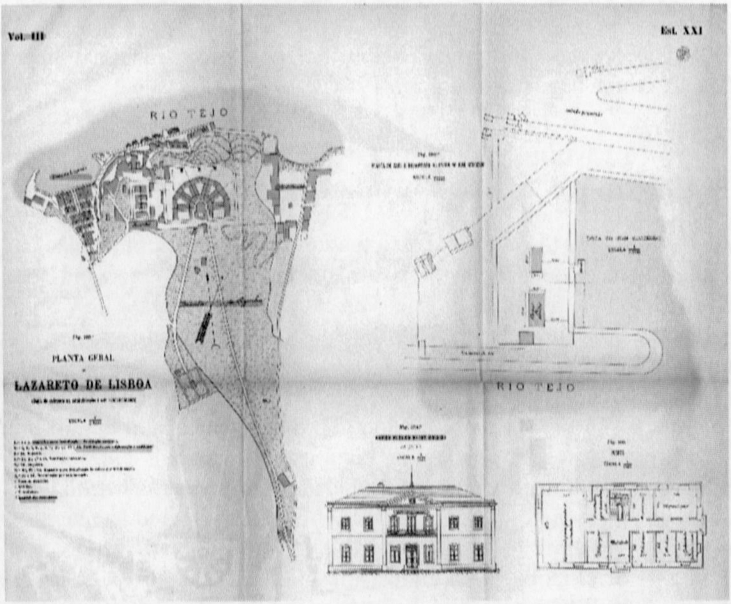

Fig. 8.9. Schematic representation of the relative positioning of the Lisbon Lazareto, at the Tagus south bank, and the Lisbon Maritime Disinfection Post, at the north (represented as Edifício de Saúde no Bom-Sucesso); from the health building shown on the right down in the previous diagram, is evident the division wall on the lower floor of the administrative building. Unknown author. Reproduced from Adolpho Loureiro's Atlas, Os portos marítimos de Portugal e ilhas adjacentes, Estampa XXI, figs. 102-103, 1907.

The health stations were placed in the 1st rank as soon as the disinfection stations had been installed. In addition to Lisbon, they included the facilities in Oporto, Ponta Delgada and Funchal. The 1st rank stations were headed by health service physicians (called chief guards), were assisted by qualified auxiliary staff (clerks, interpreters, guards and rowers) and a post for inspecting people and disinfecting merchandise, luggage and vessels. At the time, the Lisbon Health Station was still the only one with a certified lazaretto.[111] As early as 1859, during the reign of King Pedro V (1853-1861), the High Council for Public Health was instructed to urgently submit its report, projects, budgets and any other clarifications concerning the

[111] Decreto de 24 de Dezembro de 1901, 1039, 1057, 1058.

lazarettos to be built in Funchal and Horta.[112] However, just thirteen years later, a property was expropriated in Funchal for the construction of the local lazaretto, which began operating in 1901.[113]

Lisbon Maritime Disinfection Station

In 1902, a commission was appointed to choose the location and design for the construction of the maritime disinfection station in Lisbon, replacing the one that had functioned in the old lazaretto and the previous accommodation of the Lisbon health station.[114] The project considered that the Tagus would separate the lazaretto from the maritime post, the first being situated on the south bank and the second on the north bank (Fig.8.9).

The construction and installation of the maritime post was financed through a loan taken out in the Kingdom. The management and administration for the project was entrusted to an administrative commission.[115] Another commission was put in charge of proposing the means of regulating the docking of ships and the disembarkation of passengers and baggage at the new maritime station.[116]

Built at Rocha Conde de Óbidos, the maritime station of Lisbon was inaugurated in 1906 by King Carlos I (reigned from 1898 to 1908). On the tombstone placed in the building, still accessible, the following inscription reads as follows:

> In the reign of His Majesty King Carlos I, His Excellency the President of the Council and Minister of the Kingdom Ernesto Rodolfo Hintze Ribeiro, in the interests of public health, international relationships and general interests of the country, ordered the construction of this maritime disinfection station as provided by the General Regulation of Public Health Services of 21-12-1901, which opened on 5-3-1906.

The new Maritime Disinfection Station in Lisbon, as it was called at the time, covered an area of 8,500 square metres. The administrative building, where the inauguration plaque figures, was extended by a pier about 300 metres in length, allowing the simultaneous docking of three ships. Along

[112] Portaria de 14 de Julho de 1859, 345.

[113] Decreto de 29 de Maio de 1872, 94. Decreto de 19 de Julho de 1901, 292. The staff of the Funchal disinfection post would only be approved in 1994. (Decreto de 23 de Maio de 1904, 231-232).

[114] Portaria de 11 de Novembro de 1902.1095-1096.

[115] Decreto de 11 de Dezembro de 1902, 1291.

[116] Portaria de 3 de Outubro de 1905, 436.

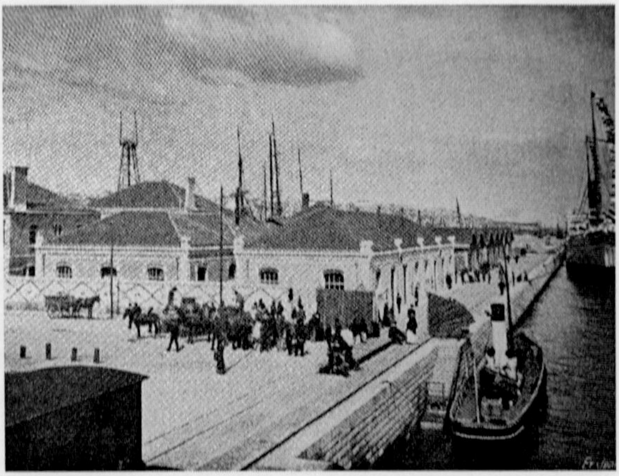

(a)

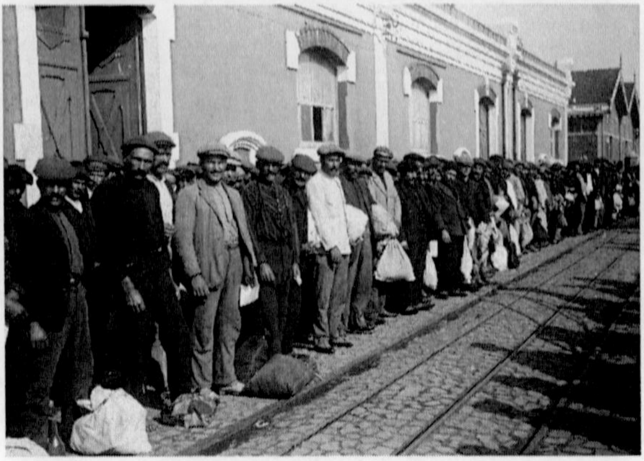

(b)

Fig. 8.10a. Lisbon Maritime Disinfection Post disembarkation pier: View from the pier. Unknown author. Reproduced from Guilherme Ennes' A Desinfecção Publica em Lisboa 1896.
8.10b. Group of fishermen from Póvoa do Varzim arriving from Brazil awaiting the health inspection, along with the Posto's facilities and warehouses, on the pier. Autor: Ferreira da Cunha. Photo: Arquivo Municipal de Lisboa.

the quay stood the buildings of a customs delegation and tax post, two large warehouses, sanitary services facilities and housing for the staff (director, physician, custom head services and two inspectors) (Fig.8.10a Fig. 8.10b).[117]

The sanitary service was provided with disinfection equipment (sulfurization chambers, steam ovens, showers and bathtubs) and prophylactic treatment [Clayton type B equipment, with pipes for the sulphurization chambers and berths. Geneste & Herscher ovens (Fig. 8.11a), Ennes formalinizers, (Fig. 8.11b), shower and bathtubs, disinfection facilities and products] and additional facilities for people, small goods and clothes were also provided. Large items of merchandise continued to be sent to the lazaretto, where no means and equipment for treatment were available, among other requirements and complementary materials (Oliveira 1911, 79-80). At that station, passengers arriving in the city began to benefit from integrated medical services, along with the Royal Bacteriological Institute and the Hygiene Laboratory,[118] no longer needing to head to the lazaretto for disinfection and quarantine.

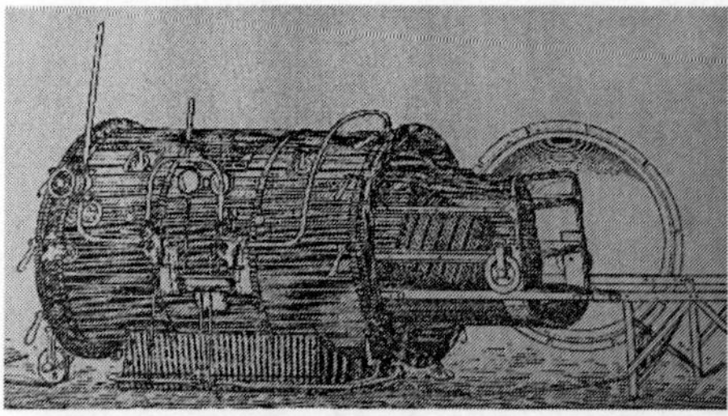
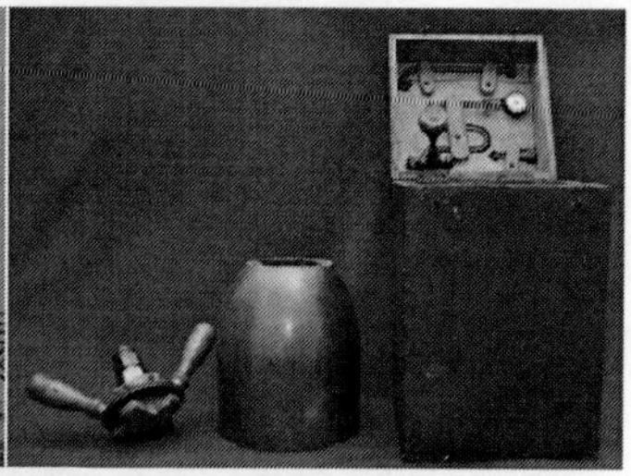

Fig. 8.11a. 8a Some equipment at the Maritime Station: (a) Geneste & Herscher greenhouse scheme. Unknown author. Reproduced from Guilherme Ennes' A Desinfecção Publica em Lisboa, 1896.
Fig. 8.11b. Photograph of Ennes formolizer. Used in formaldehyde disinfection, under pressure, contained in a transportable metallic container to which associated tubes and pressure gauges allow the spraying of houses and public spaces potentially contaminated with infectious diseases, invented by the doctor Guilherme Ennes. Author: José Guilherme Ennes. Photo credit: Health Museum, National Health Institute Doctor Ricardo Jorge. Exhibitor-Portuguese Red Cross. 1896.

---

[117] Decreto de 30 de Novembro de 1905, 607-608; Portaria de 30 de Novembro de 1905, 607-608. Brasil-Portugal, "Posto de desinfecção", Nº 162, 285,1905.
[118] Decreto de 24 de Dezembro de 1901, 1039.

Lisbon Public Disinfection Station

Following the prevailing orientation "in all civilized countries", the Government realized it was essential to provide the capital with a permanent station for mandatory public disinfection, with modern equipment, organization and personnel with suitable training to effectively fight preventable diseases, ensure defence against imported epidemics and other contagious diseases. [119]

However, correctly choosing the right place to install the Lisbon disinfection system properly proved complicated. The first provisional choice was that of the former convent of Esperança and, with some urgency, its respective fencing. Legal impediments as to the use of the building forced them to look for another location on land belonging to the Industrial Institute, which was refused. The third site was close to the convent of Santa Joana, which was also rejected because it was part of the future improvement plan for the city.

Finally, in June 1893, after 255 days of frustrating attempts to resolve an urgent public health issue, the Government made it possible to exchange the land of the convent of Santa Joana for that of Francesinhas (next to the Assembly building), then an asylum and school for dressmakers and maids (Ennes 1896, 25-26). This location had the advantage of being in the capital's centre, close to Brandão and Esperança neighbourhood and Rua João das Regras (Fig. 8.12) (Ennes 1896, 27-29).

The Public Disinfection Station project was approved in June 1893, and the works were authorized three days later, the works beginning on 10 July.

The facility consisted of eight buildings and related structures. They were divided into two conveniently isolated areas: the "impeded area" (dirty) located next to the entrance gate (Fig. 8.13a), and the "clean area" (disinfected) (Fig.8.13b). The buildings included the administration, main building (or workshops), vehicle disinfection shed, disinfectant warehouse (Fig. 8.13c), incineration oven, repair shop, well and water supply reservoir, and washrooms.

Much of the material acquired to defend the borders against the cholera epidemic, which had spread from southern France to northern Spain since 1892, was reused to equip the Post. As a complement, two more Geneste & Herscher greenhouses (one fixed and one locomotive) were initially required (Figs) and six sprayers (Figures 8.14.a and 8.14b).

---

[119] Decreto de 12 de Abril de 1894, 158.

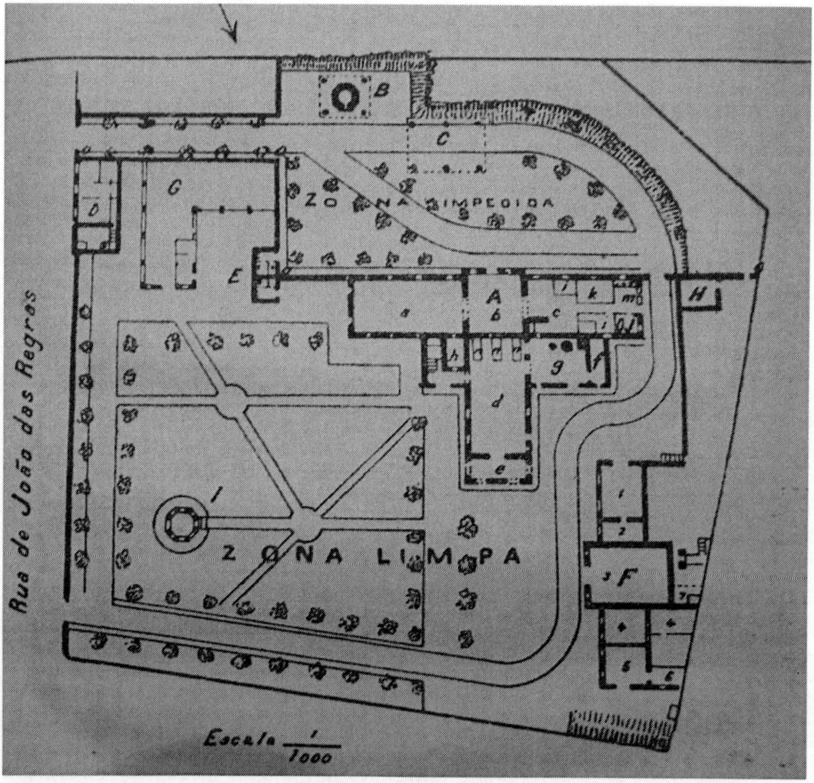

Fig. 8.12. Scheme of the Public Disinfection Post location in Lisbon, within the framework of some streets in Lisbon, and the internal layout of its main areas (dirty and clean areas) and facilities. An arrow indicates the entrance. Unknown author. Reproduced from Guilherme Ennes' A Desinfecção Publica em Lisboa, 1896.

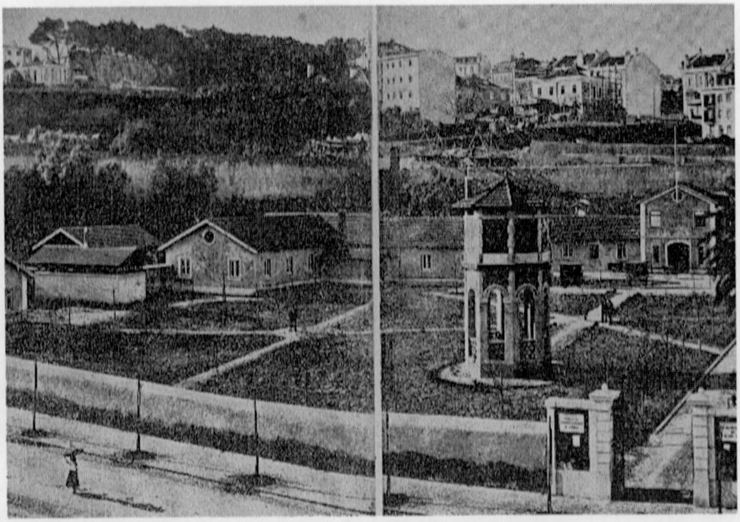

8.13a.

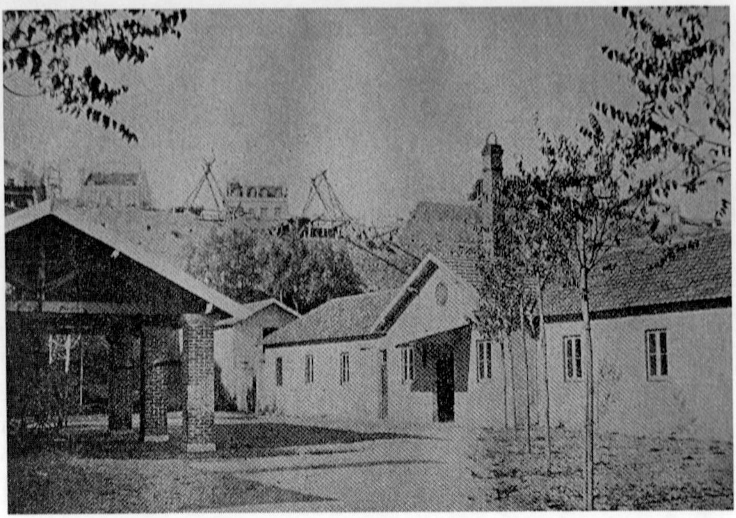

8.13b.

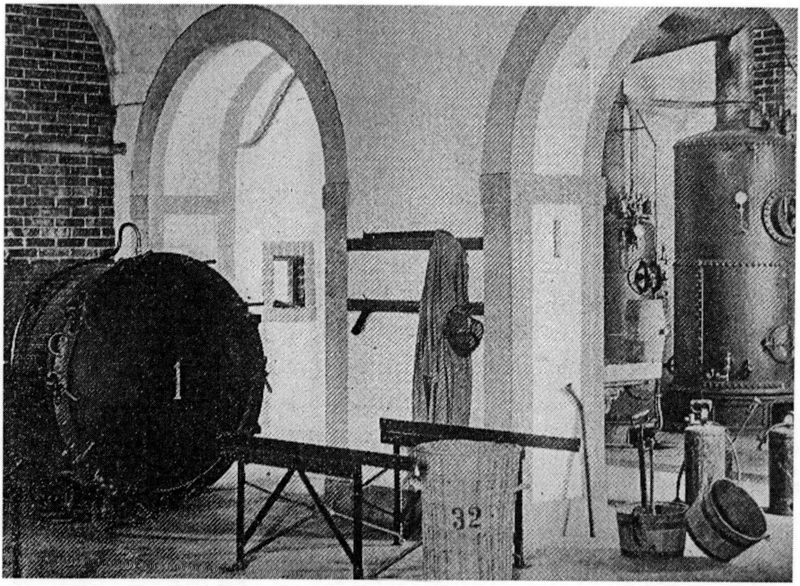

8.13c.

Fig. 8.13a. Photo of the Lisbon Public Disinfection Post, in 1894, and of some of its pavilions (a) The "dirty area" was located in the foreground; in the background, some buildings in the neighbourhood are seen. 8.13b. Image of the "clean" zone.
Fig. 8.13c. Image of the interior of the disinfection workshop. Unknown author. Reproduced from Guilherme Ennes' A Desinfecção Publica em Lisboa, 1896.

It was planned to purchase three more fixed ovens — to permanently support the disinfection of the city (for example, infectious diseases, clothes from pawnshops or rag and bone individuals) — and other material (clothes, furniture, various equipment and two vehicles for the external service). Later, it was necessary to utilize the water supply from a well of the old convent, at the "dirty area", near the installation access (Ennes 1896, 41-43).

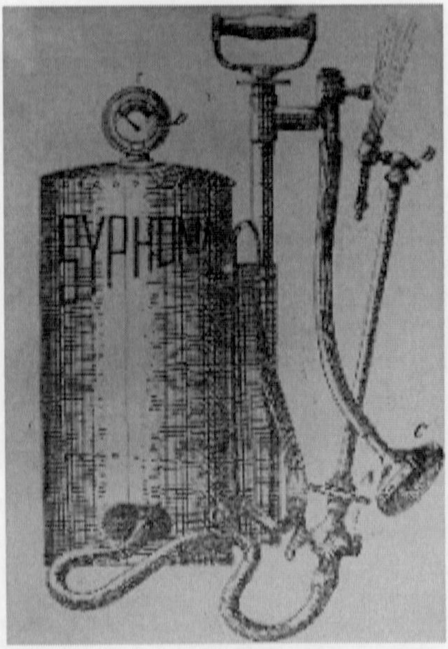

8.14a.

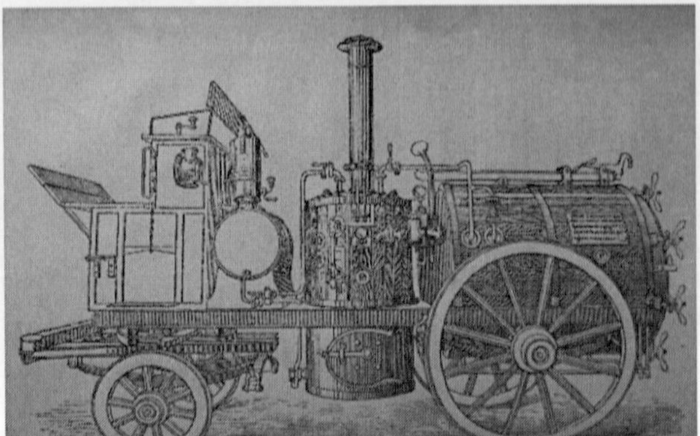

8.14b.

Fig. 8.14a. Some disinfection equipment. Scheme of a Syphonia pulverizer.
8. 14b. Scheme of a traction engine. Unknown author. Reproduced from Guilherme Ennes. A Desinfecção Publica em Lisboa. 1896.

The construction led to some local opposition, fearing the proximity of a disinfection service that could endanger the functioning of both institutions and residents. Consequently, the Government was urged to move the Post to another location. The matter was eventually clarified, pleasing all those involved (Guilherme Ennes 1896, 36-37).

The Public Disinfection Station started its fixed activity on 2 May 1894 and, domestically, a week later. Under the motto: "all communicable diseases are preventable diseases", its purpose was to promote preventive medicine activities and the disinfection of all materials, houses and other places that had been in contact with infected patients. It was mandatory to declare the epidemic diseases (e.g. typhoid fever, exanthematic typhus, tuberculosis, plague, cholera, among many other infectious and/or epidemic diseases) to the authorities (Ennes, 1901, 21-22).

The disinfection of the Lisbon municipality, both with respect to contaminated areas and clothing, shoes and other potentially contaminated objects intended for resale, was the responsibility of personnel assigned to that service. It was stipulated that such sanitary practices were to be expanded to all parts of the national territory, provided that "public disinfection services were already organized there". Finally, the sub-delegates of health who had knowledge of cases of disease or the clinicians who treated them were obliged to request those services, under penalty of disobedience.[120] A seal from the public disinfection station was required for items on sale, including second-hand rags or wool that the railway company offered for sale in Lisbon or Oporto.[121] On the same occasion, the regulation was approved and the price list for that station in Lisbon was established, also to be applied to the disinfection station in Oporto.[122] Other mainland cities were allowed to build disinfection stations.[123]

When, in an 1897-1898 report from the disinfection services, it was found that numerous cases of infectious disease (namely, smallpox and tuberculosis, including deaths from them) registered in the capital had not been notified, as prescribed in the previous decree of 12 April, the Government, reacting to these facts and other occurrences of medical negligence, decided to re-establish mandatory compliance with the established norms, under penalty of a criminal trial.[124]

The continued non-compliance with those notifications by the sub-delegates and clinicians of the municipality of Lisbon, claiming that some

---

[120] Decreto de 12 de Abril de 1894, 159.
[121] Decreto de 12 de Julho de 1894, 597.
[122] Decreto de 28 de Abril de 1894, 221. Decreto de 4 de Maio de 1894, 241.
[123] Decreto de 17 de Maio de 1901, 151.Decreto de 24 de Maio de 1902, 197.
[124] Portaria de 15 de Outubro de 1898, 736.

of the infectious diseases were benign (wrongly, as was the case with smallpox in its attenuated form), led to a new official call for strict observance of the stipulated sanitary provisions. [125]

Lisbon Sanitary Park

In 1929, the site of those facilities, expanded and reformulated, was occupied by a new institution created by the General Directorate of Health, called the *Parque Sanitário*, with its headquarters in Lisbon and a section in Oporto.[126]

The improvements introduced in this new structure favoured the prevention of epidemic diseases, as well as disinfection and deworming of every admitted patient. A programme to assist the most deprived was also organized, including washing clothes and providing access to changing rooms. A rapid transport system for medical and auxiliary personnel was created to provide home patients with an early diagnosis and all necessary subsequent assistance. For this purpose, it was necessary to acquire a fleet of vehicles suitable for the transport of infected patients, water inspection and disinfection, transport of beds, clothes and other materials necessary for the anti-epidemic battle, in addition to the movement of health and technical personnel (Figs. 15 a-e).

The leading equipment already in place at the Disinfection Station was reinforced with new units (Geneste & Herscher oven, formalization and sulfurization chamber), a changing room, deworming station, laundry, storage of transportable material for setting up emergency hospitals, collapsible tents, observation and consultation facilities, vaccine control and handling laboratories, equipment for chlorine, water purification, and a material repair workshop among other benefits. Particular attention was paid to preventing contact between objects subjected to disinfection. To this end, steam double-doored disinfection ovens were built in the walls of the rooms, each door opening into a different room, one for receiving the objects to be disinfected and the other for collecting the disinfected (José Faria 1951, 1951).

---

[125] Portaria de 22 de Abril de 1899, 83.

[126] Decreto de 18 de Outubro de 1927, pp.1995-1996; Decreto de 18 de Abril de 1929, p.975.

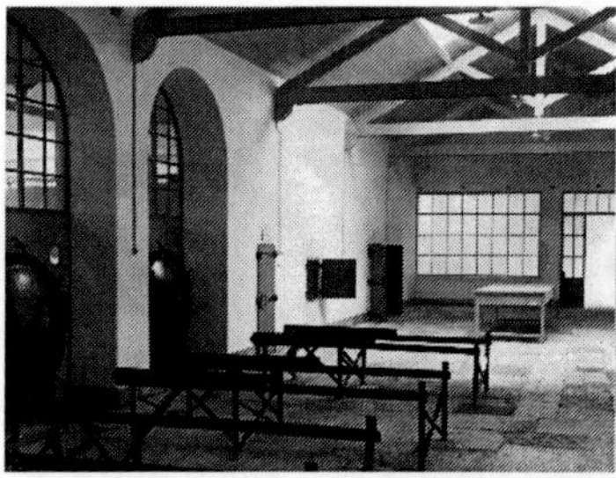

(a)

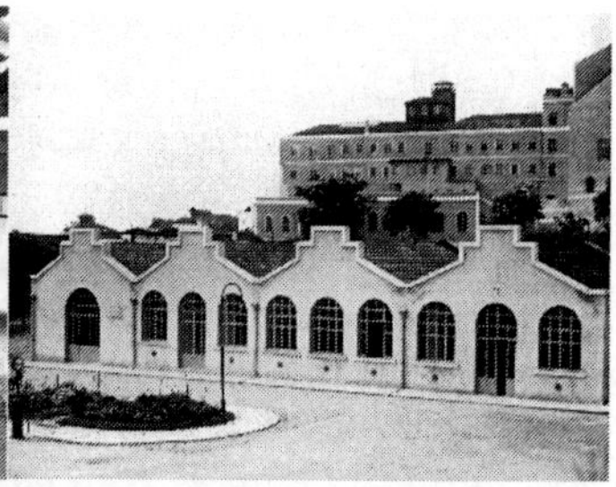

(b)

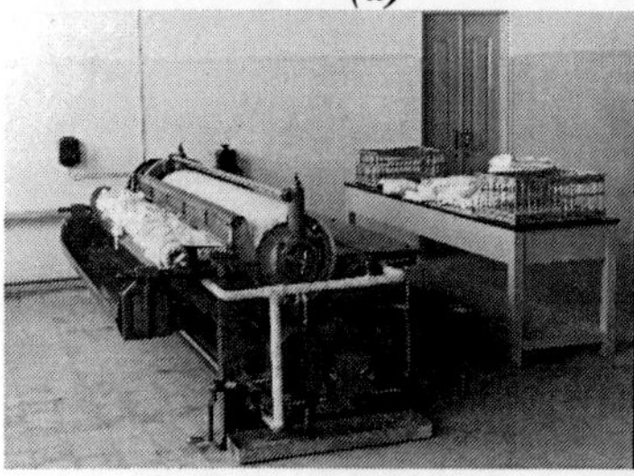

(c)

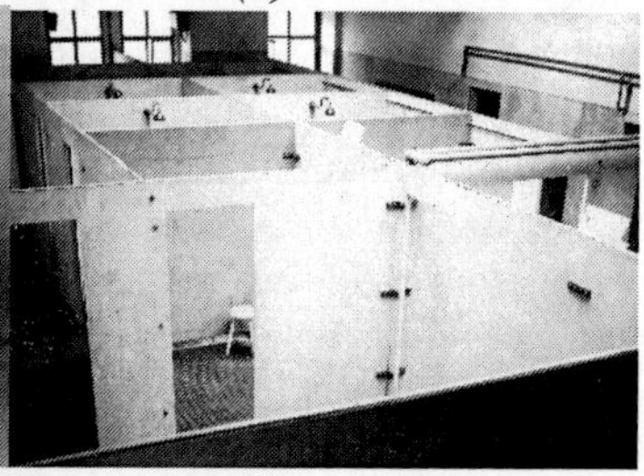

(d)

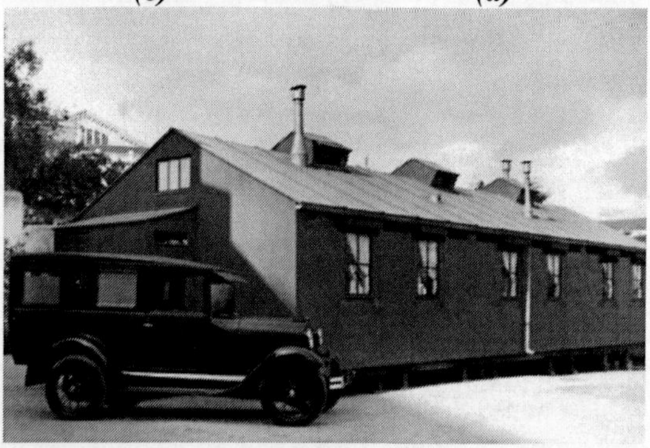

(e)

Fig. 8.15a. Lisbon Sanitary Park. Entrance of the Disinfection Greenhouses; on the left, part of two Geneste & Hercher autoclaves for disinfection and sterilization; in the centre, supports and workbenches; Fig. 8.15 b. Laundry and Hospitalization Material Warehouse. Fig. 8.15c. Ironing: ironing machine and laundry transport baskets. Fig. 8.15d. Bathhouse and Delousing; the bathhouse was divided into shower areas, and a delousing area. Fig. 8. 15e. Mobile Hospital and Car Ambulance. Unknown author. Photo: Museu da Saúde, Instituto Nacional de Saúde Doutor Ricardo Jorge.

The land and structures of this institution in Lisbon remained under the auspices of the Directorate-General for Health until 1993, when it became the new Campus of the *Instituto Superior de Economia e Gestão* (ISEG).

Conclusion

This essay presents the structure and functions performed by the Health Station, Lazaretto, Maritime Disinfection Station, Public Disinfection Station and Sanitary Park in Lisbon. Design, structure and function were based on a seventeenth-century regulation with later adaptations, extended to all the ports of the Portuguese Kingdom. Prophylactic care to prevent the spread of epidemic outbreaks in the national territory, such as lockdown and systematic disinfection of passengers (plus possible treatment of the sick, when required) and disembarked goods, resulted in the establishment of a first provisional lazaretto annexed to the port of Lisbon in the sixteenth century. Subsequent adaptations followed until the completion of a definitive lazaretto in the second half of the 19th century. As the distance between the lazaretto on the south bank of the Tagus River and the Lisbon health station on the north bank was a permanent source of discomfort and presented difficulties for the disembarked travelers and the effectiveness of the services involved, most services at the lazaretto and health station were merged in a new institution, the Lisbon Maritime Disinfection Station. The new facilities opened at the beginning of the twentieth century. The restructuring of the health services in 1901 consolidated a new development step with the construction of the Lisbon Public Disinfection Station, later renamed the Sanitary Park, to prevent and protect the entire population against a wide range of infectious diseases.

Acknowledgments

My gratitude goes to my colleague Dr. Maria do Sameiro Barroso for clarifying textual details and assisting in the production of an accurate translation. Also, I thank to the Arch. António Duarte Correia for technically improving the images used in this work.

Archival Sources and References

Arquivo histórico da câmara municipal de lisboa

Chancelaria Régia, Livro 5º de registo de consultas e decretos de D. Pedro II.
Chancelaria Régia, Livro 2º de consultas e decretos de D. João V do Senado Ocidental.
Chancelaria Régia, Livro 3º de Consultas e Decretos de D. João V, do Senado Oriental.
Chancelaria Régia, Livro 3º de consultas e decretos de D. João V do Senado Ocidental.
Chancelaria Régia, Livro 4º de consultas e decretos de D. João V do Senado Ocidental
Chancelaria Régia, Livro 5º de Consultas e Decretos de D. João V, do Senado Oriental.
Chancelaria Régia, Livro 6º de Consultas e Decretos de D. João V, do Senado Oriental.
Chancelaria Régia, Livro 15º de consultas e decretos de D. João V do Senado Ocidental.
Chancelaria Régia, Livro 18º de consultas e decretos de D. João V do Senado Ocidental.
Chancelaria Régia, Livro 8º de consultas, decretos e avisos de D. José I. Chancelaria Régia, Livro 9º de consultas, decretos e avisos de D. José I. Chancelaria Régia, Livro 17º de consultas, decretos e avisos de D. José I.
Chancelaria Régia, Livro 18º de consultas, decretos e avisos de D. José I.
Chancelaria Régia, Livro 5º de registo de avisos de D. Maria I.
Chancelaria Régia, Livro 1º de registo de decretos de D. João VI
Chancelaria Régia, Livro de consultas de 1795-1797, de D. João VI.
Provimento da Saúde, Cópia do Livro 1º do provimento da saúde.
Provimento da Saúde, Pasta n.º 2 de reais avisos expedidos das Secretarias de Estado.
Provimento da Saúde, Pasta n.º 3 de papéis remetidos das Secretarias de Estado. Provimento da Saúde, Pasta n.º 5 da Provedoria-Mor da Saúde da Corte e Reino.
Provimento da Saúde, Livro de registo de decretos, alvarás e ordens da casa da saúde.
Provimento da Saúde, Pasta n.º 6 da Intendência-Geral da Polícia da Corte e Reino.
Provimento da Saúde, Pasta n.º 7 da Corte e Província da Estremadura.

Provimento da Saúde, Pasta n.º 8 de papéis pertencentes à Província do Alentejo.
Provimento da Saúde, Livro de registo dos avisos da Secretaria de Estado à Provedoria-mor da Saúde.

Legislação Régia

Alvará de 4 de Novembro de 1800, D. João, Regente do Reino (1792-1816), Livro 1791-1801.
Carta de Lei de 10 de Fevereiro de 1844, D. Maria II, Leis e Ordenações, maço 17, n.º 2.
Decreto de 21 de Outubro de 1804, D. João, Regente do Reino (1792-1816), Livro 1802-1810.
Decreto de 20 de Outubro de 1813, Governo do Reino, Livro 1812-1814.
Decreto de 22 de Outubro de 1815, Governo do Reino, Livro 1815-1816.
Decreto de 3 de Janeiro de 1837, D. Maria II (1826-1827; 1834-1853), Livro 1837 - 1º Semestre.
Decreto de 18 de Setembro de 1844, Sem Entidade, Livro de 1844.
Decreto de 26 de Novembro de 1845, D. Maria II (1826-1827; 1834-1853), Livro 1845.
Decreto de 28 de Junho de 1851, Ministério do Reino, Livro 1851.
Decreto de 15 de Dezembro de 1851, Ministério do Reino, Livro 1851.
Decreto de 3 de Dezembro de 1868, Ministério do Reino, Livro 1868.
Decreto de 29 de Maio de 1872, Ministério das Obras Públicas, Livro 1872.
Decreto de 12 de Novembro de 1874, Ministério do Reino, Livro 1874.
Decreto de 27 de Junho de 1879, Ministério do Reino, Livro 1879.
Decreto de 4 de Outubro de 1889, Ministério do Reino, Livro 1889.
Decreto de 17 de Outubro de 1891, Ministério do Reino, Livro 1891.
Decreto de 24 de Setembro de 1892, Ministério do Reino, Livro 1892.
Decreto de 12 de Abril de 1894, Ministério do Reino, Livro 1894.
Decreto de 28 de Abril de 1894, Ministério do Reino, Livro 1894.
Decreto de 4 de Maio de 1894, Ministério do Reino, Livro 1894.
Decreto de 12 de Julho de 1894, Ministério do Reino, Livro 1894.
Decreto de 21 de Janeiro de 1897,Ministério do Reino, Livro 1897.
Decreto de 17 de Agosto de 1899, Ministério da Fazenda, Livro 1899.
Decreto de 23 de Agosto de 1899, Ministério do Reino, Livro 1899.
Decreto de 17 de Maio de 1901, Ministério do Reino, Livro 1901.
Decreto de 19 de Julho de 1901, Ministério do Reino, Livro 1901.
Decreto de 24 de Dezembro de 1901, Ministério do Reino, Livro 1901.
Decreto de 24 de Maio de 1902, Ministério do Reino, Livro 1902.
Decreto de 11 de Dezembro de 1902, Ministério do Reino, Livro 1902.

Decreto de 23 de Maio de 1904, Ministério do Reino, Livro 1904.
Decreto de 30 de Novembro de 1905, Ministério do Reino, Livro 1905.
Decreto de 18 de Outubro de 1927, Diário do Governo, I Série, Nº230.
Edital de 22 de Outubro de 1800, Junta da Saúde, Livro 1791-1801.
Edital de 8 de Outubro de 1804, Junta da Saúde, Livro 1802-1804.
Edital de 5 de Abril de 1816, Junta da Saúde, Livro 1815-1816.
Edital de 10 de Maio de 1816, Junta da Saúde, Livro 1815-1816.
Edital de 8 de Fevereiro de 1819, Provedor, Livro 1817-1820
Edital de 16 de Julho de 1853, Conselho de Saúde Pública, Livro 1853.
Edital de 9 de Setembro de 1853, Conselho de Saúde Pública, Livro 1853.
Edital de 8 de Abril de 1858, Conselho de Saúde Pública, Livro 1858.
Edital de 26 de Janeiro de 1859, Conselho de Saúde Pública, Livro 1858.
Edital de 25 de Abril de 1859, Conselho de Saúde Pública, Livro 1859.
Edital de 8 de Março de 1860, Conselho de Saúde Pública, Livro 1860.
Lei de 7 de Abril de 1845, Sem Entidade, Livro 1845.
Lei de 10 de Abril de 1874, Ministério do Reino, Livro 1874.
Lei de 6 de Abril de 1876, Ministério do Reino, Livro 1876.
Lei de 9 de Fevereiro de 1876, Ministério do Reino, Livro 1876.
Lei de 21 de Junho de 1880, Ministério do Reino, Livro 1880.
Lei de 27 de Junho de 1881, Ministério do Reino, Livro 1881.
Ofício de 15 de Setembro de 1854, Conselho de Saúde Pública, Livro 1854.
Ofício de 3 de Abril de 1858, Ministério da Marinha, Livro 1858.
Provisão de 27 de Julho de 1807, Governo do Reino, Livro 1802-1810.
Portaria de 28 de Agosto de 1813a, Governo do Reino, Livro 1812-1814.
Portaria de 28 de Agosto de 1813b, Governo do Reino, Livro 1812-1814.
Portaria de 28 de Agosto de 1813c, Governo do Reino, Livro 1812-1814.
Portaria de 29 de Julho de 1834, Secretaria de Estado dos Negócios do Reino, Livro 1833-1834.
Portaria de 18 de Maio de 1836, Sem Entidade, Livro 1836, 1º Semestre.
Portaria de 2 de Outubro de 1839, Secretaria de Estado dos Negócios da Fazenda, Livro 1839.
Portaria de 26 de Março de 1840, Secretaria de Estado dos Negócios do Reino, Livro 1840
Portaria de 15 de Julho de 1847, Ministério do Reino, Livro 1855.
Portaria de 5 de Maio de 1850, Ministério do Reino, Livro 1850.
Portaria de 6 de Fevereiro de 1854, Ministério do Reino, Livro 1854.
Portaria de 28 de Novembro de 1856, Ministério do Reino, Livro 1856.
Portaria de 12 de Maio de1858, Ministério do Reino, Livro 1858.
Portaria de 28 de Outubro de 1858, Ministério das Obras Públicas, Livro 1858.

Portaria de 14 de Julho de 1859, Ministério do Reino, Livro 1859.
Portaria de 28 de Setembro de 1860, Ministério das Obras Públicas, Livro 1860.
Portaria de 10 de Fevereiro de 1871, Ministério do Reino, Livro 1871.
Portaria de 1 de Fevereiro de 1876, Ministério do Reino, Livro 1876.
Portaria de 15 de Outubro de 1898, Ministério do Reino, Livro 1898.
Portaria de 22 de Abril de 1899, Ministério do Reino, Livro 1899,
Portaria de 11 de Novembro de 1902, Ministério das Obras Públicas, Diário do Governo nº 256 de 12 de Novembro.
Portaria de 3 de Outubro de 1905, Ministério da Marinha e Ultramar, Diário do Governo, n.º 225, de 5 de Outubro.
Regimento de 20 de Dezembro de 1693, D. Pedro II (1667-1706), Livro 1683-1700.
Regimento de 20 de Dezembro de 1693, D. Pedro II (1667-1706), Livro 1683-1700b.
Regulamento de 18 de Julho de 1807, Governo do Reino, Livro 1802-1810.
Regimento de 22 de Outubro de 1815, Governo do Reino, Livro 1815-1816.

Arquivos e Relatórios Oficiais
Anais de Saúde Pública do Reino, publicados pela Inspecção Geral dos Serviços Sanitários, Secção de Legislação, Tomo II. Lisboa: Imprensa Nacional, 1904,155-170.

Periódicos
Diário de Notícias, 11 de Novembro de 1899
Jornal de Notícias, 12 de Novembro de 1899.

References

Abreu, Laurinda. 2018. "A luta contra as invasões epidémicas em Portugal: políticas e agentes, séculos XVI-XIX". *Ler História*, 73: 93-120.
Alvarez Thomaz; Salcedo, Garcia de.1598. *Recopilaçam das cousas que conuem guardarse, no modo de preseruar à cidade de Lisboa: e os sãos, e curar os q[ue] esteuere[m] de peste.* Lisboa: Casa Sebastião Carvalho.
Bakija-Konsuo, Ana. 2018. "Lazarettos – From Isolation to Contemporary Scientific Medical Findings. Rich Medical History of Dubrovnik Written in Stone". In: Milošević, Ante, ed. *Lazaretto in Dubrovnik: The Beginning of the Quarantine Regulation in Europe*, 65-82. Dubrovnik: ALFA 2 d.o.o.

Barbosa, Inácio de Vilhena.1864. "Novo lazareto da Torre Velha". *Archivo Pittoresco: semanário ilustrado*. VI (27):209-210.

Bíblia Católica. Available online (Accessed on 31st July, 2021): https://www.liturgiacatolica.com/biblia-catolica.html

Bivar, Carlos. 1945. "O lazareto". *Gazeta dos Caminhos de Ferro*, 56 (1374):133-134.

Byrne, Joseph P.2008. *Encyclopedia of Pestilence, Pandemics, and Plagues*. Foreword by Fauci, Anthony S. Westport, Connecticut: Greenwood Press.

Cliff, Andrew D; Smallman-Raynor, Matthew R.; Stevens, Peta M. 2009. "Controlling the geographical spread of infectious disease: plague in Italy, 1347–1851". *Acta medico-historica Adriatica*, 7 (1):197-236.

Cyrus, Cynthia. 2021. "Five strategies in sixteenth-century tertiaries' prayers against pestilence". *Academia Letters*, Article 479: 1-5.

Domingues d'Oliveira, José. 1911. *Sanidade Marítima*. Porto: Typoghraphia Santos.

Ennes, Guilherme José. 1896. *A Desinfecção Publica em Lisboa*. Lisboa: Imprensa Nacional.

Ennes, Guilherme José. 1901. *Processos e Progressos da Desinfecção Publica de Lisboa*. Lisboa: Livraria Nacional e Estrangeira de José Antonio Rodrigues, ed.

Faria, Manoel Seferim de. 1740. *Notícias de Portugal*. Lisboa Occidental: Officina de Antonio Isidoro da Fonseca.

Fracastoro, Girolamo. 1893. *De Contagionibus et Contagiosis Morbis et eorum Curatione* (1546). Meunier, Léon, tradotto in francese. Paris: Société d'éditions Scientifiques.

Franco, Francisco. 1569. *Libro das enfermedades contagiosas y de la preseruation dellas*. Seuilla: Impresso por Afonso de la Barrera.

Frazâo, António. 1897. "Lazareto de Lisboa". *Branco e Negro: semanário ilustrado*, 60:112-118.

Gimbel, Lena Mackenzie. 2012. *Bawdy badges and the Black Death: late medieval apotropaic devices against the spread of the plague*. Electronic Theses and Dissertations. University of Louisville. Paper 497. (Accessed on 2nd June, 2021): https://ir.library.louisville.edu/etd/497/

Gomes, Bernardino António, filho. 1858."Apontamentos para a historia epidemiólogica Portuguesa. Ephocas das grandes epidemias que reinaram em Portugal, segundo os documentos impressos". *Gazeta Medica de Lisboa*, 6 (126):81-85.

Hippocrates. 1959. *Hippocrates. Heracleitus on the Universe*. Vol. IV. Page, T.E. *et alii*, eds. Jones W. H. S. trans. London: William Heinemann Ltd.

Isidore of Seville. 1857. *De Natura Rerum Liber (Book on the Nature of Things)*. Becker, Gustavus, ed. Berlin: Weidmann.

Jouanna, Jacques. 2012. "Hippocratic medicine and Greek tragedy". In: Scarborough, John; Van der Eijk, Philip; Hanson, Ann Ellis; Ziegler, Joseph, eds. Allies Neil, trans. *Studies in Ancient Medicine- Greek Medicine from Hippocrates to Galen: Selected Papers*. Vol. 40. Leiden: Brill.

Loureiro, Adolpho. 1907. *Os portos marítimos de Portugal e ilhas adjacentes*. Atlas. Vol. III. Lisboa: Imprensa Nacional.

Milošević, Ante. 2018. "Quarantine and lazarettos in Dubrovnik: fortuna critica et historica". *In* Milošević, Ante, ed., *Lazaretto in Dubrovnik: The Beginning of the Quarantine Regulation in Europe*. Institute for Restoration of Dubrovnik. Dubrovnik: ALFA 2 d.o.o, 167-214.

Oliveira, Eduardo Freire. 1901a. *Elementos para História do Município de Lisboa*. 1ª Parte, Tomo XI. Lisboa: Tipografia Universal.

Oliveira, Eduardo Freire. 1901b. *Elementos para História do Município de Lisboa*. 1ª Parte, Tomo XII. Lisboa: Tipografia Universal.

Oliveira, Eduardo Freire. 1904. *Elementos para História do Município de Lisboa*, 1ª Parte, Tomo XIV. Lisboa: Tipografia Universal.

Oliveira, Eduardo Freire. 1908. *Elementos para História do Município de Lisboa*. 1ª Parte, Tomo XVI. Lisboa: Tipografia Universal.

Regimento de 1693. *Collecção Chronologica da Legislação Portugueza. 1683-1700*. Compilada e Annotada por André Justino de Andrade e Silva, 1859, 333-340.Lisboa: Imprensa Nacional.

Sehdev, Paul S.2002."The origin of quarantine". *Clinical Infectious Diseases*, 35 (9):1071-1072.

Silva, António Delgado da. 1828. *Collecção de Legislação Portugueza desde a Ultima Compilação de Ordenações,1791-1801*. Lisboa: Typografia Maigrense.

Silva, João Martins e.2020. "The appearance of bubonic plague in Porto, 1899". *Vesalius*, 26 (1, e-supplement): 212-241.

Silva, Luiz Augusto Rebello da. 1860. *História de Portugal*. Vol.1. Lisboa: Imprensa Nacional.

Silva, Luiz Augusto Rebello da. 1871. *História de Portugal*. Vol.5. Lisboa: Imprensa Nacional.

Sousa, Manuel de Farya y. 1675. *Asia Portuguesa*. Tomo III. Lisboa: Officina de Antonio Craesbecck de Mello.

Sousa, Raúl Henrique Pereira de.1981. *Fortalezas de Almada e seu Termo*. Almada: Edição do Arquivo Histórico da Câmara Municipal de Almada.

Stathakopoulos, Dionysios. 2005." La peste de Justinien (541-750): questions médicales et la réponse sociale". *Médecine et Société de l'Antiquité à nos Jours*, 31 - 48. Rouen : Cahiers du GRHIS.

Stathakopoulos, Dionysios. 2007."Crime and Punhishment: the evidence of non-literary sources". *In* Little, Lester K. *Plague and The End of Antiquity*, 99-118. Cambridge: Cambridge University Press.

Ziekler, Philip. (2009). *The Black Death*. New York: Harper Perennial Modern Classics.

Further Links

Centro de Arqueologia de Almada- *Porto Brandão, a Terra e o Tejo*. Available online (Accessed on 15th February, 2020): http://www.caa.org.pt/pdf/Expo%20Porto%20Brand%C3%A3o%20Total.pdf

CHAPTER 9

JACOB DE CASTRO SARMENTO (1691-1762): A BRIEF REVIEW

CHRISTOPHER J. DUFFIN

Abstract

Jacob de Castro Sarmento was trained as a physician in Portugal, but fled the Inquisition, arriving in London in 1721. There, he integrated into the Sephardic community and became a congregant at Bevis Marks Synagogue, enjoying close relations with Rabbi David Nieto and dedicating his expertise to founding and serving the Beth Holim hospital. The first successful Jew to obtain a domestic MD from Aberdeen University, Sarmento was elected Licentiate of the Royal College of Physicians in 1725 and FRS in 1730. His scientific work included an account of variolation for smallpox in 1721, and a series of publications in Portuguese designed to introduce Newtonian science to the country of his birth. Sarmento took pains to advertise his own proprietary medicines based on "secret" recipes, such as that for *Água de Inglaterra*, the quinine-containing "Water of England", wherever possible.

Key words: Jacob de Castro Sarmento; Sephardic Jews; smallpox; Water of England; *materia medica*

Resumo

Jacob de Castro Sarmento concluiu a sua formação médica em Portugal, mas fugiu da Inquisição, chegando a Londres em 1721. Integrou-se na comunidade sefardita da cidade, tendo sido acolhido na congregação da Sinagoga Bevis Marks e mantido relações estreitas com o rabino David Nieto. Participou na fundação do hospital Beth Holim, no qual desenvolveu o seu trabalho como médico. Foi o primeiro judeu a conseguir uma licenciatura na Universidade de Aberdeen, tendo sido autorizado a exercer a medicina pelo the Royal College of Physicians em 1725, tornando-se membro efectivo em 1730. O seu trabalho científico incluiu um relato de inoculação da varíola em 1721 e uma série de publicações em português,

destinadas a introduzir a ciência newtoniana no seu país natal. Sarmento divulgou o mais que lhe foi possível os seus medicamentos patenteados com base em receitas "secretas", tais como a da Água de Inglaterra que continha a quinina como principal princípio activo.
Palavras-Chave: Jacob de Castro Sarmento; judeus sefarditas; varíola; Água de Inglaterra; *materia medica*

Introduction

Jacob de Castro Sarmento (1691-1762; Fig. 9.1) was a Portuguese émigré to early Georgian London. Trained in Portugal as a medical practitioner, he seems to have been a complex character who led a colourful life marked both by success and controversy. Rather than being entirely lost to his homeland, Sarmento made significant and pioneering contributions to Portuguese intellectual and philosophical development, as well as making an impact on the English scientific scene. He is an excellent example of an *estrangeirado* or "Europeanised intellectual" who introduced and disseminated scientific ideas into Portugal from a relatively peripheral, remote position (Simões et al. 1999, 2000; Carneiro et al. 2000). He has been the subject of several biographical studies from both Portuguese and English perspectives (e.g. Lemos 1910; d'Esaguy 1946a, 1946b; Barnett 1978-80; Andrade and Guimarães 2010).

Early life in Portugal

King D. Manuel I (sometimes referred to as "The Fortunate"; 1469-1521) passed an edict in 1496 decreeing that all Jews should convert to Christianity; if they were unable to do so they were forced to exit the country, leaving their children behind. The aim of the Inquisition was to combat heresy. On the Iberian Peninsula, the impact of this movement began in the fifteenth century. The *Tribunal del Santo Oficio de la Inquisición* or Spanish Inquisition was established in 1478. Although initially enjoying good relations with the Jews in Portugal, D. Manuel I hoped to marry Isabella of Aragon (1470-1498), a match which might potentially lead to his becoming King of Castile. Isabella agreed to the marriage only if Manuel expelled those Portuguese Jews who refused to convert to Christianity. The couple married in September 1497 and so began a protracted period of persecution of Portuguese jewry. Following Isabella's death, Manuel married her younger sister, Maria (1482-1517). Manuel petitioned Pope Leo X (Giovanni di Lorenzo de' Medici; 1475-1521) to establish the Portuguese Inquisition in 1515, but was refused. Pope Paul III

(Alessandro Farnesi; 1468-1549) eventually permitted the installation of the Inquisition, but only after Manuel had died. Manuel's son, King D. João III (1501-1557), also referred to as "The Pious", introduced the Inquisition in Portugal in 1536 (López-Salazar 2013).

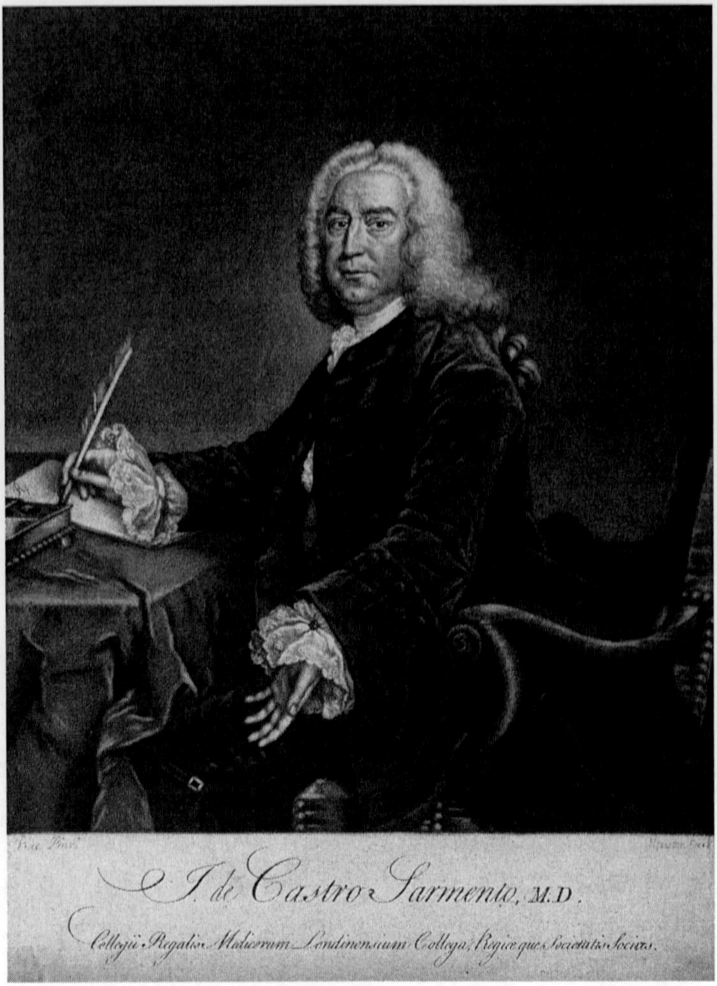
J. de Castro Sarmento, M.D.
Collegii Regalis Medicorum Londinensium Collega, Regiæque Societatis Socius.

Fig. 9.1 Jacob de Castro Sarmento (1691-1762). Mezzotint by R. Houston after R. E. Pine. Wellcome Collection, Public Domain Mark.

Thus, the establishment of the Portuguese Court of Inquisition has mostly been attributed to the religious fervour and cruelty of King D. João III (Herculano 2009; Martins 2004, 251-259). However, more recently, new research suggests that the whole process seems to have been much more complicated. At that particular time, King D. João III was too busy managing the governance of the vast empire that his father had left to him. What appears to be beyond doubt is that the Spanish kings pressed the Portuguese to follow them in persecuting the Jews. Given the close relationship between the Portuguese and Spanish royal families, the Portuguese were more-or-less obliged to accept their political views (on this subject, see, Marcocci et al., 2011; Ramos et al., 2009, 238-239).

One of the prime targets of the Portuguese Inquisition was those Portuguese Jews who had converted to Christianity, but were suspected of practicing their former Jewish religion in secret. In consequence, Jews lost many of their rights of citizenship, such as being able to hold public office. Denunciations were common and helped to engender a culture of fear. Accusations of heresy were brought before a committee for assessment. If there seemed to be grounds for proof, the arrest of the individual was followed by sequestration of property and imprisonment whilst awaiting trial before the Tribunal. Interrogation might involve torture and was designed to elicit a confession. A guilty verdict resulted in an *auto-da-fé*, the final step in the inquisitorial process. This was a highly orchestrated ritual of public penance, centred around a Catholic Mass, in which numbers of prisoners judged to be guilty were paraded, their sentences read, and sometimes immediately carried out (e.g. Mocatta 1877).

The Sarmento family was a long-established Jewish dynasty residing for many generations in the geomorphologically highly varied historic province of Trás-os-Montes e Alto Douro, situated in the north east corner of Portugal. Jacob's parents were Francisco de Castro Almeida and his second wife, Violante Mesquita (Barnett 1978-80, 84). Both were Catholic converts from Judaism, often referred to as "New Christians" (also *Conversos* or *Marranos*). The family originally lived in the city of Bragança, at the centre of a dense population of *Conversos* and thus a target for the officers of the Inquisition. It was here that Henrique de Castro, later to be known as Jacob de Castro Sarmento, the second son of Francisco but the only one from his marriage to Violante, was born. Francesco earned his living as an *estanqueiro* – a licenced seller of commodities on behalf of an authorised monopoly. The family later moved south to the town of Grandola in the Alentejo Region, in what is now the Setúbal District of south-west Portugal. This may have been in response to the pressure of persecution then actively being promoted in Trás-os-Montes. The move did not secure the family's protection, however. On 5 September 1708, both Jacob's parents were arrested by the Inquisition. Violante died, presumably in prison, before the trial could take place. In the event, Francisco was found guilty. He was processed in the *auto-da-fé* held at Évora on 20 July 1710, had his property confiscated, was imprisoned and required to do penance. Despite what must have been straightened circumstances Jacob, probably cared for by relatives, was able to pursue his education. He went to school in Mértola, near the border with Spain, in the south east of the country. From here, he progressed to the University of Évora (Colégio dos Jesuítas de Évora), some 130 km to the north north west, where he received his MA in the same year as his father's *auto-da-fé.* In 1711 he moved further north still and enrolled at the University of Coimbra (d'Esaguy 1946a). Here, Jacob eventually qualified as MD in 1717.

Jacob then embarked on his medical career, firstly by practising as a physician at Beja in the Alentejo Basin, where he mostly treated the poor, and later moving to the Algarve. Unsubstantiated accounts suggest that he might himself have been imprisoned and subject to *auto-da-fé* (Barnett 1978-80, 84-85). It is certainly true that the Inquisition was active at Beja whilst Jacob was there (Sousa-Dias 2005). Francisco de Sá et Mesquita (b. 1680-1723) was frustrated in his ambition to work as a physician, having trained in the Faculty of Medicine at Coimbra University (graduated MD in 1703), and having confessed to the Inquisition of judaizing (following Jewish practices) even though he was a "New Christian". His envy of the success of his colleagues, particularly economically, led him to denounce around 100 people to the Inquisition of Lisbon on 9 September 1720. He raised specific complaints against his fellows for meeting together to celebrate the Hebrew Festival of Weeks. No result was forthcoming from the Inquisition at Lisbon, so he lodged a further denunciation (under a different name) at the Inquisition of Évora on 9 October 1720. Amongst those whom he denounced was Pedro Dias Nunes (dates unknown), with whom Jacob was in partnership, both in Beja and the Algarve (Barnett 1978-80, 84). Nunes was eventually absolved, but it seems that Jacob, in the face of accusations against many of his friends and colleagues, took the measure of leaving the country with his wife, Isabel Inácia. This seems to have raised suspicions of his collaborating with the Inquisition. Independent investigations were carried out both in Lisbon and in London, but the accusations remained unproven (Sousa-Dias 2005, 57). The Sarmentos made their way to London in 1721, travelling via Hamburg (Goldish 1997, 653), possibly to avoid pursuit.

Bevis Marks

In 1721, when Sarmento arrived in London, he seemed fully to embrace his original religious heritage and quickly integrated into the Sephardic congregation at Bevis Marks Synagogue; he changed his name from Henrique de Castro to Jacob de Castro Sarmento. His wife changed her name to Raquel and the pair renewed their marriage vows on 10 March.

After some 200 years of increasingly intense persecution, the Edict of Expulsion issued by King Edward 1 on 18 July 1290, constituted a royal decree banishing all Jews from England. Over 350 years later, during the time of the Protectorate, Jews were permitted to return to the country. Resettlement of the Jews in England followed a period of increasing religious freedom and tolerance, and two events in particular. One was the visit of the exiled Portuguese Rabbi Manoel Dias Soeiro (also known as Menasheh ben Yossef ben Yisrae; 1604-1657) from Amsterdam in 1655; he arrived as a guest of Oliver Cromwell (1599-1658) and petitioned for the return of the Jews to England. Then, in 1656 an Iberian New Christian, Antonio Rodrigues Robles (dates unknown), requested the return of his confiscated property because he belonged "to the Hebrew Nation" rather than being Spanish, against which country war had just been declared. This coincided with a petition from other members of his community for permission to be able to gather together for worship and to acquire a burial ground for their dead. While no formal permissions were granted, Cromwell could see the economic benefits to the country and gave a verbal agreement, backed by the Council of State, allowing the Jews to return with the freedom to practise their faith. There followed a considerable influx of Jews, mostly from Portugal and Spain (Sephardic Jews), with a smaller contingent from Germany (Ashkenazi Jews). The Sephardim began worshipping in a small synagogue in Creechurch Lane from about 1663. Increasing numbers in the Congregation demanded larger premises so, in 1701, the Bevis Marks Synagogue was dedicated. It was to represent a centre of unparalleled importance in Jewish matters both in the UK and worldwide, for the next 100 years; the oldest synagogue in the UK, it is still going strong today with an unbroken period of over 300 years of religious services.

The Chief Rabbi (or *Hakham*) of the Anglo-Sephardic Community at the time when Sarmento attended the Congregation was Daniel Nieto (1654–1728), a physician and preacher originally from Leghorn (now Livorno) in Italy (Jacobs & Lipkind 1906, 302-303). A renowned intellectual, philosopher and prolific writer, Nieto's interests (in addition to medicine and theology) extended to mathematics, astronomy and poetry. He became the focal point for a group of Jewish intellectuals, of whom

Sarmento was surely one. Sarmento and Nieto clearly got on well together; Sarmento's published theological texts were all produced during Nieto's lifetime - the *Exemplar de Penitência* (three sermons in Portuguese for the Yom Kippur holiday) in 1724, and then in January 1728 a funeral sermon dedicated to Nieto (Sousa-Dias 2005, 58).

Beth Holim

The resettlement of Jews in London during the closing decades of the seventeenth century saw the establishment of a Spanish-Portuguese Sephardic community (the *Shaar Ashamaim* or "Gates of Heaven Congregation") from around 1656, and the setting up in 1687 of an associated *Hebrá* or Brotherhood whose full title was the *Hebrá de Bikur Holim e Gemilut Hasadim* (Brotherhood for Visiting the Sick and Acts of Loving Kindness) (Barnett 1978-80, 86; Lieberman 2017a, 112; Lieberman 2017b, 112). This was part of the system of *Sedaca* or charity exercised by the Congregation for the poor in the Jewish community. The roles of its members involved visiting the sick, preparing the body of the deceased and then providing for its burial. A separate *Hebrá* was founded by David Nieto in 1709 with the responsibility of caring for the sick. The two Brotherhoods eventually combined and were sustained by *sedaca* funds which paid for a doctor and a surgeon who ministered to the "ailing poor" (Lieberman 2017b, 112).

The increasingly zealous and extensive activities of the Inquisition, especially during the 1720s led to a surge in Portuguese migration to London, the Sarmentos among them. It has been estimated that about 3000 Iberian refugees, mostly from Portugal, arrived and settled in the London Sephardi community (Lieberman 2017b). The community itself helped a number of the migrants to make the journey by providing financial assistance. Whilst some of the migrants belonged to wealthy families or were (like the Sarmentos) affluent merchants or professionals who quickly became self-sufficient after their arrival, most of the refugees were severely impoverished. This dramatic influx placed increasingly heavily burdens on the *sedaca* funds and the level of provision they were expected to support. The response of the community to this burgeoning population of legitimately needy families was (Lieberman 2019) (1) to closely define which groups would be qualified to be placed on the *sedaca* roll, especially amongst the *forasteiros* (strangers or foreigners), and thus to receive support; (2) to encourage some to move, often with financial backing, to various British colonies in the New World; (3) to create voluntary subscription charities for the establishment of appropriate institutions.

One of these institutions, arguably the most effective, was the Beth Holim Hospital (House of the Sick), which was funded and set up in relatively short order, the hospital opening its doors to the poor of the Sephardic community in 1748. At a meeting of the Committee of Management which took place on 14 October 1747, it was noted that "the poor at present often want the common necessaries of life, such as covering, bedding, lodging, a nurse and proper food for their disorders" and that a proposed hospital might assist "families of middling circumstances" in gaining access to "phisick on easy terms" (Barnett 1978-80, 91). Jacob and two other Jewish physicians offered their services to the hospital for free. It was proposed that a fact-finding visit should be made to the London Infirmary (later to become the Royal London Hospital) in order better to be able to assess what provision might be appropriate. The Infirmary had been established in autumn 1740 and, at the time, occupied premises in Prescott Street, a short distance away from Bevis Marks Synagogue in Whitechapel. Feedback was very positive and it was proposed that the hospital should accommodate 20 beds. The proposal was not without controversy (and a certain amount of melodrama), however; in March 1748 Jacob received an anonymous letter raising the spectre of imminent danger to the subscribers – there was the "intention to shoot those that have been authors and set their houses on fire" (Barnett 1978-80, 91). Thankfully, the threat never materialised.

On 4 September 1748, the inaugural meeting of the "Grand Committee" of the hospital took place, where it was reported that £747/4/10 ½ had been donated by subscription of the members of the Congregation to the cause. The first staff appointments were made – a dispenser, a matron, a secretary, an apothecary, a nurse, a watchman, a housemaid and two midwives. The hospital duly opened in rented accommodation in Leman Street near Whitechapel Road. The medical duties were taken up by three Committee members-Jacob de Castro Sarmento plus Philip de la Cour (1710-1785) served as physicians, while Jacob de Castro (dates unknown; no relative to Sarmento in spite of their similar names), formerly employed as the apothecary gave his services as a surgeon free of charge.

The next step was to develop a system of carefully considered plans. Sarmento and de la Cour proposed a set of 14 regulations which they considered to be representative of the prevailing practices at a range of London hospitals, but these were never formally incorporated into the Beth Holim regulations (Lieberman 2017, 118). The governance of the hospital depended upon a series of committees (see Lieberman 2017 for details). Sarmento served on the Grand Committee (*Junta Geral*) and the Medical Committee, which involved active participation in all planning aspects of the hospital. In appreciation for the donation of their time and expertise, the members of the Medical Committee were named founders or subscribers of the hospital, their subscription fees were waived, and they were permitted to attend the meetings of the hospital directors (although their decision-making powers were limited to medical matters).

In addition to their administrative commitments and day-to-day investment of time, effort and expertise as hospital medical personnel, de Castro Sarmento and de la Cour contributed to the publication of a pharmaceutical formulary for use at Beth Holim (Berman 1960). The *Pharmacopoeia Contracta in usum Nosocomii ad Pauperes e gente Lusitanica curandos nuper instituti* ("Pharmacopoeia drawn up for the use of the hospital recently set up for the poor of the Portuguese race") contained 238 pharmaceutical receipts and was authored by "J. de C.S. and P. de L." (Sarmento and de la Cour 1749; a second edition was published in 1770). This has been hailed as the first Pharmacopoeia to be published in England for an English hospital (Barnett 1978-80: 93). The *Pharmacopoeia Londinensis*, first published by the Royal College of Physicians in 1618, had gone through nine editions by 1718 (Fowler 2018). In 1747, the Royal College of Physicians published the *Pharmacopoeia Collegii Regalis Medicorum Londinensis* "to the Prevention of such Deceits in the making and compounding medicines, wherein the Lives and Health of his Majesty's Subjects are so highly concerned" (Royal College of Physicians 1747, vi-vii). Sarmento surely knew of this publication as he is listed as one of the College *Candidati* (Royal College of Physicians 1747, xiv).

Since Sarmento was co-author of the *Pharmacopoeia Contracta* and cited in the slightly earlier *Pharmacopoeia* from the Royal College, it might be interesting to see the degree of similarity between the two. Both books begin with an introductory dedicatory letter, followed by a section on Weights and Measures. This is followed by a list of *materia medica*. Almost 95% of the items of *materia medica* (133 of a total of 138) in the *Pharmacopoeia Contracta* are also found in the *Pharmacopoeia Collegii Regalis Medicorum Londinensis.* This is not unexpected as the pool of available and recommended items of *materia medica* was reasonably limited and a high degree of similarity probably existed amongst the various national pharmacopoeia available at the time. Interestingly, the list of *materia medica* items in both cases does not necessarily correspond with the medicinal simples incorporated into the receipts which follow in the remainder of the formulary; some of these include simples not listed in the *materia medica* section.

The points of difference, although few, are also instructive. Some merely represent nomenclatural differences for identical items in the two lists, whilst others are items that conceivably hark back to Sarmento's Portuguese roots. The *Pharmacopoeia Contracta* lists *Balsamum Divi Thomae* (Balsam of St Thomas), known elsewhere as Tolu Balsam, a resinous exudate harvested by means of tapping the trunks of trees of *Myroxylon balsamum* (Family Fabaceae; South America). This is listed as *Balsamum tolutanum* in the London Pharmacopoeia. *Brasiliensis cortex* in the *Pharmacopoeia Contracta* must refer to the bark of *Cinchona brasiliensis*, a source of quinine, sometimes referred to in older literature as *China brasiliensis*. *Butuae radix* is the root of *Butea monospermae*, also a member of the Fabaceae, but this time from India; the plant is sometimes referred to as Bastard Teak or Flame-of-the-Forest. *Viscus quercinus* refers to Mistletoe that parasitises the Oak and was commonly used to treat epilepsy. Most interesting of all is Sarmento's listing of *Terra Lusitanica* or Lisbon Earth.

With regard to medical receipts, 60% of those recorded in the *Pharmacopoeia Contracta* are also found in the London Pharmacopoeia. Those restricted to the *Pharmacopoeia Contracta* include a number of waters (8), types of Bolus or large soft pill (17 in all), electuaries (11), enemas (3), gargles (2), draughts ("*Haustus*"; 8), infusions (4), Lacs or milks (4), linctuses (1), liniments (1), mixtures ("*Mistura*"; 7), pills (6), powders (4) and other occasional items such as syrups, tinctures and troches. Two of the powders contain the Portuguese Earth cited above – *Pulvis è Terra Lusitanica*. The first recipe recommends a powdered blend of *Terra Lusitanica*, gum arabic and cinnamon, while the second incorporates opium into the mix. Of the various medicinal earths in active use during the eighteenth century, the most popular were *Terra Lemnia*, *Terra Melitensis* and *Terra Silesiaca*, collected from Lemnos, Malta and Poland respectively (e.g. MacGregor 2013; Duffin 2013, 2019). *Terra Lusitanica* receives relatively infrequent mention by comparison.

The earliest mention of this medicinal earth in English pharmaceutical literature appears to have been by Samuel Dale (1659-1739; Fig. 9.2), an apothecary and physician born in the Whitechapel area but later working in Essex (Morris 1974; Burnby 2004). Dale originally published his *Pharmacologia* in 1693, "virtually a combined textbook of materia medica, pharmacology and therapeutics" (Morris 1974, 122; Dale's was the first publication to use the word "pharmacology"). It ran to several editions, some of them posthumous. *Terra Lusitanica* is introduced in his supplement to the main text in 1718 (Dale 1718, 10). Cited as "*Terra Portugallica*" or "Earth of Portugal", he indicated that it was a form of *terra sigillata* (sealed earth) impressed with the figure of a rose, and had styptic and astringent properties, being employed in cases of the bloody flux ("*in profluviis ventri valet*"). Sir John Hill (1714-1775) a keen contributor to

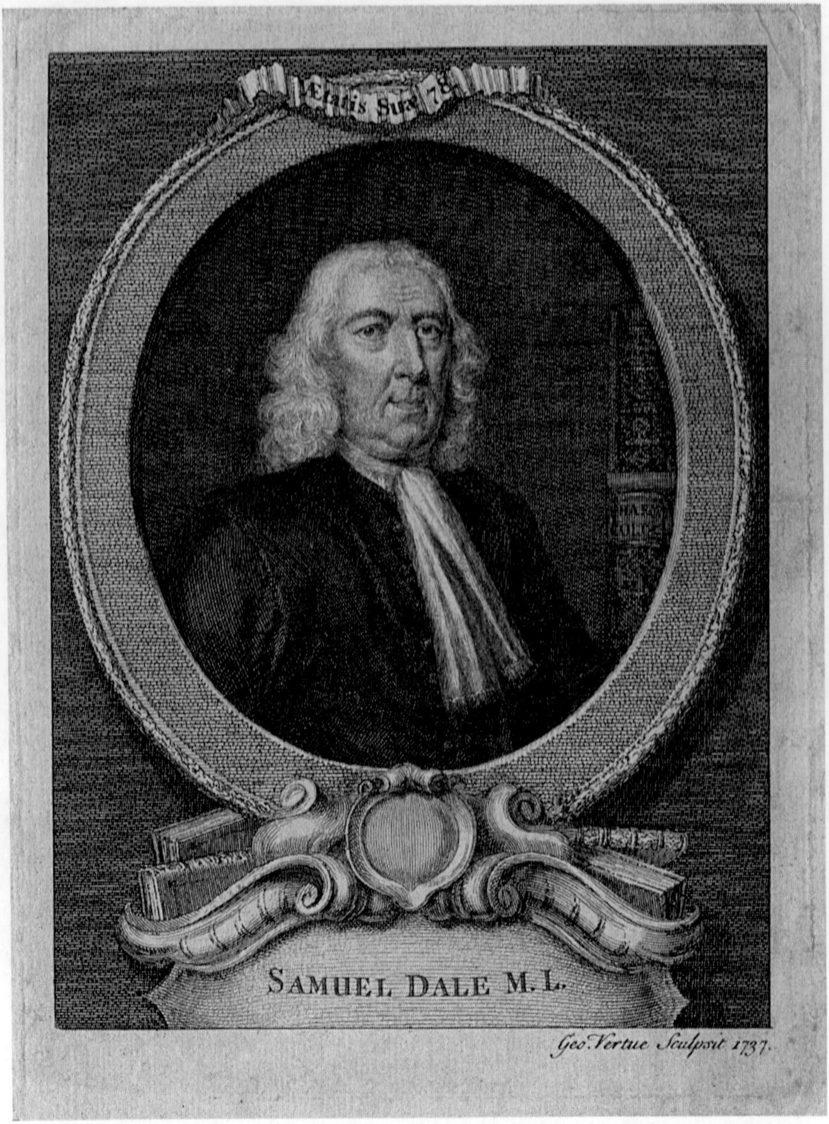

Fig. 9.2. Samuel Dale. Portrait of Samuel Dale, aged 78, line engraving 1737 by George Virtue. Wellcome Collection. Attribution 4.0 International (CC BY 4.0).

many areas of natural history and their links with the *materia medica* (Duffin 2018), later described the earth in some detail (Hill 1748, 13). Noting it to be "a very fine and valuable Earth" with a "manifest astringency", he stated that it was "dug in great plenty in the northern parts of Portugal", and was "esteemed a remedy against poisons, venomous bites, and malignant fevers" (Hill 1748, 13). In his slightly later *History of the Materia Medica*, Hill (1751, 188-189) noted that, at the time he was writing, *Terra Portugallica Rubra* was "neglected at present", but he thought it worthy of reintroduction to the goods normally stocked by an apothecary as a useful substitute for the counterfeit oriental boles then being sold. He indicates that it "is usually brought over to us made up into thin and flat Cakes, resembling small Segments of Cylinders, sealed with the Impression of a Wreathe round the Edges, and the Words *Terra Sigillata* filling up the space within" (Hill 1751, 189). Hill states further that it was long known amongst the Portuguese for curing malignant fevers and bites from venomous animals.

Hill had a complex relationship with the London-born Sephardic Jew, Emanuel Mendes da Costa (1717-1791; Duffin 2018) and who, in 1767, was caught embezzling funds from the Royal Society and consigned to a debtor's prison for a five-year sentence. Da Costa commented on two forms of *Terra Lusitanica*-one white and one red. He noted that they were found geologically adjacent to each other and mined, not in the northern parts of Portugal as claimed by Hill, but at Estremoz in the Province of Alentejo, which is in the south-eastern part of central Portugal, some 135 km due east of Lisbon. The area around Estremoz is most famous for its ornamental Palaeozoic marbles and dimension stones, which have been actively mined there since Roman times (Lopes & Martins 2015). The marbles crop out in the 45 km by 10 km, NE – SW trending Estremoz Anticline. Chemical weathering of the marbles has produced extensive deposits of a red, residual soil known as *Terra rossa* (Martins et al. 2013); this is likely the source of *Terra Lusitanica* cited by da Costa.

Da Costa (1757, 20) agrees with Hill (1751) concerning the properties of this "fine florid red" earth as an astringent, making it "an efficacious remedy for the cure of fluxes, and other distempers of the like kind". He notes that in both Spain and Portugal it was used historically as "a sovereign remedy against poisons of all kinds; and their women often chew it to correct the acids, and for a dentifrice, for which it is greatly extolled" (Da Costa 1757, 20). He also indicated that, whilst the British fleet was at anchorage in Lisbon during Queen Anne's War (1702-1713), the second in a series of French and Indian wars (effectively, the American theatre of the War of the Spanish Succession that was taking place in Europe), the forces suffered terribly from a "series of fluxes which then violently raged in the fleet". Extensive use of *Terra Lusitanica* brought considerable relief to those suffering from the debilitating conditions (Da Costa 1757, 20). Chambers (1781) notes that, later in the eighteenth century, *Terra Portugallica* was not stocked in English apothecary shops, the popular and cheaper *Bol Armoniac* or Armenian Bole having effectively replaced all similar materials. He notes further that *Terra Portugallica*, known alternatively as *Bucaros*, was also used to filter and cool water, as well as to produce earthenware.

Several of the more complex and formerly highly popular recipes in the London Pharmacopoeia, such as Andromachus' Theriac dating from the first century (e.g. Parojcic et al 2003), are omitted from the *Pharmacopoeia Contracta.* Conversely, otherwise popular recipes dropped from the London Pharmacopoeia, such as the *Confectio Alkermes*, appear in the *Pharmacopoeia Contracta,* albeit in much reduced form. The emphasis in the *Pharmacopoeia Contracta* seems to be on simplified recipes with minimal redundancy of ingredients, for which the medicaments would have been relatively easy to source (even those obtained from Portugal), and for which preparation would have been a comparatively simple process.

The early years of the Beth Holim hospital did not go smoothly. On 22 September 1748, Moses Pereyra de Castro, the clerk, was suspended for making financial errors; Jacob made up the missing sum from his own pocket. Then, on 6 May 1749, Mordechai de la Penha, the Apothecary, was suspended for "indecency" (sexual harrassment) toward a young English girl who had gone to the pharmacy to collect a medicine (Barrett 1978-80, 92; Lieberman 2017, 134). These events, combined with the fact that the votes of the governors in favour of the initial setting up of the hospital was in the majority by only 17 (for) to 13 (against), and that Sarmento and de la Cour decided that only the Sephardim should be treated (and the Ashkenazi excluded) led to a campaign of satirical criticism. An engraving (Fig. 9.3) entitled "*Jerusalem Infirmary alias A Journey to the Valley of Jehosaphat"* was published under a pseudonym; Barnett (1978-80) believes the perpetrator to have been Meyer Löw Schomberg (see below). This "ferociously scurrilous printed cartoon" depicts a meeting of the Grand Committee in which the members are seated at a table; Sarmento is depicted as Hippocrates (No 6 in the cartoon) and de la Cour as Galen (No 8). The speech bubbles are in Spanish rather than Portuguese and relate both to the admission of non-Sephardim Jews to the hospital, and to a dispute with Schomberg over the prescribing of opium to a patient. The latter event took place in 1738. Benjamin Mendes da Costa, a London merchant, had been

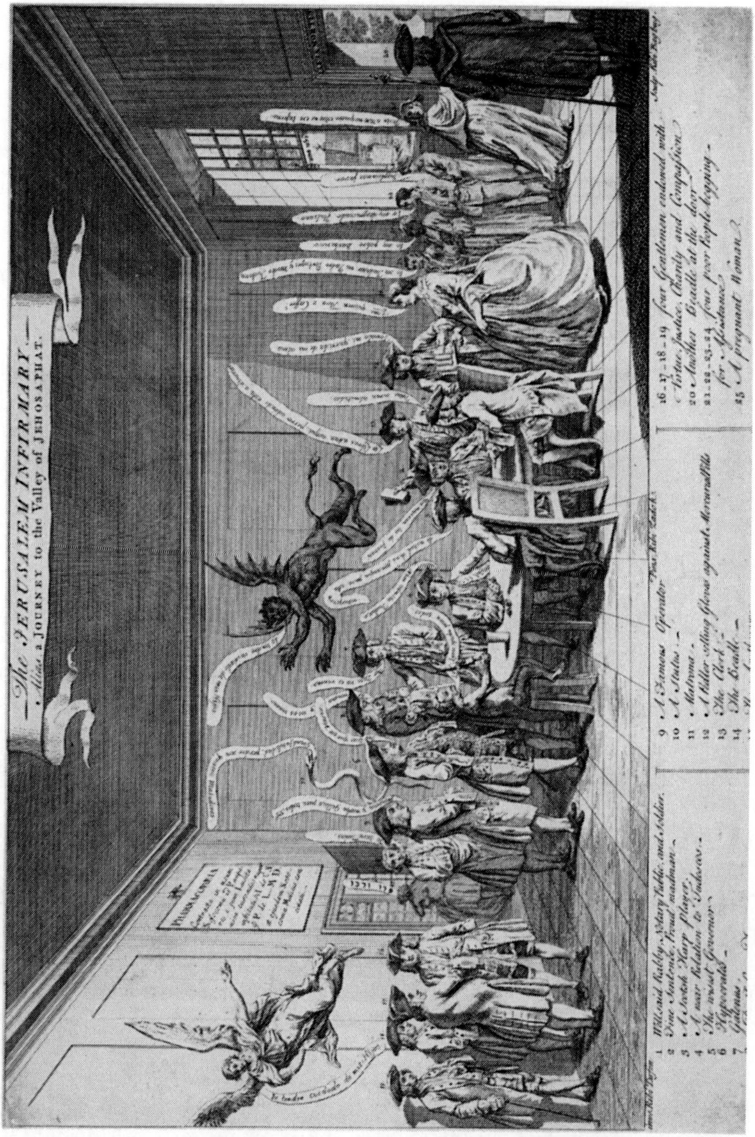

Fig. 9.3. The Jerusalem Infirmary, Alias, a Journey to the Valley of Jehosaphat. Satirical print circa 1750. © The Trustees of the British Museum.

treated by Schomberg for an extreme fever, but later requested treatment from Sarmento. Opium was prescribed for the patient but Schomberg, horrified, accused Sarmento of using a treatment which he, Schomberg, deemed to be both inappropriate and dangerous to the patient (perhaps because of difficulties in dose management and the possibility of addiction). His reputation thus being impugned, Sarmento took the complaint to the Disciplinary Committee of the Royal College of Physicians, who ruled in his favour and severely reprimanded Schomberg, ordering him to pay a fine of £4. Opium is one of the items of *materia medica* listed in the *Pharmacopoeia Contracta,* but absent from the London Pharmacopoeia. In the cartoon, a plaque on the wall depicts the title of the *Pharmacopoeia Contracta.*

A play with the same title as the cartoon was also circulated at the time. More detailed analysis of the two satirical works can be found in Barnett (1978-80, 92 ff., 104 ff.) and Rubens (1936, 119-123). The pressure seems to have preyed upon Sarmento; he attended his last Committee Meeting on 6 June 1750 and left the hospital. De la Cour also left (Collins 2019).

A physician in London

Would it be possible for the now thirty-year old, fully qualified and seemingly enthusiastic, committed physician with several years' experience of curative practice under his belt to make his way professionally in the medical world of early eighteenth-century London? Most of the fairly small number of Jewish doctors practising in London at this time had qualified abroad. Professional recognition and the freedom to practise medicine was achieved through the Royal College of Physicians, founded in 1518. Jacob became a Licentiate on 25 June 1725.

One means by which immigrant physicians could increase their social standing and acceptance as well, perhaps, as attracting potential patients, was to obtain a domestic medical degree. Jacob was something of a trailblazer in this respect. Marischal College in Aberdeen (later to combine with King's College to become the University of Aberdeen) awarded medical degrees, having had a Professor of Medicine in post since 1700. Awards of an MD degree were relatively few and far between, only 13 having been conferred when Jacob applied for consideration in 1739. The process involved the paying of a fee, which was £11/1/6 at the time of Jacob's application, but no period of residency at the College. £8 of the fee went to the Professor of Medicine. The candidate also required the support of at least two patrons who were willing to attest to the medical competence and reputation of the applicant. Jacob's supporters were of the highest standing. Sir Hans Sloane (1660-1753), a famous physician to high society in London was, at the time of Sarmento's application, serving as President of the Royal Society, following a stint as President of the Royal College of Physicians. Cromwell Mortimer (1702-1752) was a close friend of Sloane's who had studied under Herman Boerhaave (1668-1738) at Leiden and became Secretary to the Royal Society the year after supporting Sarmento's application (Gibbs 1950). Jacob's final supporter was Alexander Stewart (Collins 1984-1985, 15). Jacob was successful in his application and was awarded his Aberdeen MD. He was the first Jewish candidate to be recognised in this way; it would be another 6 years before the second Jewish medical graduate would be so honoured-Ralph Schomberg (1714-1792), one of twin physician sons of Meyer Schomberg (see below).

Sarmento must have met his eventual supporters for the Aberdonian degree at the Royal Society. Fellowship of this august and highly respected body was another means of cementing his credentials as a scientist of considerable ability. The path to Fellowship, however, was not a smooth one. He first applied in 1729; the Council Minutes for 11 December of that year record that the ballot for three new members had resulted in the admission of only two-Sarmento's application was unsuccessful (Barnett 1978-80, 103). The cause seems to have been rumours which werc circulating about his supposed collaboration with the Inquisition prior to his leaving Portugal, charges which he vigorously repudiated both in his home country and on his arrival in London. Indeed, the charge had been thoroughly investigated some 5 years earlier by the Sephardim wardens of Bevis Marks Synagogue, and Sarmento was found to be to be completely innocent of the charge and exonerated (Samuel 1959-1961, 91). The source of the complaint was Dr Meyer Löw Schomberg (1690-1761), an Ashkenazi German Jew who had studied at the University of Giessen, gaining his MD there in 1710. After moving to London in 1721 Schomberg began practising medicine and was admitted FRS on 12 January 1726, three years before Jacob's application. Sarmento was re-nominated for candidature and this time the results of the Ballot were in his favour; he was admitted FRS on 3 February 1730, in spite of letters of objection received by the Society from Schomberg and Stephen Hall (Barnett 1978-1980, 103). Schomberg was thenceforth his bitter enemy. This was not Schomberg's only dispute; he and his twin sons, Isaac and Ralph (see above) were involved in a protracted (and ultimately unsuccessful) battle with the Royal College of Physicians over the admission of Isaac to the College (Sakula 1994). Furthermore, Schomberg wrote a polemical attack-the *Emunat Omen*-seemingly directed especially towards Portuguese Jews, for perceived infractions against the

Ten Commandments, accompanied by a vigorous defence against similar accusations levelled at himself (Samuel 1959-1961).

Smallpox

Another means of establishing Sarmento's reputation and credentials as a serious medical scientist was to publish. His first publication was issued in both English and Latin versions and concerned inoculation against smallpox (Sarmento 1721, 1722; Fig. 9.4); the English version was published in London, described by one author as "the smallpox capital of England" (Williams 2010, 77) and the Latin one in Leiden.

The subject was extremely topical and not without contemporary controversy. The history of inoculation for smallpox has received considerable attention in the literature (e.g. Stearns & Pasti 1950; Behbehani 1983; Hopkins 2002; Williams 2010; Grant 2019), but Sarmento's publication is barely mentioned. A brief outline of the structure of Sarmento's work with a few contextualising notes will have to suffice here.

Sarmento's Dissertation is divided into three sections: (1) a brief history of smallpox with comments on its effects; (2) a brief review of contemporary means of treatment; (3) an account of inoculation. He wrote at a time when waves of the disease seemed annually to plague the streets of London; Sarmento described smallpox as "a foul and loathsome Distemper" (Sarmento 1721, 2). He considered that the disease was either "Epidemical", with spread depending on the "Constitution of the Air", or "Contagious" and spread by means of "Morbifick Effluvia" (pus and other materials) released from infected patients. This indicates that he followed the miasma theory of disease origins, particularly popular at the time he was writing, but dating back to classical times and holding sway until it was superseded by the germ theory in the nineteenth century (e.g. Jouanna 2012; Karamanou et al. 2012). Essentially, it was believed that corrupted (rather than life-giving and fresh) air, often identified by the presence of foul odours and issuing from geographically well-defined locations, on entering the body, spread poison to various parts of the body, especially the heart. The imbalance that this brought about led to the signs and symptoms of particular diseases, especially plague, malaria (whose name relates back to the idea of bad air) and smallpox. As a consequence, poisons accumulated at different sites in the body as various discolourations, discharges and smells, and could be released to infect both the surrounding air and, by direct contact, any who touched the patient.

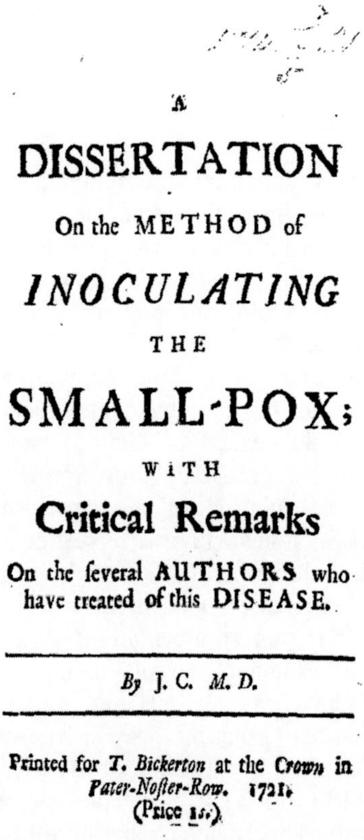

A

DISSERTATION

On the METHOD of

INOCULATING

THE

SMALL-POX;

WITH

Critical Remarks

On the ſeveral AUTHORS who have treated of this DISEASE.

By J. C. *M. D.*

Printed for *T. Bickerton* at the *Crown* in *Pater-Noſter-Row*. 1721.
(Price 1*s*.)

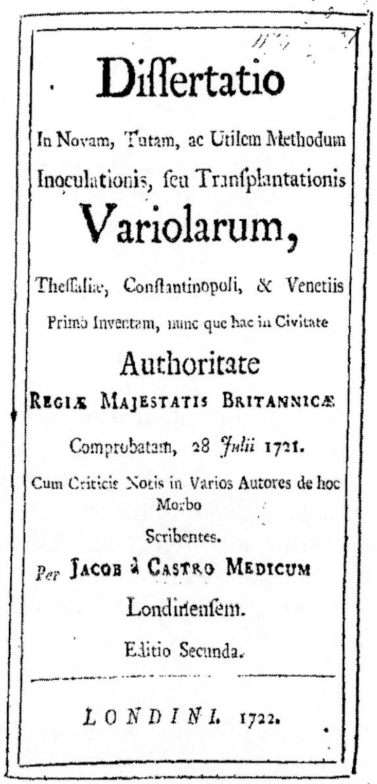

Diſſertatio

In Novam, Tutam, ac Utilem Methodum Inoculationis, ſeu Tranſplantationis

Variolarum,

Theſſaliæ, Conſtantinopoli, & Venetiis Primò Inventam, nunc que hac in Civitate

Authoritate

REGIÆ MAJESTATIS BRITANNICÆ

Comprobatam, 28 *Julii* 1721.

Cum Criticis Notis in Varios Autores de hoc Morbo Scribentes.

Per JACOB à CASTRO MEDICUM Londinenſem.

Editio Secunda.

LONDINI. 1722.

Fig. 9.4. Title pages of the 1721 (English) and 1722 (Latin) editions of Sarmento's Dissertation on Smallpox. Wellcome Collection.

Sarmento goes on to identify four different stages or "Periods" of the disease:

1. Invasion: marked by (amongst others) shivering and shaking; high temperature; whitened tongue; extreme thirst; loss of appetite; drowsiness; nasal irritation leading to sneezing; itchy and watering eyes; frequent vomiting; dry cough; respiratory difficulties; rapid pulse rate; "violent pains" in the head, back, loins and stomach; flushed appearance; convulsions in children.

2. Eruption: appearance of small pimples ("Pustules"), especially on the face, neck and chest, expanding to cover the entire body, and steadily

increasing in size; the spots are red to begin with, but gradually turn "Chrystalline" with yellowish apices; the adjacent skin swells and becomes very painful; the eyelids swell and eventually close the eyes;

3. Maturation: the peak of pustule development, accompanied by inflammation, especially in the hands.

4. Exsiccation: gradual drying and shedding of the pustules, which are replaced with "scurfy scales"; when the dried scales are shed they leave behind "deep Pock holes, and often unseemly Scars, Contractions of the skin, and Seams hind".

The succeeding section on the history of accounts of the disease is very cursory, directing the reader to the works of Mesue (c. 777-857), Rhazes (854-925) and Avicenna (c. 980-1037), with very little additional comment.

Then follows a review of the means of treatment then being employed, particularly:

1. Cold Regimen: commended by Thomas Sydenham (1624-1689) and involving the use of "gentle Diaphoretics" but, in Sarmento's estimation, resulted in contraindications which "unless timely opposed, hurry the Patient to the other World"!

2. Hot Regimen: "espous'd and Approved by all the Old Women and Nurses in the City" and advocated by Richard Morton (1637-1698) and Martin Lister (1639-1712). The aim was to "drive the Pox from the heart"; the Morbific and malignant particles were, according to the physicians, expelled from the internal to the external parts of the body.

3. The general method of Herman Boerhaave (1668-1738): this involved the extensive use of venesection, vomits and laxatives in a bid to prevent the formation of pustules. Sarmento correctly characterised this approach as a "Mal-Practice as it exposes the Patient to Prodigious Hazards" by weakening the body rather than fortifying it.

4. Oleose Regimen: as recommended by John Woodward (1665-1728) and involving the use of vomit-inducing medicines, clysters and the prescription of large quantities of oils (assuming that the "Disease takes rise in biliose Salts").

5. Mercurial Ptyalism: production of large quantities of saliva by the application of mercurial medicines, advocated by Archibald Pitcairne (1652-1713). Sarmento judged this approach "only to be used by the Judicious", it otherwise being "only a Sword in a mad Man's Hand carrying along with it immediate Death and Destruction".

6. Purgation Method: supported by John Friend (1675-1728) and Richard Mead but opposed by John Woodward, this approach relied on the application of a suite of emetics and laxatives, often combined with a special diet; Sarmento thought it had the same drawbacks as mercurial ptyalism.

Sarmento then proceeds to commend and outline a procedure of inoculation which he acknowledges was practised in Greece, Turkey and Italy. The first step was to choose a suitable donor of "Pocky matter"-a smallpox sufferer, and preferably a pre-pubescent boy. Pus was extracted from the pustules, usually from the legs and thighs, on the twelfth or thirteenth day of the disease when they were at the peak of their development (the Maturation stage). Expressed into a clean receptacle, the pus was then kept warm until the recipient was ready, having been prepared in advance for the procedure by various means "according to his particular Constitution". An incision was made with a "Launcet or Three-edged needle", usually on the arms or legs, and the blood flowing from the wound mixed with the pus from the donor. A half walnut shell was then used to cover the wound. The patient was monitored for up to 30 days in order to judge the progress of the disease and forced to adhere to a careful dietary regimen. The expectation was that the same symptoms would manifest themselves as in untreated patients but, although occasionally severe, they would generally be milder and persist for a shorter period of time. The pustules would be fewer in number, less extensively distributed over the body and not so severe. On drying, shedding of the hard scales would be far less likely to leave pock marks.

1721, the date of publication of Sarmento's *Dissertation*, was a significant year in the history of smallpox treatment; it is best seen as a watershed, rather than representing the inception of variolation. Indeed, different approaches to variolation had been practised for hundreds of years. The process of "nasal insufflation", beginning in China some time before the mid-sixteenth century and spreading from there to Japan and Russia, involved blowing powdered smallpox material (usually dried, powdered scabs harvested from patients suffering from only mild cases of the disease) up the nostrils by means of a blowpipe (Williams 2010, 60). Arabian and African approaches involved introduction of smallpox blister contents through the skin (Williams 2010, 61). By the early eighteenth century, "buying the smallpox" was an established tradition in the Haverfordwest area of Pembrokeshire in Wales; in 1700, it cost three pence to purchase the juice from twelve pustules for introduction into the recipient via small scratches in the skin (Williams 2010, 53).

Lady Mary Wortley Montagu (1689-1762; Fig. 9.5; Grundy1999), a beautiful, highly intelligent and gifted writer with ferocious drive and force of personality, lost her younger brother to smallpox in 1713 and contracted the disease herself in the closing days of 1715. Treated by Richard Mead and John Woodward, she eventually recovered but her beauty was decimated by hundreds of facial pock-marks and the loss of her eyelashes.

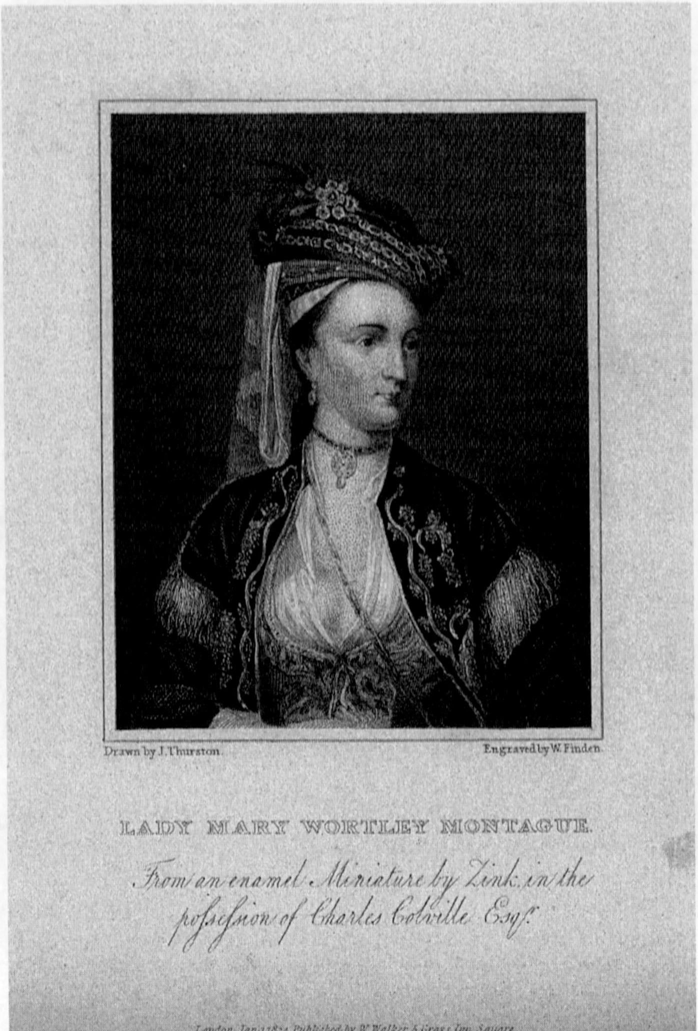
Drawn by J. Thurston
Engraved by W. Finden
LADY MARY WORTLEY MONTAGUE.
From an enamel Miniature by Zink, in the possession of Charles Colville Esqr.
London, Jan. 1. 1824. Published by W. Walker, 5 Grays Inn Square.

Fig. 9.5. Lady Wortley Montagu (1689-1762). Line engraving by W. Findon, 1824, after J. Thurston after C. F. Zincke. Wellcome Collection.

Travelling to Turkey with her husband, who had been appointed Ambassador to the Ottoman Empire, she was accompanied by Aberdonian surgeon Charles Maitland (1668-1748). Firstly at Adrianople and later at

Constantinople, she noted the lack of smallpox scars on the people with whom she came into contact, and was informed this was the result of inoculation against the disease. Writing to her friend, Sarah Chiswell on 1 April 1717, she described how older women would collect pus from smallpox blisters, store it in a nut shell, and introduce it via a scratch into the blood of an inoculee-essentially the same process as described by Sarmento in 1721. The whole process was completed *en masse* at special parties such that, each year, thousands of protective inoculations were performed. Mary determined to have her son, Edward Wortley Montagu (1713-1776), later to become a renowned traveller and writer, inoculated for the disease. Maitland and an elderly Greek nurse performed the procedure on 18 March 1718-all went well.

The Montagus returned to London in 1718 with Lady Mary keen to promote smallpox inoculation. Over the previous two decades, the Royal Society had received several communications advocating variolation but had, at best, proved to be passive regarding the information (e.g. Williams 2010; Stearns & Pasti 1950). Indeed, Lady Mary returned to "a veritable smallpox war" being actively engaged by a group of physicians (Grundy 1999, 209). A suitable opportunity for Lady Mary to demonstrate the technique she so fervently believed in, and which had been ratified by personal experience, arose during a resurgence of smallpox in London in 1721. She arranged to have her three-year old daughter Mary inoculated by Maitland in the presence of witnesses from the Royal College of Physicians. By the summer of 1721, Lady Mary had successfully evangelised for the procedure in the face of much opposition. The Princess of Wales (Caroline of Ansbach; 1683-1737) had almost lost her daughter to the disease earlier in 1721, and now a good friend of Lady Mary's, suggested to a group of senior physicians that application should be made to the king for royal approval to conduct a formal clinical trial of the procedure. Three men and three women prisoners at Newgate Prison were selected for the trial with the promise of a full pardon in respect of their participation. Charles Maitland undertook the procedures under royal license on 9 August 1721; all the prisoners survived variolation. A second trial was carried out on twelve orphans from the Parish of St James, Westminster in order to confirm the safety of the procedure when applied to the very young. Again, the results were all positive.

At the same time as these events were taking place in London, infected members of the crew of *The Seahorse* re-introduced smallpox to the population of Boston in the American Colonies when it docked on 21 April 1721. Cotton Mather (1663-1728) advocated the use of a variolation technique about which he had been informed by one of his slaves. This brought about an enormous clash of medical personalities and was the source of a highly vituperative pamphlet war; the outbreak waned toward the end of a year in which variolation had been used to protective benefit, in spite of the surrounding brouhaha (Hopkins 2002, 247 ff.; Williams 2010, 96 ff.).

Thus, Sarmento's *Dissertation* was published at the height of the flurry of activity concerning variolation and only shortly after he arrived in London. Although providing a fairly succinct summary presentation of the facts concerning smallpox as he saw them and promoting the means of inoculation which Lady Mary was about to have demonstrated to the great and the good of London medical society, he did not really add anything new to the debate. It is not clear as to how much he drew on knowledge and experience gained from his time in Portugal, and how much this was just an opportune communication.

Sarmento complains about the "ill reception" of inoculation. In his view, it was difficult to understand due to the "ill success of all other methods" (Sarmento 1721, 2). Therefore, with his contribution, he intended to convince the sceptical doctors. He gave an accurate description of the appearance, evolution, outcome and complications of the disorder with consistent semiotic details, also trying to understand its origin (Variola virus (VARV), a member of the genus *Orthopoxvirus,* was isolated in the 20th century; its' origin is still a matter of discussion). This point must have been relevant at the time since the work was translated into Latin. Besides, the inoculation carried out at that time needed improvement since the living virus of smallpox was inoculated. Despite these early successes, which also included some hazardous cases, however, most physicians of the time seemingly did not feel comfortable adopting a treatment which had still not been fully studied and proven.

Inoculation with the smallpox virus also carried a risk of fatality since variolation could potentially spread the disease; inoculated people were effectively temporary carriers of the condition.

Finally, the vaccine was greatly improved by Edward Jenner (1749-1823), a physician and scientist who also studied geology and was considered the father of immunology. He famously observed the analogy between smallpox and cowpox and proved the procedural safety of inoculating with the cowpox virus, efficaciously preventing smallpox infection, and provoking only minimal cutaneous reaction at the site of inoculation (Jenner 1801).

Água de Inglaterra

The naturally-occurring alkaloid, Quinine ($C_{20}H_{24}N_2O_2$), was chemically isolated from the bark of Cinchona trees (Fig. 9.6, 9.7) in 1820 by Pierre-Joseph Pelletier (1788 –1842), who was also a co-discoverer of strychnine, and Joseph Bienaimé Caventou (1795–1877). The genus *Cinchona* is a member of the Family Rubaceae embracing 23 or more species and is native to the tropical Andean rain forests of western South America. Bark from several species was exploited by indigenous people for its febrifugal properties and particularly as a treatment against shivering (e.g. Crawford 2014; Gachelin et al. 2017). Introduced into Europe by the Jesuits, the bark and its powdered form were known by several different names, such as Jesuit's Bark and Powder, *Cortex Peruanus* and *quina-quina*. It was quickly seen as being useful and effective in the treatment of intermittent fevers (malaria). The history of use of Peruvian Bark has been told many times (e.g. Thomson 1928; Rocco 2004).

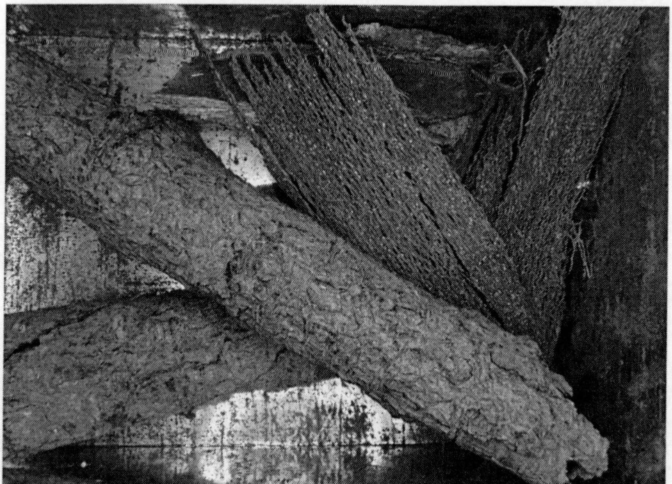

Fig. 9.6. Cinchona bark. Corbyn cabinet, Drawer 22 Column 1 Row 5, Royal Pharmaceutical Society Museum. Author's photograph.

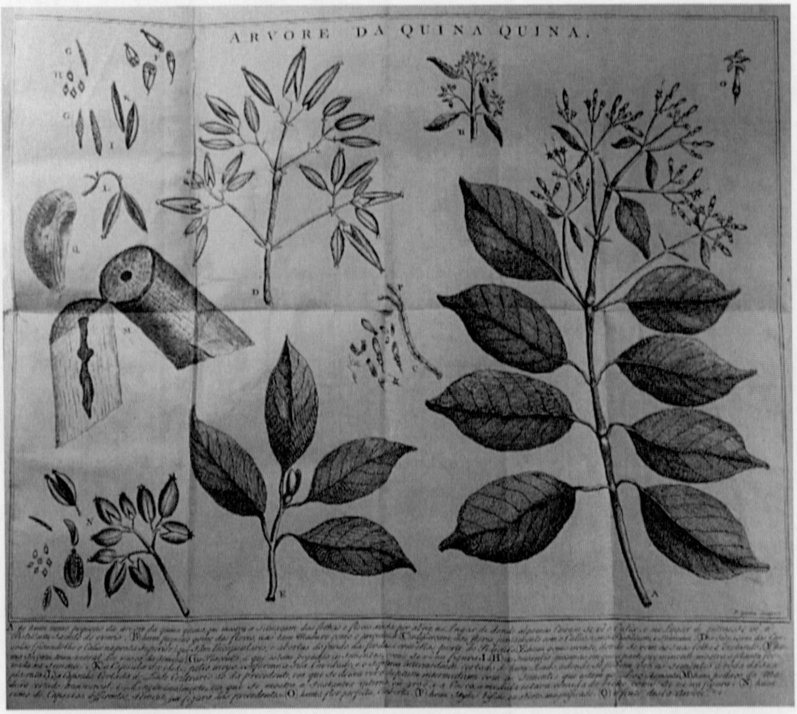

Fig. 9.7. "Quina quina". Plate from Sarmento (1756). Wellcome Collection.

Sarmento claimed proprietary rights to the secret formula for *Água de Inglaterra* (Water of England), which was actually no more than an alcoholic solution of Jesuit Bark.

Fernando (formerly Fernão) Moses Mendes (1647-1724; Perry 2004), originally from Trancoso, Beira Alta (Portugal), gained his M.D. at Montpellier in January 1668 and then emigrated to London in 1669. He became physician to Catherine of Braganza (1638-1705) and was one of the physicians who attended her husband, Charles II (1630-1685) on his deathbed. Mendes died a wealthy man; part of his fortune may have been the result of his introduction of *Água de Inglaterra* into Portugal which, at the time, was a country in which malaria was rife (d'Esaguy 1936; Figueiredo 2012). Mendes "received a handsome gift from His Serene Highness King D. Pedro II (reigned 1683-1706), on condition that he should reveal to him the secret of its composition and withhold it from the public".

As a consequence, "the inventor achieved great fame and won the opinion even of those who were opposed to Quina-quina" (Sarmento, quoted in d'Esaguy 1936, 404). Mendes' agent in Portugal was Father Manuel Dias and the "*Água de Inglaterra* de Fernando Mendes" was produced in the Rua das Rosas in Lisbon by Vicente Dias, Father Manuel's nephew, and sold by his wife, Ana Maria de Brito (Figueiredo 2012, 117). Other centres of production (Coimbra, for example) and competing preparations sprang up (such as the *Água Lusitana* of João Curvo Semedo, 1635-1719), so Mendes petitioned the king in 1724 for permission to use an authenticating seal on his waters; anyone who tried to circumvent this authentication would have to pay a fine to the Hospital de Todos os Santos (Figueiredo 2012, 117).

The concoction supposedly "did not enjoy popularity for very long, either because its results did not correspond to expectations, or on account of the sudden death of its inventor" (Machado, quoted in d'Esaguy 1936, 404). Sarmento took up Mendes' mantle and, employing what seems to have been a more acceptable recipe, marketed his version of *Água de Inglaterra* both in England and Portugal very effectively. Sarmento does not seem to have been very impressed with Mendes' recipe, describing it as "*turba, e mal preparada*" ("cloudy, and poorly prepared"; Sarmento 1758, 404) and apt to give rise to contraindications such as headache and constipation (Pinto 2011, 12). According to Sarmento, experiments which he conducted on the Jesuit's Bark allowed him to make improvements to the manufacturing process of *Água de Inglaterra*, thereby eliminating undesirable side effects. He marshalled various testimonies praising the superiority of his preparation, both in terms of therapeutic effectiveness and its ability to be tolerated without the development of unpleasant medical consequences (Pinto 2011, 12). *Água de Inglaterra* could be purchased at Jesuit pharmacies (*Botica*) of the Colégio de Santo Antão in Lisbon and the Colégio dos Jesuítas in Coimbra, until the Order of Jesus was expelled from Portugal in 1759.

Others were keen to jump on the bandwagon of such pharmaceutical economic success and the market was soon flooded with competitive counterfeits (d'Esaguy 1936, 405-406).

Sarmento was keen to keep his *Água de Inglaterra* in the public eye, and especially in the consciousness of his medical colleagues. To this end, he referred to it wherever possible in his published works. His *do Uso e Abuso das Minhas Aguas de Inglaterra* (Sarmento 1756; Fig. 9.8) was dedicated to the subject, but he also includes a section on it in the second edition of his *Materia medica physico-historico-mechanica* (Sarmento 1758, 402-410; see below for further details of this work).

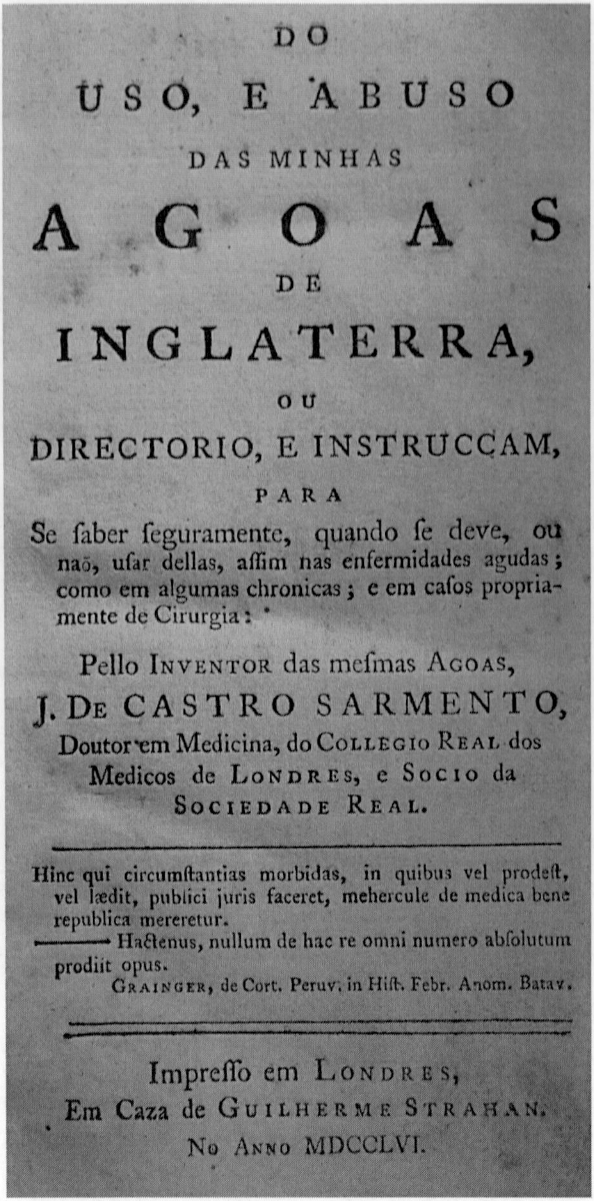

DO
USO, E ABUSO
DAS MINHAS
AGOAS
DE
INGLATERRA,
OU
DIRECTORIO, E INSTRUCCAM,
PARA
Se ſaber ſeguramente, quando ſe deve, ou naõ, uſar dellas, aſſim nas enfermidades agudas; como em algumas chronicas; e em caſos propriamente de Cirurgia:

Pello INVENTOR das meſmas AGOAS,
J. DE CASTRO SARMENTO,
Doutor em Medicina, do COLLEGIO REAL dos Medicos de LONDRES, e SOCIO da SOCIEDADE REAL.

Hinc qui circumſtantias morbidas, in quibus vel prodeſt, vel lædit, publici juris faceret, mehercule de medica bene republica mereretur.
——— Hactenus, nullum de hac re omni numero abſolutum prodiit opus.
GRAINGER, de Cort. Peruv. in Hiſt. Febr. Anom. Batav.

Impreſſo em LONDRES,
Em Caza de GUILHERME STRAHAN.
No ANNO MDCCLVI.

Fig. 9.8. Title page, Sarmento (1756). Wellcome Collection.

Sarmento's will saw the secret recipe for his *Água de Inglaterra* bequeathed to his wife and son (Henrique); in a rather odd symmetry, one of the witnesses was Edward Wortley Montagu, who had been variolated against smallpox as a young boy in Turkey (see above). This was Sarmento's third wife; Elizabeth was the Christian mistress whom he married after presenting him with an illegitimate son (a second son, Charles, was baptised in 1758) (Barnett 1978-80, 94; Sousa-Dias 2003). However, it was Sarmento's nephew, André Lopes de Castro (dates unknown) who seems to have monopolised the market for *Água de Inglaterra*, having supposedly stolen the recipe for the drink from his uncle and returned to Lisbon in 1756 (d'Esaguy 1936, 405; Figueiredo 2012, 119).

Materia medica physico-historico-mechanica

The title of Sarmento's *Materia medica* (Fig. 9.9) provides clear insight into its thrust; it was a work written for Portuguese physicians and other medical personnel, promoting the Newtonian synthesis as applied to medicine.

Sir Isaac Newton (1642-1727) published two seminal works-*The Principia* (1687) and *Opticks* (1704)-which together established a new spirit in natural philosophy based on reason, experience and utility, and which expanded from science into both politics and religion (e.g. Fehér 1990). Rather simply expressed, the Newtonian world view is one in which the complex world about us represents a mechanical system which can be described in terms of simple laws, quantitative measurement and analysed mathematically. In the words of Henrik Wulff, man could be seen in this outlook as "a complex physicochemical machine. Disease is a fault in that machine, and it is the aim of medicine to repair or prevent the fault" (Wulff 1999, 50).

Sarmento may have first encountered the Newtonian approach to science whilst studying at Coimbra but experienced something of a full baptism when he arrived in London. Joining the congregants at Bevis Marks Synagogue, as indicated above, he formed a close, disciple-like friendship with *Hakham* David Nieto, a charismatic leader and philosopher whose pro-Newtonian views had helped shape a Jewish theology syncretising religion and science (Ruderman 1995; Goldish 1997, 652-3; Sousa-Dias 2005, 57). Furthermore, Sarmento came into contact with numerous Newtonian physicians during the course of debate about variolation and his entry into the hallowed halls of the Royal Society-people like Richard Mead, John Freind and George Cheyne (1672-1743) (Brown 1987; Guerrini 1996).

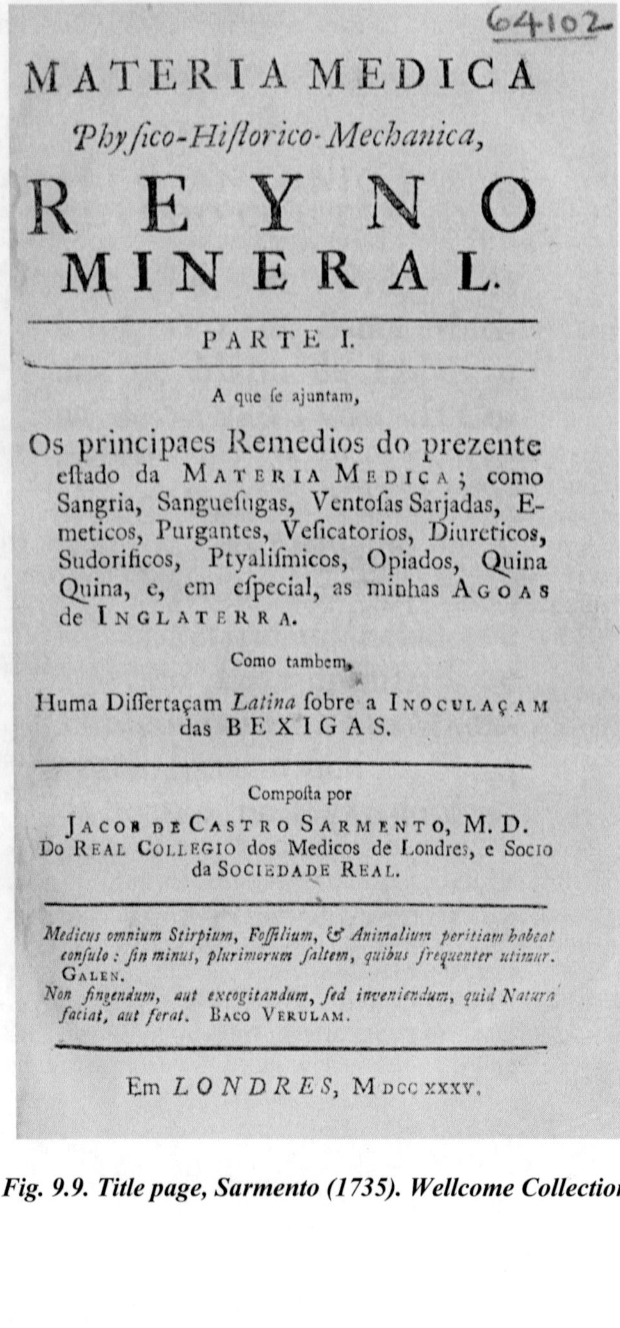
64102

MATERIA MEDICA

Phyſico-Hiſtorico-Mechanica,

REYNO

MINERAL.

PARTE I.

A que ſe ajuntam,

Os principaes Remedios do prezente eſtado da MATERIA MEDICA; como Sangria, Sangueſugas, Ventoſas Sarjadas, Emeticos, Purgantes, Veſicatorios, Diureticos, Sudorificos, Ptyaliſmicos, Opiados, Quina Quina, e, em eſpecial, as minhas AGOAS de INGLATERRA.

Como tambem,

Huma Diſſertaçam *Latina* ſobre a INOCULAÇAM das BEXIGAS.

Compoſta por

JACOB DE CASTRO SARMENTO, M. D.
Do REAL COLLEGIO dos Medicos de Londres, e Socio da SOCIEDADE REAL.

Medicus omnium Stirpium, Foſſilium, & Animalium peritiam habeat conſulo: ſin minus, plurimorum ſaltem, quibus frequenter utimur. GALEN.
Non fingendum, aut excogitandum, ſed inveniendum, quid Natura faciat, aut ferat. BACO VERULAM.

Em *LONDRES*, MDCCXXXV.

Fig. 9.9. Title page, Sarmento (1735). Wellcome Collection.

One of Sarmento's prime motives in writing the *Materia medica* was to introduce Newtonianism in a propaedeutic way to the Portuguese scientific community. Although fleeing the country for England, he kept up a lively correspondence with Portuguese Jesuit colleagues and, acting as an intermediary, communicated several of their letters to the Royal Society (see Sousa-Dias 2005 for further details). Scientific ties with his country of birth were strengthened, however, when Sarmento corresponded with Manuel Teles da Silva (1682-1736), a nobleman (*fidalgo*; 3rd Marquis of Alegrete, 4th Count of Vila Maior) belonging to the household of King D. João V ("The Magnanimous"; 1689-1750) and Secretary of the Royal Academy of History, which had been set up in 1720. The idea was mooted in 1730 to set up a botanical garden at Coimbra University, with Sarmento supplying seeds from Chelsea Physic Garden in London; in the end, the proposal came to nothing. A year later, the king contacted Sarmento through the Count of Ericeira (Francisco Xavier de Meneses; 1673–1743) concerning the reform of medical studies in Portugal, beginning with a Portuguese translation of Francis Bacon's philosophical works.

By the early decades of the eighteenth century, it was felt that Portugal was losing its grip as an imperial power and that the time was ripe for reform. Sebastião José de Carvalho e Melo, 1st Marquis of Pombal and 1st Count of Oeiras (often referred to as "Pombal"; 1699 - 1782) was a leading *estrangeirado* who, from 1738 was Portuguese Ambassador in London, and elected FRS in 1740. Recalled to Portugal in 1749, he was later a major figure in the intellectual circle centred around Ericeira seeking to introduce Newtonianism into the country. The Pombaline Reforms were designed to bring about economic stability, strength and self-sufficiency and involved extensive administrative reorganisation both domestically and colonially. Quasi-monopolistic Jesuit methodology was perceived as having a stultifying stranglehold on the education system, leading to their expulsion from the country in 1759 (see also above) and a series of educational reforms. Sarmento, with whom Pombal had interacted in London (including having Pombal protect him from British revenue authorities), was to be one of the agents of change. Indeed, Sarmento dedicated several of his publications to the instigators of Portuguese reform-the future King D. João V, Pombal, and Pombal's uncle (Marco António de Azevedo Coutinho; 1688-1750), a leading politician (de Andrade 1966, 127; Maxwell 1995, 12).

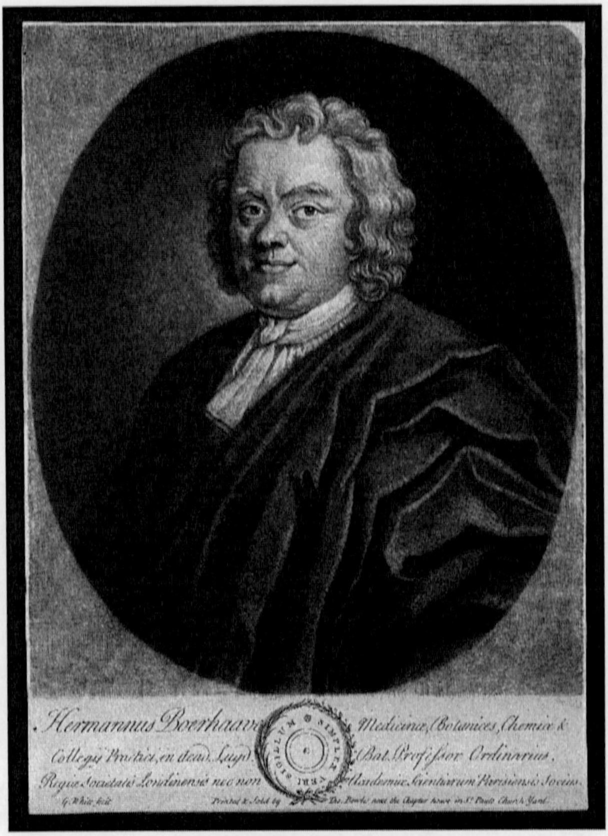
Hermannus Boerhaave Medicinae, Botanices, Chemiae &
Collegii Practici, in Acad. Lugd. Bat. Professor Ordinarius,
Regiae Societatis Londinensis nec non Academiae Scientiarum Parisiensis Socius.
SIGILLUM SIMPLEX

Fig. 9.10. Portrait of Herman Boerhaave (1668-1738). Wellcome Collection.

The first part of Sarmento's *Materia medica*, dedicated to medicines from the mineral realm, was first published in 1735. A second edition in 1758 added sections on medicinal plants and animals. Sarmento nailed his colours to the mast right from the outset. He first gave a brief historical review where he cursorily considered the work and philosophies of many highly revered physicians of the past (Hippocrates, Podicus, Aristotle, Aesculapius, Galen, Pliny, Soranus, Celsus, Antonius Musa, Theophrastus, Aetius, Oribasius, Rhazes, Abulcasis and others). He then declared in the Preface that the "falsehood" of all the systems followed by these eminent forerunners of the science of medicine, with their embedded conjectural speculation, had now been replaced by a system which depended on demonstration and evidence "aided by philosophical experiments, chymical, and anatomical" from which could be formulated underpinning Mechanical Principles and Natural Laws (Sarmento 1735, xlix ff.). He saw the genius of the Dutchman Herman Boerhaave (1668-1738; Fig. 9.10) as having produced a most "concise System of Medical Mechanics" within which "The English Hippocrates", Thomas Sydenham (1624-1689) had since made the greatest strides (Sarmento 1735, l). Sarmento declared his intention to remedy the deficiency he perceived in Portuguese medical education by writing "a rational and proper method" in the vernacular (Sarmento 1735, lii). He takes the opportunity throughout to level criticism at various Portuguese medical authors, thereby fortifying his credentials as a reforming voice sweeping away outdated notions with the new broom of Newtonianism. João Curvo Semedo (1635-1719) and Brás Luís de Abreu (1692–1756), two of the most influential Portuguese medical writers from the early decades of the eighteenth century, are singled out for special treatment (see Pinto 2011 for further details).

Sarmento covers the Mineral Kingdom in 8 chapters dealing with metals, salts, stones, earths, sulfur, semi-metals, fresh waters and mineral waters. Although not referred to in the text by name, the legacy of Paracelsus clearly exerts an influence in Sarmento's work where numerous alchemical derivatives are detailed, often with comments as to how they should be produced and what conditions they should be prescribed for. To give a couple of examples: the highly caustic escharotic artificial "stone", *Lapis infernalis* (silver nitrate, $AgNO_3$) was often used as a cauterising agent to rid the body of dermal growths (Sarmento 1735, 53; Duffin & Pymm 2015, 30-31); *Sal prunella* or *Crystal mineral* was commended by Sarmento (1735, 125-126) as a diuretic, and to treat both fevers and gonorrhoea (see Duffin 2020, 189).

Bearing in mind Sarmento's desire to stamp out "falsehoods" and to bring a rigour born of rational thought and experimental demonstration and evidence-gathering to eighteenth century Portuguese pharmacy, his section on "Stones" (*Pedras*) contains some surprising retentions from a more superstitious age in which the doctrine of signatures played a major part in the identification of potential therapeutic qualities in geological (and other) materials. For some of these entries Sarmento does comment on their fabulous reputation. Indeed, by the time the second edition of his *Materia medica* was published in 1758, many items in this section had been dropped from general use, as indicated by Sir John Hill (1714-1775) in his *History of the Materia Medica* (Hill 1751) and survived only as apothecarial curiosities. Although there is no direct evidence for Sarmento and Hill meeting in Georgian London, it is eminently possible that they did so, considering the overlap that existed between their respective interests. By way of example, Sarmento retains Amethyst as a therapy for drunkenness on the basis of its wine-like colour; *Lapis judaicus* (*Pedra Judaica*) is cited as being used in urogenital disorders (although he does comment that it is little used in England) (see Duffin 2006, 2008); haematite seems to be accepted as being useful as a haemostatic (Sarmento 1735, 156, 159, 176).

Sarmento (1735, 222 ff.) also includes a section on *Argilla Estremotia* or *Barro de Estremós* in his chapter on earths. These are alternative names for *Terra Portugallica* discussed above. After describing its qualities (vivid red colour, sticks to the tongue) and local uses (jugs and other tableware, items of jewellery), Sarmento briefly alludes to experiments which he conducted in an attempt to determine the composition of the earth. Noting its styptic and absorbent qualities, he indicates that he had used it "repeatedly with good success" in treating Flux of the Womb (*Fluxos de Ventre*-probably referring to excessive menstrual bleeding), and that his friend Richard Myddelton Massey (1678-1743) found it to be effective against Fluor Albus ("the whites"-leucorrhoea, a vaginal discharge) when administered in the form of an electuary. Contrary to the position taken in Britain (see above), Sarmento was convinced that *Argilla Estremotia* was far more efficacious than Armenian Bole. After giving instructions on how to prepare the material, Sarmento turns his critical gaze upon Francisco da Fonseca Henriques (1665-1731), personal physician to D. João V. In common with other medicinal earths, Francisco da Fonseca Henriques had apparently ascribed "Bezoartic Virtue" (Sarmento 1735, 224) to the clay from Estremoz, claiming that it had alexipharmic properties. It is certainly true that he was impressed by the supposed antitoxic powers of bezoar stones, dedicating quite a lot of space to them in his *Medicina Lusitana,* first published in 1710. Sarmento thoroughly disagreed with Fonseca's position.

During the late seventeenth century, there was a rise in popularity for "taking the waters", and numerous new spas began to emerge in Britain (Mather & Duffin 2017); "chalybeate" or iron-bearing waters were particularly popular. Sarmento seems to have had a lifelong interest in medicinal waters and dedicates Chapter VII of the *Materia medica* to their consideration. Following some general comments, he indicates certain materials which he employed as reagents to help in his assaying of various waters: certain galls, Syrup of Violets, Oil of Tartar, and a solution of silver, for example. He also briefly comments on some items of equipment which he used-Boyle's vacuum pump, hydrostatic balance, thermometer and microscope. Casting his net quite widely, he considers waters from a range of European localities, often drawing heavily on accounts published by the

Royal Society-Canterbury and Tunbridge Wells are included. He pays particular attention, as might be expected, to the waters of Caldas da Rainha ("Queen's Baths") in western central Portugal. The therapeutic hot springs there have an associated church and hospital (Hospital Termal Rainha D. Leonor or "Queen Leonor Spring Water Hospital"). The latter was founded by Eleanor of Viseu (1458 –1525; consort of D. João II) and completed in the closing years of the fifteenth century-the oldest such purpose-built institution of its kind. The Caldas da Rainha is a sulphurous spring whose waters picked up their mineral content as they passed through adjacent Triassic and Jurassic rocks. The spring is one of several that lie on the Caldas da Rainha fault line and is now a Geoheritage site (Dinis & Bernardes 2004). Francisco da Fonseca Henriques had included Caldas da Rainha in his treatment of medical waters (*Aquilegio medicinal*) published in 1726. He claimed many therapeutic virtues for the waters, including provoking menstruation, and being able to ease a wide range of nervous, urinary, digestive, rheumatic and other disorders (Fonseca Henriques 1726, 5 ff.; see also Sarmento 1735, 407 ff.). Sarmento once again criticises Fonseca Henriques, this time for listing the therapeutic applications of the waters without performing analytical tests on them (Sarmento 1758, 262).

Sarmento also takes the opportunity in his Materia medica to refer to proprietary therapies of his own design – "secret medicines" for which the means of preparation was never revealed. *Água de Inglaterra* has a section dedicated to itself and even appears in the long title of the book! He also writes about *Tinctura Styptico-Balsamica*, a solution of iron, for which he claims much therapeutic benefit in cases as wide-ranging as open wounds, internal conditions involving the blood (haemorrhage, especially from the womb, vomiting and coughing blood), diabetes, dysentery and gonorrhoea (Sarmento 1758, 63). True to his Newtonian roots and his desire to validate his statements with reference to suitable experiments, he records a particular test undertaken on 12 January 1731, in the presence of a set of witnesses, many identified by name. The test subject was a dog. A surgeon made an incision deep in the musculature at the top of the leg and hindquarters of the animal, cutting into the Crural Artery. The tincture was applied to the area and the bleeding supposedly immediately started to coagulate. This led Sarmento to speculate as to how useful his solution might prove to be as a surgical aid (Sarmento 1758, 64).

For further details of the roles of the *estrangeirado*s, including Jacob de Castro Sarmento, in the introduction and diffusion of Newtonianism in Portuguese science and education see de Carvalho (1934), de Andrade (1966), Maxwell (1995), Goldish (1997), Carneiro et al. (2000), Sousa-Dias (2005) and Pinto (2011).

Translations

Following the opening of communication with Portuguese authorities intent on instituting reforms which would reverse the "fossilizing influence of the Inquisition and the limitations of Aristotelian philosophy" (Barnett 1978-80, 87), Sarmento suggested that the work of Francis Bacon (1561-1626), foundational to the development of the scientific revolution, be made available in Portuguese. Sarmento intended to base his translation on an English translation of the original Latin text by Peter Shaw (1694-1763). In the event, the project was dropped (see Barnett 1978-80, 87-88 for further details).

Theorica Verdadeira das Mares, conforme á Philosophia do incomparavel cavalhero Isaac Newton ("The True Theory of the Tides, in accordance with the philosophy of the incomparable Sir Isaac Newton") was published by Sarmento in 1737. This was not a translation, but a volume relevant to Sarmento's aims of introducing Newtonianism to Portuguese scientific and wider society. Following a short homage to Newton, and a brief biography, Sarmento explained lunar influences on the movement of the tides, based on Newton's laws of gravity. He also apparently translated Newton's posthumously published (1728) *The Chronology of Ancient Kingdoms Amended* into Portuguese, but the manuscript was never published (Barnett 1978-80, 99).

In the 1740s, Sarmento produced two Portuguese translations of medical works by British scientists. The first was a rendition of a publication by Stephen Hales (1677-1761; Fig. 9.11), an English cleric with wide scientific interests and a penchant for experimentation and invention. Hales and Sarmento clearly knew each other; they were both Fellows of the Royal Society (Hales in 1718) and Hales records that Sarmento was a witness to his experiments on "sweetening great Quantities of stinking Cask-water in Ships" (Hales 1758, 342). The translation was of Hales' (1740) book on a series of investigations into *Mrs. Stephens's medicines for dissolving the stone.* The title clearly fulfilled Sarmento's mission of bringing works with good Newtonian methodology to the attention of Portuguese scientists, and the medical fraternity in particular. The volume relates to an interesting episode in the history of treatment of renal calculi. In brief, Mrs Joanna Stephens achieved fame through her medicinal remedies for dissolving bladder stones. This group of medicines is referred to as lithontriptics. Mrs Stephens proposed to sell her secret remedy for her proprietary medicine for the not inconsiderable sum of £5000. David Hartley (1705-1757) collected ten case histories of patients claiming to have been cured from "the stone", a condition from which he also suffered, and had benefited from being treated with her medicine (Hartley 1738). A year later, he had accumulated a total of 155 positive testimonials to the efficacy of Mrs Stephens' treatment. Public subscription had raised a total of £1356 for the publication of her recipe, and Parliament eventually awarded her the full requested sum of £5000; Stephen Hales was one of the Parliamentary Trustees appointed to assess the claims (Viseltear 1968). The recipe was revealed to consist of (Stephens 1739):

> "egg-shells and garden snails well calcined until the snails have done smoaking. The decoction was made by boiling various herbs with soap, honey and swine-cresses burnt to blackness. The pills were composed of calcined snails, wild carrot seeds, burdock seeds, ashen keys, hips and haws, all burnt to a blackness, soap and honey."

Fascinated by the claims of the various parties supporting the efficacy of Mrs Stephens' remedy and its potential to ease human suffering, several scientists undertook *in vitro* experiments to check the chemical components of the medicine and the claims of its ability to act as a lithontriptic. These scientists included David Hartley, the French physician and chemist Étienne François Geoffroy (1672 –1731) and Stephen Hales. By determining the chemical makeup of the remedy and then eliminating any superfluous materials it might be possible to determine and isolate the therapeutically active component of the mixture. Experimenting on bladder stones immersed and heated in a series of solutions, Hales initially thought that the soap was the active ingredient, but later concluded that it was the lime in the calcined egg shells. His methodology was attacked by James Parsons (1705-1770) and there were sustained accusations that Joanna Stephens' nostrum was a quack remedy (Viseltear 1968). Sarmento clearly thought that the information was worth laying before the Portuguese medical fraternity.

Sarmento's second translation during the 1740s was a volume on surgery by Samuel Sharp (1709-1778), a surgeon at Guy's Hospital in London. His *A treatise on the operations of surgery* was first published in 1739 and quickly went through a series of new editions, the 10th edition appearing in 1782. The critically acclaimed volume was the first British work dedicated exclusively to operative techniques, and Sharp himself is recognised as "an innovative surgical practitioner and communicator" (Kirkup 1996, 6). In choosing this textbook for translation, Sarmento must have benefited generations of Portuguese medical students.

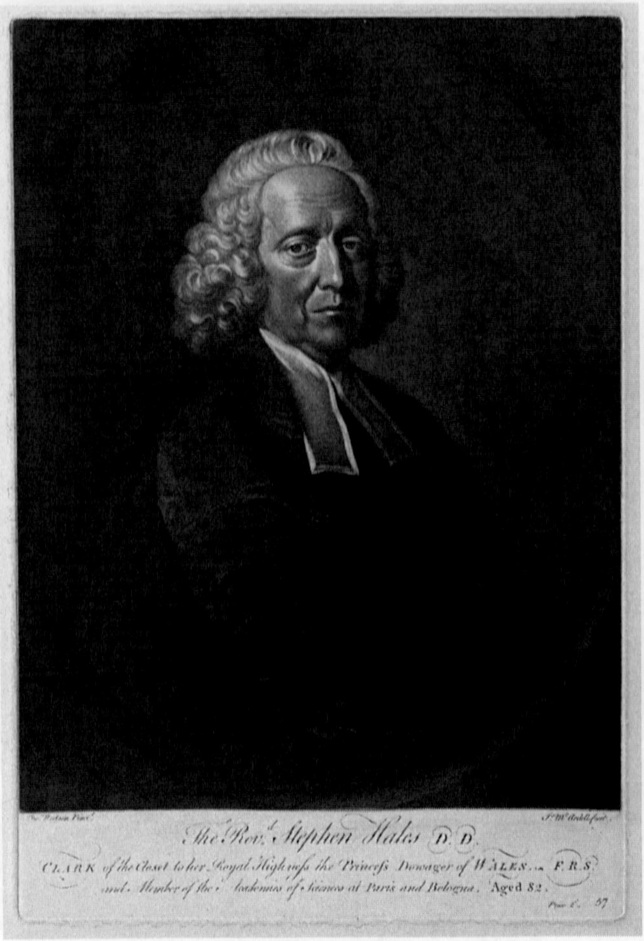
The Rev.d Stephen Hales D.D.
CLARK of the Closet to her Royal Highness the Princess Dowager of WALES. F.R.S.
and Member of the Academies of Sciences at Paris and Bologna. Aged 82.

Fig. 9.11. Portrait of Stephen Hales (1677-1761). Wellcome Collection.

Conclusions

Jacob (formerly Henrique) de Castro Sarmento lived an eventful life full of ups and downs, successes and failures, fame and notoriety. Although hounded by members of the Schomberg medical dynasty, he made worthwhile practical and supportive contributions to the medical welfare of the Sephardic Jewish community in what is now the East End of London. An active member of the Fellowship of the Royal Society, he was a pioneer of that community in terms of seeking and successfully attaining domestic recognition as a physician of note and, as a celebrated and influential *estrangeirado* helping to introduce Newtonian Science into the Portuguese medical fraternity, thereby acting as an instrument of educational reform.

Sarmento's legacy in terms of published works is marked by the earliest Pharmacopoeia prepared for an English hospital and his contribution to the early discussion of variolation in the battle against smallpox, both written for an English readership. Later in life he also wrote for Portuguese medical students and practitioners.

Overall, Sarmento overcame the difficulties he faced as a Sephardic Jew displaced by the machinations of the Portuguese Inquisition, successfully integrating himself into the active medical and scientific life of his adopted country. Cognizant of his geographical roots he later found himself able to contribute to the scientific evolution of his homeland.

Acknowledgements

I am very grateful to Maria do Sameiro Barroso for her careful reading of the manuscript and helpful suggestions for improvement, the Wellcome Collection and the Trustees of the British Museum for access to some of the many works examined here and permission to publish images from their collections. The Curator of the Museum of the Royal Pharmaceutical Society (London) also kindly allowed access to the Corbyn Cabinet and permission to use images from the photographic inventory which I made of its contents.

References

Andrade, António Alberto de. 1966. *Vernei e a cultura do seu tempo.* Coimbra: Acta Universitatis Conimbrigensis.

Andrade, António Júlio, and Guimarães, Maria Fernanda 2010. *Jacob de Castro Sarmento*, Lisboa: Nova Vega.

Barnett, Richard. 1978-80. "Dr. Jacob de Castro Sarmento and Sephardim in Medical Practice in Eighteenth-Century London". *Transactions of the Jewish Historical Society of England,* 27:84-114.

Behbehani, Abbas M. 1983. "The Smallpox Story: Life and Death of an Old Disease". *Microbiological Reviews,* 47, (4): 455-509.

Berman, Alex. 1960. "The Beth Holim Formulary of London (1749)". *American Journal of Hospital Pharmacy,* 17, (1): 23-25.

Brown, Theodore M. 1987. "Medicine in the Shadow of the Principia". *Journal of the History of Ideas,* 48, (4): 629-648.

Burnby, Juanita. 2004. "Dale, Samuel". *Oxford Dictionary of National Biography*.

Carneiro, Ana, Simões, Ana and Maria Paula Diogo. 2000. "Enlightenment Science in Portugal: The *Estrangeirados* and Their Communication Networks". *Social Studies of Science,* 30, (4): 591-619.

Carvalho, Joaquim de. 1934. "Jacob de Castro Sarmento et l'introduction des conceptions de Newton en Portugal". *Archeion,* 16, (3-4): 319-323.

Collins, Kenneth E. 1982-1986. "Jewish medical students – graduates at Edinburgh University, 1739—1862". *Jewish Historical Studies,* 29 (1982-1986): 75-96.

Collins, Kenneth E. 1984-1985. "Jewish medical students and graduates in Scotland, 1767—1859". *The Scottish Society of the History of Medicine Report of Proceedings, Session 1984-5*: 10-18.

Costa, Emanuel Mendes da. 1757. *A Natural History of Fossils.* London: L. Davis & C. Reymers.

Crawford, Matthew James. 2014. "An Empire's Extract: Chemical Manipulations of Cinchona Bark in the Eighteenth-Century Spanish Atlantic World". *Osiris,* 29, (1): 215–229.

Dale, Samuel. 1693. *Pharmacologia sen Manuductio ad Materiam Medicam.* London: Sam. Smith & Benj. Walford.

Dale, Samuel. 1718. *Pharmacologiae sen Manuductionis ad Materiam Medicam Supplementum.* London: Guil. & Joh. Innys.

Dinis, Jorge and Cristina Bernardes. 2004. "Upper Jurassic outcrops along the Caldas da Rainha Diapir, west central Portugal: a Regional Geoheritage overview". *Rivista Italiana di Paleontologia e Stratigrafia,* 110, (1): 407-415.

Duffin, Christopher J. 2006. "Lapis Judaicus or the Jew's stone: the folklore of fossil echinoid spines". *Proceedings of the Geologist's Association,* 117: 265-275.

Duffin, Christopher J. 2008. "Fossils as drugs: pharmaceutical palaeontology". *Ferrantia,* 54: 1-83.

Duffin, Christopher J. 2013. "Some early Eighteenth Century geological Materia Medica". 209-233 *In* Duffin, C.J., Moody, R.T.J. & Gardner-Thorpe, C. (eds.) *A History of Geology and Medicine.* Geological Society of London Special Publication, 375.

Duffin, Christopher. 2018. "A Dwarf on Giant's shoulders: Sir John Hill and Geology". 243-265 *In* Brant, C, & Rousseau, G. (eds.) *Fame & Fortune: Sir John Hill and London Life in the 1750s.* London: Palgrave.

Duffin, Christopher J. 2019. "Snakes' tongues, Serpents' eyes and sealed earths: Geology and Medicine in Malta". *Occasional Papers of the St John Historical Society*: 1-16.

Duffin, Christopher J. 2020. "Medicinal Quartz: *Crystallus* or Rock Crystal". 162-204 *In* Barroso, M. Sameiro do, Duffin, C.J. & Sousa, G. de (eds.): *Medical Heritage of the National Palace of Mafra*. Cambridge Scholars: Cambridge.

Duffin, Christopher J. and Rachael Pymm. 2015. "A Survey of artificial pharmaceutical 'Stones' – Part 2". *Pharmaceutical Historian,* 45, (2): 28-33.

Esaguy, Augusto d'. 1936. "Água de Inglaterra". *Bulletin of the Institute of the History of Medicine,* 4, (5): 404-408.

Esaguy, Augusto d'. 1946a. *Jacob de Castro Sarmento: Notas Relativas a Sua Videa Sua Obra.* Lisbon: Atica.

Esaguy, Augusto d'. 1946b. *A Page from the Portuguese History of Medicine: Dr. Jacob or Henrique de Castro Sarmento.* Coimbra: Instituto de Coimbra.

Fehér, Marta. 1990. "The triumphal march of a paradigm: a case study of the popularization of Newtonian Science". *Tractrix,* 2: 93-110.

Figueiredo, Patrick. 2012. "A 'Água de Inglaterra' em Portugal". 113-130 *in* Cristiana Bastos, Cristina and Renilda Barreto (eds) *A Circulação do Conhecimento Medicina, Redes e Impérios*. Lisboa: Imprensa de Ciências Sociais.

Fonseca Henriques, Francisco da. 1726. *Aquilegio medicinal, em que se dá noticia das agoas de caldas, etc. do Reyno de Portugal e dos Algarves; que ou pelas virtudes medicinaes, que tem, ou por outra alguma singularidade, saõ dignas de particular memoria.* Lisboa Occidental: Off. da Musica.

Fowler, Clare J. 2018. *Pharmacopoeia Londinensis 1618 and its descendants*. London: Royal College of Physicians.

Gachelin, Gabriel, Garner, Paul A., Ferroni, Eliana, Tröhler, U. and Iain Chalmers. 2017. "Evaluating Cinchona bark and quinine for treating and preventing malaria". *Journal of the Royal Society of Medicine,* 110, (1): 31–40.

Gibbs, F.W. 1950. "Cromwell Mortimer, F.R.S.: Secretary, Royal Society, 1730-1752". *Notes and Records of the Royal Society of London,* 7, (2): 259-263.

Goldish, Matt. 1997. "Newtonian, *Converso*, and Deist: The Lives of Jacob (Henrique) de Castro Sarmento", *Science in Context,* 10, (4): 621-675.

Grant, Alicia. 2019. *Globalisation Of Variolation: The Overlooked Origins Of Immunity For Smallpox In The 18th Century.* London: World Scientific Europe.

Grundy, Isobel. 1999. *Lady Mary Wortley Montagu.* Oxford: Oxford University Press.

Guerrini, Anita. 1996. "Newtonianism, Medicine and Religion", 293-312 In Grell, Ole Peter and Andrew Cunningham (eds) *Religio Medici. Medicine and Religion in Seventeenth-century England.* Aldershot: Scolar Press.

Hales, Stephen. 1740. *An account of some experiments and observations on Mrs. Stephens's medicines for dissolving the stone: wherein Their Dissolving Power is inquir'd into, and shown.* London: printed for T. Woodward, at the Half Moon between the Temple Gates in Fleet street; Printer to the Royal Society.

Hales, Stephen. 1758. *A treatise on ventilators. Wherein an account is given of the happy effects of many trials that have been made of them in different Ways and for different purposes; Which has occasioned their being received with general Approbation and Applause, on account of their Utility for the great Benefit of Mankind. As also Of what farther Hints and Improvements in several other useful Ways, have occurred since the Publication of the former Treatise. Part second.* London: Richard Manby.

Hartley, David. 1738. *Ten Cases of Persons Who Have Taken Mrs. Stephens's Medicines for the Stone.* London: S. Harding.

Hartley, David. 1739. *A View of the Present Evidence for and against Mrs. Stephens's Medicines, as a Solvent for the Stone. Containing a Hundred and Fifty-Five Cases with Some Experiments and Observations.* London: S. Harding et al.

Herculano, Alexandre. 2009. *História da Origem e estabelecimento da Inquisição em Portugal.* David Lopes (ed.) 19ª edição, Lisbon: Livraria Bertrand.

Hill, John. 1748. *A General Natural History: or, New and Accurate Descriptions of the Animals, Vegetables and Minerals, of the Different parts of the World.* London: Thomas Osborne.

Hill, John. 1751. *A history of the Materia Medica. Containing descriptions of all the substances used in medicine, their origin, their characters when in perfection, the signs of their decay, their chymical analysis and an account of their virtues, and of the several preparations from them now used in the shops*. London: T. Longman, C. Hitch and L. Hawes.

Hopkins, Donald R. 2002. *The greatest killer. Smallpox in history.* Chicago: University of Chicago Press.

Jacobs, Joseph & Lipkind, Goodman. 1906. "Nieto, David." In Singer, Isidore (ed.) *The Jewish Encyclopedia: A Descriptive Record of the History, Religion, Literature, and Customs of the Jewish People from the Earliest Times to the Present Day*, 9: 302-303.

Jenner, Edward. 1801. "On the Origin of the Vaccine Inoculation". *The Medical and Physical Journal,* 1801 June, 5, (28): 505-508.

Jouanna, Jacques. 2012. *Greek Medicine from Hippocrates to Galen: Selected Papers*. Leiden & Boston: Brill.

Karamanou, Marianna, Panayiotakopoulos, George, Tsoucalas, Gregory, Kousoulis, Antonis A. and George Androutsos. 2012. "From miasmas to germs: a historical approach to theories of infectious disease transmission". *Le infezioni in medicina: rivista periodica di eziologia, epidemiologia, diagnostica, clinica e terapia delle patologie infettive* 1: 52-56.

Kirkup, John. 1996. "Samuel Sharp and the Operations of Surgery, 1739". *Journal of Medical Biography,* 4, (1): 1–7.

Lemos, M. 1910. "Jacob de Castro Sarmento". *Ilustração Transmontana,* 3: 114-125.

Lieberman, Julia R. 2017a. "New Practices of Sedaca. Charity in London's Spanish and Portuguese Jewish Community during the Eighteenth Century". 105-130 In Lieberman, Julia R. and Michal Jan Rozbicki (eds.) *Charity in Jewish, Christian, and Islamic Traditions*. Lanham: Lexington Books.

Lieberman, Julia R. 2017b. "The founding of the London Bet Holim hospital in 1748 and the secularization of sedaca in the Spanish and Portuguese Jewish community in the eighteenth century". *Jewish Historical Studies,* 49, (1): 106-143.

Lieberman, Julia R. 2019. "Few wealthy and many poor: the London Sephardi Community in the eighteenth-century". *Ler Historica,* 74: 41-61.

Lopes, Luís and Martens, Ruben. 2015. "Global Heritage Stone: Estremoz Marbles, Portugal". In Pereira, D., Marker, B. R., Kramar, S., Cooper, B. J. & Schouenborg, B. E. (eds) 2015. *Global Heritage Stone: Towards International Recognition of Building and Ornamental Stones*. Geological Society, London, Special Publications 407, 57–74.

López-Salazar, Ana Isabel. 2013. "General Inquisitors and the Portuguese Crown in the Seventeenth Century: between Political Service and the Defense of the Faith (1578-1705)". *Mediterranean Studies,* 21, (2): 71-90.

MacGregor, Arthur. 2013. "Medicinal terra sigillata: a historical, geographical and typological review". 113-136 *In* Duffin, C.J., Moody, R.T.J. & Gardner-Thorpe, C. (eds.) *A History of Geology and Medicine.* Geological Society of London Special Publication 375.

Marcocci, Giuseppe. 2011. "A fundação da Inquisição em Portugal, um novo olhar", *Lusitania Sacra,* Janeiro-Junho 2011: 17-40.

Martins, Oliveira. 2004. *História de Portugal.* 21st edition. Lisboa, Guimarães Editores. [1st ed. 1879].

Martins, Ruben, Gomes, Celso, Lopes, Luís, Arroz, Maria, Santos, Dulce, Rosado, Francisco and Ana Cunha. 2013. "Application in Pottery of the Residual Soils Associated to Marbles from the Estremoz Anticlinal Region". *Key Engineering Materials,* 548: 147-156.

Mather, John and Christopher J. Duffin. 2017. "Nathaniel Hodges and the purging wells of Shooter's Hill". 35-45 *In* Duffin, C.J., Gardner-Thorpe, C. & Moody, R.T.J. (eds) *Geology and Medicine: Historical Connections.* Geological Society of London, Special Publication 452.

Maxwell, Kenneth. 1995. *Pombal, Paradox of the Enlightenment.* Cambridge: Cambridge University Press.

Mocatta, Frederic David. 1877. *The Jews of Spain and Portugal and the Inquisition*. London: Longmans, Green, and Co.

Morris, A. D. (1974). "Samuel Dale (1659-1739), Physician and Geologist". *Proceedings of the Royal Society of Medicine* 67: 120–124.

Newton, Isaac. 1728. *The chronology of ancient kingdoms amended. To which is prefixed, a short chronicle from the first memory of things in Europe, to the conquest of Persia by Alexander the Great.* London: J. Tonson, J. Osborn and T. Longman.

Parojcic, Dusanta, Stupar, Dragan and Milica Mirica. 2003. "La Thériaque : Médicament et Antidote". *Vesalius,* 9 (1): 28-32.

Perry, Norma. 2004. "Mendes, Fernando Moses (1647–1724)". ODNB.

Pinto, H. 2011. "A Materia Medica de Jacob de Castro Sarmento". 165-186 *In* Fontes da Costa, Palmira and Cardoso, Adelino (eds.), *Percursos na História do Livro Médico (1450-1800)*, Lisboa: Edições Colibri.

Ramos, Rui, Vasconcelos e Sousa, Bernardo and Monteiro, Nuno Gonçalo (eds.). 2009. *História de Portugal.* Lisboa: A Esfera dos Livros.

Rocco, Fiametta. 2004. *The Miraculous Fever-Tree. The Cure that changed the World.* London: HarperCollins.

Royal College of Physicians. 1747. *Pharmacopoeia Collegii Regalis Medicorum Londinensis.* London: T. Longman, T. Shewell and J. Nourse.

Rubens, Alfred. 1936. *Anglo-Jewish Portraits: A Biographical Catalogue of Engraved Anglo-Jewish and Colonial Portraits from the Earliest Times to the Accession of Queen Victoria.* London: Jewish Museum.

Ruderman, David B. 1995. *Jewish Thought and Scientific Discovery in Early Modern Europe.* New Haven: Yale University Press.

Sakula, Alex. 1994. "The Doctors Schomberg and the Royal College of Physicians: An Eighteenth Century Shemozzle". *Journal of Medical Biography,* 2 (2): 113–119.

Samuel, Edgar R. 1959-1961. "Dr. Meyer Schomberg's Attack on the Jews of London, 1746". *Transactions (Jewish Historical Society of England)*, 20: 83-100.

Sarmento, Jacob (Henrique) de Castro. 1721. *A Dissertation On the Method of Inoculating the Small-Pox; with Critical Remarks on the Several Authors who have treated of this Disease*. London: T. Bickerton.

Sarmento, Jacob (Henrique) de Castro. 1722. *Dissertationes In Novam, Tutam, ac Utilem Methodom Inoculationis, seu Transplantationis Variolarum. Prima Methodus Auctoritate Regii Majestatis Brittanicae Comprobata 28 Julii 1721. & publicata Cum criticis Notis in varios Autores de hoc morbo scribentes.* Lugduni Batavorum: Joh. Arnold Langerak.

Sarmento, Jacob (Henrique) de Castro. 1724. *Exemplar de Penitência, dividido en tres Discursos Predicaveis para o Dia Santo di Kapur*. Place of publication and publisher unknown.

Sarmento, Jacob (Henrique) de Castro. 1728. *Sermam Funebre as deploraveis Memorias Do Muy Reverendo, e Doutissimo Haham Asalem Morenu, A.R. David Netto; Insigne Theologo Eminente Pregador, e Cabeca da Illustre Congrega de Sahar Hassamaym.* London: publisher unknown.

Sarmento, Jacob (Henrique) de Castro. 1735. *Materia medica physico-historico-mechanica, reyno mineral. A que se ajuntam, os principaes remedios do prezente estado da Materia medica; como sangria, sanguesugas, ventosas sarjadas, emeticos, purgantes, vesicatorios, diureticos, sudorificos, ptyalismicos, opiados, quina quina, e, em especial, as minhas agoas de Inglaterra. Como tambem, huma Dissertaçam latina sobre a inoculaçam das bexigas.* London: publisher not indicated.

Sarmento, Jacob (Henrique) de Castro. 1737. *Theorica verdadeira das mares, conforme à philosophia do incomparavel cavalhero Isaac Newton; Em que se mostram, pela mais evidente, e distinta forma, os principaes Phenomenos das Marés; e se-explicam de maneira, que se fazem perceptiveis a qualquer capacidade commua, ainda que sem Principios Geometricos, e Astronomicos, de que tanto se necessita, para intelligencia do que o Illustre Newton descobrio, e nos deixou sobre este difficultosissimo Phenomeno da Naturesa. Illustrado tudo com variedade de figuras, accommodadas a os principaes Phenomenos das Marés. A que se ajunta, como introducçam no principio, huma breve relaçam da vida, e descubrimentos deste immortal, e illustre philosopho: E a o fim, em forma de Apendix, a Demonstraçam, de que a Lua se retem no seu Orbe pela força da Gravidade pelo Dr. Jacob de*

Castro Sarmento, Do Real Collegio dos Medicos de Londres, e Socio da Socie Dade Real. London: publisher unknown.

Sarmento, Jacob (Henrique) de Castro. 1742. *Relaçam de alguns experimentos, e observaçoens, feitas sobre as medicinas de Madam Stephens, para dissolver a pedra ... Ajuntasse hum compendio historico de todos os factos, des de a origem deste descobrimento ... / Traduzido, e illustrado tudo, por J[acob] de C[astro] S[armento].* London: publisher unknown. [Translation of Hales, Stephen: *An account of some experiments and observations on Mrs. Stephen's medicine for dissolving the stone* first published in 1740].

Sarmento, Jacob (Henrique) de Castro. 1746. *Tratado das operaçoens de cirurgia: com as figuras, e descripçam dos instrumentos de que nellas se faz uso; e huma introducçam sobre a natureza e methodo de tratar as feridas, abscessos e chagas / Traduzido em Portugues da quarta ediçam de S. Sharp por J. de C.S. Que ihe ajunta e accrecenta a Materia chirurgica, ou, Todas as composiçoens, e remedios da presente pratica dos cirurgioens de Inglaterra: e as coisas mais principaes na cirurgia.* London: publisher unknown. [Translation of Sharp, Samuel. *A treatise on the operations of surgery*. Probably from the 4th edition dated 1743].

Sarmento, Jacob (Henrique) de Castro. 1755. *Philosophical Transactions of the Royal Society*: 409-11.

Sarmento, Jacob (Henrique) de Castro. 1756. *Do uso, e abuso das minhas agoas de Inglaterra, ou, Directorio, e instruccam, para se saber seguramente, quando se deve, ou naõ, usar dellas, affim nas enfermidades agudas : como em algumas chronicas : e em casos propriamente de cirurgia.* London: Em caza de Guilherme Strahan.

Sarmento, Jacob (Henrique) de Castro. 1757. *Appendix ao que se acha escrito na Materia medica.* London: publisher not indicated.

Sarmento, Jacob (Henrique) de Castro. 1758. *Materia medica physico-historico-mechanica, reyno mineral. A que se ajuntam, os principaes remedios do prezente estado da Materia medica; como sangria, sanguefugas, ventosas sarjadas, emeticos, purgantes, vesicatorios, diureticos, sudorificos, ptyalismicos, opiados, quina quina, e, em especial, as minhas agoas de Inglaterra. Edicam nova, corrigida, e repurgada, a que se accrescentam por coninuacamdesta Obra, para fazela Completa, Os Reynos Vegeteval, e Animal. Parte II.* London: Guilherme Strahan.

Sharp, Samuel. 1739. *A Treatise on the Operations of Surgery, with a description and representation of the instruments used in performing them, to which is prefix'd an introduction on the nature and treatment of wounds, abcesses and ulcers*. London: J. Watts.

Simões, Ana, Carneiro, Ana and Diogo, Maria Paula. 1999. "Constructing Knowledge: Eighteenth-Century Portugal and the New Sciences". *Archimedes* 2 (1999): 1-40.

Simões, Ana, Carneiro, Ana and Diogo, Maria Paula. 2000. "Enlightenment Science in Portugal: The Estrangeirados and Their Communication Networks". *Social Studies of Science,* 30, (4): 591-619.

Sousa-Dias, José-Pedro. 2003. "Jacob de Castro Sarmento e a sua fuga para Londres em 1721". *Cadernos de Estudos Sefarditos,* 3: 187-194.

Sousa-Dias, José-Pedro. 2005. "Jacob de Castro Sarmento e a conversão à ciência moderna". *Opuscula Officinara,* 1: 55-80.

Stearns, Raymond Phineas and George Pasti. 1950. "Remarks upon the introduction of inoculation for Smallpox in England". *Bulletin for the History of Medicine,* 24, (2): 103-122.

Stephens, Joanna. 1739. "A full discovery of the medicines given by me Joanna Stephens, for the cure of the stone and gravel; and a particular account of my method of preparing and giving the same". *The London Gazette*, Saturday 16 June, 1739.

Thompson, Charles John Samuel. 1928. "The History and Lore of Cinchona". *British Medical Journal*, December 29 1928: 1188-1190.

Viseltear, Arthur J. 1968. "Joanna Stephens and the Eighteenth Century Lithontriptics: a Misplaced Chapter in the History of Therapeutics", *Bulletin of the History of Medicine,* 42, (3): 199-220.

Williams, Gareth. 2010. *Angel of Death. The Story of Smallpox.* London: Palgrave Macmillan.

Wulff, Henrik. 1999. "The concept of disease: from Newton back to Aristotle". *The Lancet*, December 1999, 354, Suppl. SIV50.

Online resources

Como Francisco de Sá e Mesquita (1680-1723) quis enganar a Inquisição e acabou no cadafalso [How Francisco de Sá e Mesquita (1680-1723) wanted to deceive the Inquisition and ended up on the scaffold]. http://arlindo-correia.com/050612.html (accessed 24 August 2020).

Chapter 10

On Fevers and Other Foes of Humankind: A Collection of Medical Case Histories by the Physician Gaspar Lopes de Chaves (1729 – 1796)

Francisco Curate and Telmo António

Abstract

Manuscripts reflecting the everyday activities of Early Modern physicians are scarce. Therefore, unpublished collections of medical case histories are major sources of knowledge about the conventional medical daily practice and the physician's relationships with patients. Between 1784 and 1795, the municipal physician of Almada, Gaspar Lopes Henriques de Chaves (1729-1796), authored a collection of medical case histories, offering experience with diseases that encompassed individual biographical details, identification and description of diseases, symptoms, and therapies. The manuscripts (years 1788, 1789 and 1792) consist of the medical histories of 127 individuals, with recorded ages between 3 and 90 years. Fevers were the most frequent type of «disease», particularly the so-called intermittent and "synoch-putrid" fevers. A significant proportion of the patients died as a perceived outcome of the conditions described. The assessment of disease symptomatology, medical therapies and environmental factors described by Gaspar de Chaves adds significant information about the practice of medicine in Portugal during the late 18th century.

Key words: History of Medicine, New Christian physicians, eighteenth century, Almada, Portugal

Resumo

Os manuscritos que reverberam a atividade quotidiana dos médicos durante a Idade Moderna são escassos, e as coleções não publicadas de casos

clínicos são, portanto, fontes importantes de conhecimento acerca da prática médica diária típica e das relações entre os médicos e os seus pacientes. Entre 1784 e 1795, o médico do Partido de Almada, Gaspar Lopes Henriques de Chaves, registou um conjunto de casos clínicos que revelam experiências de doença e englobam dados biográficos individuais, identificação e descrição de doenças, sintomas e regimes terapêuticos. Os manuscritos (dos anos de 1788, 1789 e 1792) compilam as histórias clínicas de 127 indivíduos, com idades entre os três e os 90 anos. As febres, em particular as intermitentes e as «sinoch-pútridas», constituíram o género de «doença» mais frequente. A morte, enquanto consequência conjeturada das doenças descritas, foi o destino de uma proporção significativa dos pacientes. A sintomatologia das doenças, as respetivas terapias e os fatores ambientais descritos por Gaspar de Chaves proporcionam informações relevantes ao conhecimento das práticas médicas em Portugal no final do século XVIII.
Palavras-Chave: história da medicina, médicos Cristãos-Novos, século XVIII, Almada, Portugal

Introduction

The birth of modern medicine can be envisioned not as an event, a sudden eruption of paradigmatic change, as suggested by Foucault's (1963, viii-xv) unconvincing claim that the birth of the clinic happened in the last years of the eighteenth century-but as a long process of epistemological mutation during which several medical discourses and practices coexisted (Fontes da Costa 2011, 27-28; Porter 1991; Pomata 2014, 5). In the conceivable multitudes of the past, medical practices were diverse systems of choice, where it was often difficult to distinguish between an intellectual formulation and the intrusion of folklore.

A significant feature of early modern medical discourses pertains to the distinct literary genres that featured works by European physicians, including the classical *commentarii*, *consilia* or *tractatus*, and the evolving *curationes* or *observationes* (Pomata 2010, 194). Gianna Pomata (2011, 2; 2014, 2-16) argues persuasively that these are not just literary genres but *epistemic* genres, a specific genre whose essential purposes are not the creation of meaning but the production of knowledge.

Alongside the theoretical, doctrinal, or paradigmatic issues confronted in epistemic genres such as *contradicentia medica*, *controversiae* or *disputationes medicae*, other genres-contiguous to the increasing significance of medical practice and empirical knowledge-started to appear during the early modern period (Pomata 2010; Stolberg 2013, 488). Among these latter medical writings, the *observationes* (i.e., collections of case histories, the narration of individual cases and other occurrences with medical relevance) originated in the second half of the sixteenth century, becoming a fundamental style of medical writing by the eighteenth century (Pomata 2010, 193, 199-201). The genre has a genealogy that can be traced to the ancient Greek astronomical and medical traditions, including the seven Hippocratic books of *Epidemics* that comprised more than 300 case narratives, but it was not until the late Renaissance that it became a full-fledged genre in its own right (Pomata 2014, 6).

The collections of case stories provided a new configuration for collecting, describing, and arranging the materials derived from experience and personal practice-in that way, each type seems to denote knowledge based on practice instead of doctrine (Pomata 2010, 195-196), while reinforcing and depicting the proposition that medicine displays an aptitude to adapt general principles to particular situations (Giglioni 2011, 50). As such, medical case narratives are especially cogent as testimonies of the history of the practitioner/patient relationship.

Although stemming from empirical practices, the systematic process of publication of *observationes* was mostly an endeavour of physicians with academic backgrounds – and not barbers or surgeons, the "lower echelons" of medical practice (Denipoti 2017, 2; Stolberg 2013, 489). Seminal examples of the recognition of experience in the evolution of medical practices are Antonio Benivieni's (1443-1502) *De abditis non nullis ac mirandis morborum et sanationum causis* (1507) and Amato Lusitano's (1511-1568) *Curationum medicinalium centuria prima, multiplici variaque rerum cognitione referta* (1551), both published in Florence, or Jodocus Lommius's (beginning of the sixteenth century-?) *Medicinalium observationum libri tres. Quibus notae morborum omnium, et quae de his possint haberi praesagia, judiciaque, proponuntur* (1560), printed in Antwerp.

However, sources reverberating physicians' tangible practice are still scarce (Stolberg 2019, 222). Everyday medical practices are only partially represented in the printed sources of *observationes* (and, indeed, also in collections of *curationes*); thus, collections of case stories, casebooks and practice journals that were not published are utterly relevant for increasing the knowledge about the typical physician's day-by-day activities and the physician's relations with their patients. Among these, we highlight the works of Georg Handsch (1529-1578?), Pieter van Foreest (1521-1597), Hiob Finzel (?-1582), Theodore de Mayerne (1573-1655), among many others (Dinges et al. 2016; Stolberg 2019, 2013).

In this essay, we intend to present a serial record of the practice of the Portuguese physician Gaspar Lopes de Chaves (1729-1796), concerning the years of his magisterium as town physician of Almada (Portugal). In 1784 he presented a petition to be a candidate for the town's physician at a session of the Almada City Council, with a Royal provision from Queen Maria I (1777-1816). For some years, probably between 1784 and 1795, he practised medicine as the contracted municipal physician ("Partido Médico") of Almada. During this period, Gaspar de Chaves produced a set of manuscripts, designated *Observaçoens Médico Meteorológicas* (Medical and Meteorological Observations), in which he compiled a series of daily meteorological data obtained in the town of Almada. In addition to this important collection of elements related to climatic conditions, the documents add a body of clinical observations that provide a comprehensive and in-depth view of medical practice at the dawn of the eighteenth century.

Permanency and errancy in the life of Gaspar Lopes de Chaves

Gaspar Lopes Henriques de Chaves was born in Lisbon in 1729, the son of Diogo Carvalho Henriques de Chaves (?1701-?) and Juliana Teresa (?1700-?), in a family of New Christians, or "Conversos". New Christian was a socio-religious legal designation that identified forcibly converted Jews and their descendants in the late 15th century Iberian kingdoms. New Christians were subjected to ferocious and systematic persecution by the Inquisition, with members of the community facing unrelenting harassment, repression, torture, imprisonment, and death (Borges Coelho 1987, 30, 31, 43, 118; Rowland, 175-181).

As expected, the life of Gaspar de Chaves was indelibly marked by his familial roots. In 1667, his grandfather (his namesake Gaspar Lopes Henriques [1651-1718], also a physician, and at the time no more than sixteen years old) and all his great-uncles, from Fundão and residing in Lisbon, presented themselves to the Inquisition to "confess their faults of Judaism"[1]. Voluntary submission to the Inquisition, as decreed in the Portuguese Inquisition Regiment of 1640, was a defensive strategy widely used by potential victims of persecution, allowing them to anticipate the inquisitors, admitting guilt and expressing repentance.

Concerted stories were another defensive ploy when someone from the family circle or friends was arrested. In many circumstances, people who

---

[1] Arquivo Nacional da Torre do Tombo. Tribunal do Santo Ofício. Inquisição de Lisboa, proc. 5379.

were already in prison, dead, or secure in a foreign country were accused (Saraiva 1969). At the beginning of the eighteenth century, the Inquisition unleashed another repressive wave against this family[2]. Isabel Henriques (?1644-1706), a sister of Gaspar, was "relaxed to the secular arm", a euphemism for execution in an "auto de fé". His niece, Catarina Henriques, died in prison, while Gaspar Henriques was arrested in 1703 and sentenced to life imprisonment and exile in Brazil. Apparently, the sentence was not enacted, as he was visited by a physician in 1707 while imprisoned at Limoeiro, a known prison from Lisbon. His wife, Jerónima de Chaves (1665-?1728), was also accused of Judaism and incarcerated[3]. The circumstances of the death of Gaspar Henriques, the grandfather of Gaspar Lopes Henriques de Chaves, are recounted in detail in Jacob de Castro Sarmento's (1692 – 1762) "*Appendix ao que se acha escrito na Materia medica*..." (1757, 139), in which the famous physician recalls that, in 1718, Gaspar Henriques was afflicted by hemiplegia and, consequently fatal apoplexy.

Diogo Carvalho de Chaves, a lawyer, the father of Gaspar Lopes Henriques de Chaves, married Juliana Teresa, an Old Christian who was not accepted by Diogo's parents (Herson and Gutberlet 1996, 168). She died in an unknown year but certainly before 1737. Diogo de Chaves was arrested in 1733; then, being 32 years old, he endured incarceration and torture for four years without admitting any wrongdoing[4]. He was warned "that if he died, break any limb or if it lost any sense during torment, he would be blamed and not the inquisitors": a consummate example of the physical and psychological coercion and violence exerted by the Inquisition. After being released in 1737, he remarried Rosa Joaquina (?1719-?), also a New Christian.

In October of 1751, Gaspar Lopes Henriques de Chaves enrolled for the first time at the Faculty of Medicine at the University of Coimbra[5]. Six months later, in April of 1752, he obtained a bachelor's degree in Arts (a qualification in Arts was a requirement for attending a medical school (

---

[2] Arquivo Nacional da Torre do Tombo. Tribunal do Santo Ofício, Inquisição de Lisboa, proc. 1830-1.

[3] Arquivo Nacional da Torre do Tombo. Tribunal do Santo Ofício, Inquisição de Lisboa, proc. 5379-1.

[4] Arquivo Nacional da Torre do Tombo. Tribunal do Santo Ofício. Inquisição de Lisboa, proc. 3533.

[5] Arquivo da Universidade de Coimbra. Índice de alunos da Universidade de Coimbra, proc. PT/AUC/ELU/UC-AUC/B/001-001/H/000214.

Frade and Silva 2011, 58). In May of 1757, he graduated in medicine[6], sponsored by António José da Silva (1710-1774), professor of Surgery, Method, *De Crisibus* and Avicenna (Rodrigues 1992). These latter courses illustrate the enduring relevance of Galen of Pergamon (129-*c.* 200/ *c.* 216) and Avicenna (*c.* 980-1037) in the medical teaching at Coimbra-after all, Gaspar de Chaves had graduated fifteen years before the Pombaline reform of the University of Coimbra, promoted by the Prime Minister of King D. José I (1750-1777), Sebastião José de Carvalho e Melo (1699-1782), Marquis of Pombal (Teixeira Rodrigues and Fiolhais 2013, 452).

The sweeping influence of the Society of Jesus and the Inquisition in the university played a cardinal role in the rather retrograde situation of Portuguese medical teaching and practice during the early modern period (Abreu 2017, 232; Sander 2014), but, under the auspices of King D. João III (reigned 1521-1667), some improvements were being enacted with the hiring of foreign scholars in 1537 and the introduction of the course of Anatomy in 1556 (Teixeira Rodrigues and Fiolhais 2013, 444). King D. João III in October of 1546, had already given instructions to the magistrate of the district of Coimbra and to the provider of the Royal Hospital to arrange for accession of the bodies necessary to the anatomy practice of Rodrigo de Reinoso (1494-1557), royal physician and professor of the *Prima* course in the University of Coimbra (Abreu 2010, 101).

The family, namely Gaspar Lopes Henriques de Chaves and his cousin João Carlos Mourão Pinheiro (?1725-?1798), was again the target of inquisitorial persecution in 1757. Anticipating incarceration, they appeared at the Inquisition along with Rosa Joaquina, Gaspar's stepmother, and some of her relatives. All confessed the guilt of their belonging to Judaism, and concerted histories[7]. The single most serious accusation made by Gaspar de Chaves, that of "teaching the belief in the Law of Moses", was made against a friend, João Rodrigues da Costa, by "coincidence" already a refugee in Bordeaux (France). Suspecting another repressive inquisitorial wave that would have far more severe consequences, Gaspar de Chaves and his family left the country. A letter included in his file, signed by Gaspar de Chaves and his father, Diogo, dispatched from London, accounts for his intention to move to France.

In 1776, two marriages were celebrated in the parish of Sainte-Eulalie (Bordeaux), one by "Gaspard Lopes Henriques de Chaves with Leonore de Miran", and the other by "Joseph Antoine de Carvallo de Chaves with Marie

---

[6] Arquivo da Universidade de Coimbra. Índice de alunos da Universidade de Coimbra, proc. PT/AUC/ELU/UC-AUC/B/001-001/H/000060.

[7] Arquivo Nacional da Torre do Tombo. Tribunal do Santo Ofício. Inquisição de Lisboa, proc. 3800.

Madeleine de Moirane" (Szajkowski 1970: 16). Seemingly, the two men were Gaspar de Chaves and his half-brother, José António Carvalho (?1744-?), while the women were in all probability the daughters of his cousin, João Carlos Mourão Pinheiro. The latter took refuge in France in 1765, and it is known that he had a daughter named Joana Leonor and another, Maria. In the death register of Gaspar de Chaves, dated from 1796, it is mentioned that he was married to "Dona Joanna Leonor Moirão de Xaves"[8]. Gaspar de Chaves remained in Bordeaux practicing medicine for some years. The reasons for his return to Portugal are unclear, but they are certainly related to the waning influence of the Inquisition during the second half of the eighteenth century, particularly after 1773, when the Marquis of Pombal enacted laws that granted civil rights to New Christians (Olival 2004, 153; Saraiva 1969, 310-317).

In 1784 we find Gaspar de Chaves in Almada where he attended a City Council session as a candidate for the town's physician, a position to which he was duly appointed[9]. In September of 1796, Gaspar Lopes Henriques de Chaves, physician and resident in the town of Almada, died "with the sacraments of the Church" at the age of 66 and was buried in the Church of "Santa Maria do Castello"[10]. The parish priest, Joaquim Miguel de Oliveira, was undoubtedly alluding to another church: Santa Maria do Castelo had been destroyed in 1755 during the Great Earthquake of Lisbon. Interestingly, Gaspar de Chaves was formally buried as a Christian. This implies one of two things: Gaspar de Chaves was, *de facto*, a Christian-even if from a family of New Christians-or he was assuming a Christian identity to circumvent old laws dating from the sixteenth century and prejudices that tried to exclude New Christians from medical practice, and especially from public appointments as town physicians (Abreu 2017, 233, 241, 246, 256).

A significant proportion of the victims of the Portuguese Inquisition were medical professionals, mostly New Christians accused of Judaism (Baudry 2018, 92, 98-104). Prominent Portuguese physicians of Jewish or New Christian origins also faced inquisitorial mistreatment, including Jacob de Castro Sarmento, Rodrigo de Castro (c.1546-1627/29?) and António Ribeiro Sanches (1699-1783) (Abreu 2017, 243; Giglioni 2011, 48; Pinto 2011, 165). All share a similar and dreadful narrative: personal and familial persecution by the Inquisition followed by exile. These histories and his

[8] Arquivo Distrital de Setúbal. Paróquia de Santa Maria do Castelo, Registos de Óbitos, Livro 7, f. 49.

[9] Arquivo Histórico Municipal de Almada. Câmara Municipal de Almada, Atas, Livro 32, f. 28-30.

[10] Arquivo Distrital de Setúbal. Paróquia de Santa Maria do Castelo, Registos de Óbitos, Livro 7, f. 49.

own surely afflicted Gaspar's behaviour and identity. At this point, it is relevant to point out the plural and fluid identities of Portuguese New Christians (Pulido Serrano 2011, 129, 136-138), and also that "New Christian" is not an exact synonym of "Jewish"-that was only the belief of the Inquisition (Saraiva 1969, 11,177-183; Rowland, 2010, 172,173).

A physician by public appointment

As mentioned above, Gaspar Lopes de Chaves was awarded a public appointment as municipal physician ("*Partido Médico*") of Almada in 1784. In 1758 Almada was a small town, with just over 3000 inhabitants in two urban (Santa Maria do Castelo and Santiago) and five rural parishes (Amora, Arrentela, Caparica, Corroios and Seixal). In 1835, the population was almost 9000 in just three parishes, Santa Maria do Castelo, Santiago and Caparica (Silva 2008, 71, 89).

Local council physicians were paid through municipal taxes with a fixed salary, independently of the number of consultations (Coelho 2014, 33). These physicians visited patients of any socioeconomic condition, in any municipality location, not charging assistance to the patient. This system was probably created in 1568 by order of King Sebastião I (Bandeira 1997, 1) and persevered until the alteration of the Administrative Code (1937-1940). In the last quarter of the nineteenth century, the obligation to appoint a municipal was enforced by law (Coelho 2014, 34), but the municipality of Almada could afford to hire a physician to assist the most disadvantaged populations long before that.

Gaspar de Chaves was appointed to the position in 1784, but he was dismissed in 1788, only four years later, and another doctor was appointed to take his place. The reasons for his dismissal were related to the quality of his clinical observations. In March of 1788, the judge and city counsellor, José Pedro de Sequeira, signed a term of objection, criticizing the documents produced by the physician Gaspar who should have made a description of the cases of epidemic diseases and instead just depicted the general doctrines, without any order; it was further added that he should have recorded case-histories for all cases of the diseases[11].

The physician Gaspar de Chaves appealed to Queen Maria I (reigned 1777-1816) against the decision. A government official was sent to Almada; he summoned the members of the City Council to inform them of the royal

[11] Arquivo Histórico Municipal de Almada. Termo de Impugnação ao Diário das Observações. PT/AHALM/CMALM/P-D/001/0001.

decision to reinstate Gaspar as the municipal physician[12], a position he held possibly until 1795 (there is documentary evidence for a new municipal physician, José Joaquim Alvares, starting in 1796[13]). On the same occasion, another mandate issued by the Queen was conveyed to the town officials: the acceptance of the annual medical and meteorological *Observaçoens* produced by Gaspar de Chaves. The manuscripts had been previously refused. In 1793, the *Observaçoens* were mentioned again in a council session[14].

The manuscripts curated at the Municipal Historical Archive of Almada refer to the years of 1788[15], 1789[16] and 1792[17]. Since the municipal physician was required to present the medical and meteorological observations every year, it is evident that some of the manuscripts are missing. In fact, in a 1793 council session, it is declared that the physician Gaspar Lopes Henriques de Chaves presented the two compulsory annual observations (i.e., both medical and meteorological) to the City Council and that they were accepted as such.

Case histories: people and diseases

The manuscripts produced by Gaspar de Chaves comprise two main sources of historical data: meteorological observations and medical case histories. The first contains raw meteorological data, with statistical and climatological relevance, integrating daily, monthly, and yearly records of variations in temperature, atmospheric pressure, humidity, among other parameters. The clinical observations offer an organized glimpse into the medical practices in a late eighteenth-century Portuguese town and, to a certain extent, different individuals' experiences of the presentation and

---

[12] Arquivo Histórico Municipal de Almada. Câmara Municipal de Almada, Atas, Livro 32, f. 28-30.

[13] Arquivo Histórico Municipal de Almada, Observações médicas e meteorológicas, do ano de 1796, n.º 7, PT/AHALM/CMALM/P-D/001/0005.

[14] Arquivo Histórico Municipal de Almada. Câmara Municipal de Almada, Atas, Livro 32, f. 152.

[15] Arquivo Histórico Municipal de Almada, Gaspar Lopes Henriques de Chaves. Observaçoens Médico Meteorológicas, Anno de 1788, PT/AHALM/CMALM/P-D/001/0002.

[16] Arquivo Histórico Municipal de Almada, Gaspar Lopes Henriques de Chaves. Observaçoens Médico Meteorológicas, Anno de 1789, PT/AHALM/CMALM/P-D/001/0003.

[17] Arquivo Histórico Municipal de Almada, Gaspar Lopes Henriques de Chaves. Observaçoens Médico Meteorológicas, Anno de 1792, PT/AHALM/CMALM/P-D/001/0004.

evolution of the diseases. The study of these sources is relevant because they reflect the ordinary learned medical practice in a somewhat provincial town, away from the large political, economic, and educational centres (although Almada is near Lisbon, across the river Tagus). These sources also stand as an exemplary constellation of epistemic narratives characterized by an espousal of the ancient Aristotelian logic and Galenic formulations engendering a new sensibility towards practical medicine and empirical experience.

The observations written by Gaspar de Chaves are mostly concerned with people and their maladies in baroque times. In the consulted manuscripts-from the years 1788, 1789 and 1792-he recorded almost all case histories following a conventional format that includes biographical details of the patient (name, address, age, profession, humoral temperament, among others), the various symptoms that afflicted them, as well as the therapeutic regimens and their effects on the course of the disease. Lastly, he presented the case's resolution: full recovery, partial convalescence, or death. This arrangement of information had been canonical since the heyday of practice journals and case histories during the sixteenth century (Stolberg 2019, 223-224,229). Henceforth, we present two vivid examples:

> A son of J. M., a merchant, 12 years old, phlegmatic, was attacked by a lymphatic fever, headache accompanied by diarrhoea and cough; considering the patient's young age and his very weak complexion, I prescribed him a white decoction of water with Tragacanth Gum sweetened with violaceous *Althea* [mallow] syrup. He was relieved by this because fever and headaches decreased on the sixth day; on the seventh day, perspiration and a quantity of coating on the tongue forced me to purge him; on the ninth day, he took *Manna* in a barley decoction, which caused the evacuation of great matter; and he is currently in perfect health. (Winter of 1788)[18]

> J. B., a 47-year-old woman, with a sanguine temperament, very committed to work, without any regimen, fell ill on January 12 with inflammatory fever, rough tongue, red cheeks, severe dryness, continuous thirst, fever with exacerbation over the afternoon, intense shivers, and great flatulence. I

[18] Um filho de J. M., tendeiro, de idade 12 anos, fleumático, foi atacado de uma febre linfática, dor de cabeça, acompanhando diarreia e tosse; considerando a pouca idade e ser um sujeito muito débil prescrevi o cozimento branco feito em água Tragacanto adoçada com xarope violado de Alteia, com este remédio alcançou alívio pois ao sexto dia diminuiu a febre e a dor de cabeça; ao sétimo, houve suor já aparecendo quantidade de saburra na língua que me obrigou a purgá-lo em o nono dia com Maná em cozimento de cevada, que provocou evacuação de matéria louvável, e goza atualmente de perfeita saúde.

prescribed bloodletting *larga manu*, as the case requested, and as nature found relief, it was repeated, with chicken soup saturated with four large cold seeds and emollient so that the night could refrigerate what was so flared up. From the third to the fourth day, observing the swollen abdomen, a mallow poultice was applied. Enemas caused bile evacuation; from sixth to seventh, *Morbus Regius*, I prescribed an urine enema and an anti-bilious decoction made of tamarind pulp and rhubarb sweetened with lemon syrup. She evacuated bilious matter, and almost all the symptoms calmed down because the fever that continued was constant, the fibre spasm ceased; the cheeks were less fired, urinating was easy, the tongue was less arid. From the eighth to the ninth, I prescribed a laxative infusion. From the tenth to the eleventh day, there was sweat, predominantly from bile; on the thirteenth day, there were no symptoms except for a mild headache that was gone with the broths that she started to drink more often; the good regimen during the convalescence restored her perfectly. (January of 1789)[19]

These two cases perfectly reflect Gaspar de Chaves' everyday practice, or as recorded by himself, they are a "meticulous inventory of the diseases" that affected the population of Almada, providing case evidence for individual disease and therapeutic experiences. However, the more general and theoretical ideas about medicine and different diseases are not absent. Learned quotations, for example, are relatively common, and Gaspar occasionally cites famous physicians and philosophers, including Hippocrates (*c.* 460 BC-*c.* 370 BC), Spinoza (1632-1677), Santori (1566-1633), or

---

[19] J.B., mulher de 47 anos, temperamento sanguíneo, mui dada ao trabalho, sem regímen algum, adoeceu aos 12 de Janeiro de febre inflamatória, língua áspera, faces vermelhas, secura forte, sede contínua, febre com exacerbação sobre a tarde, horripilações sensíveis, flatulência grande; preenchi a indicação que foi o sangrar *larga manu*, o caso assim o pedia, e como a natureza achasse alívio repetiu-se esta, dando por bebida água de frango saturada com as quatro sementes frias maiores, a emolição para a noite, a fim de refrigerar o que estava tão incendiado. Do terceiro para o quarto dia, observando bem o ventre meteorizado aplicou-se cataplasma de malva. Clisteres que provocaram evacuação de bílis; do sexto para o sétimo, *Morbus Regius*, prescrevi clister de urina como também o cozimento antibilioso composto de polpa de tamarindos, ruibarbo adoçado com xarope de limão, evacuou matéria biliosa e por este meio calmaram quase todos os sintomas pois a febre que persistia era sem acréscimo, o orgasmo da fibra já tinha cessado mostrando as faces menos incendiadas, urinando com facilidade, a língua menos árida, do oitavo para o novo, tisana laxativa, do décimo para o undécimo houve suor mas este predominado de bílis, ao décimo terceiro não houve coisa alguma que limitada dor de cabeça que se desvaneceu com os caldos que ia bebendo mais amiúde; e bom regímen que teve na convalescença a restabeleceu perfeitamente Arquivo Histórico Municipal de Almada, Gaspar Lopes Henriques de Chaves (Observaçoens Médico Meteorológicas, Anno de 1788, PT/AHALM/CMALM/P-D/001/0002).

Boerhaave (1668-1738). The emphasis of medical thought is still firmly grounded on tradition, far from the medical transformations that would soar in French hospitals and elsewhere in the 1800s. However, Gaspar de Chaves even ventured to influence sanitary conditions at the marketplaces, houses or a county jail, suggesting some "proto-epidemiological" principles to the Crown and its representatives:

> There are things necessary for Man to subsist perfectly well, for example, the vigilance from visiting magistrates and checking out the sold foodstuffs. It is superfluous to expose again what I have been repeating over and over, but it is good to repeat ideas that were not applied, especially in the construction of houses, to avoid humidity, the callous enemy of humankind. Concerning the jail where the Crown vassals' dwell, even if they are evildoers, it is humane to ask and persuade the magistrates imbued with righteousness and goodwill […] to hasten the construction of a canal to evacuate what is harmful both to those who are unfortunately imprisoned and to those who breathe free air. (Winter of 1789)[20].

Gaspar de Chaves was insistent in requiring much-needed constructions that would prevent the deterioration of the good atmosphere of Almada, and thus preventing gastric diseases and pernicious miasmas. He is writing after his experience (after all, he was recording a detailed account of meteorological data in Almada) and appealing to Santorio Santori, the Italian physiologist, physician, and professor, to demonstrate a relationship between some of the diseases occurring in Almada with elements of the weather.

The manuscripts comprise 127 medical histories (63 females, 59 males, and five whose sex was not mentioned). Gaspar de Chaves' practice included people of all ages except babies, ranging from three (two girls and a boy) to 90 years old (a woman). The younger and older patients were diagnosed with malarial fevers, except for the three-year-old boy, who was

---

[20] Que cousas não são necessárias para que o Homem subsista perfeitamente bem, que vigilância nos magistrados em visitar e fazer examinar os víveres que estão e devem estar em venda. É supérfluo expor o que tantas vezes tenho repetido mas que digo é bem que se repita quando não aproveitou o que se tem dito, principalmente na construção das casas para evitar a humidade, inimiga crudelíssima do género humano; a cadeia onde estão os Vassalos d'el Rei que devem–se ainda que sejam malfeitores é da humanidade pedir, intimar e persuadir aos verdadeiros Magistrados revestidos daquela probidade e bondade que se requer, (…), e se apressar à construção de um Canal pelo qual seja evacuado o que é nocivo tanto aos que estão infelizmente presos como para os que respiram ar livre Arquivo Histórico Municipal de Almada, Gaspar Lopes Henriques de Chaves (Observaçoens Médico Meteorológicas, Anno de 1789, PT/AHALM/CMALM/P-D/001/0003).

afflicted with dysentery. The younger patients recovered completely. The older woman, living in a lower area near the river Tagus, died. Gaspar de Chaves declared that her age was partly responsible for her demise. People that consulted de Chaves lived in different locations, including central and peripheral areas of the municipal territory of Almada and from disparate levels of the socioeconomic ladder. The annual output of reports was unequal, with a decrease in presented cases, from 72 in 1788 to only seventeen in 1792.

Fevers, in general, were the most frequent type of "disease" (62.2%; 79/127) in Gaspar de Chaves' practice, similarly affecting both sexes. By the end of the eighteenth century, fevers had started to become classified (Hamlin 2014, 91), but not in the feverish microcosmos of Almada. Gaspar de Chaves divided *circa* half of the fevers he observed into two broad categories: intermittent (26.6%; 21/79) and "synoch-putrid" fevers (a concept created by Galen) (24.1%; 19/79). The other half included continuous, inflammatory, puerperal, anginous, and other types of fever (48.1%; 38/79). He also mentioned fevers as symptoms of other diseases, including measles, tuberculosis, and cholera. Early medical texts intersected fever as a sign or symptom *and* fever as a disease (Hamlin 2014; Sajadi et al. 2012, 976), and until at least the nineteenth century, fever was still regarded both as part of a symptom complex and as a disease in its own right (El-Radhi 201, 11). Hippocratic-Galenic fever concepts were expressed as body temperature higher than average (Sajadi et al. 2012: 976-977). Galen of Pergamon, for example, defined fever as a primary dyscrasia caused by an excess of heat. He also fashioned a rational taxonomy of fevers, dividing them into ephemeral, hectic, and those caused by the corruption of humours. The latter are called putrid fevers and include intermittent (i.e., malarial fevers) or continuous fevers-in Galenic jargon, *synochus sive putrida* (Hamlin 2014, 48; Sajadi et al. 2012, 977).

Malarial fevers were the quintessential classic fevers, and different cultures recognized their distinct periods (Hamlin 2014, 7). Gaspar de Chaves never mentions malaria. Instead, he uses the Hippocratic terms "tertian", "quartan" or "intermittent". In this case, it is not difficult to translate the ancient terms into modern medical realities-with minimal risk of presentism and/or misguided retrospective diagnosis (Arrizabalaga 2002, 57-66). These fevers were usually justified within the paradigm of miasmas, or bad atmosphere, which corrupted the humours (Hamlin 2014, 42). Gaspar de Chaves implies that such fevers were endemic in Almada and suggests an association with the hot, calm weather and lower locations near the river. The described cases were more prevalent in the spring and summer (71.4%; 15/21). Malaria was indeed endemic in some riverside areas in Portugal until the 1950s, especially in the Mondego, Tejo and Sado basins (Saavedra 2013, 52, 54, 58).

One of the first effective treatments for malaria came from the bark of the cinchona tree (*Cinchona officinalis* Lin.; the indigenous name was Quina-Quina), which contains the alkaloid quinine (Jarcho 1993, 194; Gänger 2020, 6). Several South American cultures used the antipyretic qualities of bark from trees of the genus *Cinchona* before European contact, and the Jesuits introduced it into Europe for the treatment of malaria during the seventeenth century (Jarcho 1993, 212; Hamlin 2014, 81). *Cinchona* was also the main ingredient of the "Water of England" and Huxham's elixir, preparations used liberally by Gaspar de Chaves in the therapeutic regime of patients affected by malarial fevers. "Water of England" ("Água de Inglaterra") was a leading secret remedy, produced via a concoction of the cinchona bark in alcohol and popularized during the eighteenth century by Jacob de Castro Sarmento, a Portuguese physician who took refuge in England due to Inquisitorial persecution. Prolific references to this medicine can be found in the Portuguese Pharmacopeia between the late 1600s and early 1800s (Dias 2013; Pinto 2011, 168-169). Huxham's elixir, also known as Huxham's Tincture of cinchona bark, was a popular febrifuge devised by John Huxham (1692–1768), a provincial English physician famous for his study *Essay on Fevers* (1739). Interestingly, the Portuguese Pharmacopeia of 1794 contains a recipe for a composed tincture of cinchona or antiseptic essence of Huxham (Gänger 2020, 102).

The abstruse "synoch-putrid" fevers were also common in the observations of Gaspar de Chaves. "Putrid" fevers were a major category in western medicine for about a millennium and a half-disappearing promptly during the last quarter of the eighteenth century (Hamlin 2014, 48, 119-124). As stated before, Galen considered the fevers of the humours as putrid fevers-intermittent or continuous (Hamlin, 2014, 119; Sajadi et al., 2012: 978). However, nineteenth century nosographers would render it an archaic synonym for typhus or typhoid. Two interesting cases of "synoch-putrid" fever, both occurring in the town centre (in the "Largo do Passa Rego", currently "Rua Latino Coelho"), are partially transcribed:

> In the house of J. da C., assistant of Passarego, his whole family was attacked by a malignant fever complicated with roundworms ["lombrigas", i.e., *Ascaris lumbricoides*] of formidable length in all of them. One of his sons hit by the disease, a practising surgeon at the Hospital of São José, complained of headaches, unbearable thirst, burning eyes indicating delirium, presenting red retina, short breath, extreme anxiety, prostration and weakness in a deplorable state.

M., resident in Passarego, 40 years old, of sanguine personality, firm complexion, was afflicted by "synoch-putrid" fever, accompanied by atrocious symptoms, vomiting Poracea bile with great effort and intensity, particularly during the incremental stage of fever. I have prescribed ipecacuanha in the chamomile tea to ease the great pains in the epigastric region and applied enemas and laxatives causing viscous matter. On the third day, observing that the fibre spasm soothed, I prescribed bloodletting and offered a solvent beverage to humidify and purge the abdomen because, in this situation, as in others, it is beneficial to clear the abdomen, as it is certain that the retained substances increase the fever. (Spring of 1792).[21]

It is perhaps interesting to question the nature of the "synoch-putrid" fevers described by Gaspar de Chaves or to consider a differential diagnosis. The disease experience is socially mediated, and any diagnosis is inherently social (Arrizabalaga 2002, 56; Cunningham 2002, 15). Thus, a retrospective diagnosis is not our goal but a brief ontological discussion of the particular "synoch-putrid" fevers identified in these observations. First, these fevers are different from the other "putrid" fevers presented by Gaspar de Chaves (i.e., the malarial fevers: intermittent, tertian and quartan)-not only are the designations dissimilar, but also the symptoms and therapeutic regimes.

Most of the cases presented a natural history that included at least some of the following symptoms: anxiety, suffocation, headaches, vomiting, diarrhoea, delirium, somnolence, and torpor. As for therapeutics, bloodletting was a standard procedure in these patients (52.6%; 10/19). Cinchona-based medicines were used very infrequently, while ipecacuanha (an emetic) and cordials were prescribed more often.

---

[21] Na casa de J. da C., assistente em Passarego, toda a família deste atacada de febre maligna complicada em todos com lombrigas de formidável grandeza. Um dos seus filhos praticante de cirurgia vindo do Hospital de São José molesto queixando-se de dor de cabeça, sede insuportável, olhos incendiados indicando delírio, retina vermelha, transpiração curta, ansiedade fortíssima, prostrado e abatido de forças, estado deplorável.

M., criatura assistente em Passarego, sujeita de idade 40 anos, temperamento sanguíneo, fibra forte, foi atacada de febre sinoch pútrida, acompanhando sintomas crudelíssimos, vomitando bílis Poracea com grande esforço e ânsia, principalmente no acréscimo da febre. Prescrevi emético de Hipecacuanha em chá de Marsella-Galega, a fim de evitar as grandes dores que suportava na região Epigastric. aplicando clister, laxantes que provocavam matéria viscosa. Ao terceiro dia vendo que o orgasmo da fibra se calmava prescrevi sangria baixa dando por bebida diluente a fim de humedecer e laxar o ventre, pois nestas, como em outras, é útil estar o ventre livre, tendo-se por certo que as matérias retidas fazem maior acesso de febre Arquivo Histórico Municipal de Almada, Gaspar Lopes Henriques de Chaves (Observaçoens Médico Meteorológicas, Anno de 1792, PT/AHALM/CMALM/P-D/001/0004).

We are left, perhaps, with the typhus/typhoid dyad proposed *post factum* in the nineteenth century. Both typhus and typhoid usually present as undifferentiated febrile maladies but with different etiological agents and modes of transmission. Epidemic typhus' causal agent, *Rickettsia prowazekii*, is transmitted to human beings by body lice (endemic typhus is caused by *Rickettsia mooseri* and transmitted via the rat flea), while typhoid fever's causal agent (*Salmonella typhi*) is transmitted faecal-orally (Basnyat et al. 2021, 1; Bechah et al. 2008, 417-421).

The diagnosis was not a particular goal in eighteenth-century medicine, and epidemic typhus was often confused with typhoid when Huxham made the first distinction between the two diseases in 1739 (Bechah et al. 2008, 417). As for today, it is not always simple to distinguish between typhus and typhoid fever (Basnyat 2016, 516). Many symptoms are common to both diseases even in different stages. Similarly, the cases of "synoch-putrid" fever described by de Chaves share a number of these symptoms, making it difficult to achieve an accurate diagnosis. Still, Gaspar de Chaves provides some interesting clues. First, he associates these fevers with poverty and poor sanitation, and it is a fact that both typhus and typhoid were often viewed as fevers of poverty (Hamlin 2014, 132). More remarkably, de Chaves makes an association between these fevers and the quality of the diet-and this is the detail that makes the diagnosis of typhoid (or indeed paratyphoid, or any bacterial gastroenteritis) somewhat more probable. For example:

> Therefore, ["synoch-putrid" fever] was not and is not caused by any occult miasma, a scourge that often strikes many subjects of either sex already lying in the grave. I have already said in the other observations that the phenomena which nature offers us *nosce incognitos* (knows the unknown); because considering the poverty of the town and its surroundings, and their contribution to the nasty way of living, since usually necessity obliges people to live from the cheapest foods and, as a consequence, of inferior quality and rotten for the most part; what vicious humours! (Summer of 1788)[22].

[22] Portanto (a febre sinoch-pútrida) não foi nem é causada por miasma oculto, flagelo que muitas vezes é de tantos sujeitos de um e outro sexo que se deram a sepultura; já disse em as outras observações que os fenómenos que a natureza oferece *nosce incognito*; porque considerando a pobreza da Vila e seu termo o ter contribuído ao mau regímen de viver, pois comummente a necessidade obriga a sustentar-se do mais barato e por consequência de inferior qualidade e esta corrupta pela maior parte; que humores! (Observaçoens Médico Meteorológicas, Anno de 1788, PT/AHALM/CMALM/P-D/001/0002).

Usually, contagious diseases spread among the people deprived of all the food and clothing necessary to preserve people. The widespread use of fish oil and rotten food produces indigestions, headaches, and fever because bad food generates corrupted humours. (April of 1792)[23].

Gaspar de Chaves repeatedly mentions the inadequate sanitation of Almada and the poor individual hygiene of some patients. Finally, almost half of the "synoch-putrid" fevers occurred during the autumn, and typhoid was sometimes known as "autumnal fever". Although the term "synoch-putrid" fever undoubtedly possessed therapeutic or contextual usefulness as a shorthand for a suite of symptoms, it is still difficult to give it a definite diagnostic label.

The continuous fevers were also particularly problematic in terms of diagnosis. Some post-Boerhaavian fever theorists tried to differentiate between the many forms of continuous fever. William Cullen (1710-1790) used a single, therapeutically meaningful axis, the nervous energy, while Philippe Pinel (1745-1826) identified fevers with the adjective that depicted their most conspicuous symptom, including *typhoid*. Pierre-Charles-Alexandre Louis (1787-1872) put forward a detailed description of fevers, concomitantly co-opting ancient terms like "putrid" and new terms such as "gastro-enteritis" (Hamlin 2014, 172-173). What can be concluded from Gaspar's notes on continuous fevers? In at least two cases, the municipal physician relates continuous fevers with "synoch-putrid" fevers. In some of the cases of continuous fevers, symptoms include, among others, abdominal distention, torpor, flatulence, vomiting, headaches and diarrhoea. As for therapeutics, bloodletting was used almost universally in these patients, while ipecacuanha, opium and cinchona were rarely employed.

Debatable distinctions between fevers and/or diseases were probably not a problem-at least, in practice-for Henrique Gaspar de Chaves, as for most physicians before the nineteenth century the correct diagnosis mattered much less than the desired outcome, i.e., the cure. Most of the patients that consulted Chaves recovered from their ailments, whether tertian fever, cholera, or renal colic.

---

[23] Ordinariamente grassam as doenças contagiosas em o Povo destituído de todo aquele alimento e vestuário que é necessário para a conservação do indivíduo. Este comummente usa de azeite de peixe e de maus alimentos que produzem indigestões, perturbação de cabeça, febre, porque do mau alimento se geram maus humores (Observaçoens Médico Meteorológicas, Anno de 1792, PT/AHALM/CMALM/P-D/001/0004).

However, a substantial proportion (18.7%; 23/123) died as a perceived consequence of the diseases reported. The various fevers caused or were involved in-39.1% (9/23) of all deaths.

Other diseases, like measles and syphilis, also contributed to the death toll, measles hitting a six-year-old girl (her brother, an 8-year-old boy, and a 9-year-old girl, also had measles but recovered), the treponemal disease causing the death of a 66-year-old man. Indigestion and apoplexy, probably acute myocardial infarctions, were also associated with the deaths of two patients – an 80-year-old woman and a 70-year-old obese and valetudinarian man, respectively.

The most lethal foe of the people depicted in the case notes was pulmonary disease, probably tuberculosis (considering, in some cases, the archaic term "phthisis", and in others the symptomatology), accounting for 39.1% of all deaths (9/23) and killing nine out of eleven patients diagnosed with it (81.8%). Tuberculosis (TB), commonly identified as phthisis, scrofula, or consumption before the nineteenth century (the term "tuberculosis" was coined in the middle of the 19th century by Johann Lukas Schönlein [1793-1864]), is an infectious and contagious disease caused by *Mycobacterium tuberculosis,* currently affecting nearly two billion people worldwide). By the eighteenth century, TB was rampant in Western Europe, with a yearly mortality rate as high as 900 deaths per 100,000 inhabitants (Barberis et al. 2017, 10). No wonder, then, that TB was consistently described as the "white plague" or "captain of all these men of death", and nowadays as a "serial killer" (Barberis et al. 2017, 10; Santos and Roberts 2006, 38). In the indubitable experiences of the people described in the cases by Gaspar de Chaves, a pulmonary illness that we can identify-perhaps incorrectly, but most likely not-as tuberculosis showed an astounding mortality rate, also accompanied by a spectacle of pain, suffering and loss:

> P., the wife of J. C., resident in Caparica, age 50, bilious temperament, (…), mother of many children, was subject to defluxions and challenging to be cured entirely, because of the feebleness and laxity of the lungs, so that any strange air made her cold. She came from Lisbon to take the air of Sobreda, near São Macário. She fell seriously ill with a low fever, some sweating, breathing difficulty, which increased in proportion to the fever, strongly reacting, presenting reddened face, purulent expectoration, a symptom that usually accompanies phthisis, an incurable disease as we know. (…). Someone administered only laxatives and emetics, lemon balm water, and «Quina»; (…) she came to Sobreda in the last stage of pneumonia. What could I do but palliate and not give any hope of survival where there were so many symptoms that the doctor would predict death with the least of them? (…) The patient whose history I'm recording, always afflicted with

fever and purulent sputum, (...) died on the first of September. (…) her eldest son died of the same illness, and her daughters suffered from their body constitution, being quite thin, with a narrow chest, already showing what would victimize them (March through September of 1789)[24].

Conclusion

The medical case histories compiled by Gaspar Lopes de Chaves, the municipal physician of Almada (Portugal) from 1784 until 1795, are deeply rooted in a textual tradition that developed over a long period of time, from antiquity to modern medicine (Pomata 2014). The unpublished *Observaçoens Médico Meteorológicas* provide a withered but utterly consequential glance into the everyday clinical practice in what was then a small town-located in the southern margin of the Tagus River, on the opposite side of the river and deceptively close to Lisbon, the Portuguese capital. Stealing past the windows of the blissfully dead, the physician saturates his *observationes* with intricate experiences of the disease, summoning a delicate tracery of symptoms and therapeutics and what were once real, suffering people. In the manuscripts by Gaspar de Chaves, and glossing Foucault's (1963: 85) words, the illnesses of some are transformed into the knowledge of others.

---

[24] P., mulher de J. C., assistente em Caparica, idade de 50 anos, temperamento bilioso, (…), mãe de muitos filhos, sujeita a defluxos e estes difíceis em ser curados radicalmente, porque mostrava a debilidade e frouxidão dos bofes, e qualquer ar estranho a constipava, veio da cidade de Lisboa a tomar ares em o sítio da Sobreda, junto a São Macário, procedido de ter caído gravemente doente de febre lenta, suor parcial, dificuldade no respirar, aumentando-se esta à proporção que a febre exacerbava, estímulo forte, faces rubicundas, expetoração purulenta, sintoma que pelo comum acompanha uma Phtisis, mal incurável como se sabe. (…). Administraram tão somente catárticos e vomitório por bebida, água *melis*, foram de parecer que tomasse quina; (…); com este veio para o sítio da Sobreda já no último estádio de Pulmonia. Que podia eu fazer senão paliar, e não dando esperanças absolutamente de vida onde havia tantos sintomas que o menor deles o médico prognosticaria morte? (…) A doente de que faço história sempre com febre, escarro purulento, (…) morreu nos primeiros de setembro (…) já o filho primogénito deste mesmo mal de que faleceu e suas filhas sofreram por constituição e serem bastantemente magras, peito estreito, mostrando já do que hão de ser vítimas (Observaçoens Médico Meteorológicas, Anno de 1789, PT/AHALM/CMALM/P-D/001/0003).

References

Abreu, Laurinda. 2010. "A Organização e Regulação Das Profissões Médicas No Portugal Moderno: Entre as Orientações Da Coroa e Os Interesses Privados." *In Arte Médica e Imagem Do Corpo: De Hipócrates Ao Final Do Século XVIII Médica e Imagem Do Corpo: De Hipócrates Ao Final Do Século XVIII*, edited by Adelino Cardoso, António Braz de Oliveira, and Manuel Silvério Marques, 97–122. Lisboa: Biblioteca Nacional de Portugal.

Abreu, Laurinda. 2017. "Tensions between the Físico-Mor and the University of Coimbra: The Accreditation of Medical Practitioners in Ancien-Regime Portugal." *Social History of Medicine,* 31 (2): 231–57.

Arrizabalaga, Jon. 2002. "Problematizing Retrospective Diagnosis in the History of Disease." *Asclepio,* 54 (1): 51–70.

Bandeira, Ana Maria Leitão. 1997. "Catálogo Dos Processos de Habilitação a Partidos Médicos e Boticários." *Boletim Do Arquivo Da Universidade de Coimbra* XV–XVI: 353–516.

Barberis, I., N.L. Bragazzi, M. Galluzzo, and M. Martini. 2017. "The History of Tuberculosis: From the First Historical Records to the Isolation of Koch's Bacillus." *Journal of Preventive Medicine and Public Health*, 58: E9–12. https://doi.org/10.5005/jp/books/14180_2.

Basnyat, Buddha. 2016. "Typhoid versus Typhus Fever in Post-Earthquake Nepal." *The Lancet Global Health,* 4 (8): e516–17. https://doi.org/10.1016/S2214-109X(16)30094-8.

Basnyat, Buddha, Farah Naz Qamar, Priscilla Rupali, Tahmeed Ahmed, and Christopher M. Parry. 2021. "Enteric Fever." *The British Medical J*ournal https://doi.org/10.1136/bmj.n437.

Baudry, Hervé. 2018. "Medicine and the Inquisition in Portugal (Sixteenth and Seventeenth Centuries): People and Books." *Early Science and Medicine,* 23 (1–2): 92–113. https://doi.org/10.1163/15733823-02312P06.

Bechah, Yassina, Christian Capo, Jean Louis Mege, and Didier Raoult. 2008. "Epidemic Typhus." *The Lancet Infectious Diseases,* 8 (7): 417–26. https://doi.org/10.1016/S1473-3099(08)70150-6.

Borges Coelho, António. 1987. *Inquisição de Évora: Dos Primórdios a 1668*. Lisboa: Caminho.

Castro Sarmento, Jacob. 1757. *Appendix Ao Que Se Acha Escrito Na Materia Medica*. Londres: Livraria d'Alcobaça.

Coelho, José Abílio. 2014. "Facultativos Dos Partidos Municipais: Cuidados Médicos Prestados Aos Doentes Pobres Nos Concelhos e Nos Hospitais." In *Anais Do IV Encontro Internacional de História*

Colonial, 15:148–62. Belém: Editora Açaí.

Cunningham, Andrew. 2002. "Identifying Disease in the Past: Cutting the Gordian Knot." *Asclepio,* 54 (1): 13–34. https://doi.org/10.3989/asclepio.2002.v54.i1.133.

Denipoti, Cláudio. 2017. "Medical Translators and the Idea of Translation in Portugal in the Late Eighteenth Century: The Case of Books on Medicine." *Historia, Ciencias, Saude - Manguinhos,* 24 (4): 913–31. https://doi.org/10.1590/S0104-59702017000500004.

Dias, José Pedro Sousa. 2013. *A Água de Inglaterra: Paludismo e Terapêutica Em Portugal No Século XVIII*. Lisboa: Caleidoscópio.

Dinges, Martin, Kay Peter Jankrift, Sabine Schlegelmilch, and Michael Stolberg. 2016. *Medical Practice, 1600-1900.* Leiden: Brill. https://doi.org/10.1163/9789004303324.

El-Radhi, A. 2011. "The Role of Fever in the Past and Present." *Medical Journal of Islamic World Academy of Sciences,* 19 (1): 9–14.

Fontes da Costa, Palmira. 2011. "Os Livros e a Ordem Do Saber Médico." In *Percursos Na História Do Livro Médico, (1450 - 1800)*, 13–32. Lisboa: Edições Colibri.

Foucault, Michel. 1963. *Naissance de La Clinique*. Paris: Presses Universitaires de France.

Frade, Florbela Veiga, and Sandra Neves Silva. 2011. "Medicina e Política Em Dois Físicos Judeus Portugueses de Hamburgo: Rodrigo de Castro e o Medicus Politicus (1614), e Manuel Bocarro Rosales e o Status Astrologicus (1644)." *Sefarad,* 71 (1): 51–94. https://doi.org/10.3989/sefarad.011.003.

Gänger, Stephanie. 2020. *A Singular Remedy: Cinchona Across the Atlantic World, 1751–1820*. Cambridge: Cambridge University Press.

Giglioni, Guido. 2011. "Reality and Metaphors in the Language of Renaissance Medicine: The Case of Rodrigo de Castro." In *Percursos Na História Do Livro Médico (1450 - 1800)*, 45–58. Lisboa: Edições Colibri.

Hamlin, Christopher. 2014. *More than Hot: A Short History of Fever*. Baltimore: Johns Hopkins University Press. https://doi.org/10.5860/choice.187910.

Herson, Bella, and Jutta Gutberlet. 1996. *Cristãos-Novos e Seus Descendentes Na Medicina Brasileira, 1500-1850*. São Paulo: Edusp.

Jarcho, Saul. 1993. *Quinine's Predecessor: Francesco Torti and the Early History of Cinchona*. Baltimore: Johns Hopkins University Press.

Olival, Fernanda. 2004. "Rigor e Interesses: Os Estatutos de Limpeza de Sangue Em Portugal." *Cadernos de Estudos Sefarditas* 4: 151–82.

Pinto, Hélio. 2011. "A Materia Medica de Jacob de Castro Sarmento." In

Percursos Na História Do Livro Médico (1450 - 1800), 165–86. Lisboa: Edições Colibri.

Pomata, Gianna. 2010. "Sharing Cases: The Observationes in Early Modern Medicine." *Early Science and Medicine,* 15 (3): 193–236. https://doi.org/10.1163/157338210X493932.

Pomata, Gianna. 2011. "A Word of the Empirics: The Ancient Concept of Observation and Its Recovery in Early Modern Medicine." *Annals of Science*, 68 (1): 1–25. https://doi.org/10.1080/00033790.2010.495039.

Pomata, Gianna. 2014. "The Medical Case Narrative: Distant Reading of an Epistemic Genre." *Literature and Medicine,* 32 (1): 1–23. https://doi.org/10.1353/lm.2014.0010.

Porter, Roy. 1991. "History of the Body." 206-32, In *New Perspectives on Historical Writing*, edited by P. Burke. Oxford: Polity Press.

Pulido Serrano, Juan Ignacio. 2011. "Plural Identities: The Portuguese New Christians." *Jewish History,* 25 (2): 129–51. https://doi.org/10.1007/s10835-010-9133-8.

Rodrigues, Augusto. 1992. *Memoria Professorum Universitatis Conimbrigensis 1772-1937*. Coimbra: Arquivo da Universidade de Coimbra.

Rowland, Robert. 2010. "Cristãos-Novos, Marranos e Judeus No Espelho Da Inquisição." Topoi (Rio de Janeiro) 11 (20): 172–88. https://doi.org/10.1590/2237-101x011020012.

Saavedra, Mónica. 2013. "Malária, Mosquitos e Ruralidade No Portugal Do Século XX." *Etnográfica,* 17: 51–76. https://doi.org/10.4000/etnografica.2545.

Sajadi, Mohammad M., Reza Bonabi, Mohamad Reza M. Sajadi, and Philip A. MacKowiak. 2012. "Akhawaynī and the First Fever Curve." *Clinical Infectious Diseases,* 55 (7): 976–80. https://doi.org/10.1093/cid/cis596.

Sander, Christoph. 2014. "Medical Topics in the de Anima Commentary of Coimbra (1598) and the Jesuits' Attitude towards Medicine in Education and Natural Philosophy." *Early Science and Medicine,* 19 (1): 76–101. https://doi.org/10.1163/15733823-00191p03.

Santos, Ana Luísa, and Charlotte Ann Roberts. 2006. "Anatomy of a Serial Killer: Differential Diagnosis of Tuberculosis Based on Rib Lesions of Adult Individuals from the Coimbra Identified Skeletal Collection, Portugal." *American Journal of Physical Anthropology*, 130 (1): 38–49. https://doi.org/10.1002/ajpa.20160.

Saraiva, António José. 1969. *Inquisição e Cristãos-Novos*. Porto: Editorial Inova.

Silva, Francisco Manuel Valadares e. 2008. "Ruralidade Em Almada e Seixal Nos Séculos XVIII e XIX." Lisboa: Universidade Aberta.

Stolberg, Michael. 2013. "Empiricism in Sixteenth-Century Medical Practice." *Early Science and Medicine,* 18 (6): 487–516. https://doi.org/10.1163/15733823-0186p0001.

Stolberg, Michael. 2019. "A Sixteenth-Century Physician and His Patients: The Practice Journal of Hiob Finzel, 1565-1589." *Social History of Medicine,* 32 (2): 221–40. https://doi.org/10.1093/shm/hkx063.

Szajkowski, Z. 1970. *Jews and the French Revolutions of 1789, 1830 and 1848*. New York: Ktav Publishing House.

Teixeira Rodrigues, Isilda, and Carlos Fiolhais. 2013. "O Ensino Da Medicina Na Universidade de Coimbra No Século XVI." *Historia, Ciencias, Saude - Manguinhos* 20 (2): 435–56. https://doi.org/10.1590/S0104-59702013000200005.

CHAPTER 11

TWO CENTURIES SINCE THE ISOLATION OF CINCHONINE: BERNARDINO ANTÓNIO GOMES'S NETWORKS (1768-1823)

JOÃO RUI PITA, MARIA GUILHERME SEMEDO AND ANA LEONOR PEREIRA

Abstract

In the 19th century, the South American vegetable drug cinchona bark was a popular treatment for intermittent fevers. The chemical study of cinchona bark consequently became an important field of research. In 1810, the Portuguese physician Bernardino António Gomes (1768-1823) isolated cinchonine from cinchona bark. In the work *Ensaio sobre o Cinchonino e sobre a sua influencia na virtude da quina e d'outras cascas* (1812) Gomes describes his experimental protocol and results. It was published in Portuguese and English. The isolation was highly disputed in Portugal, but it became known by the international scientific community. This work engaged the French scientists Pelletier and Caventou in the study of cinchona bark. Their research on the "grey" cinchona bark was based upon the method used by Gomes to isolate cinchonine. In 1820, Pelletier and Caventou isolated quinine, the alkaloid that later became the mainstay in malaria treatment until the mid-twentieth century.

Key words: Bernardino António Gomes (1768-1823), cinchonine, quinine, cinchona bark, history of science

Resumo

No século XIX, a droga vegetal sul-americana quina era um popular tratamento para as febres intermitentes. Em consequência, o estudo químico da quina tornou-se num importante campo de pesquisa. Em 1810, o médico português Bernardino António Gomes (1768-1823) isolou a cinchonina a partir da quina. Na obra *Ensaio sobre o Cinchonino e sobre a sua influencia na virtude da quina e d'outras cascas* (1812), Gomes descreve o seu procedimento experimental e resultados. A obra foi publicada em português e inglês. O isolamento foi muito disputado em Portugal, mas tornou-se conhecido pela comunidade científica internacional. Este trabalho envolveu os cientistas franceses Pelletier e Caventou no estudo da quina. A sua pesquisa sobre a quina "cinzenta" foi baseada no método usado por Gomes para isolar a cinchonina. Em 1820, Pelletier e Caventou isolam a quinina, o alcalóide que mais tarde se tornou o principal tratamento para a malária até meados do século XX.

Palavras-chave: Bernardino António Gomes (1768-1823), cinchonina, quinina, quina, história da ciência

Introduction

In the nineteenth century, as in the eighteenth century, cinchona bark was a very popular vegetable drug used to treat intermittent fevers. Progress achieved in the field of chemistry at the beginning of the nineteenth century enabled the isolation of several active principles from vegetable drugs. This was also the case for cinchona bark from which quinine was extracted in 1820. However, years earlier, the Portuguese physician Bernardino António Gomes (1768-1823) (Fig. 11.1) extracted cinchonine from the bark of the cinchona tree. Gomes described his experimental protocol and results in his work *Ensaio sobre o Cinchonino e sobre a sua influencia na virtude da quina e d'outras cascas* (1812). It was published in Portuguese and English. The isolation of this active ingredient was very controversial in Portugal, but the information rapidly spread throughout the international scientific community. This discovery was paramount for the study of the cinchona bark and the extraction of quinine in 1820, the alkaloid that became the main therapy for malaria until the mid-twentieth century.

It is now two centuries since quinine was isolated (1820), approximately 210 years since cinchonine was extracted (1810) from cinchona bark and approximately two hundred and fifty years since the birth of Bernardino António Gomes (1768). The authors highlight in this essay the importance for the history of medicine and pharmacy of the chemical studies conducted by this Portuguese physician and scientist, whose work culminated in the isolation of cinchonine.

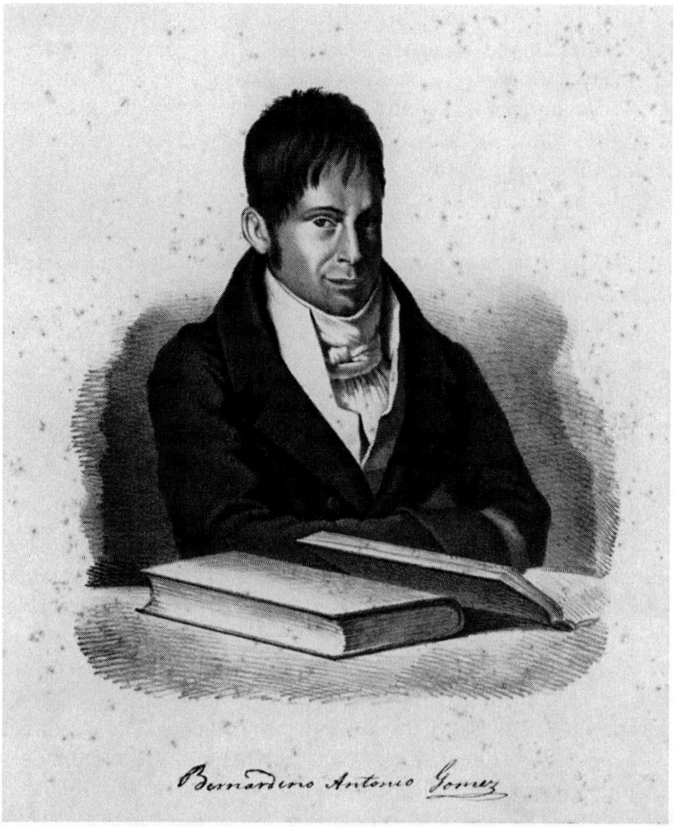

Fig. 11.1. Bernardino António Gomes (1768-1823). Biblioteca Nacional de Portugal. Lisboa (E-311-V).

Bernardino António Gomes: biographical outline

Bernardino António Gomes was born in 1768 in Paredes de Coura, a town in the north of Portugal, in the Minho region near Spain. In 1793 he graduated in Medicine at the University of Coimbra. It should be noted that twenty years earlier, in 1772, the University had undergone deep-seated reforms decreed by the Marquis of Pombal (the chief minister to the King D. José who reigned 1750-1777). These reforms enhanced the teaching of experimental chemistry, which may have been propitious for the education of Bernardino António Gomes in the subject. After he graduated, B. A.

Gomes began working as a physician in the city of Aveiro in the centre of Portugal. Sometime later he joined the Portuguese Navy as a physician. He settled in Lisbon. In 1797 he went to live in Brazil until returning to Lisbon in 1801. B. A. Gomes began working at the Military Hospital in Lisbon in 1804, and in 1810, due to health and other reasons, he turned exclusively to private practice. He was a prestigious physician.

He was back in Brazil in 1817, after being appointed the physician of Princess Leopoldine of Austria (1797-1826), who was engaged to D. Pedro (1798-1834), the future Emperor of Brazil, and went to live in Rio de Janeiro. Gomes carried out his duties as physician of the Portuguese Navy with great skill and played an important role in combatting the typhus epidemic that afflicted a Portuguese squadron in Gibraltar.

In addition to medicine and public health, he had particular interests in botany and chemistry. He was physician of the Royal Chambers, which illustrates his reputation as a doctor. He also founded the *Instituição Vacínica da Academia Real das Ciências de Lisboa* in 1812, an institution that sought to disseminate Jenner's smallpox vaccine in Portugal. His concern about smallpox is an indication of how he kept up to date with public health developments. In 1812 he was made knight of the Order of Christ and permanent member of the Royal Academy of Sciences of Lisbon (Subtil, 2017, 40, 42).

Bernardino António Gomes was a striking figure in the Portuguese history of medicine. He bequeathed to us many written accounts. He was a physician and scientist of remarkable erudition. He mastered French, English and Latin and his proficiency in languages enabled him to read prominent foreign authors.

Bernardino António Gomes fostered some medical innovations in Portugal for the treatment of typhus and the disinfection of letters. He was particularly interested in dermatology and is regarded as the first Portuguese dermatologist. He published several medical works on illnesses that cause skin manifestations, such as leprosy and framboesia (tropical infection caused by *T. pertenue*). B. A. Gomes also assessed the treatment methods of other physicians by conducting clinical trials of sorts to determine whether the recommended treatment was effective. Such was the case with the research he carried out into the anthelminthic properties of the pomegranate tree described in the book *Memoria sobre a virtude tænifuga da romeira* (1822). The works he published were generally based on his experience and observations.

In addition to practising the medical profession and promoting public health, he conducted other studies, namely in botany and chemistry. He worked in Brazil for several years. This encouraged him to perform a range of internationally recognised botanical studies of the ipecacuanha and other less well-known Brazilian plants. He became particularly well-known for research that resulted in the isolation of cinchonine in 1810. Cinchonine was the first known alkaloid of the cinchona bark and one of the first alkaloids obtained from a plant. Cinchona bark provided the basis for preparing febrifugal herbal remedies used to treat intermittent fevers, which medical historiography has associated with malaria (Oaks Jr. et al. 1991). At the time, there was no tradition of performing innovative scientific research in Portugal. It should be recalled that in 1820 French scientists Joseph Pelletier (1788-1842) and Joseph-Bienaimé Caventou (1795-1877) extracted quinine from cinchona bark. Furthermore, developments in the field of chemistry in the late 18th and early 19th centuries enabled the isolation of several active ingredients from plants. Bernardino António Gomes was perfectly aligned with international achievements. The following were some of the early discoveries in this field: narcotine (Derosne 1803), morphine (Serturner 1805), emetine (Pelletier and Magendie 1817), veratrine (Meisner 1818), strychnine (Pelletier and Caventou 1818), brucine (Pelletier and Caventou 1819), caffeine (Runge 1820), quinine (Pelletier and Caventou 1820), and atropine (Mein 1831).

B. A. Gomes had a son who was also called Bernardino António Gomes (1806-1877). His son was a prominent physician and scientist, who published several books on general medicine and other more specific texts, for example on health care, psychiatry, pharmacology and hygiene. He was also a supporter of liberalism. Bernardino António Gomes' son had two sons, each of whom excelled in other branches of knowledge in Portugal: Bernardino Barros Gomes (1839-1910) in botany, forestry and agriculture; Henrique Barros Gomes (1843-1898) studied mathematics, astronomy and geography, and also performed important political activity as a member of the national parliament and minister in several ministries.

The discovery and isolation of cinchonine

The cinchona tree is a medicinal plant famous for its antimalarial properties. It is indigenous to the South American forests of the Andes in Peru, Bolivia, Ecuador, Colombia and Venezuela (Costa 1944, 16). It was possibly used in the 16th century as a remedy against humidity and cold weather (Andrés Turrión 2005, 133; Crespo 1997, 347). In the seventeenth century Cinchona was already exported to Europe (Crawford 2016, 10-11), but information on the plant was scarce and contradictory. In 1738, Charles-Marie de La Condamine (1701-1774) published the first scientific description of the plant, which he called *quinquina* (Condamine 1738). The name was derived from the Quechua word "quina quina" (Honigsbaum 2003, 23). In 1742, Linnaeus created the genus *Cinchona* (Linnaeus 1742, 527).

In the early nineteenth century cinchona bark had become a popular treatment for intermittent fever (Gachelin et al. 2017, 73), namely the so-called tertian and quartan fevers (Sarmento 1756, xxiii) that can be caused by malaria. However, the cinchona tree only grew spontaneously in some parts of South America (Costa 1944, 16). Consequently, in the second half of the nineteenth century several European nations believed that these plants were becoming scarce and, moved by economic and health interests, they tried to cultivate the plant in their African and Asian colonies (Costa 1944, 21-42; Brockway 2002, 104, 111-113).

Chemical research on cinchona bark became an important line of research. It sought, among other things, to discover the principles of the activity of the cinchona bark against fever (Seguin 1804; Vauquelin 1806, 162; Gomes 1812a, 213). In 1803, the Scottish physician Andrew Duncan Junior (1773-1832) detected in the cinchona bark a substance he called cinchonin (Duncan Junior 1803, 228). In France, several chemists, such as Armand Seguin (1765-1835) and Louis-Nicolas Vauquelin (1763-1829), also conducted chemical studies of the cinchona bark (Seguin 1804, Vauquelin 1806).

The government in Portugal was interested in finding cinchona bark alternatives in its overseas territories, namely Brazil, then a Portuguese colony. In 1804, a royal charter authorised the chief physician of the Kingdom (i.e. the person in charge of health management and health services in Portugal), Francisco Tavares (1750-1812), to commission "the necessary tests and inquiries" of the Brazilian bitter barks in Portuguese hospitals (Royal Charter in *Jornal de Coimbra*, 1814a, 282). The intention was to find out whether these barks had the same febrifugal properties as the cinchona bark from Peru (Royal Charter in *Jornal de Coimbra* 1814a, 282). Consequently, several samples of potentially febrifugal barks were sent from Brazil to Portugal to be analysed (Noticia 1857, 13).

In Coimbra, the chemist Tomé Rodrigues Sobral (1759-1829), who taught at the University of Coimbra and was the director of the university chemistry lab, was commissioned to perform the chemical analyses on the samples of Brazilian barks (Costa 1944, 92; Amorim da Costa 2015, 1003).

Bernardino Gomes was among the scientists who studied these barks in Lisbon (Noticia 1857, 13). Gomes used these barks in his clinical practice at the military and navy hospitals, especially in the treatment of intermittent fevers (Gomes, 1812a 212-213). Bernardino Gomes noted that not all samples had febrifugal properties. Consequently, he decided to conduct chemical tests to compare "cinchona barks from the Spanish Americas" to the Brazilian barks, thinking that he might be able to detect the element responsible for the febrifugal activity in the cinchona bark from Peru (Gomes 1812a, 213). The study resulted in the isolation of cinchonine by Bernardino António Gomes, in 1810.

Bernardino António Gomes had learnt about Dr Duncan Junior's study of "cinchonin". Thus, by performing chemical analyses on cinchona bark, he created an experimental process that enabled him to isolate cinchonine. The experimental protocol, the findings and the conclusions of the isolation work are described in *Ensaio sobre o Cinchonino e sobre a sua influencia na virtude da quina e d'outras cascas* (1812) (Gomes 1812a).

The *Ensaio sobre o cinchonino* was delivered at a general meeting of the Royal Academy of Sciences of Lisbon on July 7, 1810 (Silva 2015, 252). The paper was translated and published in English in two periodicals, *The Edinburgh Medical and Surgical Journal* (Gomes 1811) and the *Medical and Physical Journal* (Gomes 1812b)[1]. As a consequence of the French invasions (Silva 2015, 185), *Ensaio sobre o cinchonino* was published in Portuguese only 2 years later, in *Memórias da Academia Real das Ciências de Lisboa* of the Royal Academy.

In *Ensaio sobre o cinchonino*, Bernardino Gomes suggests that cinchonine might be the substance in cinchona bark accounting for its febrifugal properties. However, he asks whether cinchonine is febrifugal by itself, or is only "an essential part of the febrifuge principle" (Gomes 1812a, 214).

On 22 May 1811, the Secretary of State for War Affairs and the Navy also charged the Royal Academy of Sciences to appoint a committee to study the Brazilian "cinchona barks" (Silva 2015, 253). The committee, of which Bernardino Gomes was a member, completed its analysis on 18 July 1811 (Silva et al. 1814, 118). The research was reported in *Experiencias Chymicas, sobre a Quina do Rio de Janeiro comparada com outras* (1814).

Cinchonine's isolation triggered an intense discussion between Gomes and the editors of the *Jornal de Coimbra*, the only medical journal existing in Portugal at the time (Noticia 1857, 17). The articles in this controversy were published from 1812 to 1819. The editors of the *Jornal de Coimbra*, Ângelo Ferreira Dinis (1768-1848), Jerónimo Joaquim de Figueiredo (1772-1828) and José Feliciano de Castilho (1769-1826), who also taught at the University of Coimbra, challenged the experimental procedure and the purity of the reagents (Redactores 1812a, 451; Castilho 1814b, 228), and

[1] The paper was fully translated into English except for a small portion in section 9, in which Gomes exhorted the doctors who worked in Portuguese hospitals, particularly military hospitals, to conduct additional clinical experiments with cinchona bark, to further clarify cinchonine's febrifugal activity.

they were not convinced that cinchonine actually existed (Redactores 1812b, 91-92; Castilho 1817, 218).

Nonetheless, the isolation of cinchonine by Gomes was an important event in the history of chemistry, as it later contributed to the isolation of quinine by Joseph Pelletier and Joseph-Bienaimé Caventou in 1820.

International effects and the input of Bernardino António Gomes to isolating quinine

In France, Vauquelin, whom Gomes had asked for advice on cinchonine (according to José Feliciano de Castilho), announced that Bernardino António Gomes had isolated cinchonine (Castilho 1817, 219). Vauquelin informed the chemist Charles Laubert (1762-1834) about the isolation of cinchonine.

In 1816, Laubert described Gomes's experimental procedure in one of his works (Laubert 1816, 295-296). Laubert stated: "I was pleasantly surprised when I read Mr. Gomes's memoirs, because I saw that the crystal material I found in cinchona bark had already been found by this chemist, who confirmed my experiment and encouraged me to look at the crystals as a particular substance" (Laubert 1816, 296).

Meanwhile, several scientists mentioned the work that had been carried out to isolate cinchonine, namely the Scottish physician Andrew Duncan Junior in 1813 (Duncan Junior 1813, 95-96), the French physician (1768-1837) in 1817, who underlined that the matter that Laubert had ingeniously isolated was no more than "cinchonin" that the "wise chemist" Mr. Gomes (Alibert 1817, 45) had extracted; and the French chemist Louis-Jacques Thénard (1777-1857) stated that Dr Gomes from Lisbon "had managed to obtain the bitter ingredient of crystallised cinchona" which he called "cinchonin" (Thenard 1818, 379).

Later, Pelletier and Caventou also performed chemical analyses on cinchona bark based on Gomes's experimental procedure, and they isolated quinine in 1820 (Pelletier and Caventou 1820).

Quinine replaced cinchona bark in the therapy. In 1820 quinine was clinically tested to treat intermittent fevers (Double 1820; Webb Junior 2009, 102). Several European countries and the United States of America also quickly began producing quinine. Pelletier set up his own quinine-producing company (Webb Junior 2009, 103-104).

In the work that describes the isolation of quinine *Des Recherches chimiques sur le Quinquinas*, Pelletier and Caventou acknowledge that the Portuguese physician was the first to have extracted cinchonine (Pelletier and Caventou 1820, 363). They also report having used the experimental procedure of Gomes to search for cinchonine "as reported by M. Lauber [sic], who found out about it through Mr. Vauquelin, as described in Mr. Thenard's *Traité de Chimie*" (Pelletier and Caventou 1820, 291). Therefore, Pelletier and Caventou did not learn about the experimental procedure directly from Gomes, but rather through the *Traité de Chimie* by Thenard.

Why did Pelletier and Caventou conduct new research into the cinchona bark? According to Pelletier and Caventou:

> "The discovery of plant alkalis [substances with basic chemical properties, i.e. with a pH above 7] (...) explains a series of irregularities found in the analysis of plants. Salifiable organic bases have such unique properties, they are so often the active ingredient of the plants that contain them, that it is only natural to look for them in the bark of the cinchona tree: indeed, if cinchonine, discovered by Mr. Gomes in the grey cinchona is, as the physician reassures, the substance through which its bark acts in the animal economy, although the scientist states that it is neither acid nor alkaline, would it not have been necessary to examine whether a mistake was committed in the last preparation phase? These are the reflections that gave us the idea to undertake new research into the cinchona bark: as soon as we embarked on this journey, we took our work beyond our initial proposition" (Pelletier and Caventou, 1820, 290-291)[2]

Pelletier and Caventou also suggested that the name "cinchonin" that Gomes had given to the substance he had isolated be changed to "cinchonine". Since cinchonine is a base, it should be feminine, like other "salifiable" organic bases (Pelletier and Caventou 1820, 294-295).

For years after quinine was isolated, the contribution of Gomes to Pelletier and Caventou's research was highlighted in several works.

In 1835, the *Dictionnaire de Médecine et de Chirurgie Pratiques* referred to Gomes, Reuss and Duncan's work and how it fostered new research, namely by Pelletier and Caventou (Andral et al. 1835, 47).

---

[2] Original citation: "La découverte des alcalis végétaux fait époque dans la science; elle explique une suite d'anomalies qui se rencontraient dans l'analyse végétale. Les bases salifiables organiques ont des propriétés si particulières, elles sont si constamment la matière active des végétaux qui les recèlent, qu'il était naturel de les rechercher dans les quinquinas: d'ailleurs, si la cinchonine, découverte par M. Gomès dans le quinquina gris, est, comme l'assure ce médecin, la substance en vertu de laquelle cette écorce agit sur l'économie animale, bien que ce savant assure qu'elle n'est ni acide ni alcaline, n'était-il pas nécessaire d'examiner s'il n'y avait pas erreur dans la dernière partie de sa préparation? Telles sont les réflexions qui nous ont suggéré l'idée d'entreprendre de nouvelles recherches sur les quinquinas: une fois entrés dans cette carrière, nous avons poussé nos travaux au-delà du but que nous nous étions d'abord proposé" (Pelletier and Caventou 1820, 290-291).

F.-V. Mérat (1780-1851) and Adrien Jacques de Lens (1786-1846) in *Dictionnaire Universel de Matière Médicale, et de Thérapeutique Générale* also acknowledged Gomes's contributions. Mérat and Lens stated that Pelletier and Caventou in their analyses of the cinchona bark, which culminated in the isolation of quinine, were mostly guided by the work conducted by Gomes and Reuss (Mérat and Lens 1837, 28).

Furthermore, in 1889, B. Dupuy (1838-1917) declared that when Gomes discovered in the grey cinchona a "crystallizable matter", that aroused Pelletier and Caventou's curiosity to conduct chemical research into cinchona bark. Dupuy also states that the French scientists used the experimental procedures of Gomes to obtain cinchonine, and then showed that cinchonine was alkaline using their "common method for purification" (Dupuy 1889, 41-42).

Conclusion

As explained above, although several people contributed cumulatively to the isolation of quinine, the role of Gomes is highlighted by Pelletier and Caventou in their work *Des Recherches chimiques sur le Quinquinas* (1820), in which they describe the isolation of quinine and cinchonine.

The isolation of cinchonine by Bernardino António Gomes caught the attention of the international scientific community and was disseminated in several countries. Gomes concluded that cinchonine was possibly the substance responsible for the febrifugal activity of the cinchona bark. Furthermore, he did not identify cinchonine as a base. These conclusions, in addition to the later discovery that plants could contain basic substances, which were also often the active ingredients of the plants, inspired Pelletier and Caventou to conduct new research into cinchona bark. This culminated in the isolation of the most important alkaloid in cinchona bark, quinine.

It is thus demonstrated that Bernardino António Gomes's revelation was a major development at the national and international level. Furthermore, it fostered the development of several networks of scientific relations.

References

Alibert, J. L. 1817. *Nouveaux Élémens de Thérapeutique et de Matière Médicale*. Fourth Edition, Vol. I, Paris: Crapelet.

Amorim da Costa, António Marinho. 2015. "Thomé Rodrigues Sobral (1759-1829) e a virtude febrífuga de um grande número de quinas". *Quimica Nova*, 38 (7): 1002-1007. doi: 10.5935/0100-4042.20150114 (accessed on 21th January 2020).

Andral [et al] – *Dictionnaire de Médecine et de Chirurgie Pratiques*. Vol.14. Paris: Mequignon-Marvis, J.-B. Baillière, 1835.

Andrés Turrión, María Luisa de. 2005. "Las polémicas de la quina" Vol. I, 133-134. In: Puerto Sarmiento J, ed., *Ciencia y técnica en latinoamérica en el período virreinal*, [s.l]: CESCE.

Brockway, L. H. 2002. *Science and Colonial Expansion. The Role of the British Royal Botanic Gardens*, New Haven & London: Yale University Press.

Cabral, Célia, Pereira, Ana-Leonor and Pita, João Rui. 2015. "Pharmacy, quina and quinine in Portugal, 18th-20th centuries". *Circumscribere: International Journal for the History of Science*, 16: 138–153.

Castilho, José Feliciano de. 1817. "Resposta de José Feliciano de Castilho a um escrito de Bernardino Antonio Gomes, publicado no *Investigador Portuguez* em Inglaterra, Num. LXVII. 260". *Jornal de Coimbra,* [10] 52 (1): 217-254.

Castilho, José Feliciano de. 1814a. "Reflexões de José Feliciano de Castilho, sôbre um Escrito de Bernardino Antonio Gomes, publicado no *Investigador Portuguez* em Inglaterra, Num. XXII. p. 206". *Jornal de Coimbra*, 6 (29) (Parte 1): 277-287.

Castilho, José Feliciano de. 1814b. "Reflexões de José Feliciano de Castilho sôbre um Escrito de Bernardino Antonio Gomes". *Jornal de Coimbra*, 7 (35) (Parte 1): 201-240.

Condamine, C. M. de la. 1738. "Sur l'arbre du Quinquina". *Mémoires de l'Académie Royale de Sciences de Paris*: 226–243.

Costa, Aloísio Fernandes. 1944. *O problema das quinas*, Lisboa: Cosmos. Biblioteca Cosmos.

Crawford, Matthew James. 2016. *The Andean Wonder Drug: Cinchona Bark and Imperial Science in the Spanish Atlantic, 1630-1800*, Pittsburgh: University of Pittsburgh Press.

Crespo, Fernando I. Ortiz. 1997. "Monardes y Fragoso: Dos protobotánicos del Siglo XVI que se ocuparon de las plantas del Nuevo Mundo y las implicaciones de sus escritos sobre la introducción europea de la corteza del árbol de «quina» (Cinchona)". 347-360. *In* Rios M, Pedersen H. B., eds., *Uso y Manejo de Recursos Vegetales. Memorias del Segundo Simposio Ecuatoriano de Etnobotánica y Botánica Económica*. Quito: Ediciones Abya-Yala.

Double F. J. 1820. "Considérations thérapeutiques sur une nouvelle préparation de quinquina". *Revue médicale 6ème livraison*:130–152.

Duncan Junior, Andrew. 1803. "Letter from ANDREW DUNCAN, M. D. F. R. S. E. containing Experiments and Observations on Cinchona, tending particularly to shew that it does not contain Gelatine". *Nicholson's Journal* 6 (December): 225-228.

Duncan Junior, Andrew. 1813. *The Edinburgh New Dispensatory*. Seventh Edition, Edinburgh: Bell & Bradfute.

Dupuy, B. 1889. *Alcaloïdes. Histoire, propriètés chimiques et physiques. Extraction, action physiologique, effects thérapeutiques. Toxicologie, Observations. Usage em médecine, Formules, etc.* Vol. I, Paris and Bruxelles: [Rongier].

Gachelin, G., Garner, P., Ferroni, E., Tröhler, U., and Chalmers, I. 2017. "Evaluating Cinchona bark and quinine for treating and preventing malaria". *Journal of the Royal Society of Medicine*, 110 (2): 73–82.

[Gomes, Bernardino António]. 1857. *NOTICIA da vida e trabalhos scientificos do medico Bernardino Antonio Gomes*, Lisboa: Typographia da Academia Real das Sciencias.

Gomes, Bernardinus Anthony. 1811. "AN ESSAY upon Cinchonin, and its Influence upon the Virtue of Peruvian Bark, and other Barks". *The Edinburgh Medical and Surgical Journal,* 7 (28): 420-431.

Gomes, Bernardino António 1812a. "Ensaio sobre o Cinchonino, e sobre a sua influencia na virtude da quina, e d'outras cascas". *Memorias da Academia Real das Sciencias de Lisboa,* 3 (1): 201-216.

Gomes, Bernardinus Anthony. 1812b. "AN ESSAY upon Cinchonin, and its Influence upon the Virtue of Peruvian Bark, and other Barks". *Medical and Physical Journal,* 27: 295-306.

Honigsbaum, Mark. 2003. *The fever trail: in search of the cure for malaria*, New York: Picador.

Laubert. 1816. "Sur l'écorce du Cinchona condaminea, Humb. et Bonpl., Cascarilla de Loxa des Espagnols". *Journal de pharmacie et des sciences accessoires*, 2 (7): 289–296.

Linnaeus, Carl. 1742. *Genera Plantarum*, Second Edition, [s.l.]: Lugduni Batavorum.

Pelletier and Caventou. 1820. "Des Recherches chimiques sur le Quinquinas". *Annales de Chimie et de Physique*, 15: 289–318; 337–365.

Mérat, J.-F. and A. J. Lens. 1837. *Dictionnaire unversel de matière médicale et de thérapeutique générale.* Vol. IV, Bruxelles: Société Belge de Librairie.

Oaks Jr., S. C., Mitchell, V. S., Pearson, G. W., & Carpenter, C. C. J. (1991). *Malaria: Obstacles and Opportunities*. (C. for the S. on M. P. and C. D. of I. Health, Ed.), National A, Washington, D.C.

Pereira, Ana Leonor and Pita, João Rui. 2001. "Bernardino António Gomes, Pai (1768-1823). O isolamento do cinchonino". *In Vivo*. 2 (6): 44-45.

Pereira, Ana Leonor and Pita, João Rui. 1994. "Ciências". *In* Mattoso, José (dir.), *História de Portugal – O Liberalismo (1807-1890)*, Vol. 5, 652-667. Lisboa: Editorial Estampa.

Pita, João Rui. 2007. *História da farmácia*. Third edition, Coimbra: Minerva Coimbra.

Redactores do J. de C. 1812a. "Resposta á réplica segunda e ultima do Sr. B. A. Gomes". *Jornal de Coimbra*, 2 (12): 449-451.

Redactores. 1812b. "MEMORIA sôbre as Quinas em geral; e ensaio em particular de algumas mais usadas, comparando a Brasiliense. Analysada, em Notas, pelos Redactores". *Jornal de Coimbra,* 2 (8): 90-102.

Sarmento, Jacob de Castro. 1756. *Do Uso e Abuso das minhas Agoas de Inglaterra, ou Directorio, e Instruccam, para Se saber seguramente, quando se deve, ou não, usar dellas, assim nas enfermidades agudas; como em algumas chronicas; e em casos propriamente de Cirurgia*, Londres: Caza de Guilherme Strahan.

Seguin. 1804. "Abstract of a Memoir on the Febrifuge Principle of Cinchona". *The Medical and physical journal*, 11 (61): 215–217. Available online: https://www.ncbi.nlm.nih.gov/pmc/articles/PMC5669646/?page=1 (accessed 16 September, 2020)

Silva, J. A. T. R. da, 2015. *A Academia Real das Ciências de Lisboa (1779-1834): ciências e hibridismo numa periferia europeia.* Dissertação de Doutoramento Faculdade de Ciências da Universidade de Lisboa.

Thenard, L. J. 1818. *Traité de Chimie Élémentaire, Théorique et Pratique*. Second Edition, Vol. III, Paris: Crochard.

Silva, J. B. A. e, Trigozo, S. F. de M., Croft, J., and B. A. Gomes. 1814. "Experiencias Chymicas, sobre a Quina do Rio de Janeiro comparada com outras". *Memorias de Mathematica e Physica da Academia Real das Sciencias de Lisboa*. 3 (2): 96–118.

Subtil, Carlos. 2017. *Bernardino António Gomes: Ilustre médico iluminista nascido em Paredes de Coura*, Paredes de Coura: Câmara Municipal de Paredes de Coura.

Vauquelin. 1806. "Expériences Sur les diverses espèces de Quinquina". *Annales de chimie ou recueil de mémoires concernant la chimie et les arts qui en dependente, et spécialement la pharmacie*: 113-169.

Webb Jr., J. L. A. 2009. *Humanity's Burden. A Global History of Malaria*. Cambridge: Cambridge University Press.

CHAPTER 12

PNEUMONIC INFLUENZA (SPANISH FLU) IN PORTUGAL

ANTÓNIO TRABULO

Abstract

At a time when our planet has been hit again by a viral pandemic, it seems appropriate to remember the catastrophe triggered by the Pneumonic Influenza (Spanish flu) of 1918-1919 and, if possible, to learn something from the memories. We will focus mainly on the implications of Pneumonic Influenza in Portugal, paying symbolical tribute to the tens of thousands of casualties recorded in our country, and remembering Amadeo de Souza Cardoso (1887-1918), one of the most illustrious Portuguese contemporary artists, taken away by the pandemic.
Key words: Epidemic diseases; Spanish flu in Portugal; Amadeo de Sousa Cardoso

Resumo

Na altura em que o nosso planeta volta a ser abalado por uma pandemia viral, parece oportuno recordar a catástrofe desencadeada pela Gripe Pneumónica de 1918-1919 e, se possível, retirar das memórias alguns ensinamentos. Trataremos, em especial, das implicações da Pneumónica em Portugal. Homenageamos simbolicamente as dezenas de milhar de vítimas mortais registadas no nosso país descrevendo, de forma breve, a vida do português mais ilustre que o vírus ceifou: o pintor Amadeo de Souza Cardoso (1887-1918).
Palavras-chave: Epidemias; Gripe espanhola em Portugal; Amadeo de Sousa Cardoso

Introduction

2018 marked the centenary of the onset of the Pneumonic Influenza (Spanish flu), the deadliest pandemic in human history, caused by Influenza, a virus of the H1N1 subtype, infecting 500 million people globally when the world population was around 1.6 billion (Vagneron 2018, 21-43). Almost a third of the planet's inhabitants fell ill (Sobral 2001, 45-65). Estimates of global casualties range from 20 to 100 million people. (Sequeira 2001, 49-55, Pereira 2019, 55-86, Johnson and Mueller 2002, 105-115). Some historians point to the number of casualties compared to the sum of civilian and military casualties recorded in the set of the two Great Wars (Sobral 2001, 45-65). In a single year, Pneumonic Influenza probably harvested a third of the number of lives claimed by the plague in six centuries of history (Sequeira 2001, 49-55). The mortality rate varied depending on the countries affected, the waves of the epidemic, and the observational criteria. Johnson and Mueller (2002, 105-115) point to a mortality rate of 2.5 to 5 per cent worldwide. It was higher in the second wave, reaching 6 to 8 per cent, and approaching 20 per cent in some regions. In the United States, Native American populations were thoroughly devastated.

The geographical origin of the so-called "Spanish flu" continues to be discussed. What is known, however, is that it did not start in Spain. The explanation for the nickname is simple (Sequeira 2001, 49-55). Spain was one of the few countries that maintained neutrality during World War I and, for that reason, one of the few countries where the press was free to report the epidemics. It was known that, even so far from the region of the armed conflict, thousands and thousands of people were falling ill and dying. The belligerent countries avoided over-alarming national public opinion, censoring the news.

The first reliable record comes from Kansas, in the centre of the USA. The disease was first identified in a Haskell County military camp in January 1918. (Sequeira 2001, 49-55). Soon afterwards, the virus was carried by American soldiers. Pneumonics travelled by sea. In Europe, the first cases were recorded in April 1918, occurring in French, English and American soldiers at ports of embarkation in France (Sequeira 2001, 49-55). This is the prevailing opinion. However, some argue that the pandemic started earlier, in French and English military installations (Killingray 2009, 41-61). Others admit the possibility that the flu might have had a multicentric origin, with independent foci in Asia, Europe and the USA. The pneumonic flu virus travelled throughout the world for eighteen months, from March 1918 to August 1919.

In September of that year, two French bacteriologists Charles Nicolle (1866-1036) and René Dujarric suggested the viral origin of the flu. A “filterable” microbe, so tiny that it passed through the best filters, was responsible for transmission (Andrade 2018, 67-92; https://www.history of vaccines.org/node/2381, accessed 25 July 2021). In 1931, Richard Shop isolated the swine influenza virus. In 1933, the English physicians Wilson Smith, Christopher Andrews and Patrick Laidlow attributed the human ‘flu to the influenza virus (Andrade 2018, 67-92). The influenza virus in humans was isolated in 1939. Pneumonia was caused by a strain of the Influenza A virus, subtype H1N1 (Sequeira 2001, 49-55; Sobral 2018, 45-66, Morens and Fauci, 2027, 1018).

The influenza virus is an orthomyxovirus with two essential types of surface glycoproteins: hemagglutinin and neuraminidase (Sequeira 2001, 49-55). The variation in the antigenicity of these glycoproteins allows Influenza to present itself in new forms almost every year. More significant variations occur from time to time, the so-called “antigenic shift” (Sequeira 2001, 49-55). The immune system defence is based upon humoral immunity by producing antibodies against antigens. The antibody-mediated immunity is supported by cellular immunity, under the charge of T lymphocytes, natural killer cells and macrophages (Sequeira 2001, 49-55).

According to Francisco George, a Public Health specialist, flu pandemics are always different from previous outbreaks, every pandemic being followed by annual epidemics caused by related viral strains, like a dynasty. In 2005, the genetic sequencing of the 1918 influenza virus was announced from studies in corpses buried in the frozen fields of northern Europe (Sequeira 2001, 49-55).

Children and the elderly are often the most vulnerable to epidemics. However, Pneumonic Influenza hit the young sectors essentially, predominantly those aged between 20 and 40. Studies in mice suggested that deaths occurred when the immune system overreacted to the virus, with excessive release of cytokines. These cytokine “storms” may have precipitated lung involvement and death in young adults (Andrade 2018, 67-92).

Evolution of the Pneumonic Influenza in Portugal

In Portugal, calculations of total deaths vary between 100,000 (Sequeira 2001, 49-55) and more than 130,000 (Bandeira 2009, 131-154, Sobral 2018, 45-65). These numbers are in stark contrast to the 8,000 dead Portuguese soldiers registered in the First World War, the 9,000 fallen during the 16 years of the colonial wars and the 10,550 attributed to AIDS over the 30 years of the endemic period (Abreu 2018, 93-120). Pneumonics increased during the years 1918 and 1919. Its progress was not regular, evolving in three successive waves (Sequeira 2001, 49-55). The first was the most benign and ran until August 1918; the second was the deadliest. It settled during the cold months of autumn and winter. Portugal is said to have recorded one of the highest mortality rates in Europe. The calculations vary between 9.8 per thousand inhabitants (Sobral 2018, 45-65) and 22 per thousand inhabitants (Bandeira 2009, 131-154). In neighbouring Spain, deaths were around 13 per thousand. The third wave ran from April to May 1919.

The flu pandemic presented rare virulence and aggressiveness, killing quickly, sometimes in two or three days, people presenting haemorrhagic symptoms. The association of severe bacterial respiratory complications was frequent. The elderly are often more vulnerable to epidemics. This was not the case with Pneumonics, which which preferentially hit the young sectors of the population, especially those aged between 20 and 40.

In Portugal, children under two years of age and young adults were most affected. Half the deaths are recorded in the 20 to 40-year-old age group (Andrade 2018, 67-92) and 55 per cent in those between 15 and 39 years of age (Sequeira 2001, 49-55). However, it is possible that some of those deaths were falsely attributed to the flu.

The measures taken against the pandemic were similar to those learned from the centuries-old experience of combating Exanthematic Typhus[1] and the Bubonic Plague: mandatory bathing, disinfection of clothes and housing, isolation of patients and their contacts. In addition, there was mandatory notification of infections and the division of larger cities into sanitary areas, with restrictions on circulation between neighbourhoods. The use of masks and frequent hand washing was recommended. Public spaces were disinfected with formaldehyde, creolin and other products. On 2 October 1918, the direction of the H.C.L. (Lisbon Civil Hospitals) prohibited visits to hospitalized patients (Andrade, 2018, 67-92).

The first known cases occurred during May 1918 in Vila Viçosa. They were brought from Spain by Portuguese seasonal workers from Badajoz and Olivença (Sequeira 2001, 49-55). However, the points of entry of the virus into our country may have been multiple, related to the return of soldiers from fighting in France (Andrade 2018, 67-92). In Oporto, some cases were already registered in early March.

The flu spread rapidly across Alentejo, arriving in Lisbon in June. In a short time, it spread across the country. In Madeira, it started in mid-

[1] https://apps.who.int/iris/handle/10665/237828 accessed 18 August 2022.

September, having been introduced by passengers on the ship Mormugão. One week later, it reached the Azores, transmitted by patients who travelled by sea from Bordeaux to Ponta Delgada (Andrade 2018, 67-92).

When some cases of fulminant pneumonia occurred in Vila Nova de Gaia in August (Sequeira 2001, 49-55), some people feared facing an outbreak of bubonic plague, of which there was a recent memory. An outbreak of epidemic plague had occurred in the region at the end of the 19th century (Pereira 2019, 57). The health authorities clarified that it was flu, but the population will have gained nothing from the change. This marked the beginning of the second wave of the flu. It only lasted for a few months, but the mortality rate was higher than in the first wave. Lisbon, Oporto and Viseu were the most badly affected districts (Bandeira 2009, 131-154).

The highest mortality rates did not occur in the most populous countries of the continent. Benavente was the village most affected by the epidemic, with seven per cent of the affected patients dying. Among the cities, the most affected were Covilhã and Leiria (Bandeira 2009, 131-154; Pereira 2019, 55-86). The mortality rate was higher in women (54 per cent of the total deaths), compared to other countries (Sobral 2018, 45-65).

In a chapter of a still unpublished book, Rogério Palma Rodrigues, an orthopaedic doctor, reports on the effects of the second wave of Pneumonic Influenza in patients hospitalized at the Outão Sanatorium (near Setúbal).

In November 1918, 57 young ladies admitted to the Sanatorium for various forms of extrapulmonary tuberculosis and other diverse pathologies were affected by the "Spanish" flu (at the time, Outão received only female patients). Most were from the Lisbon District. Four patients died, corresponding to a seven per cent mortality rate. The first patient diagnosed was from Ameixial (Estremoz) and survived the 'flu (Rodrigues, Chapter "A gripe pneumónica no Sanatório do Outão" (Fig. 12.1).

At the time, the first multipurpose vaccines were tested. Some came to be used in late 1918 with limited success. In 1920 (the numbers for 1918 are not known) there were 2,580 medical doctors in Portugal (1/2,338 inhabitants) and 1,577 pharmacies (1/3,825 inhabitants), mainly concentrated in large cities. They were scarce in peripheral regions, such as Algarve. Mobilisation of many doctors for the war in Flanders worsened the country's health situation (Sobral 2018, 45-65).

Ricardo Jorge (1858-1939) (Fig. 12.2), director of the then Central Hygiene Institute, played an important role, although not always consensual, in the fight against influenza. He had become known for his intervention in the outbreak of bubonic plague in Oporto in July 1899.

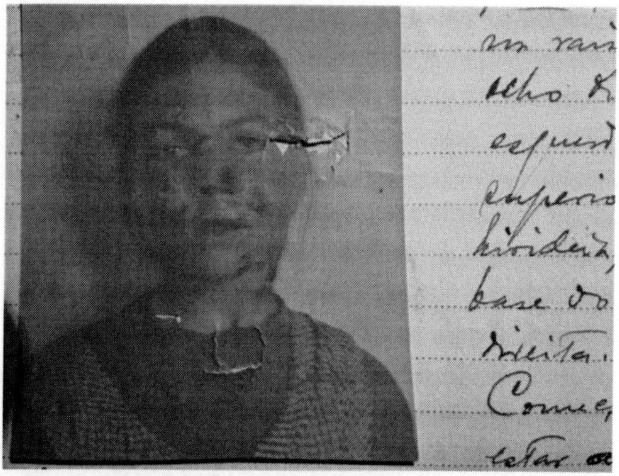

Fig. 12.1. 14-year-old girl suffering from tuberculosis of cervical tuberculosis lymphadenitis (scrofula) and cutaneous tuberculosis. Rodrigues, Rogério Palma. Outão-Meio século de trabalhos e de memórias. A gripe pneumónica no Sanatório Marítimo do Outão.

When Pneumonic Influenza entered the country, he was Director-General of Health and appointed General-Commissioner by the Government to the fight against the 'flu epidemic. On 18 June 2018, he presented a report to the Hygiene Superior Council referring to "the new peninsular incursion of influenza" (Pereira 2019, 55-86). Ricardo Jorge mandated the notification of all diagnosed cases, sought to prevent the movement of military forces and the migrations of seasonal agricultural workers, and endeavoured to contain increases in drug prices at pharmacies. He suspended school activities, banned visits to hospitals and prohibited fairs and pilgrimages. However, he was also concerned with the economy and mental health of the Portuguese people. The factories continued working. The schools, cafes, concert halls, churches and public transports were not closed (Andrade 2018, 67-92). Beds for the sick were lacking. In Lisbon, Liceu Camões and the convent of Trinas were transformed into hospitals. As in other countries, young children and young adults were the hardest hit.

The clinical picture of the Pneumonic flu was similar to that of today's flu: fever, headache, myalgia, pharyngeal soreness, rhinorrhea and, occasionally, conjunctivitis. In most cases, the disease progressed well, healing in three to five days. The most feared complication was primary pneumonia with foamy and haemoptoic sputum. It often caused acute respiratory failure syndromes, killing the patient in a day or two. Occasionally, other organs and systems were invaded. Myocarditis and encephalitis were common, and, probably associated with the use of salicylates (Reye's syndrome).

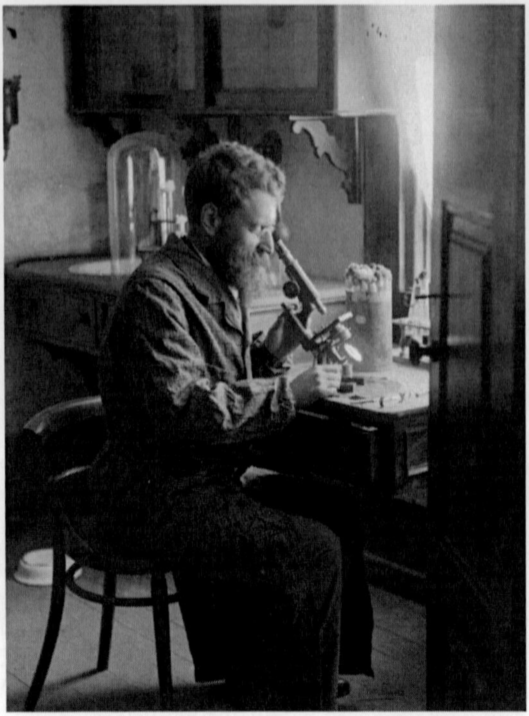

Fig. 12.2. Ricardo Jorge in the Municipal Bacteriological Lab in Oporto. Date: Before 1899, Municipal Archives from Oporto.

Ill fortune was in plain sight. Every day funerals were held for people on the same street and even from the house next door. The epidemic raged across all social classes. Bakers, milkmen, doctors and gravediggers died. Church bells were ringing almost continuously. At some point, some fell silent as local authorities considered they contributed too much to prevailing social alarm.

Death became trivialized. Coffins were missing, and many bodies were buried in mass graves, wrapped in burlap. Here is a transcription of the dramatic telegram that the Civil Governor of Faro addressed to the President of the Republic and published by the newspaper "O Século" on 14 October 1918:

> Hon. Mr President of the Republic. Belém. Lisbon. Severely ill, I´m asking you to protect Algarve. Epidemic wipes out entire villages, with cemeteries already complete, with burials in shallow graves. There is ~~a~~ lack of medicines, rice, sugar, candles, oil, pasta, butter, potatoes, and there has been no bread [...]. Orderly, people come asking me for bread, and children roam in the streets crying with hunger. The General Director of Supplies ordered requisition of all potatoes from Monchique, the only producing municipality that no longer has potatoes for half of the district. I plead your protection in helping so much misery. At any moment, people fall on the street with disease and hunger. Fishing boats are stopping working due to the lack of people. There is no fish.

Although there are notable differences in hygiene and diet, in the opinion of many researchers, the flu impacted all social classes (Sobral 2018, 45-65). Others, such as Ricardo Jorge, considered that the poorest were the most affected by the disease.

What advice could be given to help the sick? Some of the suggestions are still current today: staying at home, resting and having a light diet. Chicken broths and menthol gargles were also recommended. Therapy was symptomatic (Andrade 2018, 67-92). Fever was reduced with solutions of quinine and salicylates. The cough was treated with sodium benzoate and ammonium acetate syrups (Sequeira 2001, 49-55). In the most severe cases, injections of arsenical solutions, caffeine and adrenaline were used.

Some authors argue that some deaths from influenza might have been associated with poisoning with aspirin, recommended in doses of up to 30 grams per day, and capable of provoking haemorrhage. However, mortality was also high in regions where the population had no access to this drug like in other undeveloped countries.

Malnutrition and the lack of hygiene caused by the war, and human agglomerations in the military camps and the cities undoubtedly contributed a lot in Europe. The overcrowding of hospitals will have facilitated the outbreak of bacterial superinfections, responsible for many deaths. Older people were spared, somewhat, because of their previous contact with viruses related to this one, and which had been in circulation decades previously (in the 1890 pandemic).

Sidónio Pais (President of the Portuguese Republic from May 9, 1918-December 14, 1918), called "President-King" by the Poet Fernando Pessoa (1888-1935), was personally committed to fighting the pandemic, making a political flag out of the flu.

Influenza viruses mutate rapidly, probably evolving into less lethal strains. As the highly deadly variants end up with their host in a short time, they cannot spread so quickly. It is a process of natural selection.

Among tens of thousands of strangers, the flu took the lives of several prominent figures of Portuguese society: the painter Amadeu de Souza Cardoso (1887-1918) the "shepherd of Fátima" Francisco Marto (1908-1919), the pianist and composer António Fragoso (1897-1918) and the founder of the Sporting Football Club, José Alvalade (1885-1918). We will dedicate some space to the painter Amadeo de Souza Cardoso.

Amadeo de Souza Cardoso

Amadeo de Sousa-Cardoso (1897-1918) (Fig. 12.3) belonged to the age group most heavily punished by the Pneumonic flu. Born in Manhufe (Mancelos) on 14 November 1897, into a family of wealthy farmers, he studied first in Amarante and then in Coimbra before enrolling in the preparatory drawing course at the Royal Academy of Fine Arts in Lisbon in 1905. The following year, he moved to Paris, where he resided for around eight years, coming to Portugal only for short visits. He lived in the well-known Montparnasse quarter, a ghetto for international artists and intellectuals.

During his prolonged stay in Paris, Amadeo de Sousa Cardoso was acquainted with some of the most impressive names in painting and sculpture of the time. Another Amedeo (Modigliani) (1884-1920) became his close friend. In March 1911, they held an exhibition together in Amadeo´s atelier, in the neighbourhood of the Quai d'Orsay. Celebrities from the world of culture and art, such as Max Jacob (1876-1944), Guillaume Apollinaire (1880-1918), who also died of the pandemic flu, and Pablo Picasso (1881-1973), signed the book of honour (Alfaro 2010, 25).

Anyone who looks at Amadeo's works today is impressed by the vitality conveyed by his paint brush. There, we can trace his drive to experiment, his ambition, good taste, desire for affirmation and great harmony in the mixture of colours. Here and there, the artist gives the impression of groping, as if walking blindfolded through a little-known path. He painted hundreds of pictures, producing the best ones around 1917. His early death, his origin in a peripheral country, and his great stylistic versatility delayed his recognition as an artistic genius.

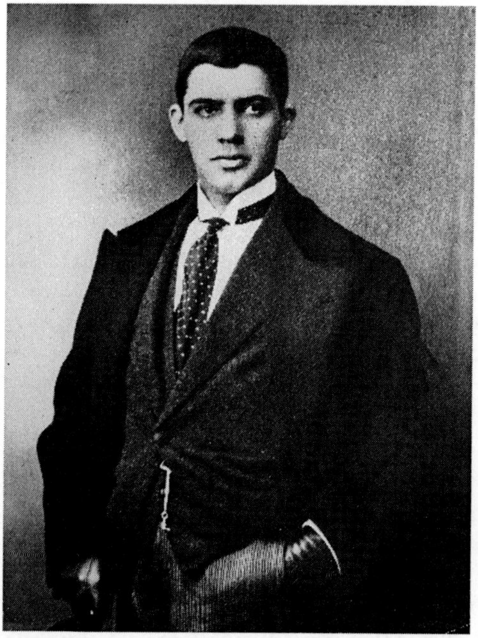

Fig. 12.3. Portrait of Amadeo de Souza Cardoso. Date: Before 1918. Art Library Fundação Calouste Gulbenkian. Wikimedia Commons.

The Portuguese took years to recognize the exceptional character of his work. Today the quality of his painting is compared by some to the best of his time. Amarante named its Municipal Museum "Amadeo de Souza Cardoso", in which many of his excellent paintings are now on display. One of his intriguing paintings depicts a medical doctor (Fig. 12.4).

The title is unknown, and it is not a portrait. It seems to be a reflection by Amadeo on a medical doctor as someone who auscultates his interior self.

Art took its toll on Amadeo's epidermis. The inks used in artistic painting varied according to the times but often contained products inducing cutaneous sensitization. Oil paints often included flaxseed oil and poppy, walnut and sunflower seeds, diluted and cleaned out with volatile solvents, which also induced skin irritation (Travassos et al. 2014, 277-280).

Amadeo experimented with several techniques, including wax, gouache, enamel and wax as well as other materials, but he preferred oil (Alfaro, 2010, 58). During the last years of his life, even before Pneumonics, the artist was prevented from painting. His skin disease affected his hands and face and was regarded at the time as eczema, possibly dermatitis related to an allergy to the components of the paints he used. A doctor even accompanied the painter to the Baths of Taipas where he sought relief (Travassos 2014, 277-280), apparently without much success.

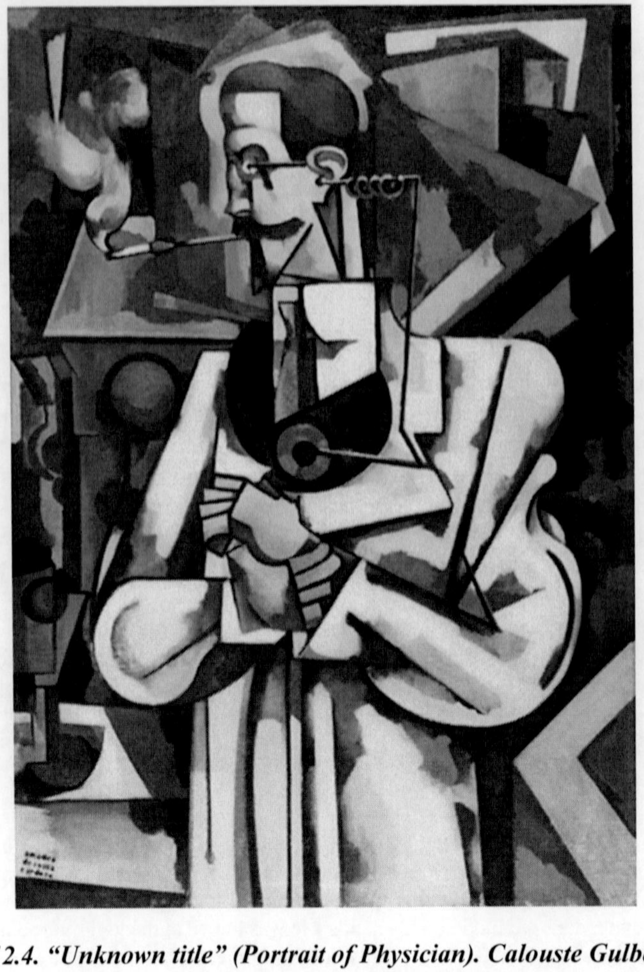

Fig. 12.4. "Unknown title" (Portrait of Physician). Calouste Gulbenkian Museum, Lisbon, Portugal. Wikimedia Commons.

Pneumonics burst into Espinho and took many young lives. Amadeo's disease followed a rapid course. Fever, accompanied by asthenia and body pain, was quickly followed by severe cough and haemoptoic expectoration and dyspnoea a couple of days later. To protect himself, Amadeo took refuge in Espinho, where the family owned a holiday home. In early October 1918, he wrote his last known letter to his brother António, from which we transcribe some excerpts:

> My dear António:
> Sending some news from us which are as follows: Gracita remains in the same state. She has not gotten worse, but the improvements are not giving her rest. Last night, the thermometer showed a very high temperature. Today, at the time of writing, it has been dropping: 39, 39 and a half. I have a terrible cold. From time to time, I feel brutal oppression in my chest. I have been throwing myself at Port wine as a precaution. I do not know what is telling me that there will be a significant change in my family's life. I am pessimistic, I hope!
> Your very dedicated brother hugs you,
> Amadeo
> (Cardoso in Alfaro 2010, 79).

This letter was written three weeks before his death. The painter feared pneumonics, but, at that time, he had not yet fallen ill. Precise medical information from his last days is not available in his documentary archive, entrusted to the Calouste Gulbenkian Foundation in the late 1980s by his widow, Lucie de Sousa Cardoso, and by his friend, Paulo Ferreira. Amadeo was struck by the most severe form of the disease. His last night was recreated by the journalist José Miguel Gaspar in *Jornal de Notícias* on the centenary of his death on 21st May 2018[2].

The painter died around 9 am on 25 October. He would have celebrated his 31st birthday less than a month after his death. Some days before, his sister Maria da Graça had died. No one knows how much he still might have contributed to Portuguese and World Art.

---

[2] Oppressed, sweating by fatigue and suffocation, his skin very pale, his head bursting, his lips blue. Amadeo, burning with fever, was shivering, his pulse throbbing as if his heart was climbing up to the head, coughed over and over until he saw thick, dark red blood on his hands. He was in bed at the lookout room, where he painted at the Souza-Cardoso family holiday home, in Espinho, by the sea breeze. Illness hovered in the room. He could hardly breathe- two days earlier, severe flu-like bronchopneumonia had come up - and he wanted to call a priest who came at dawn. The day was breaking, the holy anointing was prayed, and Amadeo's lungs, damaged inside, shrouded and sucked, imploded, and he died at 9 am on October 25, 1918. (1https://www.jn.pt/artes/a-ultima-noite-de-amadeo-souza-cardoso-sobre-a-terra-foi-a-tremer-12224820.html accessed March 21 2021).

Acknowledgments

The author thanks Rogério Palma Rodrigues, Orthopaedist and former Director of the Outão Sanatorium, for the information kindly taken from his unpublished manuscript and Dr Maria do Sameiro Barroso for the English translation of this essay.

References

Abreu, Laurinda. 2018. “A luta contra as invasões epidémicas em Portugal: políticas e agentes, séculos XVI-XIX” 93-120. Em: *Revisitar a Pneumónica de 1918-1919*. Lisboa: ISCTE-IUL.

Alfaro, Catarina. 2010. Amadeo de Sousa Cardoso, Pintores Portugueses, Matosinhos: Edições Quidnovi.

Andrade, Helena Rebelo de & Felismino, David. 2018. “A pandemia de gripe de 1918-1919: um desafio à ciência médica no princípio do século XX.” *Ler História,* 73: 67-92.

Bandeira, Mário Leston. 2009. “A sobremortalidade de 1918 em Portugal: análise demográfica.” 131-154. *In A Pandemia Esquecida: Olhares comparados sobre a Pneumónica (1918-1919)* organização de José Manuel Sobral; Luísa Lima; Paula Sousa Castro, Paulo Silveira. Lisboa: Imprensa de Ciências Sociais.

Johnson, Nial and Mueller, Juergen. 2002. “Updating the Accounts: global mortality of the 1918-1920 “Spanish” Influenza Pandemic”. *Bulletin of the History of Medicine,* 76 (1): 105-15.
https://www.historyofvaccines.org/node/2381 accessed 24-1-2022.

Killingray, David. 2009. “A pandemia de gripe de 1918-19: causas, evolução e Consequências” 41-61. *In* J. M. Sobral e al. (eds), *A pandemia esquecida: olhares comparados sobre a Pneumónica (1918/19)*. Lisboa: Imprensa de Ciências Sociais.

Morens, D. and Fauci, Anthony S. 2007. “Inluenza Pandemic: Insights for the 21st Century”. *The Journal for Infectious Diseases,* 195 (7) :1018-28.

Pereira, Rui. 2019. “Ricardo Jorge, o mal-amado A organização dos serviços de saúde militar no quadro da Grande Guerra e da Gripe Pneumónica” 55-85. *In Centenário da Gripe Pneumónica. A pandemia em retrospetiva. Portugal, 1918- 1919. Ciclo de conferências (maio a setembro de 2019,* coordenação de Helena da Silva, Rui M. Pereira e Filomena Bandeira, Lisboa: IGAS.

Reid, Ann H., Taubenberger, Jeffery K and Fanning, Thomas G. 2001. "The 1918 Spanish influenza: integrating history and biology". *Microbes and Infection,* 3 (1): 81−87.

Rodrigues, Rogério Palma. Unpublished manuscript. *Outão-Meio século de trabalhos e de memórias. A gripe pneumónica no Sanatório Marítimo do Outão.*

Sequeira, Álvaro. 2001. "A pneumónica, Spanish influenza." *História da Medicina,* 8 (1): 49-55.

Smith, Wilson; Andrewes, CH, Laidlaw P.P. and Timbury, Morag C. 1995. "A virus obtained from influenza patients" *Medical Virology* https://doi.org/10.1002/rmv.1980050402 reproduced from *The Lancet,* 1933: 66-68.

Sobral, José Manuel e Lima, Maria Luísa. 2018. "A epidemia da pneumónica em Portugal no seu tempo histórico" 45-66. *In* Abreu, Laurinda & Simões, José Vicente (eds) *Ler História. Dossier: Revisitar a Pneumónica de 1918-1919* nº73: 21-43.

Travassos, Ana Rita, Almeida, Soares de, Marinho, Rui, 2014. "A Medicina na Obra de Amadeo de Sousa Cardoso." *Acta Médica Portuguesa,* 27 (2): 277-280.

Vagneron, Frédéric. 2018. "La grippe espagnole: une historiographie centenaire Revisitée.", *Ler História,* 73: 21-43.

CHAPTER 13

DR. MARIA ROPALA CICKERSKY (1881-1973), THE FIRST ROMANIAN WOMAN FORENSIC PHYSICIAN AND HER PORTUGUESE ECHO

DANA BARAN

Abstract

Maria Ropala Cickersky (1881-1973) was the first female forensic physician in South-Eastern and Western Europe, and one of the earliest worldwide[1]. Even though she defended her doctoral thesis in forensic medicine in 1907, Dr. Cickersky really started her career in this field in 1919, as an assistant professor at the Department of Forensic Medicine of the Faculty of Medicine at Iași University (Romania). From 1920 Dr. Cickersky-Ropala also worked as a forensic physician at the Court of Justice of Iași. In 1927, she specialized in forensic medicine and psychiatry in Paris with the celebrated Professors Victor Balthazard and Henri Claude, respectively. After 1930, she directed the Laboratory of Forensic Medicine of the Faculty of Medicine of Iași. A foreign corresponding member of the French Society of Forensic Medicine since 1924, she published her investigations in specialist journals, mostly in France. In 1939 she was appointed lecturer at the Iasi University-Chair of Forensic Medicine. In 1936, the Portuguese assistant professor Carlos Ribeiro da Silva Lopes, from the Oporto Faculty of Medicine and Institute of Forensic Medicine, mentioned the promotional role of Romanian forensic scientists in his doctoral thesis. He emphasised Maria Ropala`s paper *Les caprices des projectiles*, a study already cited by the Spanish Professor António Piga in

[1] Under various circumstances, her forename was written Maria or Marie, and her family name became Cicherschi, Ciherschi, Cikerski, Cecherschi, Cikerschi or Cickersky; after her marriage to Dr. Emil Ropala in 1908, she signed Maria/Marie Cickersky Ropala or simply Maria Ropala.The form Dr. Marie Ropala Cickersky usually appears in French periodicals.

1928. Thus, during her lifetime, Maria Ropala also gained visibility in Iberian medicine.
Key words: Ropala Cicherschi, female doctor, forensics, Da Silva Lopes

Resumo
Maria Ropala Cickersky (1881-1973) foi a primeira médica forense do Sudeste da Europa Ocidental e uma das primeiras em todo o mundo. Apesar de ter defendido sua tese de doutoramento em medicina forense em 1907, a Dra. Cickersky, na realidade, iniciou sua carreira nesta área em 1919, como assistente do Departamento de Medicina Legal da Faculdade de Medicina da Universidade de Iași (Roménia). A partir de 1920, também trabalhou como médica forense no Tribunal de Justiça de Iași. Em 1927, especializou-se em medicina forense e psiquiatria em Paris com os célebres professores Victor Balthazard e Henri Claude, respectivamente. A partir de 1930, dirigiu o Laboratório de Medicina Legal da Faculdade de Medicina de Iași. Membro correspondente estrangeiro da Sociedade Francesa de Medicina Legal desde 1924, publicou os seus estudos em revistas especializadas, principalmente na França. Em 1939, foi nomeada professora na Universidade Iași – Cátedra de Medicina Forense. Em 1936, o professor português Carlos Ribeiro da Silva Lopes da Faculdade de Medicina do Porto e Instituto de Medicina Legal referiu o papel dos cientistas forenses romenos na sua tese de doutoramento. Destacou o artigo de Maria Ropala *Les caprices des projectiles*, num estudo já citado pelo professor espanhol António Piga em 1928. Assim, em vida, Maria Ropala adquiriu também visibilidade na medicina ibérica.
Palavras chave: Ropala Cicherschi, médica, Medicina forense, Da Silva Lopes

An epoch of technological progress and feminine emancipation

The dawn of the twentieth century saw forensic medicine developing on a much more modern basis, closely connected with both new technologies and the recent application of the exact sciences to medicine. At that time, forensic medicine was not fully recognised as a distinct speciality internationally. Feminine and/or feminist emancipation was a sign of the epoch. Female doctors were gradually conquering medical areas previously considered *par excellence* to be dominated by, or to be the sole preserve of male doctors, and making valuable contributions to progress in such fields. Consequently, forensic medicine and psychiatry became increasingly complex and accurate. Romanian medical historiography considers Dr.

Maria Ropala Cicherschi to be the first woman forensic doctor in Romania and South-Eastern and Western Europe, and probably only the second in the world. After basic training in Iaşi, Romania, she further specialized in Paris (Maftei 1985, 225). This assertion as to her primacy must be thoroughly documented, as several women became involved in forensic practice, research and teaching at almost the same time. Indeed, until recently (Nazarov 2011, 58), Maria Ropala Cickersky was acknowledged as the first female forensic doctor in Europe and possibly even in the world.

Here is Dr. Ropala`s confession, testifying in an original handwritten text that, in the 1960s, she was officially considered in her country to be the first female forensic doctor in Europe (Fig. 13.1.):

> "To my dear niece Gaby,
> Aunt Marcel
> Former Forensic Physician
> Court of Justice of Iasi - 1920
> University lecturer
> The first woman forensic doctor in Europe -1968
> Ropala Cikersky - Romania" (Fig. 13.1) (Baran 2016, 192)

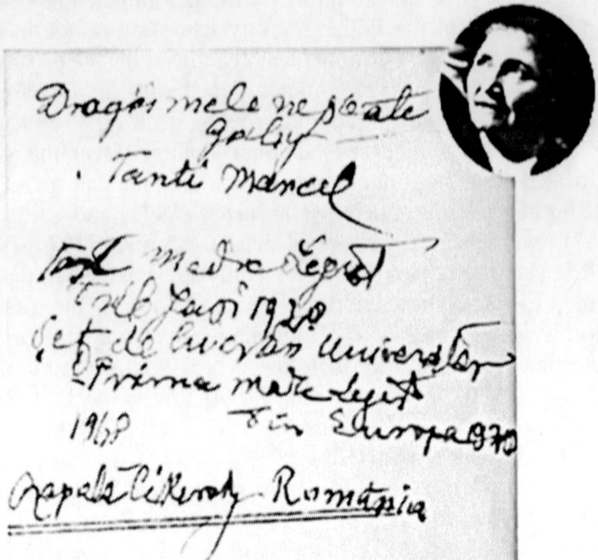

Fig. 13.1. The photograph Maria Ropala offered to her niece, Gaby, in 1968, stating on the reverse that she was the first woman forensic doctor in Europe (autograph text). (Courtesy of Maria Ropala`s nephews).

But Anna Smyslova (1876-1918?), in 1904, graduated from the Medical School in 1904 and then received her doctoral degree at Sankt Petersburg in 1909 (Nazarov 2011, 58; Klevno and Nazarov 2017, 265). Even though her doctoral thesis was defended two years after that of Maria Cickersky, Smyslova continued to work uninterruptedly in this field and probably deserves the title of the first woman forensic physician in European history. From 1904 to 1918, Smyslova was a lecturer at the Departments of Forensic Medicine of the Women`s Medical Institute, of the Grand Duchess Elena Pavlovna`s Clinical Institute and of the Private University of Petersburg Psychoneurological Institute. Some publications have outlined the pioneering role of a female Russian forensic doctor, Anna Mikhailovna Smyslova.

Biographical landmarks of Maria Cickersky

The school and the general horizon of ideas

Maria Cicherschi was born in Iasi, on 18 December 1881, to the family of Franz Cickersky[2], a mechanical engineer. Franz's father, Filip Cickersky, belonged to a branch of the Polish nobility who took refuge in Romania (Moldavia) after one of the mid-nineteenth century Polish Uprisings.

In 1901, Maria Cickersky completed her studies at "Oltea Doamna" High School in the Moldavian capital, a recognized girls' college, today known as the "Mihai Eminescu" National College. Over the years, the School educated some important contributors to Romanian social, cultural and scientific life, such as Lucia Mantu (1888–1971) and Otilia Cazimir (1894-1967), two sensitive writers; also Ella Negruzzi (1876–1948), the first female lawyer in Romania and among only a few in the world practising at that time; Elena Densusianu Puscariu (1875-1966), the first female physician-university professor in Romania, and among the first, if not actually the first woman in the world to become a university professor of ophthalmology (1920); Maria Franche (1890-1989), the first Romanian woman professor of infectious diseases and director of the "Isolation" Hospital in Iași; Maria Briese (1894-1969), the first woman professor of Endocrinology at the Iași Faculty of Medicine and coordinator of the Endocrinology Clinic, founded in 1948; Asia Ballif Chipail (1915-2001), daughter to psychiatry professor Leon Ballif, the first woman professor of pediatric clinic in Iași, her hometown; Marioara Tanasescu Niculescu, who finished High School in 1932, daughter to professor of surgery Ion

[2] Franz Cickersky`s birth and death dates are not precisely known.

Tanasescu (1875-1954), a valuable woman researcher in the field of haematology (her professional pathway interfered with that of Maria Ropala, when, from 1 October 1939 to February 1941, Marioara Niculescu was a substitute teaching assistant in the Laboratory of the Institute of Forensic Medicine); and last but not least, the exceptional chemist Raluca Ripan (1894 -1972), the first woman member of the Romanian Academy, another brilliant woman to have graduated from the same College, crowning an impressive galaxy of pioneering ladies successfully involved in various fields of expertise.

In Iași, the city where progressive ideas flourished around the *Contemporanul* ("The Contemporary") newspaper at the end of the nineteenth century, teachers and students of the famous "Oltea Doamna" High School were among the animators of women`s emancipation, militating, by the very force of their own example, for official recognition and respect of their legitimate rights to human and professional fulfillment. Among the figures who illustrated the "Oltea Doamna" College and its atmosphere during Maria Cickersky`s school years were Maria Butzureanu Lambrino (1870-1919), teacher of pedagogy (1884-1886), an activist for the emancipation of women through culture; Ana Conta Kernbach (1865-1921), then the only woman in the country to have graduated from the École Normale Supérieure in Paris, doctor of ethics, teacher of logic and psychology (1885-1895); Isabela Andrei Sadoveanu (1870-1941), pedagogue and publicist, actively dedicated to the feminist cause, teacher of philosophy and pedagogy (1890-1894); Maria Amfilochi Xenopol (1861-1939*),* a particularly enterprising principal of the High School (1888-1902), and a teacher of history and philosophy.

University studies and academic destiny

Maria Cickersky remained in Iași, undertaking her university studies from 1901 to 1907. In 1907, she defended her doctoral thesis entitled *Contribuțiune la studiul biologiei și criminalității femenine (Din punctul de vedere medico-legal)* ("Contribution to the biological study of female criminality from the forensic point of view) (Fig. 13.2.). Supervised by Professor Dr. George Bogdan (1859-1930), head and chair of the Forensic Medicine and dean of the Faculty of Medicine, the thesis focused on the issue of female psychology and delinquency, a topical subject of considerable concern at that time.

Consequently, in 1907, Dr. Cickersky was appointed university assistant to the Chair of Bacteriology of the Faculty of Medicine, a position she held for only a short time (1907-1908). In those days Bacteriology was represented in Iași by Dr. Emil Puscariu (1859-1928), a former collaborator with the famous Professor Dr. Victor Babes (1854-1926) from Bucharest, and a prominent interdisciplinary researcher in domains such as anatomopathology and vaccinology (see, for example, Puscariu`s anti-rabies vaccine; Puscariu and Vesesco 1895, 210). In terms of his academic position, Emil (Knight of) Puscariu was a substitute professor of Bacteriology, full professor of Histology and head of this latter Department.

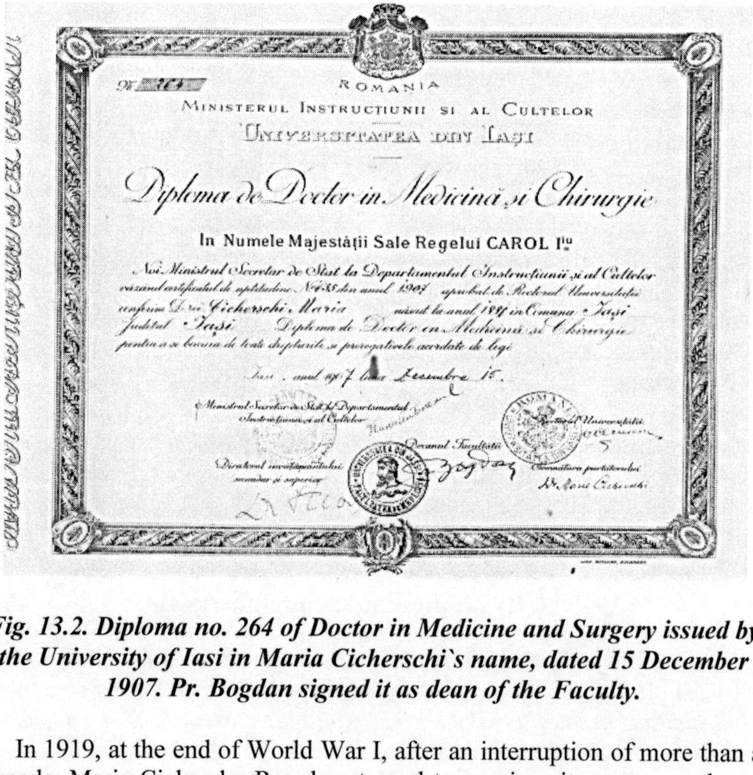

ROMANIA
MINISTERUL INSTRUCTIUNII ȘI AL CULTELOR
UNIVERSITATEA DIN IAȘI
Diploma de Doctor in Medicină și Chirurgie
In Numele Majestății Sale Regelui CAROL I-lu
Noi Ministrul Secretar de Stat la Departamentul Instrucțiunii și al Cultelor
văzând certificatul de aptitudine ... din anul 1907 aprobat de Rectorul Universității
conferim D-rei Cicherschi Maria născută la anul 1881 in Comuna Iași
Județul Iași Diploma de Doctor in Medicină și Chirurgie
pentru a se bucura de toate drepturile și prerogativele acordate de legi
Iași, anul 1907 luna Decembre 15.
Ministrul Secretar de Stat la Departamentul Instrucțiunii și al Cultelor
Rectorul Universității
Decanul Facultății
Directorul învățământului secundar și superior
Semnătura posesorului
Dr. Maria Cicherschi

Fig. 13.2. Diploma no. 264 of Doctor in Medicine and Surgery issued by the University of Iasi in Maria Cicherschi`s name, dated 15 December 1907. Pr. Bogdan signed it as dean of the Faculty.

In 1919, at the end of World War I, after an interruption of more than a decade, Maria Cickersky Ropala returned to a university career, and was appointed assistant professor at the Department of Forensic Medicine of the Faculty of Medicine of the University of Iași, directed by Professor George Bogdan. Dr. Bogdan himself was a founding father of Romanian forensic medicine and deontology education, a foreign corresponding member of the French Society of Forensic Medicine, and a former disciple in Paris of Paul Camille Hippolyte Brouardel (1837-1906), a reference name in the history of forensics. Brouardel had directed Bogdan`s doctoral thesis, defended in

1885. Belonging to the Faculty of Medicine, the Department provided by then the teaching of Forensic Medicine both for the fourth-year students of the Faculty of Law, and the fifthyear students of the Faculty of Medicine. From 1920, Dr. Ropala also worked as a forensic physician at the Iași Court of Justice. She followed in her Master`s footsteps, as Professor Bogdan was the first forensic doctor of the Prosecutor's Office of Moldavia, and, since 1892, of the Courthouse and the Court of Appeal of Iași. The notions of bacteriology that Ropala was familiar with, along with her medical experience in times of peace and war must have been very useful to her under those circumstances. In October 1923, George Bogdan offered a photo of his to Maria with an encouraging dedication on its reverse: "To my distinguished collaborator, with particular affection for her special support in our painful work." If Professor Bogdan helped Ropala's activity, legend has it that it was Professor Mina Minovici (1858-1933) from Bucharest, another outstanding and founding personality of Romanian forensic medicine, who dissuaded her to proceed further in this field as, according to him and the prejudices of the day, it was an endeavour unsuitable for a lady doctor. In any case, Dr. Ropala was already acknowledged as a forensic expert (Bologa, Bratescu, Dutescu & Milcu 1972, 408; Baran 2016, 6) (Fig.13.3a. Fig.13.3b.).

In 1935, when the supposed relics of Prince Dimitrie Cantemir (1673-1723) were brought back to Iași in Romania from Russia, Dr. Ropala was asked to identify them (Baran, 2016, 117).

In 1924, Dr. Maria Ropala Cickersky was accepted as a foreign corresponding member of the French Society of Forensic Medicine in Paris and, in 1927, following recommendation by Professor Bogdan, she further specialized there in both forensic medicine and psychiatry, working with the famed professors Victor Balthazard and Henri Claude, respectively.

Once back home, she helped Professor Bogdan edit the first Romanian Forensic Medicine handbook and published some of her papers in specialty journals, most of which were French.

After her mentor's death in 1930, she took over the management of the Forensic Laboratory of the Iași Faculty of Medicine as full director, while continuing to fulfill her teaching, practical and research duties.

Paradoxically, it was only on 4 July 1939 that Maria Ropala was promoted to senior lecturer at the Chair of Forensic Medicine, just a few years before she retired. This was the highest academic position that Maria Cicherschi held and it somehow characterised the various obstacles prevalent in the years during which she lived and worked-obstacles which thwarted women's progress in their academic careers, especially in forensic medicine.

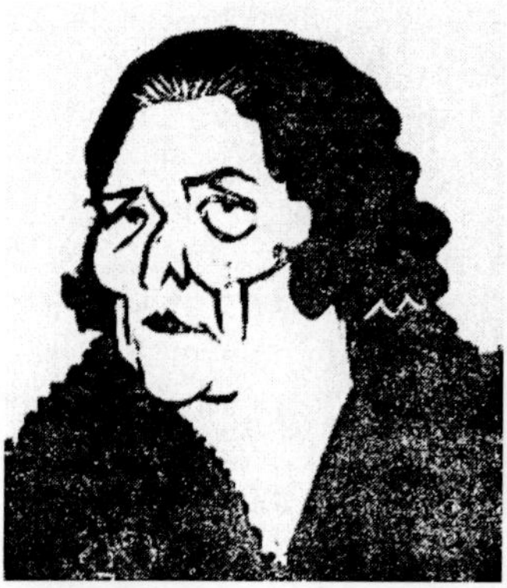

a.

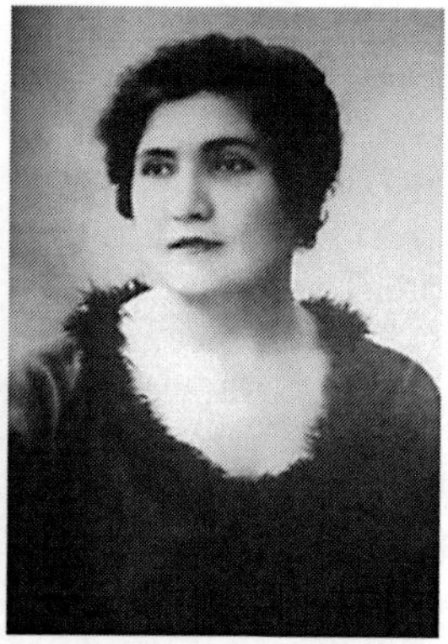

b.

Fig.13.3a. Dr. Ropala's caricature illustrating a humorous "Forensic Report" in a local magazine (The World), April 14th, 1935.
Fig. 13.5b. Maria Cickersky Ropala's photo.

Succeeding Professor Bogdan, the direction of the Forensic Medicine Department was temporarily taken over (1931-1933) by Professor Grigore T. Popa (1892-1948) from the Chair of Anatomy, and then by Dr. Nicolae Balan (1886-1966), from the Chair of Pathological Anatomy, who eventually was appointed full professor and head of the Chair of Forensic Medicine (1933).

Consequently, Dr. Cickersky Ropala continued to maintain a rather low profile reflecting the general prevailing mentality and possibly her own compliance with this status.

She was officially retired in 1941 having reached the required age limit. Yet, due to the consequences of World War II, Maria Ropala prolonged her stay at the Chair until 1945, when, after more than 26 years in the service of forensic medicine, she left Iasi for Bucharest, to join her daughter`s family (Baran 2016, 98).

Following a short-lived period of discredit by the communist regime (1948-1958), in the 1960s she once again enjoyed recognition of her pioneering merits in Romanian Forensic Medicine. The fall into disfavor was possibly related to her social position but, most likely, to the interference of forensic medicine with some ideological and political aspects, too. However, she finally conquered, both for herself and for future generations of women, a new medical domain, contributing to the further improvement of the status of women in medical science in Romania (Fig.13.1). It came as a token of social and scientific rehabilitation (Maftei 1985, 225; Baran 2016, 100). Fortunately, she led a sufficiently long life as to be able to rejoice in this situation, eventually dying in Bucharest on 10 August 1973, at the age of 92.

Interestingly, nowadays, the Romanian male/female ratio in forensic medicine tends to be dominated by woman doctors.

Looking into details

Woman, doctor and citizen

In 1907, the year of her graduation from the Faculty, Maria Cickersky got engaged to Dr. Emil Ropala, a skilled surgeon, whom she married a year later (1908). Soon she gave birth to a daughter-Carmen. These events meant that, for a while, she abandoned the University. Together with her husband she worked for ten years (1908-1918) as a general practitioner in various regions of Romania. Maria Ropala participated in the Second Balkan War (1913) and during the First World War she was mobilized to the frontline in Moldavia, and in Iași, where she cared for wounded and diseased patients, and became involved in combating the many severe epidemics that ravaged the country.

A beautiful and elegant woman, intelligent and sensitive by nature, she always appreciated art, music (especially opera), literature (especially theatre), and she loved to travel. She also expressed her creativity by composing epigrams and poetry. The examples of her predecessors, thanks to whom her destiny itself was assured, stood before her. In addition to his complex medical erudition and expertise, Professor Bogdan, for instance, also embodied the humanist doctor, having expressed his artistic creativity in writing short stories, and having participated in the activities of the "Lutetia" Circle for Franco-Romanian Studies in Iași. A devoted Francophile and Francophone intellectual, son of a French mother, he equally presided over "Lutetia" for a while. The same was true for Professor Grigore T. Popa, a substitute professor of Forensic Medicine immediately after George Bogdan`s death: he was a noteworthy scientist, but also a writer with a militant and active social conscience, reflecting the spirit of physicians of that time. Perhaps their "artistic choice" was also their soul`s compensatory reaction to the often unforgiving, harsh demands of their profession, which aroused their aesthetic need and, at the same time, their ethical attitude.

The first Romanian woman forensic doctor: specialization and pioneering

Professor George Bogdan's disciple and close collaborator, Maria Cickersky Ropala, was sent to specialize in the French capital in 1927 (Fig. 13.4.).

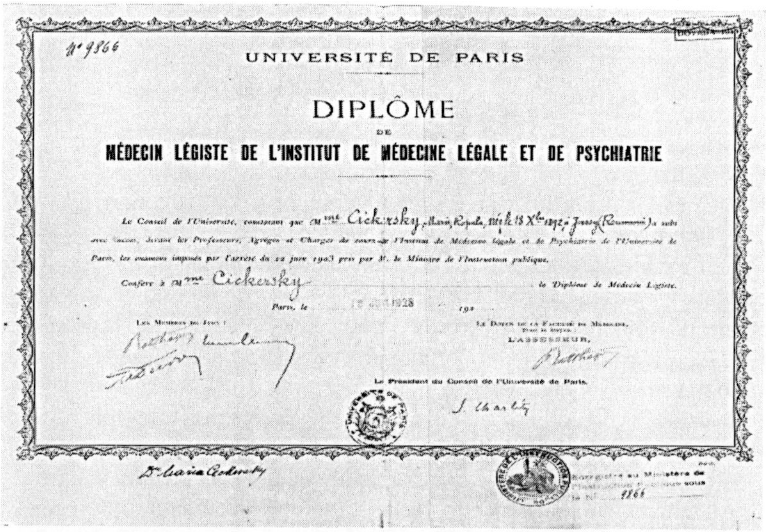
N° 9866

UNIVERSITÉ DE PARIS

DIPLÔME

DE

MÉDECIN LÉGISTE DE L'INSTITUT DE MÉDECINE LÉGALE ET DE PSYCHIATRIE

Le Conseil de l'Université, constatant que Mme Cickersky, Maria Ropala, née le 18 Xbre 1892 à Jassy (Roumanie) a subi avec succès, devant les Professeurs, Agrégés et Chargés de cours de l'Institut de Médecine légale et de Psychiatrie de l'Université de Paris, les examens imposés par l'arrêté du 22 juin 1903 pris par M. le Ministre de l'Instruction publique.

Confère à Mme Cickersky le Diplôme de Médecin Légiste.

Paris, le 18 JUIN 1928

Les Membres du Jury :

Le Doyen de la Faculté de Médecine,

L'ASSESSEUR,

Le Président du Conseil de l'Université de Paris.

Dr Maria Cickersky

Fig. 13.4. Diploma of Forensic Physician of the Institute of Forensic Medicine and Psychiatry in Paris issued by the University of Paris in Maria Ropala`s name on 18 June, 1928. (Courtesy of Maria Ropala's nephews).

She was received by Professor Victor Balthazard (1872-1950) from the Sorbonne, one of the most important forensic doctors of the twentieth century and a descendant of Brouardel (1837-1906). A friend of the Romanians, Balthazard was an honorary member of the Romanian Academy (1919). In iatro-historiography he is noted for several achievements: researches undertaken with the physicist Pierre Curie (1859-1906) and his colleague from the Sorbonne, the pathologist Charles Bouchard (1831-1915), on the physiological repercussions of radium / radon emanations in mice and guinea pigs, immediately after natural radioactivity was discovered; implementation of original investigation methods; individualized examination of fingerprints; performing the first forensic analyses of hair; noteworthy contributions to forensic ballistics, but also his approaches to professional deontology. Together with his wife, Marcelle Lambert, a doctor of science, Professor Balthazard published several papers, including his successful and pioneering monograph on "The hair of man and animals. Applications to forensic expertise and fur expertise" (Lambert and Balthazard 1910).

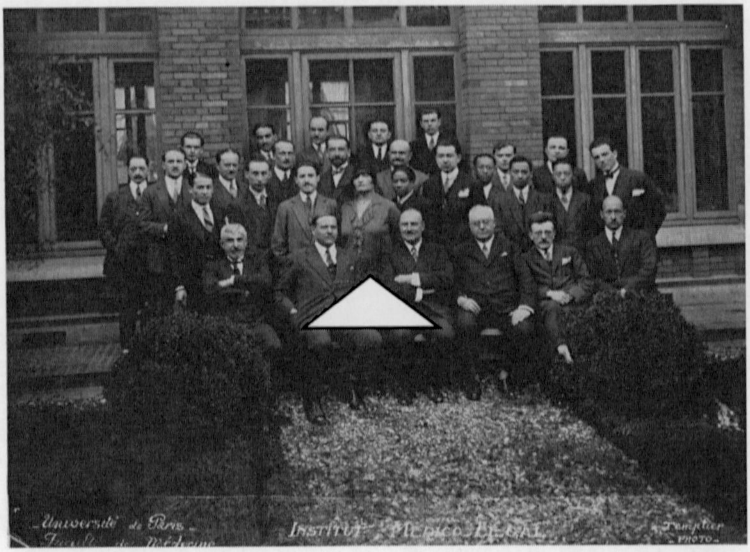

Fig. 13.5. Paris University. Faculty of Medicine. Institute of Forensic Medicine. Maria Cicherschy Ropala (white arrow), the only woman amidst her colleagues, exclusively men. (Courtesy of Maria Ropala`s nephews)

Also in Paris, at the "Sainte Anne" Hospital, Maria Ropala entered the labyrinth of forensic psychiatry, initiated by another world authority in the field: Professor Henri Claude (1869-1945), who worked there from 1922 to 1939. A talented psychiatrist and neurologist, a follower of organo-dynamism and psychobiology, Henri Charles Jules Claude introduced Freud's theories into French medicine. Whilst not a psychoanalyst himself, he created the first laboratory of psychoanalysis and psychotherapy and authored a treatise on Forensic Psychiatry (Claude 1932). Psychoanalysis indeed proved to be closely correlated with female psychology and psychopathology, allowing a different way of understanding them and their connection to forensics. On 18 June 1928 the Institute of Forensic Medicine and Psychiatry of the Faculty of Medicine conferred on her the Diploma of Forensic Physician of the University of Paris (Fig. 13.4.).

At the beginning of the twentieth century, of course, specialist courses in forensic medicine were given in the major universities of Europe, but they seemed to be primarily intended for men, colder-blooded beings. However, in a centre like Paris, Maria Ropala established herself as the first female doctor who had the ambition and eventually succeeded to practice and qualify at a higher level in forensic medicine (Fig. 13.5.).

Paradoxically, before ending her specialization in Paris, on the basis of her scientific merit she had already been elected as a foreign corresponding member of the Society of Forensic Medicine in France in 1924 (Annuaire, 1924, 10) and maintained this quality throughout her carreer.

After returning to the country, Dr. Cickersky Ropala continued to combine her activity at the Faculty Department with that of forensic doctor of the Iași Court.

In fact, the academic vocation of almost all forensic doctors closely integrated both legal and clinical applications (Scripcaru 1982, 181).

Scientific papers

Doctoral thesis in medicine and surgery: feminine biology and criminality

The first forensic analysis undertaken by Maria Cicherschi was her own thesis for a doctorate in medicine and surgery. Entitled "Contribution to the study of female biology and criminality (From the forensic point of view)", the thesis was an original analysis: "In Romania no work has been reported in this direction. Also, I could not obtain any Romanian criminology statistics to insert in my paper"-she mentioned (Cicherschi 1907, 4). Only one study by Professor Bogdan existed at the time-*O pagina de anthropologie criminala* ("A Page of Criminal Anthropology") (1894), presented at the University of Iași as an opening lesson of the academic year 1894-1895. Another investigation by Professor Mina Minovici-*Remarques sur la criminalité féminine en Roumanie* ("Observations on feminine criminality in Romania") was edited in *Archives d'Anthropologie Criminelle et de Psychologie Normale et Pathologique*, the same year as Cicherschi`s doctoral defense-1907 (Minovici 1907). Maria Cicherschi managed to construct a framework for the problem of female criminality in the world, such as it was known, understood and studied by then, dealing with aspects of both general and special criminality. Behavioural problems of "the eternal feminine" fascinated contemporary scholars. Reviewing the speciality literature, Dr. Cickersky agreed with the opinions of some European authorities, but also included data from the local specialized literature.

The influence that the predominant ideas exerted at the time was clearly outlined: sexual differences on the scale of biological evolution; differences and complementarities, superiority versus inferiority in characterizing the two genders, and in normal versus criminal individuals. Supposedly at the lowest level of zoological development, the woman would have been superior to man, whereas later, on the evolutionary ladder the ratio reached equality before finally being reversed: "From the above we see that the woman is superior to the man in the first steps of the zoological ladder; but as we ascend higher into the zoological world, we see that the man equals and surpasses the female. But his superiority is established in the class of mammals. However, in species where the male is inferior in height and strength, he possesses variations and structures superior to the female." Consequently, "the higher we go in the zoological tree, the better we see that the man equals the woman and comes to surpass her" (Cicherschi 1907, 7).

Craniology and stigmas

Data from personal research related to anthropometry and craniology were integrated in the Thesis, which was quite an updated, quantified, approach to forensics: "Curves. Studying the proportion of the different parts of the fronto-occipital curve (reduced to 100) and of the anterior horizontal one considering 100 as the horizontal curve, we found in criminal women (…) (values) which show us the opposite of what is claimed that there is no size in the subcerebral curve of the criminal women." … "In the craniofacial structure a number of abnormalities and stigmas of degeneration have to be noted. Cranial capacity, shape, size, along with the shape, size and position of the ears and eyes, and the general aspect of the teeth were used to distinguish between healthy persons with eugenic features, and criminal individuals, women in this case. Inborn physical defects often expressed feeblemindedness, too" (Cicherschi 1907, 38).

Evolution and heredity

In parallel, Dr. Cicherschi debated on the relationship between evolution, heredity, adaptation capacity and environment dynamics, referring to both Darwin and Spencer: "the man whose struggle for life, with the continuous variations and adaptations within the living environment, contributed to the variations of his organs and functions"; or: "the fact that the prostitute woman has more numerous characters is explained by the fact that, as prostitution existed since ancient times, the woman preserved the retrograde characters, currently presenting, through atavism, the mentioned characters." The bio-psycho-social inferiority of the woman would be manifested "due to her innate vicious inclinations" (...) "One of the most important factors that directly influence criminality is heredity." (…) "From what we have said we see that individuals in such condition will surely pass on to their descendants' stigmas of degeneration, evil instincts and brutal passions" (Cicherschi 1907, 49). Congenital or inherited traits versus acquired, environmentally determined ones represented a point of interest because they potentially offered social and economic solutions to the problems of both criminality and deliquency, which, to a certain extent, depended on education and living standards, and hence a wealthier state of mind (Cicherschi 1907, 35).

Even though according to Lombroso, for example, criminals were defective people belonging to "more primitive races" (Lombroso 1896), insofar as their humanisation process was concerned, Dr. Cickersky obviously supported complementary concepts of human development that linked behavioural genetics to phenotypical correlations, to put it in modern terms: faith, habits, and role models always counted.

Religion, mentality, moral sense

According to Maria Cickersky, religiosity was specific to women, more suggestible than men, and who are important characters in most religions, where they are, by far, the dominant sex. Besides, women's religiosity would be tightly related to sexuality, and lack of both intelligence and social autonomy. "According to Loyseau – the doctoral candidate argued –, there is a close connection between a woman's sexual abnormalities and religious mania, especially in puberty." Furthermore: "Religiosity is organic in women, having its origin in their psychological state. We know that the woman is very accessible to suggestion. (…) Religion is a suggestion because none of us have seen the deities or their miracles: whoever is more accessible to this suggestion will become more religious." Religiosity and rationality seemed to be inversely proportional: "Seeing her inability to dominate these phenomena, she looked up at an unknown and unseen superhuman power. But the civilized man, through his superior intelligence, will and knowledge, succeeding to master the forces of nature and life events, relying only on his energy, will and intelligence, feeling in control of himself, seeing various successes due only to himself, began to become less accessible to the suggestion of a supreme power and as a consequence his religiosity declined" (Cicherschi 1907, 19),

Identically, religion would be closely linked to a moral sense that is different in women, and both religion and morality would be explained by a combination of lower female intelligence and psychic disorders: "in Lombroso's opinion, man possesses a superior native intelligence thanks to his minor participation in the reproduction and preservation of the species. There is an antagonism between reproductive functions and intellectual functions." This would explain why, submitted to a more intense organic wear and tear and family occupations, "the woman remained at a lower intelligence level" (Cicherschi 1907, 25).

Education and humanization

"The fruit of culture"-Dr. Cickersky reckoned-"was the submission of the animal system to the conscious system, i.e. refraining from animal instincts, impulses and passions. But as soon as a pathological process weakens the activity of the higher, moderating and regulating centres, the lower centres of instincts and impulses become leaders, transforming the individual into an animal with a human face, yielding to the lowest instincts, impulses and passions. This is observed in cases of degeneration, like congenital criminality" (Cicherschi 1907, 22).

Nutrition and basic instincts

"Nutrition is such an important vital act that the body itself has automatic indicators like, for instance: hunger, thirst and satiety that manifest themselves chronometrically whenever the body demands nutrition and cease when the feeling of fullness occurs. Yet this so important vital act is dominated, restrained, sent in the background and even neglected by the civilized man, while forming the essence of life for the uneducated man. This is the case of a peasant from Botosani County who killed his comrade, following his refusal to give him bread for his hungry children" (Cicherschi 1907, 47).

Chronobiology and meteropathology

The doctoral student noted both elements of chronobiology and meteorosensitivity, emphasizing the existence of periodic, mostly seasonal, pathological behaviors: "Statistical data on the various types of crime committed at various times of the year show that attacks on property predominate in winter and autumn, while those against the individual abound in spring and summer and this is easily explained by knowing that winter creates difficulties in the circumstances of existence, bringing over with it misery and therefore the violation of the vital conditions of society." The biological rhythm should probably have an impact: "Ferri claims that crimes are more numerous in hot summers."

Meteorological phenomena also have an influence on criminal organizations. The directors of prisons as well as of madhouses tell us that, before the storms, the women-detainees are very prone to irritations, excitements and disorders" (Cicherschi 1907, 31).

Psychoanalysis, hysteria and menstruation

Besides some other pathologies, hysteria was a frequent diagnosis in Parisian clinics at the crossroads of the nineteenth and twentieth centuries. Alienists and neurologists thought it might have had a hereditary basis and was compared to epilepsy. Both hysteria and epilepsy might have been linked to criminality "through fleeting emotivity", grave psychic disturbances, sexual problems and suggestibility (hypnotic suggestion, suggestion, autosuggestion). Elements of Freudian psychoanalysis were explicitly formulated in Cickersky's dissertation, proving the acquisition of new interpretations, just launched after 1895: "Other times motherhood merges with sexuality giving rise to incest, then the woman loves her offspring not as a child but as a lover. This is because maternal love has a sexual basis". In the spirit of the time, hysteria occupied an entire subchapter of the Thesis, being directly correlated with criminal acts (Cicherschi 1907, 54). It was the same hysteria that Charcot had insistently dealt with, applying hypnosis as a treatment, a therapy his student, Sigmund Freud, the father of psychoanalysis, reconsidered and performed on a regular basis. About hysteria Maria Cicherschi wrote, among other things: "Another product of degeneration is Hysteria. (…) Hysterics are very liable to influence by suggestion and self-suggestion. Hysterism is quite widespread and preferably in women. Their number is very large. It manifests itself even in childhood" (Cicherschi 1907, 54). In its turn, the menstrual cycle was involved in complementary biological explanations. In his doctoral thesis (1889), Dr. Séverin Icard (1860-1939) had already set up a classification of eight menstrual psychoses: kleptomania, pyromania, dipsomania, religious delirium, as well as multiple and varied psychoses (Icard 1889, 143). He concurrently defined sexual behaviour troubles and homicide tendencies possibly induced by the menstrual cycle (Icard 1889, 185).

Undoubtedly, once expelled from Paradise as a sinner, the woman lost her balance, equality and social status. Supposedly the same happened to men. However, she concluded: "in all countries, the number of criminal women is much lower than that of criminal men" (Cicherschi 1907, 3).

Degeneration, prostitution, inborn criminality

Among the causes responsible for female criminality, lack of education, inadequate environment, primary instinctuality, heredity, alcoholism, and degeneration were invoked in the foreground. "One of the common crimes in wild women`s criminality is abortion and infanticide". "Wild women are very cruel, but less so than men. They have a great pleasure in torturing the enemy." (..) "Congenital prostitutes, who are related to inborn criminals", "both have the same early inclination for evil, the same lack of moral sense, and the same indifference to public opinion. They are the source of attraction for criminals."(…)"Their moral sense is completely erased, unaware of their guilt and unable to distinguish between good and evil, just as they are unable to tell the difference between what is noble and what is degrading." Feeblemindedness, and sexual behaviour, prostitution above all, resulted to be more significantly related to criminality (Cicherschi 1907, 28).

Social conditioning and sanitary misery

"The struggle for existence and the obstacles in front of the most urgent needs turn the man from the lower classes into a selfish man with vulgar instincts who would not hesitate to use a knife, were he not restrained by fear of imprisonment and fear of sinning" (Cicherschi, 1907, 35).

Finally: "Misery with its hideous procession conquers the field of honour. Its faithful vassals such as Vice, Syphilis, Drunkenness, Tuberculosis and Pelagra invest new soldiers with the order of degeneration, creating the class of innate criminals" (Cicherschi 1907, 35).

In conclusion

Maria Cickersky`s thesis perfectly illustrated the main contemporary ideological trends and opinions when considering feminine criminality and delinquency at the dawn of the twentieth century. The overall medical *zeitgeist* was revealed, discussed and partially assumed. Some of the solutions proposed still seem valid today: training, integration, rather than brutal repression, education. "Female criminality could be reduced if women were given a more sober education, in which altruism played a major role; and for the woman who committed the crime or murder, a new system of detention should exist, because penitentiaries, prisons etc endanger woman's morality worse than they correct it." (…) "Prisons are real schools of criminality" (Cicherschi 1907, 32). From this point of view, forensic medicine has to exert a sanogenetic action in society, yielding not only diagnoses and punishments, but complex explanations, social measures and judicial clarifications, all at the same time. This principle was in keeping with a motto of the French school of criminal anthropology engraved on Alexandre Lacassagne`s medal (1913), that in 1924 Professor Mina Minovici adopted and proclaimed as a precept of Romanian forensics: "*Medicina dux auxiliumque justitiae*" ("Medicine, conductor and helper of Justice") (Normand 2004).

Forensic Medicine Handbook and some scientific articles

Professor Bogdan`s Forensic Medicine Handbook

Together with Dr. George Bogdan, her Master, Dr. Ropala investigated a series of injuries including blows, infanticide, abortion, sudden death, and attacks on public morality, to which forensic reports were added. She helped Professor Bogdan edit the five volumes of the first Romanian course of forensic medicine (Scripcaru 1982, 189). The author dedicated his treatise to Dr. Victor Balthazard, Professor of Forensic Medicine at the Faculty of Paris; Dr. Étienne Martin, Professor of Forensic Medicine at the Faculty of Lyon; Dr. Eugène Stockis, Professor of Forensic Medicine at the Faculty of Liège; and Dr. Mina Minovici, Professor of Forensic Medicine at Faculty of Medicine of Bucharest. George Bogdan's Textbook was enthusiastically welcomed by specialists in his own country and in Europe and praised by Mina Minovici (Bucharest), Stockis (Liège) and Balthazard (Paris), among others.

Volume I (Bogdan 1921) focused on "Attacks on health and life by wounds and blows"; volume II (Bogdan 1922) pointed to aspects related to "Attacks on good morals"; volume III (Bogdan 1924) dealt with "Pregnancy, birth, abortion, infanticide and medical deontology"; volume IV (Bogdan 1925) paid attention to "Death and sudden death". The fourth volume was written together with Séverin Icard, a well-known French forensic specialist, member of the Academy of Medicine in Paris and of the Institute of France, but also a well-known numismatist from Marseilles, author of several reference works on real and apparent death, as well as on the souls of those who die (Icard 1860; 1897; 1929). Séverin Icard had also deepened the peculiarities of female psychology and behaviour in relation to the menstrual cycle from a standpoint still marked by prejudices considered especially in its relationship with morality and forensics (L'état psychique de la femme pendant la période menstruelle…) (Icard 1889; 1890). Icard`s conception inspired some theories of Cesare Lombroso (1835-1909), the father of forensic anthropology, such as they appeared, for example, in *The criminal woman, the prostitute and the normal woman* (Lombroso and Ferrero 1896). In an era marked by the school of Jean Martin Charcot (1825-1893), hysteria-a dominant contemporary medical theme-mainly illustrated a manifestation of "impure blood" and controversial female sexuality.

After Professor George Bogdan`s death (December 1930), Maria Ropala published the manuscript of the fifth and final volume of his treatise of forensic medicine, in which the topic of "Asphyxias" was developed (Scripcaru 1982, 190).

Maria Cickersky Ropala`s Scientific Articles

The investigations undertaken by Dr. Maria Cickersky Ropala, alone or in collaboration with Professor Bogdan, reflect the main theoretical orientations of the time, but also the main types of problems that occurred in practice. Besides several doctoral theses which she conducted, Dr. Ropala published a series of scientific articles. In *Annales d'Hygiène Publique et de Médecine Légale* (Paris), she published the papers "Pericardo-pulmonary symphysis. Sudden death" in 1920, and in 1922 "The whims of projectiles". In 1922, in *Annales de Médecine Légale, de Criminologie et Police Scientifique* (Paris), she published "Two interesting autopsies", and in 1923, "Contribution to the study of sudden death. Consequence of arteropathies and coronarites". The papers were signed "by Dr. Marie Ropala Cickersky, Assistant of the Course of Forensic Medicine. Forensic doctor of the Jassi Court (Romania)". In 1925, Dr. Ropala authored "Contributions to the study of asphyxia from a forensic point of view" (Scripcaru 1982, 183).

"Pericardo-pulmonary symphysis. Sudden death"

The article "Pericardo-pulmonary symphysis. Sudden death" brought to attention the pleuro-pericardial symphysis-a potential cause of sudden death, in the vision of Professor Bogdan, to whom the author often refers (Ropala 1920, 292). Pericardo-pulmonary adhesions, sometimes affecting the anterior mediastinum, too, are described in three different situations: a 35-year-old man, who died suddenly before entering the Courtroom whilst on trial for theft; a 70-year-old woman whom the neighbours found dead in an advanced state of putrefaction; a 14-year-old boy killed by the accidental explosion of a grenade. There were no data on any of the victims attesting to any previous cardio-respiratory suffering. The lungs were characterized by increased stasis, volume, and consistency. The pericardo-pulmonary symphysis was expressed by apparently fibrinous false membranes, with calcification areas and ossification plates that linked together the pleura and the pericardium. Dr. Ropala attributed their demise to impaired lung function due to this "accretio cordis", a morbid entity that-in her opinion-gave the verdict of "*cor ultimum moriens*" and not of "*cor primum moriens*", as most authors were tempted to believe (Ropala 1920, 291).

"The Whims of Projectiles"

The study "The Whims of Projectiles" *(Les caprices des projectiles)* was also presented by Professor Georg Strassmann (Berlin) as a short "Report" in the *Deutsche Zeitschrift für die gesamte gerichtliche Medizin*, inserted in thc chapter on 'Injuries. Violent death from physical causes' (Strassmann 1924, 181). The article focused on a topic of ballistics, an aspect dear to Professor Balthazard, and presented two circumstances in which the projectile trajectory was completely unpredictable, "bizarre", according to the author's expression. The first situation, the case of a 25-year-old Polish man (Maximilian Krausosky), was a suicide by firearm, autopsied after 36 hours. The revolver bullet, applied precordially, had entered the left intercostal space, in the sub-nipple region, perforated the pericardium and exclusively the anterior wall of the left ventricle. The heart was thought to be in systole, as the 9 mm calibre projectile had affected the middle sigmoid of the aortic valve, which appeared black-purple and swollen; it had then entered the systemic bloodstream and, completely piercing the aortic wall, fixed itself on the second lumbar vertebra, where the bullet was found.

The second case, a 22-year-old woman (Elena Olariu), was also an accidental death by firearm. It occurred six hours after the emergency laparotomy was performed after a revolver had inadvertently discharged, about 80 cm from the victim, the projectile hitting her in the abdomen, on an oblique trajectory, oriented from bottom to top. The entrance orifice was observed at 1 cm to the left of the umbilicus, the peritoneum and the sutured loops were congestive, with vascular arborizations, while the stomach was perforated in two places: near the cardiac orifice, and near the pylorus, respectively. Crossing the greater curvature of the stomach, the bullet had penetrated the transverse colon and descended into the ascending colon, stopping in a faecal bolus where it was spotted in the examination. The affective participation of the forensic doctor is not missing: "Continuing the autopsy, we were terribly surprised" – she said – or "a revolver discharged (the bullet…that) came to strike the unfortunate lady" (Cickersky Ropala 1922a, 226). Concluding the communication Dr. Ropala paid homage to her Master: "These two trajectories show once again that projectiles do not always follow the regular paths described in all the classical treatises, but they sometimes make an exception to the general rule, as it is so well supported by our learned Master, Professor Bogdan, in his beautiful book on blows and wounds published last year[3]" (Ropala 1922 a, 228).

"Two interesting autopsies"

The article "Two interesting autopsies" (*Deux autopsies intéressantes*) by "Dr. Marie Ropala Cickersky, Assistant in the Course of Forensic Medicine at the Faculty of Medicine of Jassy-Romania. Forensic doctor of the Court of Iasi", was published in *Annales de Médecine Légale, de Criminologie et de Police Scientifique*, in January 1922. Two comparable cases of sudden death were reported, which occurred in approximately the same period. The first autopsy in a woman aged 35-40 indicated two different but associated lesions: (1) rupture of the gallbladder wall, accompanied by the discharge of bile into the peritoneal cavity; (2) ulceration of the tricuspid valve on both sides, associated with rupture of two papillary muscles in the right heart. The direct cause of death was considered to be the heart damage. In the second case, in a 52-year-old man who died during a brawl, the autopsy revealed absolutely comparable heart damage as in the previous case but affecting the left side of the heart: mitral valve ulceration and rupture of the papillary muscles. These injuries were thought to have been the direct cause of his sudden death, and not the quarrel (Ropala 1922 b, 43).

"Contribution to the study of sudden death. Consequence of arteropathies and coronarites"

The paper "*Contribution à l'étude de la mort subite. Suite d'artéropathies et coronarites*" investigated four cases, illustrating various degrees and locations of atheromatous disease, which, under precise conditions, led to sudden death. The precipitating factors of the final drama had been physical effort, conflict situations accompanied or not by physical violence, intellectual and emotional stressors. Heredity was also indicated among

[3] G. Bogdan`s handbook previously mentioned, first volume, (Wounds and Blows), 1921.

predisposing factors. In the four ambiguous situations, Dr. Ropala tipped the scales in favour of internal causes, such as generalized arterial and coronary suffering. Consistent with Séverin Icard's ideas, sudden death was in reality the "unexpected" result of morbid processes that, sometimes unknown, had long evolved in the body. This study was also presented by Professor Karl Meixner (Vienna) as a "Report" in the *Deutsche Zeitschrift für die gesamte gerichtliche Medizin* (Meixner 1924, 205). Here is the translation of the Report (Summary): "1. A 35-year-old man collapses unconscious while loading some bags. The necropsy shows the torsion of one of the two cusps of the mitral valve and the rupture of two muscle bundles in the left ventricle, coronary arteries strongly narrowed by atheromatosis, the left one completely closed by a yellowish-reddish embolus (?). Atheroma with degeneration of systemic arteries. The author excludes the possibility of a work accident. 2. A 65-year-old man who had repeated attacks of angina pectoris (stenocardia) (following mechanical trauma of the left hemithorax) dies suddenly. The left and right coronary arteries were rigid and obstructed. 3. A hotelier about 65 year old is punched in the chest by his younger wife during a marital conflict and dies shortly afterwards. No other lesions were noticed. The left coronary artery was on a large area obliterated by a thrombus. Atheromas were observed on the curvature of the systemic arteries. 4. In a man who died after a strong emotion, an atheroma of the aorta was found with obliteration of both coronary arteries. The man's mother also had frequent heart attacks, and died suddenly, as well. His grandfather at the age of 58 had suddenly died on learning that a grandchild had been born to him. Corpses of his mother and grandfather had not been necropsically examined."

In this paper, Ropala discussed every forensic aspect against a very complex bibliographical-historical background. She evoked Orfila, Devergie, Tardieu, Brouardel, Toinot, Balthazard, Barié, Potain, Vaquez and Œstreich, along with Romanian experts-G. Bogdan, M. Minovici, N. Stoenescu-who investigated arteropathies, coronarites, work accidents and medical conditions of traumatic origin. Commenting on heredity in heart diseases, she mentioned Gilbert and Baudoin, forerunners of the hypothesis of the hereditary sudden death, and Vibert (Ropala 1923, 508).

Maria Cickersky Ropala, Romanian forensic medicine and their Portuguese echo

In 1936, a Portuguese university assistant, Dr. Carlos Ribeiro da Silva Lopes of the Faculty of Medicine and Institute of Forensic Medicine of Oporto, mentioned several Romanian contributions to forensic medicine in his doctoral thesis entitled "*Homicídio e Suïcídio. Seu diagóstico nos ferimentos por armas de fogo curtas*". Da Silva Lopes brought to attention some pioneering personalities of Romanian forensic medicine and their roles in the overall progress of forensics. Thus, he pinpointed the outstanding contribution of Professor Mina Minovici, one of the fathers of Romanian forensic medicine, in strengthening the technical police: "There are no Technical Police Laboratories in Portugal - true science to which Hanns, Gross, Bertillon, Stockis, Bayle, Galton, Ottolenghi, Reiss, Vucetich, Lacassagne, Balthazard, Locard and Minovici, among others, have contributed a lot" (Da Silva Lopes 1936, 21). Minovici was equally the founder of the first Institute of Forensic Medicine in the world. This happened in Bucharest in 1898. Bibliographical references in the thesis also included papers by Dr. Neculai Balan, professor of Forensic Medicine in Iasi, by Dr. Mihail Kernbach, professor of Forensic Medicine in Cluj, future head of the Department of Forensic Medicine at the Faculty of Medicine of Iasi, and by jurist Constantin Zguriadescu of Bucharest (Da Silva Lopes, 1936, 130). Dr. Balan, was Professor Bogdan`s successor at the Iasi Faculty of Medicine. Lopes cited two of his studies undertaken with two important French collaborators-René Piédelièvre and Pierre Étienne Martin-and published in Paris. Two studies by Dr. Mihail Kernbach were equally specified, having appeared in the *Annales de Médecine Légale de Criminologie et de Police Judiciaire* (Kernbach 1927, S1) and in *Revue Internationale de Criminalistique* (Kernbach 1932, 108), respectively (Da Silva Lopes 1936, 140). As to Zguriadescu`s volume on the Technical Police and Scientific Forensic Investigation (Zguriadesco 1913), Lopes indicated a bookreview he consulted, included in the *Archives Internationales de Médecine Légale* (Da Silva Lopes 1936, 147).

The Romanian Technical Police already had such a tradition: in 1896, the first School of Scientific Police was established and in 1893 in the city of Craiova Nicolae I. Alexiu's "Handbook for the judicial police officer" appeared.

Quoting Professor António Piga y Pascual, a famous Spanish forensic specialist and academician, Da Silva Lopes also referred to one of Maria Ropala`s articles-*Les caprices des projectiles* (*The Whims of Projectiles*) (Ropala Cickersky 1922), whose observations and comments he had taken from Professor Piga`s treatise on "Emergency Forensic Medicine" (Piga 1928).

Professor António Piga's book discussed Dr. Ropala`s study and her conclusions. Commenting on various migratory bullets in the circulatory system as a result of the blood flow, António Piga cited a "very notable" situation described by Ropala "in which the bullet penetrated the fifth left intercostal space below the nipple, and passed through the pericardium, crossing the left ventricle. The heart was in systole. The projectile, drawn by the blood stream, perforated the aorta at the level of the second lumbar and there it remained fixed". Lopes instead considered that "in his view", this was an "incomprehensible case", concluding, however, that: "All of these observations show the difficulty that sometimes exists in finding the bullet during the autopsies and in establishing the position of the weapon that injured the individual" (Da Silva Lopes 1936, 93).

Hence Romanian forensic medicine was placed among the avant-garde schools of the world, integrating itself into the international scientific movement of the epoch.

Years after, appointed full professor of Forensic Medicine and Forensic Toxicology, Carlos Ribeiro da Silva Lopes (1906-1997) also directed for a while the Museum of the History of Medicine of the Faculty of Medicine in Oporto.

A tradition that continues

Maria Cickersky Ropala appears in the history of Romanian medicine as the first lady-forensic doctor not only in her country, but also in South-Eastern and Western Europe, although her personality is often eclipsed or forgotten. The medical-historical context of her epoch reveals its notable importance since the ideas and conceptions born at the beginning of the twentieth century, in the atmosphere of great feminist claims, forged not only the scientific bases of the old truths, but enabled other theories and heresies to be generated regarding the woman's status, physiology and mental pathology, dominated by hysteria. Woman`s sexuality was rediscovered and redimensioned.

Maria Cickersky Ropala's emancipation itself was limited: although intelligent, diligent and dedicated to forensic expertise, she remained, throughout her entire life, in her Master`s shadow, failing, not daring, and, perhaps, not being allowed, to fully manifest and professionally accomplish her personality.

In keeping with this historical landmark, under completely different circumstances, Romanian forensic medicine came to be illustrated in Iași by the first woman forensic doctor to acquire the highest academic position, in 2002, when Dr. Monica Plahteanu was appointed full professor of Forensic Medicine and head of this Department at the Institute of Medicine and Pharmacy of Iași. Presently, in 2020, the Forensic Institute of Iași, e.g., is directed by a woman forensic expert, as well.

In December 2019, in Maria Ropala's honor, a conference hall was inaugurated bearing her name in the "Nicolae Leon" building of the "Grigore T. Popa" University of Medicine and Pharmacy of Iași.

These data on the national and international context of forensic medicine at the beginning of the twentieth century could better explain how a Romanian lady-doctor from Iași was admitted to acknowledged professional societies, being one of the very first woman forensic doctors in the world. Since its beginning Romanian forensic medicine, directly connected to the French tradition, represented indeed a prestigious school, already recognized at that time in Europe and beyond.

References

Annuaire. 1924. *Annales de Médecine Légale, Criminologie et Police Scientifique,* 10: 244.

Baran, Dana. 2016. *Maria Ropala Cickersky, prima femeie medic legist (Maria Ropala Cickersky, the First Woman Forensic Doctor*). Iași: "Gr. T. Popa" Publishing House-University of Medicine and Pharmacy of Iași.

Bogdan, George. 1921. *Atentate în contra sanatatii si a vietei prin raniri si loviri din punctul de vedere juridic si medico-legal (Attacks on health and life by wounds and blows from the legal and forensic point of view*) (vol.1). Bucuresti: Editura Cartea Romaneasca.

Bogdan, George. 1922. *Atentatele contra bunelor moravuri din punctul de vedere juridic si medico-legal (Attacks on morality from the legal and forensic point of view)* (vol. II). Bucuresti: Editura Cartea Romaneasca.

Bogdan, George. 1924. *Sarcina-nasterea, avortul - pruncuciderea si deontologia medicala din punctul de vedere juridic si medico-legal (Pregnancy-birth, abortion-infanticide and medical deontology from the legal and forensic point of view*) (vol.III). Iași: Tipografia H. Goldner.

Bogdan, George. 1925. *Moartea si moartea subita (Death and Sudden Death*) (vol. IV). Iași: Tipografia H. Goldner.

Bologa, Valeriu Lucian, Gheorghe Bratescu, Benone Dutescu and Stefan Marius Milcu. 1972. *Istoria Medicinei Romanesti*. Bucuresti: Editura Medicala, 408.

Cicherschi, Maria. 1907. *Contributiune la studiul biologiei si criminalitatii feminine (Din punctul de vedere medico-legal*). Teza pentru doctorat in medicina si chirurgie. Prezentata si sustinuta in Iunie 1907 (Nr. 266). (Contribution to the study of female biology and criminality (From a forensic point of view). Doctoral thesis in medicine and surgery. Presented and defended in June 1907. Iași: H. Goldner Printing House.

Claude, Henri. 1932. *Psychiatrie Médico-Légale*. Paris: Gustave Doin et Cie. Éditeurs.

Da Silva Lopes, Carlos Ribeiro. 1936. *Homicídio e Suïcídio. Seu diagóstico nos ferimentos por armas de fogo curtas.* Porto: Imprensa Nacional de J. Vasconcelos. http://hdl.handle.net/10216/61792.

Icard, Séverin. 1889. L'état psychique de la femme pendant la période menstruelle, considéré plus spécialement dans ses rapports avec la morale et la médecine légale. Paris: Thèse de médecine.

Icard, Séverin. 1890. *La femme pendant la période menstruelle: étude de psychologie morbide et de médecine légale*. Paris: Félix Alcan Éditeur.

Icard, Séverin. 1897. *La mort réelle et la mort apparente* (Real death and apparent death). Paris: Félix Alcan Éditeur.

Icard, Séverin. 1907. *Le signe de la mort réelle en l'absence du médecin: la constatation et le certificat automatiques des décès, procédé de la réaction sulfhydrique*. Paris: A. Maloine.

Icard, Séverin. 1929. *L'âme des mourants*. Paris: Bibliothèque Eudiaque – Henri Durville Éditeur.

Kernbach, Mihail. 1927. "Une nouvelle contribution à l'élimination des erreurs dans la détermination des groupes sanguins". *Annales de Médecine Légale, de Criminologie et de Police Scientifique,* 1:1-7.

Kernbach, Mihail. 1932. "Trois observations médico-légales avec 131 applications criminalistiques". *Bibliothèque de la Revue Internationale de Criminalistique,* 2: 108-119.

Klevno, Vladimir Aleksandrovich and Viktor Yuryevich Nazarov. 2017. *History of Russian Forensic Medicine*. In Burkhard Madea (ed) *History of Forensic Medicine*. Berlin: Lehmans Media.

Lambert, Marcelle and Balthazard, Victor. 1910. *Le poil de l'homme et des animaux.* Paris: G. Steinheil.

Lombroso, Cesare. 1896. "L`uomo delinquente". *Bocca,* 1: 33-34.

Maftei, Ionel. 1985. *Ropala Cicherschi, Maria (1881-1973), medic legist.* (*Personalities of Iasi*). vol. V. Iasi, 225-226.

Meixner, Karl. 1924. "Referate. Plötzlicher Tod aus innerer Ursache. Cickersky, Marie-Ropala: Contribution à l'étude de la mort subite. Suite d'artéropathies et coronarites". (*Zur Kenntnis des plötzlichen Todes infolge von Erkrankung der Kranzschlagadern*), *Deutsche Zeitschrift für die gesamte gerichtliche Medizin,* 4 (1): 205.

Minovici, Mina. 1907. "Remarques sur la criminalité féminine en Roumanie". *Archives d'Anthropologie Criminelle et de Psychologie Normale et Pathologique,* 22: 565-664.

Nazarov, Viktor Yuryevich. 2011. ("Anna Mikhailovna Smyslova - the first Russian woman forensic medical expert"). *Sudebno-meditsinskaia ekspertiza,* 54 (5): 58-60.

Normand, Jean. 2004. Alexandre Lacassagne, un pédagogue original, *Millénaire 3. La prospective de la Métropole.* www.millenaire3.com

Piédelièvre, Balan and Etienne-Martin, Pierre. 1931. "L'hémorragie sous-dermique par tiraillement dans les orifices d'entrée des projectiles". *Annales de Médecine Légale, de Criminologie et de Police Scientifique,* 12 (1): 569-575.

Piédelièvre, Balan and Etienne-Martin, Pierre. 1931. "Blessure d'un fœtus dans la cavité utérine par coup de feu". *Annales de Médecine Légale, de Criminologie et de Police Scientifique,* 12 (1): 575-577.

Piga, Antonio. 1928. *Medicina Legal de Urgencia (La Autopsia Judicial*). Madrid: Ediciones Mercurio.

Puscariu, Emil, and Mircea Vesesco. 1895. Essais de vaccination antirabique avec le virus atténué par la chaleur. *Annales de l`Institut Pasteur,* 9: 210-213.

Ropala Cickersky, Marie. 1920. "Symphyse péricardo-pulmonaire. Mort subite". *Annales d'Hygiène Publique et de Médecine Légale,* (4) 34: 283-292.

Ropala Cickersky, Marie. 1922a. "Les caprices des projectiles". *Annales d'Hygiène Publique et de Médecine Légale,* (4) 38: 225-228.

Ropala Cickersky, Marie. 1922b. "Deux autopsies intéressantes". *Annales de Médecine Légale, Criminologie et Police Scientifique,* 2 (1): 43-44.

Ropala Cickersky, Maria. 1923. "Contribution à l'étude de la mort subite. Suite d'artéropathies et coronarites", *Annales de Médecine Légale, de Criminologie et de Police Scientifique,* 3 (8): 508-516.

Scripcaru, Gheorghe. 1982. "Un secol de invatamant, cercetare si asistenta medico-legala la Iasi" (A century of forensic education, research and assistance in Iasi). *Revista Medico-Chirurgicala a Societatii de Medici si Naturalisti din Iasi,* 86 (1): 181-193.

Strassmann, Georg. 1924. Referate. Verletzungen. Gewattsamer Tod aus physikalischer Ursache. Cickersky, Marie Ropala: "Les caprices des projectiles". (Die Launen der Kugeln), *Deutsche Zeitschrift für die gesamte gerichtliche Medizin,* 3 (1): 181.

Zguriadescu, Constantin. 1913. *Politia tehnica si ancheta judiciara stiintifica (Technical police and scientific judicial investigation*)(Bucuresti: *Tipografia*) Universala Iancu Ionescu. Refer. in Archives Internationales de Médecine Légale. Liège, 1913, Vol. IV, Fasc. 3.

CHAPTER 14

FERNANDO DE ALMEIDA (1903-1979) - THE STORY OF THE DOCTOR WHO WAS ONE OF THE GREATEST PORTUGUESE ARCHAEOLOGISTS

CAROLINA MOREIRA

Abstract: Fernando de Almeida (1903-1979) is a little-known name in Portuguese Medicine and, in particular, at the Faculty of Medicine of Lisbon, where he graduated and taught. As such, he has received far less recognition than names such as Egas Moniz (1874-1955), Reynaldo dos Santos (1880-1970) or Henrique de Vilhena (1879-1958) have. Much greater is his recognition in the area of History and Archaeology. This led to the birth of the Final Master's Work "Fernando de Almeida-Physician and Archaeologist", which serves as the basis for this article, to revive the memory of his contribution to Medicine. Shortly after graduating in Medicine, he started teaching Anatomy and carrying out research in this area in connection with the Institute of Anatomy of the Faculty of Medicine of Lisbon. Also noteworthy was his contribution to Neurology and research in collaboration with Egas Moniz, the most significant name in Portuguese Neurology in the 20th century, perpetuated above all by the discovery of cerebral angiography, which was first performed on a living human being in 1927. This collaboration resulted in a total of five articles on the application of this angiographic technique. Fernando de Almeida specialized in Obstetrics and Gynecology, having worked at the Dr. Alfredo da Costa Maternity Hospital for various years. When he was 51, he graduated in Historical and Philosophical Sciences from the Faculty of Letters of Lisbon, starting a new career in History and Archaeology, just as or even more successful than the previous one, thus proving that a doctor is much more than someone who only knows about medicine.

Key words: Egas Moniz; Anatomy; Neurology: Cerebral Angiography: Archaeology

Resumo: Fernando de Almeida é um nome pouco conhecido na Medicina portuguesa e, em particular, na Faculdade de Medicina de Lisboa, onde se formou e leccionou, ficando assim muito distante do reconhecimento que nomes como Egas Moniz (1874-1955), Reynaldo dos Santos (1880-1970) ou Henrique de Vilhena (1879-1958), alcançaram. Muito maior é o seu reconhecimento na área da História e Arqueologia. Com o objectivo de reavivar a memória sobre o seu contributo para a Medicina, nasceu o Trabalho Final de Mestrado "D. Fernando de Almeida – Médico e Arqueólogo", que serve de base a este artigo. Pouco após a sua licenciatura em Medicina, D. Fernando, começou a leccionar a Cadeira de Anatomia e a desenvolver investigações na área em ligação ao Instituto de Anatomia da Faculdade de Medicina de Lisboa. De destacar ainda o seu contributo para a Neurologia e as investigações em colaboração com Egas Moniz, nome maior da neurologia portuguesa do século XX, perpetuado sobretudo pela descoberta da angiografia cerebral, pela primeira vez executada em 1927 no homem vivo, continuou a desenvolver esta técnica e a aperfeiçoá-la. Alguns desses estudos, cinco no total, contaram com o apoio de Fernando de Almeida, que teria ainda tempo, durante a sua carreira, para se especializar em ginecologia-obstetrícia e, aos 51 anos, licenciar-se em Ciências Históricas e Filosóficas pela Faculdade de Letras de Lisboa, iniciando uma nova carreira na História e na Arqueologia, tão ou mais bem-sucedida do que a anterior, provando assim que um médico é muito mais que alguém que só sabe de medicina.
Palavras chave: Egas Moniz; Anatomia: Neurologia; Angiografia cerebral; Archaeology

Introduction

Fernando de Almeida was born on 28 November 1903 in Fundão and graduated in Medicine from the Faculty of Medicine of Lisbon in 1927. During his graduation year, he began collaborating as a volunteer teaching assistant at the Institute of Anatomy, directed by Prof. Henrique de Vilhena (1879-1958) and at the Surgery Service, directed by Prof. Reynaldo dos Santos (1880-1970). This taste for teaching would accompany him throughout his life. His first articles appeared in the area of Anatomy and Neurology. As a teaching assistant at the Institute of Anatomy, he produced several articles resulting from his dissections. Between 1932 and 1933 he published five articles in the field of Neurology in collaboration with Egas

Moniz (1874-1955), on the topic of the application of the cerebral angiography technique. At this time, he started his specialization, as an intern, in Obstetrics and Gynecology, at the Dr. Alfredo da Costa Maternity Hospital, which he concluded in 1940. He would be a specialist at that Hospital until 1948, when he became Head of the Out-Patient Services at the Maternal Institute. He would occupy this position for 10 years, until 1958. From that year until 1966, he would act as Assistant Clinical Inspector for the Board of the Maternal Institute, at a time when he had almost completely abandoned clinical practice.

In 1949, at the age of 46, he decided to take a course in Historical and Philosophical Sciences at the Faculty of Arts in Lisbon, finishing his degree in 1954. His career in this area extended for 30 years until the end of his life and was to be of great importance and contribute to the advancement of knowledge, especially regarding the High Middle Ages in Portugal.

In total, throughout his life, Fernando de Almeida wrote 143 papers, 50 in the field of Medicine and 93 in the areas of History and Archaeology.

Early Life and Initial Training

Fernando de Almeida or, to give him his full name, Fernando António de Almeida e Silva Saldanha, was born in Fundão, Castelo Branco, on 28 November 1903. He was the son of Fernando António de Nazaré de Almeida e Silva de Saldanha (1873-1942), a doctor in Fundão, and Maria do Carmo de Figueiredo Falcão Frazão Saldanha (1877-1933) (Fig. 14.1.).

Little or nothing is known about his childhood, only that he was always in contact with Medicine and some of its practitioners because of his father, who obtained his degree in Medicine from the University of Coimbra, where he was a classmate and friend of Egas Moniz, both having completed the course in 1899. This relationship persisted beyond the course, with Egas Moniz being chosen to be Fernando's godfather.

After completing his high school studies and medical preparations in Coimbra, he enrolled at the Faculty of Medicine of Lisbon, where he graduated in 1927 with a final classification of 16 ("Good with Distinction"). In that same year, he began to work as a volunteer teaching assistant at the Institute of Anatomy, headed by Professor Henrique de Vilhena and in the Surgery Service, headed by Prof. Reynaldo dos Santos at the Arroios Hospital. In the following two years, he would deepen his studies by doing two postgraduate courses: one in Hydrology and Climatology and the other in Sanitary Medicine.

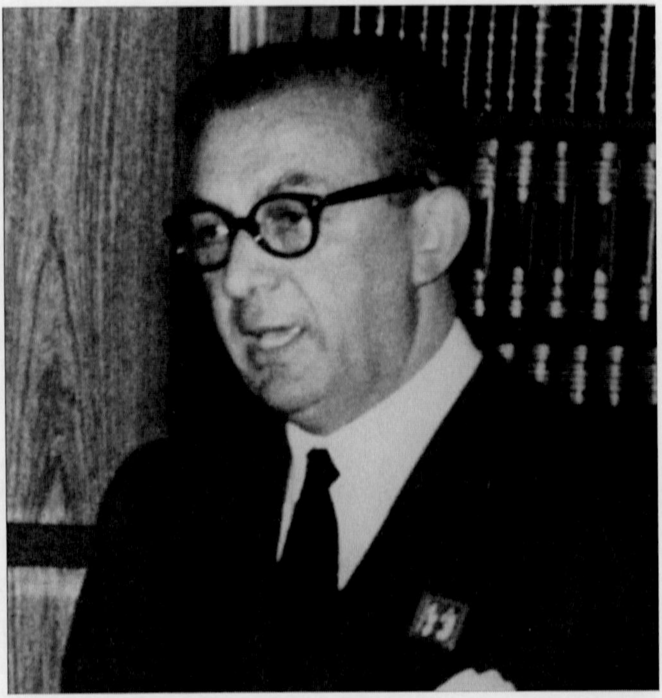

Fig. 14.1. Fernando de Almeida. Photo reproduced with permission of Dr. Luís Raposo.

First steps as a Doctor, Professor and Researcher

In 1929 he started working as an Intern at the Lisbon Civil Hospitals. In the same year, he took on duties as an Anatomy Teaching Assistant at the Faculty of Medicine of Lisbon, a position he would hold until 1937, when he started to teach on the Surgery Module.

In 1930, he took on the additional position of Professor of Anatomy and Physiology at the School of Physical Education. That same year, in the Inaugural Lesson for this Course, he explained the importance of Anatomy to new students for obtaining true knowledge of the human body, ending with the following advice: "not only do not neglect Anatomy, the basis of any study on the human body, but give it the consideration it deserves due to its many centuries of existence and look upon it as an ever new science, albeit an old one" (Almeida 1931a).

In an almost prophetic manner of harking back to a distant time, Fernando de Almeida included in his presentation not only the historical bases of the evolution of the study of Anatomy but also various notes that included considerable knowledge of areas other than just Medicine such as the story of Erasistratus, a physician to the court of King Seleucus, and how he obtained royal authorization to dissect corpses for the sake of scientific knowledge.

This brief lecture, given when Fernando de Almeida was still a young man aged 27, already showed a natural inclination towards teaching and an interest in History.

Scientific work at the Institute of Anatomy

While he was associated with the Institute of Anatomy of the Faculty of Medicine (1927-1937), he produced various articles on the anatomical description of various organs and systems. He compiled observations of various anatomical variations from dissections in an article he called *Notes on descriptive anatomy* (*Notas de anatomia descritiva*), published in 1931, with 7 cases of muscle variations (Almeida 1931b). In 1935, he published a second series of notes, adding new observations and bringing together vascular and urogenital apparatus variations in addition to anatomical muscular ones (Almeida 1936a).

In a publication entitled *Une anomalie rare du Foie*, resulting from a communication held at the 28th meeting of the Association of Anatomists and the Portuguese Anatomical Society, in 1933 (Almeida 1934b), he describes a dissection of a corpse where a rare anomaly was found which, according to Fernando de Almeida, had not already been described in the literature. In a 65-year-old man who died of a stroke, he observed a liver with two almost independent lobes, connected only by a strip of avascular tissue. Each lobe had its pedicle and, under a microscope, the structure was similar to that of a normal liver. Fernando wrote: “I could say that this corpse has two livers” concluding that it was a rare arrangement which was difficult to explain (Almeida 1934b).

In *Sur L'Irrigation d'a reine en fer-à-cheval* (Almeida 1934a), he reported observations made on a corpse with a horseshoe kidney. The article provided a detailed description of the vascularization of this kidney, including the origin, path and termination of each of the main arteries and veins. He concluded that, while the right portion was irrigated by 4 arteries, on the left there was only one (Fig. 14.2). This would make an intervention in the right kidney, such as a nephrectomy, more complex than the left.

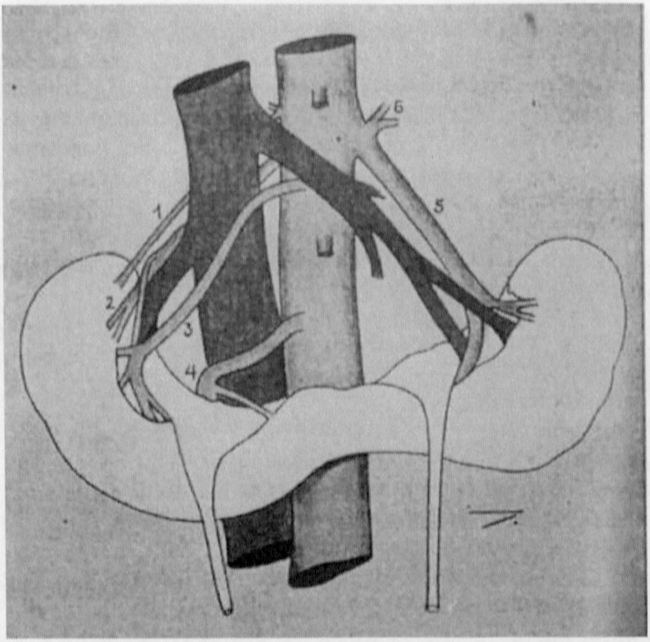

Fig. 14.2. Schematic representation of the horseshoe kidney, described by Fernando de Almeida. In: Sur L'Irrigation d'a reine en fer-à-cheval, Arquivo de Anatomia e Antropologia, 1934.

He would also have the opportunity to publish two notes *On the anatomy of the presacral nerve (Sobre a anatomia do nervo pré-sagrado).* The first, presented at the second meeting of the Portuguese Anatomical Society in 1934, was based on 37 cadaver dissections and concluded by summarizing that the presacral nerve is a plexus that forms at the level of the emergence of the inferior mesenteric artery and ends by forking 25 mm above the promontory. In the most frequently observed arrangement (64%), the plexus meshes were quite tight, giving them the appearance of tape. He also found that in the constitution of the presacral nerve, nerve fibers come from the lumbar ganglia, intermesenteric plexuses, periaortic and inferior mesenteric artery. He concluded by agreeing with the proposal to change the name from “presacral nerve" to “inter-iliac plexus” as argued for by Delmas and Laux in 1933 (Almeida 1936b). The following year, at the third meeting of the Portuguese Anatomical Society, he presented the result of the dissection of 17 more corpses, thus bringing the total number of observations to 54. The new observations confirmed the results previously presented (Almeida 1937).

Of the fifty articles he wrote on Medicine, fifteen were published in the *Archives of Anatomy and Anthropology*, appearing in volumes XIII, XIV, XVI, XVII, XVIII and XXIII, including (in addition to the works mentioned above) other research in the area of neuroanatomy, more specifically on cerebral vascularization. He published articles in the areas of Neurology (some in collaboration with Egas Moniz) and in the areas of his specialty: Gynecology and Obstetrics, and also on intestinal peristalsis in Surgery journals in other national and foreign journals.

In the field of Anatomy, the Diplomas of the award for Systematic Anatomy and Topographic Anatomy that he received and his positions as founding member of the Portuguese Anatomical Society and of the Portuguese-Spanish-American Anatomical Society (Almeida 1966) stand out.

Scientific work in the field of Neurology

His prolific scientific work began almost immediately after graduating, alongside his Anatomy teaching, and perhaps for this reason his first publications were on anatomical topics, as mentioned above.

Most of these initial works would also be in the field of the Nervous System, more specifically in the description of cerebral circulation, forming a total of 13 publications.

In one of his first articles, entitled *Note sur les collatéralles de I'artère communicante cérébrale antérieure* (Almeida 1931c), he proposed two types of classification of the collateral arteries of the Anterior Communicating Artery: one regarding the diameter of the vessels (thin, medium and thick) and another, regarding their path (anterior, superior and posterior).

Shortly afterwards, he published an extensive descriptive work which had the aim of "studying the variations of the Middle Cerebral Artery and its collateral arteries, on the surface of the brain" (Almeida 1932). He did this by studying the brains of 50 cadaver brains, supplied by the Lisbon Civil Hospitals, and 250 arterial encephalographs which formed part of the collection of the Neurology Service of the School Hospital, made available by Egas Moniz, and he also made use of these observations for several of his articles.

Another publication followed, this time presenting a detailed description of the distribution of the Anterior Cerebral and Anterior Communicating Arteries on the surface of the brain (Almeida 1933).

In 1935, he published a summary of a paper presented at the International Congress of Neurology, in London, on the technique developed by Egas Moniz and consequent discoveries and the most important advances concerning knowledge of the anatomy of the brain (Almeida 1935).

Other works included commented and illustrated observations, resulting from dissections carried out in his practical classes, showing various elements of human anatomy, from muscles, vessels and nerves to organs such as the liver and kidney.

Also noteworthy was the publication in 1944 of an article on cerebral circulation, at a time when most of his scientific research and work was already taking place in the area of Gynaecology and Obstetrics: *Considerations on the distribution of the Middle and Anterior Cerebral Arteries on the surface of the brain of term newborns* (Almeida 1944) thus joining his previous experience in Neurology with his more recent area of interest.

Collaboration with Egas Moniz

In Almeida's earliest works, a close relationship with Egas Moniz, his supporter, has already been noted, and involved the provision of arterial encephalographs for a more complete study of cerebral circulation, supplementing his cadaver dissections, for the study of anatomy *in vivo*. Even closer collaboration would result in five joint articles, out of a total of 13 devoted to the theme of cerebral circulation. Three of these five articles also involved the collaboration of Abel Alves.

Two of these: *Visibility of the deep veins of the brain to X-Rays* (*Visibilidade aos Raios X das veias profundas do cérebro*) (Moniz 1932c) and *The venous sinuses of the dura mater, their visibility to X-rays* (*Os seios venosos da dura-máter, sua visibilidade aos Raios X*) (Moniz 1932b), were published in the journal *Lisboa Médica* in 1932, and, in a way, are complementary. In the first article the authors sought, both with phlebography *in vivo* and from corpses, to describe the deep veins of the brain, more specifically the Vein of Galen and the Basilar Vein, analyzing the path of each one and their branches. The article insisted on the importance of a complete study of brain circulation and of the venous sinuses, in particular the Right Sinus and the Lower Longitudinal Sinus because, due to their position, they could serve as a reference point for certain diagnostic investigations in the case of brain tumours.

The other article began by explaining the technique of arterial encephalography through the use of Thorotrast, which "opened new horizons for the visibility of the vessels of the brain through X-rays" (Moniz

1932b). Its observations focused on the sinuses of the dura-mater, in particular the Straight Sinus and the Lower Longitudinal Sinus. To sum up, 10 to 12 cc of Thorotrast were injected in the Common Carotid Artery and then angiographic images were obtained (Fig. 14.2-A); two seconds later a new radiograph was obtained (Fig.14.2-B), making it possible to visualize the cerebral venous network (first phase phlebography). By increasing the contrast dose and waiting a few more seconds, it was possible to perform a "second phase" phlebography and visualize the sinuses (Fig. 14.2-C). One of the great difficulties pointed out by the authors was finding the balance between the injection time and the time taken to remove the film to capture the Thorotrast in the intended structures. Another impediment to perfect visualization of the sinuses was the mixture of opaque blood from one hemisphere with the blood from the opposite hemisphere (without contrast), which reduced the quality of visualization of the Lower Longitudinal Sinus, as it received half opacified blood, and it was shown to be easier to assess on *in vivo* radiographs than in corpses (in this case, the injection of the contrast was applied simultaneously to the two Internal Jugular Veins). The article also mentions that they found discrepancies between what they observed and the descriptions of anatomy treatises, such as that of *Testut* (Testut 1891), with regard to the trajectory of the sinuses, and put forward two explanations: the first mentioned that when studying the brain, in removing it from the skull, its natural suspension is lost, in the Tentorium Cerebelli and in the Falx Cerebri. The other factor that changed the position of the sinus in the corpse compared to the *in vivo* one is the alteration of the hydraulic pressure of the cerebrospinal fluid in the cerebral ventricular system after death.

Previous publications, along with some additional research, led to an article entitled *Straight Sinus and Lower Longitudinal Sinus* (*Seio Recto e Seio Longitudinal Inferior*) (Moniz 1932d), published in 1932 which constituted an extensive, exclusively anatomical work, where the authors focused on studying the direction of the Straight Sinus and the Inferior Longitudinal Sinus, concluding that, because they are the continuation of each other in a regular curve, they should be considered as a single sinus. The article concluded that the phlebographic images disagreed with the anatomical schemata and ended by saying: "To sum up, alongside the *static anatomy* of the corpse, we should produce another anatomy, which we can classify as *dynamic*, obtained from the living, in the light of the functional activity of the organs that death often adulterates, through changing their position and changing their relationships." (Moniz 1932d). They thus demonstrated the need for clinical practice, and for the rigor of anatomy itself, to use techniques such as those that Egas Moniz was developing and refining to enable *in vivo* study (Fig. 14.3).

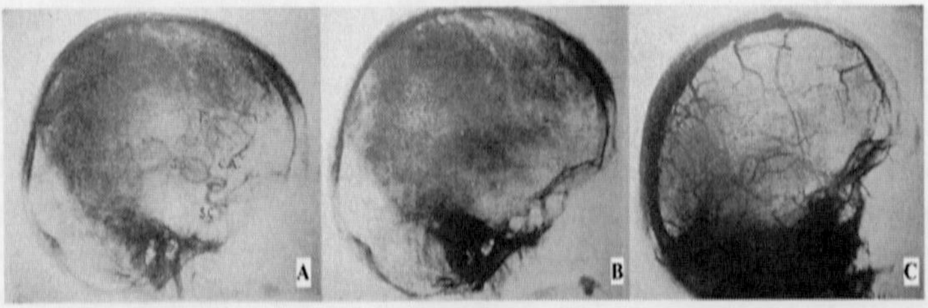

Fig. 14.3. The venous sinuses of the dura mater, their visibility to X-rays ("Os seios venosos da dura-mater, sua visibilidade aos raios X"). Egas Moniz (in collaboration with Abel Alves and Fernando de Almeida), Lisboa Médica, June 1932.

La Visibilité des Sinus de la dure-mêre par l'épreuve encéphalographique (Moniz 1932a), published in *La Presse Médicale* in 1932, compared the arrangement of the veins of the brain in a corpse with that in a living body. Although the material used by the authors was slightly different from the articles previously mentioned, the conclusions were identical.

In *Le Sinus Droitet I'Ampoule de Galien opacifiés par la voie du Tronc Basilaire* (Moniz 1933), the authors provided an extensive and detailed description of the arterial and venous circulation of the brain, concluding that there is a strong venous circulation in the Basilar Artery, in such a way that it opacifies other structures, thus demonstrating the importance of the circulation of the midbrain and the postero-inferior part of the Occipital Lobe, derived from the Basilar Artery.

This collaboration, although brief, proved to be prolific and allowed Fernando de Almeida to work with Egas Moniz and to actively participate in the research of the individual who is still to the present day considered the most important figure from Medicine in Portugal. In addition, it gave him the possibility to train himself in the scientific method that he would later successfully apply to Archaeology.

A remarkable medical career

He continued to write and publish articles in the area of Anatomy and in his area of specialty. In 1937, he started working as a member of the Surgery teaching staff at the Faculty of Medicine of Lisbon, and successful applied for a tenured position in 1938. He was professor of this subject until 1942.

He completed his internship in Obstetrics and Gynecology in 1940, at the Dr. Alfredo da Costa Maternity Hospital, where he remained until 1948. In the following year he started working as Head of External Services at the Maternal Institute, where he remained until 1958. From that year until 1966, he was the Assistant Clinical Inspector for the Board of the Maternal Institute. In 1966 he entered into an indefinite leave status, dedicating himself entirely to his successful career as an archaeologist from that moment onwards.

As a gynecologist and obstetrician he produced a substantial number of publications in the area, from the aforementioned article on cerebral circulation in neonates (Almeida 1944), as well as several clinical cases of rare pathologies he operated on, reviews of contemporary literature on topics such as abortion, sterility and endometriosis and he also published on the application of techniques such as anesthesia during childbirth or hysterosalpingography.

From his full medical career, special mention should be made of his specialist internships, as a scholarship holder, in somc of the best clinics and maternity hospitals in France (Paris, 1931 and 1939) and Italy (Modena, Turin, Bologna and Milan) in 1936; the diplomas and awards received in systemic anatomy and topographical Anatomy; participation in numerous national and international congresses; and also, his contribution as co-founder and member of various scientific associations, such as the Portuguese Anatomical Society, the Portuguese-Spanish-American Anatomical Society and the Portuguese Obstetrics and Gynecology Society. (Almeida 1966).

Change of life

In 1973, at the time of his retirement as director of the National Archeology Museum, he wrote about the reason that led him to a career change: "My interest in historical issues dates back to high school. (…) These tendencies of mine were known to friends. That was how, having gone to spend a holiday at the home of a very friendly family, on arrival I met a group of boys who were staying there. And right at the entrance, they asked me to enroll in the Faculty of Arts of Lisbon, together with them, because everyone had decided to do the same. And as I was interested in these matters, I would have to follow them" (Raposo 2003). He would, in fact, enroll in the course of Historical and Philosophical Sciences at the Faculty of Arts of the University of Lisbon, but only in 1949, graduating in 1954, with a final grade of 15 (out of 20), submitting for his undergraduate thesis: "Egypt: History and Archaeology", which was published by the Faculty.

In 1955, he started the systematic archaeological study of Idanha-a-Velha (*Civitas Igaeditanorum*), relatively close to his place of birth, Fundão, and in 1957 he accepted the post of second Teaching Assistant in the History Section of the Faculty of Arts.

He completed his doctorate in Archaeology and Art History in 1962 with the thesis "Visigothic Art in Portugal", thus becoming the first PhD holder in this field in Portugal. This work was published in *O Arqueólogo Português* (The Portuguese Archaeologist) and obtained the 1963 Calouste Gulbenkian Foundation Prize for Archaeology.

After applying for the post in 1967, he obtained the position of Professor of Archaeology and Art History at the Faculty of Arts in Lisbon and became the first Teaching Assistant in the History Section. He would go on to become the Director of this Faculty between 1969 and 1973.

In the meantime, he had taken up the post of Director of the National Museum of Archaeology and Ethnology in 1967 and started a new series of the journal *O Arqueólogo Português*, founded by José Leite de Vasconcellos (1585-1941), which led to six volumes being published on an occasional basis until 1973-the year of his retirement.

He held other positions of equal importance, namely Director of the Archaeological Museum of Odrinhas, Director of the Regional Museum of Castelo Branco, and Member of the Archeology Subsection and the Museology Subsection of the National Board of Education.

In 1958 he was awarded the position of Secretary-General of the 1st National Archaeology Congress, held in Lisbon (Santos 1985).

He was a member of several national and international scientific associations, of which the Portuguese Academy of History stands out; the Association of Portuguese Archaeologists (of which he was President); the Portuguese Institute of Archeology, History and Ethnography and was a correspondent for the Royal Academy of History (Madrid).

He led and undertook excavations in various parts of the country: Idanha-a-Velha, Mirobriga (Santiago do Cacém), S. Miguel de Odrinhas, Roman Theatre of Lisbon, Paleo-Christian Temple of S. Girão (Nazaré), Tróia (Setúbal), Roman Ruins of Cerro da Villa (Quarteira) and also Zambujal (Torres Vedras).

With his dynamism and enthusiasm, he encouraged students to participate in excavations. "We set up a true practical school in the field, where many, many students from the Faculty of Arts took their first steps in the always difficult and often ungrateful area of Archaeology, and some of them were definitely fascinated by this" (Cardoso 2005).

If his scientific work as a doctor was already remarkable, then in the area of Archaeology and Art History it was truly extraordinary, with the writing of almost a hundred articles, most of them about Late Antiquity and the High Middle Ages.

He died in Lisbon on 29 January 1979, and was transferred to the Alcaide cemetery on 9 June of the same year.

Legacy in Archaeology

Fernando de Almeida left an "indelible mark on various strata of the History of Portuguese Archaeology" (Profano 2017). This was not limited to the publishing of inventories. On the one hand, he cultivated monographic studies, on the other, "he drew up a conceptual operational model in the History of Art and Archaeology, by systematizing, into three large stylistic nuclei (Suévic, Lusitanian and Olissiponense), the growing heritage dating from the 4th to the 7th century within Portugal" (Fernandes 2003). To him "we owe the first true, systematic inventory of Visigothic Art in our country" (Fernandes 2003).

In relation to the excavation of Egitania (Idanha-a-Velha), "it managed, thus, to have reborn from ashes and oblivion, a city that returned to the light of day, constituting the first great successful Portuguese project in Urban Archaeology, with which, only many years later, was there another that could be compared: I am referring to Bracara Augusta." (Cardoso 2005).

By encouraging the participation of students and young researchers in their excavations and allowing access by them to the collections of the National Museum of Archaeology, this provided opportunities to a whole new generation with which to create science and advance the knowledge of the History of our Country. With his work and openness to younger members, he gave a future to the past.

After his death, the family donated his bibliographic collection to the Francisco Tavares Proença Júnior Museum in Castelo Branco, which in 1985 created a library bearing his name.

Other tributes followed, such as the celebrations in the year commemorating the centenary of his birth at the Association of Portuguese Archaeologists and at the Portuguese Academy of History, both in Lisbon, on 27 November 2003; at the Municipality of Fundão, in association with the neighboring parish of Alcaide, on the following day; and, in 2004, in Castelo Branco, by the Society of Friends of the Francisco Tavares Proença Júnior Museum, with the colloquium "Remembering Fernando de Almeida," which was enriched by an exhibition entitled "The journeys of a lifetime" in August (Silva 2004).

The name of Prof. Fernando de Almeida has, since 28 November 2003, been publicly commemorated in the town of Alcaide through a small monument in his honour.

Conclusion

Much remains to be said about the life and work of Fernando de Almeida. Everything I found written about this fascinating man concerns his contribution to History and Archaeology in Portugal. Although everyone devotes a few lines to Fernando de Almeida's medical background, none of the articles deepens his contribution to Medicine.

From the fifty publications he wrote in the field of Medicine, I decided to highlight the writings in collaboration with Egas Moniz. The application of angiography to visualize arterial and venous circulation, both in a living body and in the cadaver, enabled the observation and description of the vessels in their real position and to find several inaccuracies in earlier anatomical treatises on their paths and arrangement. He concluded that observation by dissection implied removing the brain from the skull, which ended up altering its anatomy and hence the inconsistencies in textbooks. He then dedicated himself to collecting the largest possible number of angiographic images and correctly describing cerebral circulation given the opinion that the correct identification of the structures was essential for clinical practice and for the diagnosis of brain tumours.

Life would later take him to other passions, or rather, he took his life to a new project, History and Archaeology, and if he was already successful as a doctor, then in this new phase he would reach a level of success only reserved for a few.

A manuscript prepared by Fernando de Almeida reflects his vision and way of drawing a parallel between Anatomy and Archaeology, and this starts by stating that there is a common element between these two sciences: Humanity. "While in Anatomy you study bones, joints and muscles, in Archaeology you study walls, stones, shards, vessels, streets, corridors" (Raposo 2003). If, in Medicine he had the mission to reconstruct the physical man, in Archaeology he had the mission to reconstruct monuments and memories.

In his image, I made it my mission to rebuild his memory in the house which trained him, allowing everything he achieved to be an example to us all that in life it is never too late.

Acknowledgements

I thank Dr. Luís Raposo, former Director of the National Museum of Archaeology in Lisbon the kind permission to reproduce the photo from Fernando de Almeida.

References

Almeida, Fernando de. 1931a. "Lição inaugural da Cadeira de Anatomia da Escola Superior de Educação Física." *Arquivos de Anatomia e Antropologia*, 14 (1): 527-532.

Almeida, Fernando de. 1931b. "Notas de Anatomia Descritiva (1.ª série)." *Arquivos de Anatomia e Antropologia,* 14 (1): 81–89.

Almeida, Fernando de. 1931c. "Note sur les collatérales de I'artère communicante cérébrale antérieure." *Arquivos de Anatomia e Antropologia,* 13 (4): 551-553.

Almeida, Fernando de. 1932. "Distribuição, na superfície do cérebro, da artéria Sílvica nos portugueses de condição humilde." *Arquivos de Anatomia e Antropologia,* 14 (2): 489-521.

Almeida, Fernando de. 1933. "Distribuição, na superfície do cérebro, das artérias Cerebral anterior e Comunicante anterior nos portugueses de condição humilde." *Arquivos de Anatomia e Antropologia*, 16: 323- 353.

Almeida, Fernando de. 1934a. "Sur I'irrigation d'un Rein enfer-à-cheval." *Arquivos de Anatomia e Antropologia,* 16: 167-170.

Almeida, Fernando de. 1934b. "Une anomalie rare du Foie." *Arquivos de Anatomia e Antropologia,* 16: 33-35.

Almeida, Fernando de. 1935. "Arteriographies et phlebographies normales du cerveau." *Revue Neurologique*, no. 4: 624-625.

Almeida, Fernando de. 1936a. "Notas de Anatomia Descritiva (2.ª série)." *Arquivos de Anatomia e Antropologia,* 17: 225-234.

Almeida, Fernando de. 1936b. "Sobre a anatomia do nervo Pré-sagrado: Nota prévia I." *Arquivos de Anatomia e Antropologia,* 17: 9-13.

Almeida, Fernando de. 1937. "Novas observações sobre a anatomia do nervo Pré-sagrado: Nota prévia II." *Arquivos de Anatomia e Antropologia,* 18: 15-16.

Almeida, Fernando de. F. 1944. "Considerações sobre a distribuição das artérias Sílvica e Cerebral anterior na superfície do cérebro de recém-nascidos de termo." *Arquivos de Anatomia e Antropologia,* 23: 299-305.

Almeida, Fernando de. 1966. *Curriculum Vitae*. Lisboa Cardoso, João L. 2005. "Fernando de Almeida: breve evocação no centenário do seu nascimento." *Ebvrobriga*, no 3 (Primavera/Verão): 22-27.

Fernandes, Paulo A. 2003. "O contributo de Fernando de Almeida para o estudo da Alta Idade Média em Portugal". *Revista Arqueologia e História*, 55: 205-213.

Moniz, Egas, Abel Alves e Fernando de Almeida. 1932a. "La visibilité des sinus de la dure-mère par l'eupreve encéphalographique". *Press Médicale*, 80: 1499-1516.

Moniz, Egas, Abel Alves e Fernando de Almeida. 1932b. "Os seios venosos da dura-mater, sua visibilidade aos raios X." *Lisboa Médica,* 9: 523-534.

Moniz, Egas, Abel Alves e Fernando de Almeida. 1932c. "Visibilidade aos Raios X das veias profundas do cérebro". *Lisboa Médica,* 9: 587-594.

Moniz, Egas, Fernando de Almeida. 1932d. "Seio recto e seio longitudinal inferior." *Folia Anatomica Universitatis Coninbrigensis,* 7: 1-35.

Moniz, Egas, Fernando de Almeida. 1933. "Le sinus droit et l'ampoule de Galien opacifiés par la voie du tronc basilaire." *Lisboa Médica,* 10 (10): 587-593.

Profano, João. 2017. "Biografia de Fernando de Almeida." 31-40 *In* Ramos, Isabel M.S. & de Pablos, Jorge M (eds): *Arqueología No Invasiva, Projecto Idave. Egitania Idanha-a- Velha. Portugal*. España: Auditores de Energía y Medio Ambiente.

Raposo, Luís. 2003. "A acção de Fernando de Almeida na direcção do Museu Nacional de Arqueologia e Etnologia." *O Arqueólogo Português,* 4 (21): 13-64.

Santos, Manuel. F. dos. 1985. *Elogio do Prof. Doutor Fernando de Almeida.* Lisboa: Academia Portuguesa da História.

Silva, Joaquim C. da. 2004. "Evocação/Memória de alguns Médicos Notáveis da Beira Interior – Concelho do Fundão (III): O Prof. Doutor Fernando de Almeida". *Medicina na Beira Interior da Pré-História ao Século XXI-Cadernos da Cultura*, no. 18 (Novembro): 60-68.

Testut, L. 1891. *Traité d'anatomie humaine. Tome deuxième, Angéiologie, névrologie*. Paris: Octave Doin.

INDEX

Aberdeen Bestiary, 131, 132, 133, 183
abortion, 173, 547, 549, 556, 570
acute myocardial infarctions, 494
Adrian von Mynsicht, 144, 146, 163, 168, 170, 172, 179
Água de Inglaterra, 423, 424, 450, 451, 452, 453, 455, 462, 468, 490, 497
Albertus Magnus, 92, 100, 112, 113, 114, 139, 166, 174, 175, 182, 194, 195, 202, 253, 292
Al-Biruni, 116
Albrecht, 228, 230, 291
Alchemy, 176, 192, 291
Alexander Yersin, 213
Alexis of Piedmont, 159
Alfonso X, 123, 125, 175, 185
Alhazen, 227
Amadeo de Sousa Cardoso, 515, 524, 528, 529
Amato Lusitano, 478
ambassador, 315, 325
amber, 95, 120, 149, 154, 163, 168, 170, 177, 190
Ambroise Paré, 150
amethyst, 95, 255
Amulets, 140, 157
Andre du Laurens, 252
Andreas Vesalius, 67, 89, 283
Antiquity, 210, 214, 228, 230, 252, 255, 286, 291, 298, 422, 572
Antonio Benivieni, 478
António Fragoso, 524
António José da Silva, 481
António Piga, 531, 554
António Ribeiro Sanches, 483
Apollo, 34, 215
Apothecaries' shops, 101
Archaeology, 28, 44, 55, 61, 64, 66, 69, 559, 560, 562, 570, 571, 572, 573, 574
Aristotle, 107, 115, 116, 193, 194, 227, 459, 475
Ark of the Covenant, 203, 204, 210, 213, 217
Armenian Bole, 437, 460
Arnoldus Saxo, 110, 200
Art History, 571, 572
Asclepius, 20, 29, 30, 31, 34, 61, 62, 70, 89, 215
Asia, 72, 116, 298, 303, 305, 350, 359, 421, 517, 534
Athanasius Kircher's, 212
Augusta, 10, 20, 21, 22, 23, 25, 28, 29, 37, 38, 39, 42, 43, 44, 49, 50, 53, 57, 58, 60, 61, 63, 64, 88, 573
authorities, 106, 107, 116, 135, 137, 322, 327, 337, 353, 354, 358, 363, 364, 365, 398, 411, 457, 462, 519, 522, 543
auto-da-fé,, 427
Avicenna, 147, 215, 444, 481
Azores archipelago, 337
Bacteriology, 535
bacterium, 298, 301
baggage, 342, 351, 402
balance, 53, 70, 74, 75, 96, 461, 547, 568
baldness, 175
Ballif Chipail, 534
bandages, 40, 81
barber-surgeons, 68
barrenness, 173
Bartolomeo da San Concordio, 234
baths, 6, 7, 8, 21, 37, 45, 47, 48, 49, 50, 52, 58, 59

Belém, 307, 309, 310, 311, 312, 316, 317, 321, 322, 324, 336, 337, 338, 339, 341, 357, 359, 364, 365, 366, 367, 371, 373, 382, 385, 387, 388, 395, 497, 523
Belém and S. Julião Towers, 317
Benito Daça de Valdes, 246
Bernard de Gordon, 234
Bernardine of Siena, 241
Bernardino António Gomes, 387, 500, 501, 502, 503, 504, 505, 507, 508, 511, 513, 514
beryl, 95, 138, 228, 233, 236
Bevis Marks Synagogue, 423, 429, 431, 441, 455
Bezoar, 150, 152, 157, 163, 168, 174
Black Death, 211, 298, 304, 347, 352, 420, 422
blindness, 253, 254
bloodletting, 35, 486, 491, 492, 494
board, 305, 306, 308, 319, 320, 329, 338, 339, 341, 342, 343, 360, 365
Board of the Maternal Institute, 561, 570
bone elevators, 37
bone levers, 37
Bow scissors, 37
Boyle's vacuum pump, 461
Bracae, 25
Bracaros, 20, 21, 25, 26
Bracas, 25
Brazil, 100, 322, 350, 360, 361, 385, 397, 403, 480, 503, 504, 506
Bruce-Chwatt, 164, 186
būbō, 301
buboes, 156, 207, 211, 215, 301, 305, 398
bubonic plague, 203, 210, 212, 220, 298, 303, 304, 398
Caelius Aurelianus, 52, 62
Camillus Leonardus, 136
Campana Plaque, 70
captain, *310*, *315*, *319*, *320*, *328*, *359*, *361*, *382*, *494*
Cardinal Hugo of Provence, 236, 237
Caricatures, 258
Caroselli, 217, 218, 220
Cascais, 308, 312, 317, 320, 321, 331, 337, 394
Case histories, 485
Catherine of Habsburg, 276
catheters, 37
cauteries, 37, 59, 77, 80, 87
Caventou, 450, 500, 501, 504, 508, 509, 510, 511, 513
Celsus, 34, 40, 41, 52, 58, 59, 62, 80, 89, 459
Central Hygiene Institute, 520
Cerebral angiography, 560
certificate, 312, 319, 339, 340, 360, 364, 362, 365
Charcot, 547, 550
Charles Bouchard, 541
Charles I, 164
Charles V, 67, 138, 276
childbirth, 92, 119, 173, 181, 570
chisels, 37, 59
cholera, 172, 300, 338, 340, 341, 367, 392, 406, 411, 489, 494
chronobiology, 546
chrysolite, 95, 100
chrysoprase, 95
Cicero, 4, 18, 34, 62
cinchona bark, 490, 500, 501, 502, 504, 505, 506, 507, 508, 509, 510, 511
Colombia, 93, 99, 138, 178, 193, 505
Colombian emeralds, 99, 101
commission, 205, 216, 392, 396, 401, 402, 506
Computerized Axial Tomography, 82, 83, 84
Concave lenses, 280
conjunctivitis, 521
Conrad Leib, 241
consul, 315, 318, 320, 324, 333

contagion, 156, 208, 210, 287, 288, 298, 313, 316, 317, 318, 319, 321, 322, 323, 327, 329, 330, 335, 336, 337, 338, 344, 352, 353, 357, 362, 363, 371, 384, 385
Contagious diseases, 301
convex lenses, 224, 225, 228, 233, 246
coral, 95, 143, 145, 149, 154, 157, 168, 170, 174, 177, 179, 255, 286
Cordial medicines, 165
cordon sanitaire, 354, 364
Costa ben Luca, 115
countries, 32, 122, 214, 236, 298, 308, 309, 322, 328, 337, 340, 341, 350, 354, 358, 363, 371, 387, 405, 509, 511, 516, 519, 521, 523, 547
Crab's Eyes, 163
craniology, 543
crew, 299, 305, 306, 308, 310, 315, 319, 320, 323, 336, 337, 338, 340, 342, 353, 357, 358, 359, 363, 384, 385, 393, 448
criminality, 535, 542, 544, 546, 547, 548, 557
crystal balsamaria, 70, 79
crystalline, 94, 251, 252, 288, 289
Cylindrical cases, 81
Cylindrical lenses, 283
cytokine "storms", 517
D. Diogo de Sousa, 20, 21, 22, 24, 37, 38, 55, 60, 64, 65, 66, 69, 75, 76, 83, 85, 88, 89, 90, 308
D. Duarte, 305, 306
D. João III, 101, 103, 276, 309, 312, 425, 426, 481
Dagon, 203, 204, 206, 210, 221
Damião de Góis, 267
delirium, 491, 492, 547
Demons, 260
Diabetes, 173
diamonds, 95, 106, 216
diarrhoea, 162, 169, 213, 486, 492, 494
Digital Radiography, 55, 82, 83, 85
Dioscorides, 106, 107
disease, 9, 52, 71, 114, 118, 126, 137, 140, 142, 143, 151, 153, 157, 172, 173, 180, 195, 199, 203, 204, 205, 207, 209, 210, 211, 212, 213, 214, 215, 298, 301, 302, 303, 305, 306, 308, 316, 319, 320, 322, 325, 327, 329, 337, 342, 352, 353, 354, 355, 356, 357, 361, 369, 385, 411, 412, 420, 442, 444, 445, 446, 448, 449, 470, 475, 476, 486, 487, 489, 491, 494, 495, 496, 516, 521, 523, 526, 527, 552
disinfection, 317, 325, 343, 350, 354, 359, 387, 393, 394, 395, 399, 400, 401, 402, 404, 405, 406, 409, 410, 411, 412, 413, 414, 415, 504, 518
docking, 299, 309, 337, 354, 402
Doctor Schnabel, 287, 288, 289
Dr. Alfredo da Costa Maternity Hospital, 560, 561, 570
Dr. Emil Puscariu, 535
dressings, 40
ear probes, 36
earths, 94, 195, 434, 459, 460, 468
Egas Moniz, 559, 560, 561, 562, 566, 567, 569, 574
electuaries, 95, 253, 255, 433
emerald, 92, 95, 97, 99, 100, 101, 105, 108, 109, 111, 112, 113, 114, 115, 116, 117, 118, 119, 121, 122, 123, 124, 125, 126, 127, 135, 136, 137, 140, 142, 143, 144, 145, 147, 148, 149, 150, 151, 152, 154, 157, 162, 163, 164, 165, 166, 167, 168, 169, 170, 171, 172, 174, 175, 177, 178, 179, 180, 181, 182, 184

Emperor, 5, 9, 10, 20, 25, 28, 59, 67, 72, 109, 143, 227, 258, 276, 503
encephalitis, 521
Endovellicus, *6, 8*
Epidemic typhus, 492
epilepsy, 92, 112, 114, 115, 116, 117, 118, 122, 125, 131, 135, 139, 140, 141, 142, 143, 144, 145, 433, 546
equipment, 26, 55, 84, 337, 404, 405, 409, 410, 412, 461
estrangeirado, 424, 457, 466
Euclid, 227
Europe, 36, 72, 92, 171, 191, 211, 214, 220, 224, 230, 233, 234, 245, 287, 292, 298, 304, 305, 318, 322, 352, 419, 421, 437, 450, 469, 471, 472, 490, 494, 505, 516, 517, 518, 523, 530, 532, 533, 542, 549, 555, 556
Exanthematic Typhus, 518
expenses, 356, 363, 375, 378, 395, 397
ex-voto, 7, 9, 11, 16, 70, 7*1*
eye medicines, 78
eyed needle, 66, 77, 81, 88
eyeglasses, 137, 225, 227, 228, 230, 231, 233, 234, 235, 236, 237, 245, 247, 249, 250, 260, 261, 265, 276, 277, 279, 284, 285, 290
Fabrizio Valguarnera, 216
Faculty of Medicine of Iaşi, 530
farsightedness, 226
feminist emancipation, 532
Fernando de Almeida, 559, 560, 561, 562, 563, 564, 565, 569, 572, 573, 574, 575, 576
Fernando Mendes, 452
Fernando Pessoa, 523
fevers, 92, 163, 177, 192, 436, 450, 460, 476, 488, 489, 490, 491, 492, 493, 494, 500, 501, 504, 505, 506, 509
First Book of Samuel, 203, 204
físico, 312
folding glasses, 234
Forensic Medicine, 530, 533, 534, 535, 536, 537, 538, 539, 540, 541, 542, 549, 550, 552, 553, 554, 555, 556, 557
forts, 354
fossils, 94, 190
Francesco Petrarca, 235, 285
Francisco Marto, 524
Friar Allessandro della Spina, 234
Friar José de Siguënza, 267
Funchal, 366, 401
Funerary banquets, 50
Gaius Julius Solinus, 109
Galen, 34, 35, 52, 53, 54, 62, 68, 90, 106, 107, 188, 252, 259, 353, 421, 438, 459, 470, 481, 489, 490, 567
ganglionic engorgements, 298, 301
Garcia de Orta, 100, 102, 103, 104, 114, 119, 138, 191, 194
Gaspar Lopes de Chaves, 476, 479, 483, 496
gem electuary, 92, 119, 162
Gem Electuary, 93, 179, 189
Georg Handsch, 479
George Bate, 164, 186
Georgius Agricola, 114, 142, 185
Giovanni Baldinucci, 209
glossopetrae, 179
Goa Stone, 92, 93, 158, 179, 186
Goldsmith's Street, 101
Graeco-Roman heritage, 88
Grave goods, *21*
Gregório Lopes, 273
grooming tools, 21, 38, 44, 58, 60, 88
guards, 310, 319, 320, 322, 329, 330, 359, 360, 364, 366, 373, 380, 382, 385, 400, 401
Guy de Chauliac, 236, 294
Hadrian, 6, 11, 59
haemoptoic sputum, 521

handle, 2, 18, 21, 30, 31, 38, 39, 40, 41, 47, 48, 49, 54, 57, 58, 59, 74, 76, 81, 85, 229, 518, 557
Hans Weiditz, 285, 286
health, 1, 3, 5, 6, 7, 9, 10, 11, 12, 15, 16, 17, 29, 40, 47, 52, 58, 59, 61, 70, 89, 135, 150, 176, 188, 201, 205, 208, 299, 310, 312, 313, 315, 316, 317, 318, 319, 320, 321, 322, 323, 324, 325, 327, 328, 329, 330, 331, 332, 333, 335, 336, 337, 338, 339, 340, 341, 342, 343, 350, 352, 353, 355, 356, 357, 358, 359, 360, 361, 362, 364, 365, 366, 367, 368, 373, 375, 379, 381, 382, 383, 384, 385, 386, 387, 388, 392, 393, 394, 395, 396, 398, 399, 401, 402, 403, 405, 411, 412, 415, 486, 503, 504, 505, 506, 519, 520, 521, 549, 556
Health Station, 356, 401, 414
Hebetation, 170
Henri Claude, 530, 531, 537, 541
Henrique de Vilhena, 559, 560, 561, 562
Herman Boerhaave, 441, 444, 458, 459
Herodicus of Selymbria, 47
Hieronimus Bosch, 265, 266, 269
Hieronymus Fracastoro, 215
Hildegard von Bingen, 120, 121, 180, 201
Hiob Finzel, 479, 499
Hippocrates, 33, 47, 48, 61, 65, 81, 87, 88, 90, 353, 420, 421, 438, 459, 470, 487
Historical and Philosophical Sciences, 560, 561, 571
History of Art and Archaeology, 573
hooks, 37, 241
horns, 140, 144, 179, 260, 261
Hortus Sanitatis, 134, 135, 136, 171, 187, 188
hospital, 325, 353, 355, 393, 394, 398, 423, 424, 431, 432, 437, 440, 461, 466, 470
humoral immunity, 517
Hyginus, 34
hysteria, 546, 550, 555
Iasi University-Chair of Forensic Medicine, 530
Igreja Matriz de S. Miguel from Freixo de Espada à Cinta, 271
indigenous deities, 1, 17
infanticide, 547, 549, 556
infirmary, 371, 375, 378, 381, 387, 394
influenza virus, 517
inoculation, 442, 445, 448, 449, 450, 474
Inquisition, 101, 103, 147, 423, 425, 426, 427, 428, 430, 441, 462, 466, 471, 475, 479, 480, 481, 482, 483, 497
inscription, 1, 2, 4, 5, 10, 17, 20, 29, 58, 71, 234, 402
installation, 353, 385, 402, 409, 425
ipecacuanha, 491, 492, 494, 504
Isidore of Seville, 110, 111, 185, 227, 293, 352, 420
island of Madeira, 309
isolation, 265, 325, 354, 355, 369, 391, 392, 394, 395, 396, 399, 500, 501, 502, 504, 505, 507, 508, 509, 510, 511, 518
jacinth, 95, 149, 160, 164, 165, 174, 177
Jacob de Castro Sarmento, 423, 424, 426, 427, 429, 431, 462, 466, 467, 468, 470, 472, 473, 474, 480, 483, 490, 498
Jan van der Straet, 247, 248, 249, 251, 280, 282
Jane Sharp, 173, 174
jasper, 95
Jean-Auguste Dominique Ingres, 219
Jesus among the Doctors, 271

Jews, 101, 212, 423, 425, 427, 429, 430, 438, 442, 471, 472, 479, 499
Johann Lukas Schönlein, 494
Johannes Kepler, 251
Johannes Mesuë, 92, 93, 119, 179
John Milton, 262
John Peckham, 228
John Tanner, 171
Jonstonus, 150, 151, 174, 175, 193
Jordan of Pisa, 233
José Leite de Vasconcellos, 28, 571
Justinian plague, 211
King D. Afonso V, 224, 277
King D. Afonso VI, 315
King D. Carlos I, 342
King D. Fernando II, 218
King D. Filipe III, 267
King D. João I, 306
King D. João II, 277, 307
King D. João V, 328, 457, 458
King D. João VI, 337
King D. José I, 331, 481
King D. Luis I, 342
King D. Manuel I, 267, 308, 425
King D. Pedro II, 318, 324, 452
King D. Pedro V, 340, 360
King D. Sebastião, 312
King Edward 1, 429
King Filipe II, 246, 267
King Henry V, 252
Kingdom, 129, 277, 298, 306, 308, 309, 312, 313, 315, 321, 322, 323, 325, 326, 327, 328, 329, 330, 331, 332, 333, 335, 337, 338, 339, 340, 342, 343, 350, 356, 357, 360, 362, 363, 364, 365, 366, 367, 379, 381, 383, 386, 387, 392, 396, 398, 399, 402, 415, 459, 506
Kitasato Shibasaburō, 213
Konrad von Megenberg, 113
Konrad von Würzburg, 229, 292
Kunstkammern, 67, 90, 102
Lady Mary Wortley Montagu, 446, 469
Lapis judaicus, 460
lazaretto, 338, 340, 341, 343, 344, 350, 351, 355, 358, 359, 360, 361, 366, 368, 369, 370, 371, 372, 373, 375, 376, 378, 379, 380, 381, 382, 383, 384, 385, 386, 387, 389, 390, 391, 392, 393, 395, 396, 397, 398, 399, 400, 401, 404, 415
Leonardo da Vinci, 286
leprosy, 135, 171, 355, 504
Leprosy, 171, 181
ligatures, 40
liniments, 95, 433
Lisbon, 2, 9, 23, 28, 44, 55, 61, 63, 82, 83, 101, 103, 105, 182, 194, 203, 216, 218, 267, 268, 269, 273, 283, 290, 298, 305, 306, 307, 308, 309, 310, 311, 312, 313, 314, 315, 317, 318, 319, 320, 321, 322, 323, 325, 329, 331, 332, 333, 334, 335, 336, 339, 343, 350, 351, 356, 357, 360, 361, 365, 368, 369, 371, 373, 375, 379, 381, 383, 384, 385, 386, 392, 393, 395, 397, 398, 399, 400, 401, 402, 403, 405, 407, 409, 411, 412, 414, 428, 433, 436, 452, 455, 468, 469, 479, 480, 483, 485, 495, 496, 503, 504, 506, 507, 508, 519, 520, 521, 523, 524, 526, 559, 561, 562, 563, 566, 570, 571, 572, 573, 574
Lisbon Public Disinfection Station, 400, 405, 415
Lisbon Sanitary Park, 412, 414
lithotomy, 35, 37
lohochs, 95
Lombroso, 544, 545, 549, 558
Lorenz Scholz von Rosenau, 143
Ludger tom Ring the Elder, 241, 244
magnifying lenses, 226, 229
Maimonides, 147, 196
malachite, 92, 100, 254

Manuel Alvares Carapeto, 216
Marco Polo, 230
Maria Cickersky, 533, 534, 535, 536, 538, 539, 540, 544, 548, 550, 553, 555
Maria Franche, 534
Maria Ropala Cickersky, 530, 531, 532, 537, 556
Marioara Tanasescu Niculescu, 534
maritime, 305, 324, 333, 342, 343, 354, 357, 364, 368, 398, 399, 401, 402
Maritime Disinfection Station, 350, 401, 402, 414
Marquis of Pombal, 381, 385, 457, 481, 482, 503
Martin Schongauer, 238, 239
Martins Sarmento, 26, 28
master, 11, 15, 59, 241, 297, 310, 322, 337, 358, 545
Master of Heiligenkreuz, 240
Master of the Saint Bartholomew, 241, 243, 297
materia medica, 95, 103, 135, 136, 137, 158, 178, 188, 199, 423, 424, 433, 434, 436, 440
mayor of Lisbon council, 315
Measles, 173, 181
Medical Optics, 251
medicine, 33, 34, 37, 47, 48, 53, 56, 58, 59, 60, 61, 62, 67, 68, 70, 74, 75, 81, 90, 94, 95, 102, 103, 104, 117, 121, 140, 142, 143, 148, 149, 151, 162, 163, 165, 166, 170, 173, 177, 185, 186, 192, 194, 195, 196, 215, 302, 411, 420, 430, 437, 440, 441, 455, 459, 463, 464, 470, 473, 476, 477, 478, 479, 481, 482, 485, 487, 490, 492, 496, 502, 503, 504, 505, 530, 532, 536, 537, 538, 539, 542, 548, 549, 550, 553, 555, 556, 557, 560
melancholy, 93, 165, 166, 174
merchandise, 310, 315, 321, 324, 326, 350, 354, 356, 359, 366, 369, 371, 373, 380, 382, 383, 385, 393, 395, 396, 401, 404
Mercurial Ptyalism, 445
meteorosensitivity, 546
miasma theory, 442
Michael Ettmüller, 153, 172
Michael Sweerts, 220, 223
microscope, 461, 564
Mina Minovici, 537, 543, 548, 549, 554
mithridatium, 162
Monastery of Jesus from Aveiro, 224, 277
Monocles, 233
mortars, 77, 78
Moses, 147, 187, 196, 212, 261, 262, 437, 451, 472, 482
Murano glass, 233
Museum of Aveiro, 186, 224, 277, 278, 279, 290
myalgia, 521
Myocarditis, 521
myopia, 280, 283, 284
Nail-cleaners, 44
National Archeology Museum, 571
National Palace of Mafra, 190, 198, 275, 276, 291, 468
Near and Middle East, 298
Necropolis, 38, 57, 58
Neurology, 200, 560, 561, 566, 567
Nicolas Culpeper, 137, 139, 142
Nicolas le Fèbure, 169
Nicolás Monardes, 149, 186
North Africa, 298, 305, 330, 354, 359
nose pinch glasses, 246
nuns, 245, 277, 278, 279
Obstetrics and Gynecology, 560, 561, 570
ocular disorders, 93
oil flasks, 36, 48
ointments, 95, 153
Old Testament, 203, 213, 260, 261, 355
Oliver Cromwell, 164, 429
Oltea Doamna, 534, 535

operations, 21, 34, 35, 37, 40, 41, 59, 191, 196, 464, 474
Oporto, 22, 304, 305, 308, 519, 520, 522
outposts, 354
Paço de Arcos, 325, 332, 335, 337, 364, 374
painter Gerard David, 271
Palaeoradiology, 66
pandemic, 17, 211, 222, 298, 303, 304, 305, 343, 350, 515, 516, 517, 518, 523, 524
Paracelsus, 153, 154, 156, 176, 188, 192, 197, 200, 459
passengers, 299, 315, 321, 327, 338, 340, 341, 342, 343, 350, 351, 353, 355, 357, 359, 364, 393, 396, 397, 398, 402, 404, 415, 519
Paul-Louis Simond, 222, 302
pearls, 95, 117, 149, 154, 157, 164, 168, 252
Pelletier, 450, 500, 501, 504, 508, 509, 510, 511, 513
pestilence, 140, 152, 193, 197, 201, 211, 220, 303, 305, 361, 420
pestilences, 122, 160, 204, 223, 300, 362
Peter Bruegel the Elder, 246
Pharmacopoeia Bateana, 164
Pharmacopoeia Contracta, 432, 433, 437, 440
Pharmacopoeia Londinensis, 160, 162, 198, 432, 468
pharmacy, 59, 61, 66, 69, 70, 74, 75, 77, 88, 89, 197, 437, 460, 502
pharyngeal soreness, 521
Philippe Pinel, 493
Philistines, 203, 204, 206, 210, 212, 213, 214, 215, 217, 219, 222, 223
physicians, 29, 34, 35, 39, 40, 58, 59, 68, 88, 143, 151, 153, 189, 197, 210, 226, 250, 259, 287, 363, 366, 367, 401, 431, 440, 444, 448, 449, 452, 455, 459, 476, 477, 478, 483, 484, 487, 494, 504, 517, 539
physiology of vision, 252
Pierre-Charles-Alexandre Louis, 493
Pieter van Foreest, 479
Pietro d'Abano, 147, 180
Pietro Tommasi, 113, 148, 201
pills, 95, 152, 172, 253, 433, 463
pilot, 321, 337
plague, 29, 93, 120, 122, 136, 143, 151, 153, 156, 157, 159, 163, 164, 176, 177, 201, 203, 204, 205, 206, 207, 208, 209, 210, 211, 212, 213, 214, 215, 216, 220, 221, 222, 223, 287, 288, 289, 298, 300, 301, 302, 303, 304, 305, 306, 307, 308, 309, 313, 314, 315, 316, 317, 318, 319, 320, 321, 322, 323, 325, 326, 327, 328, 329, 330, 331, 332, 333, 334, 335, 336, 337, 338, 340, 341, 343, 347, 348, 349, 350, 351, 352, 353, 354, 355, 356, 357, 358, 360, 361, 362, 363, 364, 367, 370, 371, 373, 375, 379, 381, 384, 385, 386, 398, 399, 411, 420, 421, 442, 494, 516, 519, 520
plague epidemics, 298
Platearius, 165, 170
Plinius the Elder, 30
pneumonic, 303, 305, 517
Pneumonic Influenza, 515, 516, 517, 518, 519, 521
Polyptych of the Virgin, 271
Ponta Delgada, 366, 401, 519
Pope Leo X, 280, 281, 425
poppy, 70, 72, 73, 525
port of Lisbon, 307, 308, 316, 318, 319, 322, 332, 337, 338, 342, 350, 351, 352, 358, 360, 364, 366, 367, 368, 371, 381, 383, 388, 415
Porto Brandão, 338, 388, 393, 422

ports, 299, 305, 312, 313, 317, 319, 320, 321, 323, 325, 326, 327, 328, 329, 330, 331, 332, 333, 334, 335, 337, 338, 340, 341, 342, 343, 350, 351, 356, 357, 358, 360, 361, 363, 364, 365, 366, 367, 368, 373, 381, 382, 386, 390, 396, 399, 400, 415, 516
Portuguese, 3, 4, 6, 10, 18, 20, 26, 28, 39, 49, 61, 66, 92, 100, 101, 103, 105, 158, 185, 188, 216, 218, 220, 271, 272, 273, 276, 277, 298, 305, 311, 313, 321, 322, 323, 325, 331, 332, 335, 336, 339, 340, 343, 350, 351, 353, 356, 357, 361, 365, 379, 380, 384, 386, 392, 397, 405, 415, 423, 424, 425, 426, 427, 429, 430, 432, 433, 434, 436, 438, 442, 455, 457, 459, 460, 462, 463, 464, 466, 468, 470, 471, 479, 480, 481, 483, 485, 490, 496, 498, 500, 501, 502, 503, 504, 506, 507, 509, 515, 518, 519, 521, 523, 524, 525, 528, 530, 531, 553, 559, 564, 565, 566, 570, 571, 572, 573
Portuguese empire, 277
Portuguese monarchs, 271, 298, 343, 350
precautions, 307, 308, 322, 326, 328, 330, 333, 339, 350, 356, 357, 363, 382
precious and semi-precious stones, 94, 95, 107, 120, 165, 182
Presbyopia, 225
Prevention, 193, 221, 299, 432
Princess Joanna, 224
prisoners, 379, 380, 386, 427, 448
probe case, 66, 81, 82, 83, 85, 87, 88
probes, 36, 37, 41, 43, 56, 59, 74, 76, 77, 78, 79, 80, 81, 82, 84, 85
Professor Câmara Pestana, 398
Professor Ricardo Jorge, 399
protection, 5, 6, 153, 285, 286, 325, 329, 336, 363, 368, 381, 385, 427, 523
protective equipment, 284, 287
Pseudo-Aristotle, 92, 115, 116, 118, 119, 124, 175
psychoanalysis, 542, 546
psychoses, 547
Public Disinfection Station, 405, 411, 414
pustules, 444, 445, 446
quarantine, 306, 313, 316, 317, 318, 322, 324, 325, 328, 329, 330, 331, 332, 333, 334, 337, 338, 339, 340, 341, 342, 344, 351, 352, 354, 355, 357, 358, 359, 360, 362, 365, 366, 367, 369, 370, 381, 393, 396, 397, 399, 400, 404, 421
Queen Dona Maria I, 335
Queen Dona Maria II, 338
Queen Maria I, 479, 484
Quinine, 450, 498, 508
Rabanus Maurus Magnentius, 110
Rabbi David Nieto, 423
Reading magnifiers, *227*, *230*
Rectangular boxes, 81
refractive errors, 252, 254
regulation, 325, 339, 342, 343, 356, 360, 361, 362, 363, 365, 367, 368, 386, 399, 411, 414
Renaissance, 4, 22, 67, 198, 252, 266, 277, 280, 286, 293, 295, 478, 498
renal colic, 494
repair, 55, 320, 340, 373, 375, 376, 378, 381, 406, 413, 455
retractors, 37, 80
Reye's syndrome, 521
Reynaldo dos Santos, 271, 559, 560, 561, 562
rivet spectacles, 233, 236, 237, 238, 240, 245, 246
Robert Midgley, 163
rocks, minerals, 94
Rodrigo de Castro, 483, 498